A CLINICIAN'S GUIDE

Endocrine and Metabolic Medical Emergencies

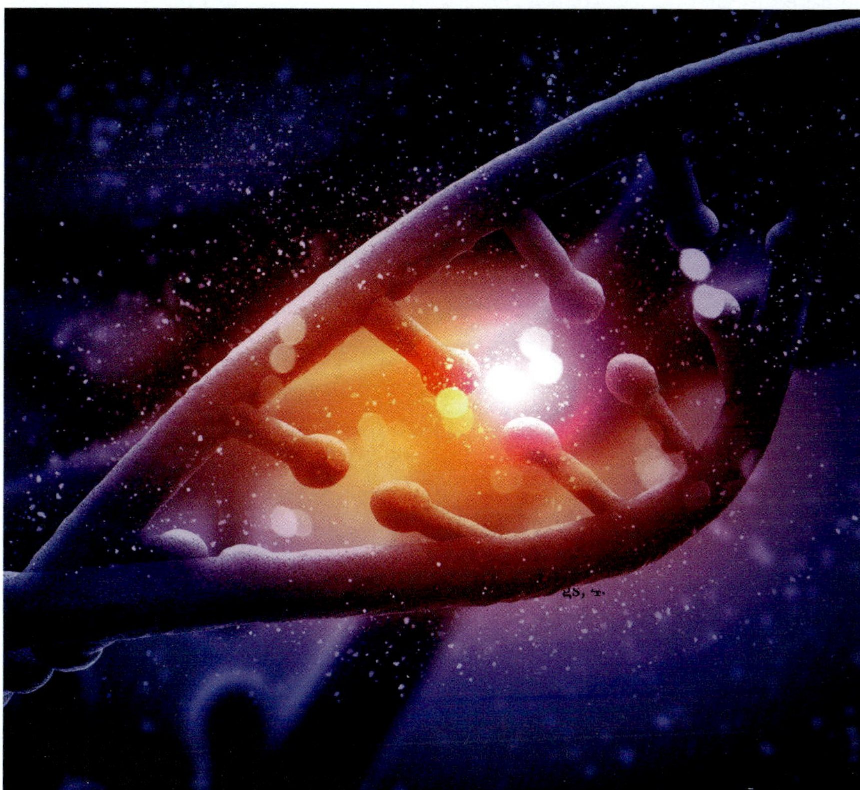

Glenn Matfin, Editor
MSc (Oxon), MB ChB, FACE, FACP, FRCP

ENDOCRINE PRESS
an imprint of the Endocrine Society

ENDOCRINE PRESS, Washington, DC

ENDOCRINE PRESS
an imprint of the Endocrine Society

press.endocrine.org

The Endocrine Society is the world's largest, oldest, and most active organization working to advance the clinical practice of endocrinology and hormone research. Founded in 1916, the Society now has more than 17,000 global members across a range of disciplines.

The Society has earned an international reputation for excellence in the quality of its peer-reviewed journals, educational resources, meetings, and programs that improve public health through the practice and science of endocrinology.

Endocrine Press Books reflects new and emerging areas in endocrinology. Endocrine Press provides researchers, clinical practitioners, and allied health professionals with access to trustworthy content on endocrine disorders.

Editor:
Glenn Matfin, MSc (Oxon), MB ChB, FACE, FACP, FRCP

Oversight Editor:
Paul Robertson, MD

ISBN: 978-1-936704-77-4
eISBN: 978-1-936704-81-1
Library of Congress Control Number: 2014938607

A CLINICIAN'S GUIDE

Endocrine and Metabolic Medical Emergencies

Glenn Matfin, Editor
MSc (Oxon), MB ChB, FACE, FACP, FRCP

Contents

Contributors

BOOK EDITOR
Glenn Matfin
National Health Service
London, UK

FOREWORD
J Larry Jameson
University of Pennsylvania
Philadelphia, PA

SECTION I:
John Wass
Churchill Hospital
Oxford, UK

Sir Richard Thompson
Royal College of Physicians
London, UK

Paul J Frost
Cardiff University
Cardiff, UK

Matthew P Wise
University Hospital of
Wales, Cardiff, UK

SECTION II:
David B Sacks
National Institutes of Health
Bethesda, MD

Penny M Clark
University Hospitals
Birmingham NHS
Birmingham, UK

Julian H Barth
St James' University
Hospital, Leeds, UK

Greet Van den Berghe
University of Leuven (KU
Leuven), Leuven, Belgium

Eva Boonen
University of Leuven (KU
Leuven), Leuven, Belgium

SECTION III:
Johannes D Veldhuis
Mayo Clinic, Rochester, MN

Anita Banerjee
Guy's and St Thomas'
Hospital, London, UK

Catherine Williamson
King's College London
London, UK

Chelsea McMahon
Garvan Institute of Medical
Research, Darlinghurst,
Australia

Katherine Samaras
Garvan Institute of Medical
Research, Darlinghurst,
Australia

SECTION IV:
Edward R Laws, Jr
Brigham and Women's
Hospital, Boston, MA

Ursula B Kaiser
Brigham and Women's
Hospital, Boston, MA

Nicholas A Tritos
Massachusetts General
Hospital, Boston, MA

Anne Klibanski
Massachusetts General
Hospital, Boston, MA

Mark Vanderpump
Royal Free Hampstead NHS
Trust, London, UK

Aikaterini Theodoraki
Royal Free Hampstead NHS
Trust, London, UK

Mark E Molitch
Northwestern University
Chicago, IL

SECTION V:
Hossein Gharib
Mayo Clinic Rochester, MN

James V Hennessey
Beth Israel Deaconess
Medical Center, Boston, MA

Natasha Kasid
Joslin Diabetes Center
Boston, MA

Henry B Burch
Walter Reed National
Military Medical Center
Bethesda, MD

Alicia L Warnock
Walter Reed National
Military Medical Center
Bethesda, MD

David S Cooper
The Johns Hopkins
University School of
Medicine, Baltimore, MD

Fausto Bogazzi
Università di Pisa, Pisa, Italy

Luigi Bartalena
Ospedale di Circolo
Varese, Italy

Luca Tomisti
University of Pisa
Pisa, Italy

Enio Martino
Ospedale Cisanello
Pisa, Italy

Shih-Hua Lin
Tri-Service General
Hospital, Taipei, Taiwan

Chih-Jen Cheng
Tri-Service General
Hospital, Taipei, Taiwan

Rebecca S Bahn
Mayo Clinic, Rochester, MN

James A Garrity
Mayo Clinic, Rochester, MN

Michael E Menefee
Mayo Clinic, Jacksonville, FL

Robert C Smallridge
Mayo Clinic, Jacksonville, FL

SECTION VI:
Paul M Stewart
University of Leeds
Leeds, UK

Ashley B Grossman
Churchill Hospital
Oxford, UK

Krystallenia I Alexandraki
Athens Medical School
Athens, Greece

Graeme Eisenhofer
University Hospital
Dresden, Germany

Jacques W M Lenders
Radboud University
Nijmegen Medical Centre
Nijmegen, Netherlands

Andrzej Januszewicz,
Institute of Cardiology
Warsaw, Poland

Christina Pamporaki
University Hospital
Dresden, Germany

SECTION VII:
John P Bilezikian
Columbia University
College of Physicians and
Surgeons, New York, NY

Richard Quinton
Royal Victoria Infirmary
Newcastle-upon-Tyne,
Newcastle, UK

Muhammad Asam
Royal Victoria Infirmary
Newcastle-upon-Tyne,
Newscastle, UK

Glenn Matfin
National Health Service
London, UK

William D Fraser
University of East Anglia
Norwich, UK

Arnold J Felsenfeld
VA Greater Los Angeles
Healthcare System
Los Angeles, CA

Barton S Levine
UCLA School of Medicine
Los Angeles, CA

Nelson B Watts
Mercy Health Osteoporosis
and Bone Health Services
Cincinnati, OH

Dima L Diab
UC Medical Center Stetson
Center, Cincinnati, OH

Ethel S Siris
New York-Presbyterian
Hospital, New York, NY

Dorothy A Fink
New York-Presbyterian
Hospital, New York, NY

David S Goldfarb
Department Veterans
Affairs Medical Center
New York, NY

Hasan Fattah
Department Veterans
Affairs Medical Center
New York, NY

SECTION VIII:
Kjell Oberg
Uppsala University Hospital
Uppsala, Sweden

Jamie Goldman
Moffitt Cancer Center
Tampa, FL

Jonathan Strosberg
Moffitt Cancer Center
Tampa, FL

SECTION IX:
Richard M Bergenstal
International Diabetes
Center at Park Nicollet
Minneapolis, MN

Shaukat Sadikot
International Diabetes Federation, Mumbai, India

Stephen N Davis
University of Maryland Medical Center
Baltimore, MD

Elizabeth M Lamos
University of Maryland School of Medicine
Baltimore, MD

Lisa M Younk
University of Maryland School of Medicine
Baltimore, MD

Ketan Dhatariya
Norfolk and Norwich University Hospital
Norwich, UK

Mark W Savage
Bendigo Health
Bendigo, Australia

Adrian Scott
Northern General Hospital
Sheffield, UK

Glenn Matfin
National Health Service
London, UK

Mike Sampson
Norfolk and Norwich University Hospital
Norwich, UK

Wen Xu
Sun Yat-sen University
Guangdong, China

David R Owens
Swansea University
Swansea, UK

Jianping Weng
Sun Yat-sen University
Guangdong, China

Guillermo E Umpierrez
Emory University
Atlanta, GA

Susan Braithwaite
University of Illinois Hospital & Health Sciences System, Chicago, IL

Curtiss Cook
Mayo Clinic
Scottsdale, AZ

Osama Hamdy
Joslin Diabetes Center
Boston, MA

Martin J Abrahamson
Joslin Diabetes Center
Boston, MA

Alissa R Segal
Joslin Diabetes Center
Boston, MA

M Molly McMahon
Mayo Clinic, Rochester, MN

John M Miles
Mayo Clinic, Rochester, MN

David Baldwin
Rush University Medical Center, Chicago, IL

Benjamin A Lipsky
University of Oxford
Oxford, UK

Karim Gariani
University Hospitals of Geneva, Geneva, Switzerland

Ilker Uckay
University Hospitals of Geneva, Geneva, Switzerland

Natasha Kasid
Joslin Diabetes Center
Boston, MA

Florence Brown
Joslin Diabetes Center
Boston, MA

SECTION X:

Daniel G Bichet
Hôpital du Sacré-Coeur de Montréal, Québec, Canada

Christopher J Thompson
Beaumont Hospital
Dublin, Ireland

Mark J Hannon
Georgetown University
Washington, DC

Joseph G Verbalis
Georgetown University
Washington, DC

SECTION XI:

Robert H Eckel
University Hospital
Denver, CO

Michael A Via
Beth Israel Medical Center
New York, NY

Jeff I Mechanick
Mount Sinai Hospital
New York, NY

Nick Finer
University College London Hospital, London, UK

Andrea Pucci
University College London Hospital, London, UK

John D Brunzell
University of Washington
Seattle, WA

Alan Chait
University of Washington
Seattle, WA

Paul D Thompson
Hartford Hospital
Hartford, CT

Carmelo V Venero
University of Tennessee Medical Center
Knoxville, TN

SECTION XII:

T M Cox
Cambridge University Hospitals, Cambridge, UK

Elaine Murphy
National Hospital for Neurology and Neurosurgery, London, UK

Robin H Lachmann
National Hospital for Neurology and Neurosurgery, London, UK

Foreword

The field of endocrinology is constantly evolving, reflecting the rapid pace of change in medicine and science more generally. In its earliest stages, endocrinology defined the clinical features of acromegaly, Graves' disease, myxedema, Cushing's syndrome, and diabetes mellitus. This era was followed by the discovery of hormones and a renaissance catalyzed by radioimmunoassays (RIAs). These measurements allowed rigorous determinations of circulating hormones and an understanding of complex hormonal feedback mechanisms. The last few decades have witnessed a more sophisticated understanding of perturbations of homeostasis in which we better diagnose disorders such as primary hyperparathyroidism, subclinical hyperthyroidism, and impaired glucose tolerance.

Endocrine and Metabolic Medical Emergencies was conceived by Glenn Matfin, an endocrinologist with extensive clinical experience in different countries and in areas relevant to the topics covered in the text. He and his coauthors recognized a paradigm shift in the field of endocrinology and metabolism. Namely, our patients rarely present with endocrine disease in isolation. Rather, hormonal disorders occur in combination with other conditions such as critical illness or HIV/AIDS, which directly or through their treatments precipitate endocrine disease or illicit physiological responses that alter hormonal pathways. Hospitalized patients are also increasingly complex and critically ill. This setting is rife with stress-related hormonal responses and is rarely appropriate for the methodical evaluation of endocrine conditions. Consequently, in the hospital setting, the emphasis has shifted to acute management of endocrine emergencies such as hypoglycemia, hyponatremia, adrenal insufficiency, thyroid storm, and pituitary apoplexy.

The essence of medical texts is to transfer knowledge and improve clinical care. This text expands the repertoire of traditional endocrine emergencies to a myriad of other conditions that require urgent attention to optimize clinical outcomes. *Endocrine and Metabolic Medical Emergencies* is a timely resource for managing today's complex inpatients with endocrine abnormalities. Each chapter is written by an expert who reviews a common situation encountered by the practicing endocrinologist. Thus, we are now armed with innovative chapters such as "Endocrine and Metabolic Testing in Acute Medical and Critical Illness" and "Management of Insulin Pumps in Hospitalized Patients." We are indebted to these authors for their innovative contributions to the medical literature.

J Larry Jameson, MD, PhD
Philadelphia, PA

Preface

The specialty of endocrinology and metabolism is no longer at the fringes of medicine and now includes some of the most common conditions and serious public health challenges facing both high- and low-income countries. Prevalent endocrine and metabolic conditions include obesity and diabetes, thyroid disorders, and metabolic bone diseases.

Acute medical care is a major focus for many healthcare providers and funders, and patients with endocrine and metabolic emergencies constitute a large proportion of this workload. In addition, many patients are not ideally managed because of the lack of excellent, up-to-date, practical guidance. The purpose of *Endocrine and Metabolic Medical Emergencies* is to help fill this gap by updating and collating existing knowledge on the management of numerous everyday endocrine and metabolic emergencies facing clinicians everywhere. The authors of each chapter are acknowledged experts in their respective areas. This book provides a highly practical and useful reference compendium of the experts' personal approaches to each problem. The contents cover many of the common (and not so common) endocrine and metabolic emergencies. In addition, some of the thorny issues that are especially taxing to the clinician or areas not so often addressed in publications (such as the management of insulin pumps or U-500 insulin in the inpatient setting) are covered. Each chapter is written to stand alone, and the chapters can be read at any time and in any sequence.

The book is divided into several sections. The first section covers acute medical care. This section starts with a discussion by Sir Richard Thompson (President of the Royal College of Physicians) and the distinguished endocrinologist John Wass of the challenges and opportunities of delivering acute medical care in the current healthcare environment. This provides the context within which endocrine and metabolic emergency care occurs. The second section focuses on the effects of acute medical and critical illness on the endocrine and metabolic systems and the impact of these changes and other factors on endocrine investigations in this setting. Several special populations of patients are then discussed, including the unique impact of aging, pregnancy, and HIV/AIDS on emergent endocrine and metabolic disorder presentation and management. The remaining sections cover various different endocrine and metabolic systems, including pituitary; thyroid; adrenal; calcium, phosphate, and metabolic bone diseases; neuroendocrine tumors; glucose; sodium; obesity and clinical lipidology; and inherited metabolic disorders.

I would like to thank J Larry Jameson for writing the Foreword. In his current and previous multifaceted roles, Dr Jameson understands the complex challenges faced by clinicians in delivering care for patients presenting with endocrine and metabolic emergencies. My thanks also go to Bill Young, whom I first approached with the concept for the book when he was serving as president of the Endocrine Society. I would also like to acknowledge the tremendous effort by the authors. Despite very tight deadlines and having numerous other commitments, they generously shared their time and expertise in writing these excellent chapters. I owe special thanks to Maxine Aldred, Director of Books Development at the Endocrine Society, who has worked tirelessly and effectively on this project. I also want to thank the staff of the publications department for bringing this superb volume to fruition.

Last but not least, I owe special thanks to the reader. Your commitment to delivering excellent patient care while maintaining (and even expanding) your knowledge using resources such as this book are to be applauded—it's not easy! Your feedback is always welcome.

Glenn Matfin, MSc (Oxon), MB ChB, FACE, FACP, FRCP
Editor, Endocrine and Metabolic Medical Emergencies

SECTION I

Acute Medical Care

SECTION INTRODUCTION

Acute Medical Care

A Crisis with Solutions

John Wass and Sir Richard Thompson

There is a crisis in acute medical care for multifarious reasons. For example, the life expectancy at birth in the United Kingdom is now 12 years longer than at the inception of the National Health Service (NHS) in 1948 and people aged over 60 years now make up nearly a quarter of Britain's population. Half of them have a chronic illness, and this proportion will increase as the number of people aged 85 years or older doubles in the next 20 years. Nearly two thirds of patients admitted to the hospital are over 65 years old, and around 25% of these patients have a diagnosis of dementia.

Furthermore, the average length of stay in acute care in the United Kingdom in 2010 was 7.7 days, which is significantly higher than Australia (5.1), the Netherlands (5.8), and the United States (4.9). Lastly, there is an increase in mortality of around 10% among patients admitted on weekends. Although the reasons are complex, there is an association between the presence of senior doctors and improved clinical outcome for patients. Other problems exist as well. Junior doctors are working shorter hours, and there is sometimes a lack of communication at handover. There is an increase in demand for medical care, and emergency care departments are increasingly busy. Medical registrars and other trainees are under increased pressure (1), and there is evidence that trainees do not get the mentorship or training that they deserve because of increasing demands on senior staff.

SOLUTIONS/OPPORTUNITIES

This together with the UK Francis Enquiry on the Mid Staffordshire NHS Foundation Trust (2) highlighting, among other things, that patients were not at the center of care showed that fundamental change was necessary in the running of the NHS (3) and in particular the organization of medical care in hospitals.

Against this background (ie, rising acute medical admissions, increasingly older and frailer patients with complex illnesses and multiple morbidities, systemic failures of care, poor patient experience, and a medical workforce crisis) the future hospital commission (4) was set up by the Royal College of Physicians under the chairmanship of Sir Michael Rawlins and published in September 2013. It set out 11 core principles for hospitals of the future (Table I-1). The first principle is that of putting patients first. Patients should be treated with compassion and dignity. They should be involved in decisions on their condition. A new model of care is needed, and the suggestion (already taken up by several Trusts in the United Kingdom) is that there should be a medical division led by a chief of medicine (similar to the current practice in the United States) as

Table I-1. Core Principles of Patient Care (Future Hospital Commission)

1.	Fundamental standards of care must always be met
2.	Patient experience is valued as much as clinical effectiveness
3.	Responsibility for each patient's care is clear and communicated
4.	Patients have effective and timely access to care, including appointments, tests, treatment, and moves out of hospital
5.	Patients do not move wards unless this is necessary for their clinical care
6.	Robust arrangements for the transfer of care are in place
7.	Good communication with and about patients is the norm
8.	Care is designed to facilitate self-care and health promotion
9.	Services are tailored to meet the needs of individual patients, including vulnerable patients
10.	All patients have a care plan that reflects their individual clinical and support needs
11.	Staff are supported to deliver safe, compassionate care and committed to improving quality

the senior doctor responsible for making sure working practices facilitate collaborative, patient-centered care, and that teams work together toward common goals and in the best interest of patients. Effective leadership is, therefore, essential.

Seven-day care is important, too, and there should be coverage 24 hours a day, 7 days a week. This is particularly because, as above, patients often present with multiple illnesses requiring a range of support. This aspect, too, is being taken up in many hospitals in the United Kingdom, but there are sometimes problems with the smaller hospitals being able to provide coverage.

There is an important consequence of this: There need to be more doctors trained in generalist medicine, including acute medicine, internal medicine, and enhanced and intensive care. This does not mean that specialist care is less important or less of a priority. It will remain essential, and indeed the degree of expertise available in the specialties is ever increasing. Accredited training in aspects of super specialist care should be available and will enhance further the quality of specialist input. This will be time-consuming and expensive to do but is important to maintain specialist expertise.

Patient safety is key, and the Royal College of Physicians, along with many other national and international organizations, is looking at ways to improve patient safety. Why can't the medical profession have the success with safety that airlines do?

Our trainees are important and should, as far as possible, work in stable medical teams that educate and have time to educate the next generation. Patient care should cross the boundaries of primary and secondary care with care pathways designed for each of the morbidities that a patient experiences. Regrettably the NHS at the moment has walls between primary and secondary care that actively need to be broken down and this is already happening in many specialties. In this regard, effective communication is key.

Although there are challenges for the future of patient care—and these have never been greater—there are also solutions, and we as a profession need to lead like Henry V from the front. The medical profession must not be as contumacious and reactionary as it can be. Although written predominantly from a UK perspective, the challenges and opportunities outlined here will resonate with all stakeholders involved in delivering high-quality, patient-centered, cost-effective, acute medical care globally.

ACKNOWLEDGMENTS

The authors have nothing to disclose.

REFERENCES

1. **Hospitals on the edge? The time for action.** London: Royal College of Physicians; 2012.
2. **Report of the Mid Staffordshire NHS Foundation Trust Public Enquiry chaired by Robert Francis QC.** London: Stationary Office; 2013.
3. **Black N.** Can England's NHS survive? *N Eng J Med.* 2013;369:1–3.
4. **Future Hospital Commission.** Caring for medical patients. London: Royal College of Physicians; 2013.

CHAPTER 1

Early Management of Acute Medical Emergencies

Paul J Frost and Matthew P Wise

ABSTRACT

Acute medical emergencies can arise at any time, and effective early management depends on prompt recognition, good teamwork, and the methodical application of the Airway, Breathing, Circulation, Disability, and Exposure (ABCDE) approach.

INTRODUCTION

Acute medical emergencies are those illnesses that can cause organ failures and death within minutes to hours of their presentation. These illnesses present with little warning, and affected patients are usually distressed, frightened, and, often, uncooperative. These episodes can occur in any hospital location, and the ability of available staff to deal with them may vary considerably. Given these circumstances, it is unsurprising that management errors occur, resulting in failures of care and poor outcomes (1). Effective, early management of acute medical emergencies requires prompt recognition, immediate correction of life-threatening physiological abnormalities, and rapid diagnosis and treatment of the underlying condition. Endocrine and metabolic disorders are common causes of acute medical emergencies.

RECOGNITION OF MEDICAL EMERGENCIES

Medical emergencies are usually recognized by clinical signs of severe cardiorespiratory or neurological insufficiency. In a large, multinational, observational study, serious physiological deterioration, most frequently hypotension and a fall in the Glasgow Coma Score, was documented in 60% of patients prior to cardiac arrest, death, or intensive care unit (ICU) admission (2). Although the underlying diagnosis may initially be elusive, the clinical signs that accompany a medical emergency are readily identified and include tachycardia or bradycardia, hypotension, cold peripheries, oliguria, cyanosis, tachypnea or bradypnea, seizures, agitation, confusion, and coma (Table 1-1). These signs are usually detected by simple, bedside observations, such as pulse, blood pressure, respiratory rate, peripheral oxygen saturations, temperature, and level of consciousness. In the United Kingdom, these bedside observations have been used to develop a National Early Warning Score (NEWS). NEWS is derived by aggregating points assigned to increasing deviations from the normal range in each observation (3). This score is linked to a graded response strategy, such that acutely ill patients who score high are immediately reviewed by an appropriately trained, rapid response team (3). Although intuitively sensible, convincing evidence that rapid response systems like NEWS are effective in preventing adverse outcomes, such as death or intensive care admission, is currently lacking (4–6). Deficiencies in rapid response systems include the fact that observations may

Table 1-1. Medical Emergency: Possible Clinical Signs

Skin: mottled; sweaty; cyanosis; warm and vasodilated or cold peripheries.
Neurological: agitation; confusion; depressed level of consciousness; seizures; localizing signs.
Respiratory: stridor; grunting; drooling; use of accessory muscles; tracheal tug; intercostal in-drawing; nasal flaring; respiratory rate (RR) >25 breaths/min or <8 breaths/min; audible wheeze or silent chest.
Cardiovascular: capillary refill time >2 seconds; pulse >150 beats/min or <50 beats/min; low volume pulse; absent peripheral pulses; systolic blood pressure <90 mm Hg; mean arterial pressure (MAP) <70 mm Hg; postural hypotension; urine output <0.5 mL/kg/hr or anuria.

not be reliably taken and scores may be miscalculated (7, 8). Moreover, the sensitivity and specificity of the NEWS as a test for acute illness will be affected by patient-specific factors, such as age, drug therapy, and comorbidity. For example, a severe gastrointestinal bleed may not cause a high NEWS in a previously hypertensive patient treated with beta blockers because blood pressure and pulse rate may remain in the "normal range" despite significant hypovolemia. Recognition of the emergency nature of these sorts of presentations remains dependent on a high degree of clinical suspicion informed by clinical experience. Nonetheless, over recent years rapid response systems have been adopted by hospitals worldwide as the default mechanism for the recognition and immediate management of deteriorating patients and medical emergencies (9). Once alerted to a medical emergency, the challenge to the responsible clinician is to make the diagnosis while providing supportive care, so that effective treatment can be administered. While most clinicians are familiar with an Airway, Breathing, and Circulation (ABC) approach, these activities may be best coordinated using an Airway, Breathing, Circulation, Disability, and Exposure (ABCDE) approach. Applying this approach at the bedside requires that the attending clinician organizes available staff into an effective team. This leadership role is largely understated in widely publicized resuscitation guidelines and yet is crucial to achieving good outcomes. Crisis resource management (CRM) has been defined as *the ability to translate the knowledge of what needs to be done into effective treatment activity in the complex and real world of medical treatment* (10). It is important that clinicians managing medical emergencies are familiar with CRM principles and adhere to them whenever possible.

THE ABCDE APPROACH

It is axiomatic that outcomes from medical emergencies are improved by early diagnosis and treatment. For example, prompt reperfusion can reduce infarct size and prolong life in myocardial infarction and stroke; while early, effective antibiotics improve survival in septic shock (11–13). However, before a diagnosis is reached these patients may die from severe physiological disturbances such as hypoxemia and shock (14). The ABCDE approach can be seen as a mechanism to preserve life, while a diagnosis is sought so that definitive treatment can be administered (15). The process starts at the bedside with a preliminary assessment of the patient's general condition; this swift assessment focuses on the presence of clinical signs associated with life-threatening cardiorespiratory and/or neurological insufficiency (Table 1-1).

Much of this preliminary assessment can be completed by observation of the patient, inspection of the clinical observation charts, and brief discussion with the bedside nurse. At the conclusion of this assessment it may be obvious that the patient is moribund or "peri-arrest" and that the "cardiac arrest" or "rapid response team" should be called. In the United Kingdom, the National Health Service (NHS) Institute for Innovation and Improvement has recommended the situation, background, assessment, and recommendation (SBAR) method for referring acutely ill patients (Table 1-2) (16). Regardless of the hospital system in place, once an emergency is recognized, assistance should be requested immediately. Rarely can these situations be effectively managed by a single practitioner. At this juncture the team (or individual clinician awaiting the arrival of assistance) should establish basic monitoring (eg, electrocardiography

Table 1-2. Situation, Background, Assessment, and Recommendation Communication Tool

Situation	Identify yourself (name, role, location), the person you are speaking to, and the patient; state reason for call and urgency. ***Example:*** *My name is Dr Frost. I am the house officer (resident) on ward 6. Are you the on-call critical care clinician? I am with Mrs Smith, a 65-year-old woman who is in extremis with oxygen saturations of 78%.*
Background	Briefly relate history, including date of admission, diagnosis, and current management ***Example:*** *Mrs Smith is a previously healthy woman who 1 week ago was admitted after having a stroke. She is currently undergoing rehabilitation.*
Assessment	State your working diagnosis. ***Example:*** *I think Mrs Smith has respiratory failure secondary to a severe hospital-acquired pneumonia.*
Recommendation	State the request. ***Example:*** *I think Mrs Smith will likely need endotracheal and mechanical ventilation. Please attend the ward immediately.*

[ECG], pulse oximetry, and blood pressure) and calmly and methodically work through the ABCDE approach, correcting life-threatening physiological disturbances as they are discovered. Other measures such as point-of-care blood glucose testing should also be performed as clinically indicated.

Airway Assessment and Management

Upper airway obstruction (UAO) must be diagnosed and treated quickly; complete obstruction will lead to cardiac arrest within minutes, while partial obstruction can impair ventilation and cause hypoxemia. UAO may be recognized by impaired or absent speech, stridor, grunting, drooling, severe respiratory distress, paradoxical chest wall movement ("see-saw" movements), prominent neck veins, facial swelling, and absent breath sounds. In general terms the aim of management is to provide a secure, patent airway but specific therapy will be determined by the underlying cause.

When the diagnosis is obvious, interventions to clear and support the airway can proceed immediately; for example, oral-pharyngeal inspection and removal of an easily accessible foreign body, or application of simple, airway-opening maneuvers, such as a chin-lift or jaw-thrust, for coma. When the diagnosis is unclear, manipulation of the airway and insertion of airway adjuncts should be avoided because these interventions may precipitate complete UAO; for example, in the setting of epiglottitis. Generally, if conscious, patients with UAO should be allowed to assume the position in which they find it most comfortable to breathe. Forcing these patients into the recovery or supine position can precipitate cardiac arrest. All patients with UAO should be assessed by an anesthetist because endotracheal intubation is frequently required to secure the airway definitively. Occasionally the airway can only be secured by a surgical technique such as cricothyroidotomy or tracheostomy. Computed tomography (CT) of the neck and chest and/or flexible bronchoscopy may be required for diagnosis of the underlying cause of the UAO but for safety, the airway should be secured prior to these investigations being undertaken.

Breathing Assessment and Management

Once the airway is deemed to be safe or secured then breathing should be assessed for signs of respiratory insufficiency (Table 1-1). Auscultation is important both diagnostically and as a means to assess response to treatment—bronchial breath sounds may help confirm the diagnosis of pneumonia, while the detection of breath sounds following drainage of a pneumothorax suggests that the lung has reinflated.

Peripheral oxygen saturations should be routinely measured in all patients with respiratory distress, and hypoxemia should be rapidly corrected. A wide variety of oxygen delivery devices are available, but in the setting of acute illness the most appropriate device to use is a non-rebreathing face mask with reservoir and one-way valve. When connected to wall oxygen at a flow rate of 15 L/min this device may provide an inspired oxygen concentration (FiO_2) of up to 90%. Expert consensus guidance suggests that in the setting of critical illness oxygen saturation targets should generally be 94%–98% (17). In some patients with chronic obstructive pulmonary disease (COPD) and carbon dioxide retention, supplemental oxygen therapy is associated with worsening hypercapnia and respiratory failure and inspired oxygen should be titrated to achieve saturations of 88%–92%, and noninvasive ventilation (NIV) should be considered (17).

Mechanical ventilation should be considered for those patients with reversible disease and persistent failure of oxygenation and/or ventilation (ie, carbon dioxide clearance). NIV is particularly indicated in patients with COPD and respiratory acidosis (pH 7.25–7.35) and hypercapnic respiratory failure secondary to chest wall deformity or neuromuscular disease. Generally invasive ventilation (ie, tracheal intubation) is indicated in those patients with respiratory failure and impaired consciousness or copious pulmonary secretions (18).

Circulatory Assessment and Management

Once appropriate steps have been taken to address any breathing difficulties attention should be directed toward the assessment and management of circulatory insufficiency (Table 1-1). Acute or chronic fluid loss is usually followed by peripheral vasoconstriction and a compensatory tachycardia in order to preserve perfusion of vital organs. There is a wide spectrum of ability among patients to compensate for fluid loss—unsurprisingly, young, fit patients can compensate for greater fluid loss than older patients, particularly those with significant cardiovascular comorbidity. Typically, after 30%–40% of circulating volume has been lost decompensation occurs, manifested by marked hypotension and multiorgan dysfunction, characteristic of shock (14). Treatment of shock requires the restoration of an effective circulating blood volume to reverse decompensation and restore organ perfusion. This process depends on diagnosis of the underlying condition so that specific therapies can be administered. A useful aide-mémoire for the differential diagnosis of shock is to classify this condition into 4 groups according to the main mechanism of decompensation (ie, hypovolemia; cardiogenic; obstructive [eg, pulmonary embolism, cardiac tamponade]; or distributive [eg, severe sepsis, anaphylaxis]) (14).

As always, accurate history is the most important determinant of the diagnosis, physical examination, aside from confirming the presence of a shock state, may be less rewarding, particularly in advanced disease. Patients with shock require urgent resuscitation, a useful mnemonic to describe the important components is the VIP rule: ventilate (oxygen administration), infuse (fluid resuscitation), and pump (administration of vasoactive agents) (14). Generally, patients with shock require intravenous (IV) fluid resuscitation; a caveat to this are those patients with pulmonary edema as gas exchange may deteriorate in these individuals. If there is diagnostic uncertainty, a fluid challenge can be helpful in identifying those patients who are likely to be fluid responsive. A fluid challenge can be delivered by administering 250 mL of IV fluid over 2 minutes—hypovolemic patients will show an improvement in their blood pressure and pulse rate (19).

There has been considerable debate in the literature as to the optimal resuscitation fluid—over the years a variety of fluids including crystalloids, colloids, and human albumin solutions have been used and a number of problems identified. Current evidence would seem to support the use of balanced electrolyte solutions such as Ringer's lactate or Hartmann's solution as appropriate first-line resuscitation fluids. Regardless of the type of resuscitation fluid selected, frequent patient reassessment against relevant clinical end points, such as peripheral perfusion, pulse, blood pressure, and urine output is essential so that therapy can be titrated and inadvertent fluid and electrolyte overload can be averted. Hyperlactatemia (>1.5 mmol/L) is also typically present in acute circulatory failure and can be monitored (14). Vasoactive drugs may be necessary if blood pressure and cardiac output remain low; these patients need to be transferred to the ICU for further management.

Disability Assessment and Management

Neurological dysfunction is frequently implicated in medical emergencies and is due either to primary neurological disease or arises as a consequence of non-neurological illnesses. For example, coma may arise as a consequence of an intracerebral hemorrhage, severe hypoglycemia, severe hyponatremia, or severe circulatory shock. Disability refers to emergency neurological assessment and management and starts with a basic assessment of level of consciousness. AVPU and the Glasgow Coma Scale (GCS) are two systems that standardize the assessment of consciousness. AVPU is simple to remember and apply: A, the patient is alert; V, the patient only responds to voice; P, the patient only responds to pain; and U, the patient is unresponsive. The GCS provides a more detailed description of consciousness in terms of eye opening, verbal response, and motor response and can be summarized using an aggregate numerical score ranging from 3, deeply unconscious, to 15, alert and cooperative. An individual patient is best described using the Glasgow Coma Scale rather than the Glasgow Coma Score, which was originally designed for audit and research purposes (20). On the Glasgow Coma Scale patients are arbitrarily defined as being in a coma if they can perform no better than eye opening to pain (E2), incomprehensible sounds (V2), and withdraw to a painful stimulus (M4). Generally, if the Glasgow Coma Score is <8/15, or if the patient only responds to pain, or is unresponsive on the AVPU scale, the ability of the patient to maintain a patent airway might be impaired. This can cause partial airway obstruction, reduced ventilation, and an increased vulnerability to pulmonary aspiration. Adherence to the ABCDE approach should ensure that the airway is secured in these patients (see Airway Assessment and Management above). There is a wide differential diagnosis for coma, and its evaluation requires a comprehensive history, general physical examination, and neurological assessment (Table 1-3).

Exposure

The ABCDE approach concludes with E (exposure), which is a prompt to complete a full physical examination. At this stage, life-threatening abnormalities have been addressed and the patient is better able to tolerate and cooperate with the demands of the examination.

DEFINITIVE DIAGNOSIS AND TREATMENT

For medical emergencies, the traditional path to diagnosis (ie, history, physical examination, and investigation) is modified and integrated with the ABCDE approach. Diagnostic synthesis and the ABCDE approach should be viewed as complementary and simultaneous processes (Figure 1-1).

History

The patient should not be needlessly exhausted by detailed interrogation; much of the relevant history can be gleaned from medical records, nursing staff, or relatives. It is important, however, to inquire as to the presence and characteristics of any pain; not only is this a cardinal diagnostic symptom, it also will need to be relieved. It is likely that clinicians use both nonanalytical (pattern recognition) and analytical methods in formulating

Table 1-3. Causes of Coma—Aide-Mémoire IF SOMNOLENT

Infection
Fits
Stroke
Overdose: alcohol, tricyclic antidepressants, benzodiazepines, etc.
Metabolic: Uremia, hepatic encephalopathy, hyponatremia, hypernatremia, hypercapnia
Neoplasm: Primary or secondary brain tumors
Oxygen deficiency: postcardiac arrest; near drowning
Low temperature: low blood pressure
Endocrine: hypoglycemia, hyperglycemia, hypopituitarism, hypothyroidism, hypercalcemia, Addison's disease
Narcotics
Trauma

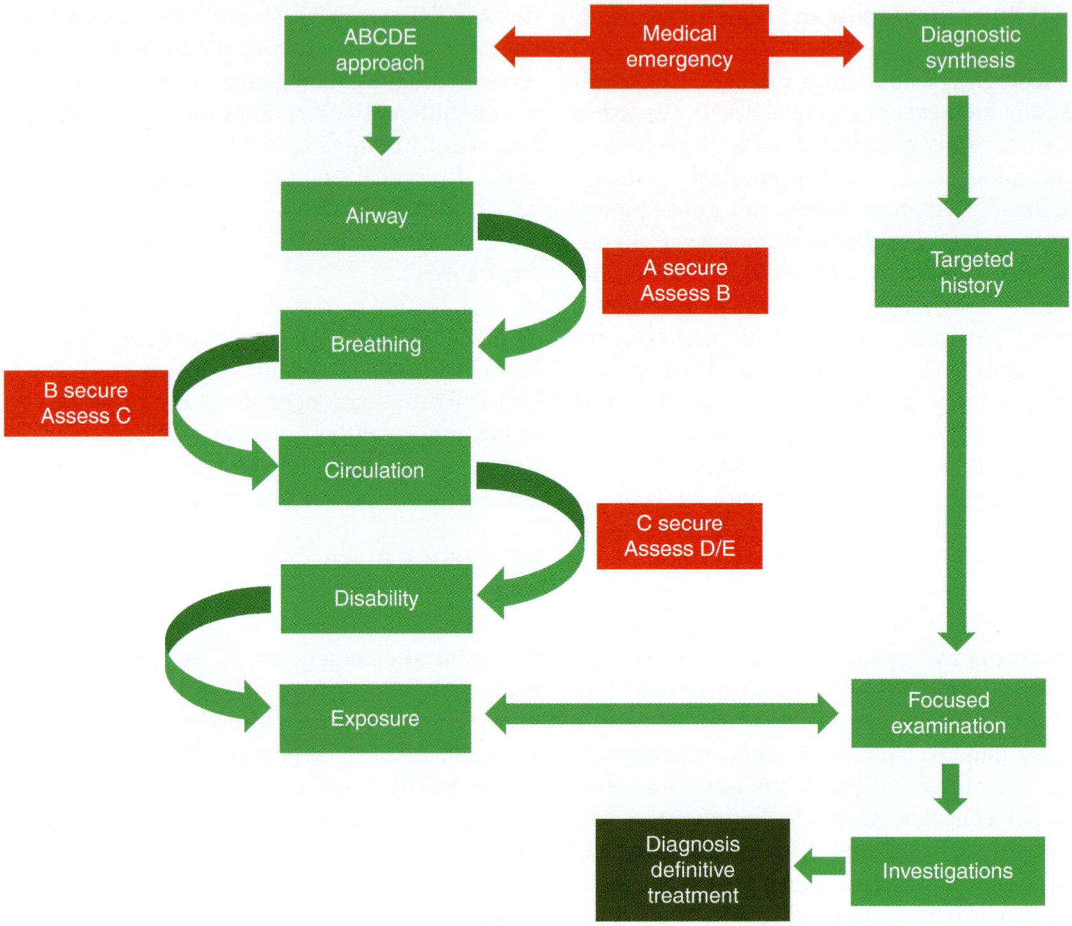

Figure 1-1. The ABCDE approach and diagnostic synthesis are complementary and simultaneous processes.

a diagnosis. This process has been termed iterative diagnosis and is prone to well-recognized cognitive errors (17). Diagnostic errors usually arise because of overreliance on pattern recognition and intuition rather than analytical reasoning. Diagnostic uncertainty should be managed by mental reversion to a highly analytical approach, rigorously analyzing available data against diagnostic hypotheses. In the setting of severe shock, the aide-mémoire above (ie, hypovolemia, cardiogenic, obstructive, or distributive) provides the full range of diagnostic possibilities against which available clinical data can be analyzed.

Physical Examination

Physical examination is completed at the conclusion of the ABCDE approach and is focused on those systems likely to be diagnostically helpful. For example, a comprehensive abdominal examination is essential in a patient with peritonitis and shock but not immediately required in a patient with an acute myocardial infarction. The physical examination should be modified to minimize patient exertion and the deleterious effects of repositioning. It is important to note that breathing difficulties and hypoxemia are exacerbated by movement from the semirecumbent to supine position, particularly in obese patients (21).

Investigations

These are guided by diagnostic impressions, but basic blood tests such as arterial or venous blood gases, complete (full) blood counts, blood urea nitrogen (BUN) or urea, electrolytes, blood glucose, and blood cultures are usually helpful.

Illness severity can be assessed with a blood lactate—one prospective study reported an 83% mortality in patients with a blood lactate of >5 mmol/L (22); while bedside investigations such as ECG, plain radiography, and echocardiography may be diagnostic.

It may be necessary to transfer patients for other tests such as CT. In these circumstances, patients should be stabilized as much as possible and the transfers undertaken by suitably trained personnel. It is important to consider the risks and benefits of all investigations, as overinvestigation may delay definitive treatment.

Treatment

Generally, medical emergencies will be managed in an emergency department, acute medical unit (AMU), or equivalent, as well as more advanced step-up facilities such as high dependency unit (HDU) or ICU. Many therapies such as blood and blood products, drugs (eg, antimicrobials, antiplatelet agents, analgesics, diuretics), and, of course, oxygen and IV fluid should be given at the bedside prior to transfer to HDU or ICU if required. International guidelines have recommended the administration of broad-spectrum antibiotics within 1 hour of recognizing severe sepsis or septic shock (23).

ICU admission is indicated for patients who require organ support, most commonly mechanical ventilation and close nursing observation. The decision to admit a patient into the ICU is informed primarily by clinical factors, such as the potential reversibility of the illness, and the wishes of the patient or their surrogates. Old age in itself is not a reason to refuse ICU admission, but old age undoubtedly reduces physiological reserve and is more likely to be accompanied by serious comorbidity. Severity-of-illness scoring systems such as the acute physiology and chronic health evaluation II (APACHE II) and the simplified acute physiology score (SAPS) are used to estimate hospital mortality for groups of patients and cannot be used to predict individual outcomes. Moreover, these systems do not provide any information about longer term survival; for example, 6–12 months following critical illness, or quality of life or functional status. Frailty is a multifaceted syndrome characterized by a demise in physical and cognitive reserves and increasing vulnerability (24). Although yet to be evaluated in critically ill patients, it has been suggested that clinical measures of frailty may help identify those elderly patients who would most benefit from ICU admission (25).

Medical emergencies should not be confused with the natural process of dying. The distinction is not always straightforward, but where there is clear evidence of terminal illness, such as advanced cancer, the treatment imperatives are comfort and dignity not aggressive resuscitation.

CONCLUSIONS

Acute medical emergencies can arise at any time and effective early management depends on prompt recognition, good teamwork, and the methodical application of the ABCDE approach.

ACKNOWLEDGMENTS

The authors have nothing to disclose.

REFERENCES

1. **National Confidential Enquiry into Patient Outcome and Death.** An acute problem? 2005. http://www.ncepod.org.uk/2005report/index.html.
2. **Kause J, Smith G, Prytherch D, et al.** A comparison of antecedents to cardiac arrests, deaths and emergency intensive care admissions in Australia, New Zealand and the United Kingdom—the ACADEMIA study. *Resuscitation.* 2004;62:275–282.
3. **Royal College of Physicians.** National early warning score (NEWS). http://www.rcplondon.ac.uk/resources/national-early-warning-score-news.
4. **McGaughey J, Alderdice F, Fowler R, Kapila A, Mayhew A, Moutray M.** Outreach and Early Warning Systems (EWS) for the prevention of intensive care admission and death of critically ill adult patients on general hospital wards. *Cochrane Database Syst Rev.* 2007;18(3):CD005529.
5. **Chan PS, Jain R, Nallmothu BK, Berg RA, Sasson C.** Rapid response teams: a systematic review and meta-analysis. *Arch Intern Med.* 2010;11;170(1):18–26.
6. **McNeill G, Bryden D.** Resuscitation. Do either early warning systems or emergency response teams improve hospital patient survival? A systematic review. *Resuscitation.* 2013;84(12):1652–1667.
7. **Gordon CF, Beckett DJ.** Significant deficiencies in the overnight use of a Standardised Early Warning

Scoring system in a teaching hospital. *Scott Med J.* 2011;56:15–18.

8. **Smith T, Den Hartog D, Moerman T, Patka P, Van Lieshout EM, Schep NW.** Accuracy of an expanded early warning score for patients in general and trauma surgery wards. *Br J Surg.* 2012;99:192–197.
9. **Litvak E, Pronovost PJ.** Rethinking rapid response teams. *JAMA.* 2010;304(12):1375–1376.
10. **Rall M, Gaba D.** Human performance and patient safety. In: Miller R, ed. *Miller's Anesthesia.* 6th ed. Philadelphia, PA: Elsevier Churchill Livingstone; 2005;3021–3072.
11. **Vemulapalli S, Zhou Y, Gutberlet M, et al.** Importance of total ischemic time and preprocedural infarct-related artery blood flow in predicting infarct size in patients with anterior wall myocardial infarction (from the CRISP-AMI Trial). *Am J Cardiol.* 2013;112(7):911–917.
12. **Wardlaw JM, Murray V, Berge E, Del Zoppo GJ.** Thrombolysis for acute ischaemic stroke. *Cochrane Database Syst Rev.* 2009;(4):CD000213.
13. **Kumar A, Roberts D, Wood KE, et al.** Duration of hypotension before initiation of effective antimicrobial therapy is the critical determinant of survival in human septic shock. *Crit Care Med.* 2006;34:1589–1596.
14. **Vincent J-L, De Backer D.** Circulatory shock. *N Engl J Med.* 2013;369:1726–1734.
15. **Frost PJ, Wise MP.** Early management of acutely ill ward patients. *BMJ.* 2012;345:e5677.
16. **NHS institute for innovation and improvement.** SBAR: Situation, background, assessment, recommendation. http://www.institute.nhs.uk/qualityandserviceimprovementtools/qualityandserviceimprovementtools/sbar-situation-background-assessment-recommendation.html.
17. **O'Driscoll BR, Howard LS, Davison AG; British Thoracic Society.** BTS guideline for emergency oxygen use in adult patients. *Thorax.* 2008;63(suppl 6):vi, 1–68.
18. **British Thoracic Society Standards of Care Committee.** Non-invasive ventilation in acute respiratory failure. *Thorax.* 2002;57(3):192–211.
19. **Cecconi M, Parsons AK, Rhodes A.** What is a fluid challenge? *Curr Opin Crit Care.* 2011; 17(3):290–295.
20. **Barlow P.** A practical review of the Glasgow Coma Scale and Score. *Surgeon.* 2012;10(2):114–119.
21. **Altermatt FR, Muñoz HR, Delfino AE, Cortínez LI.** Pre-oxygenation in the obese patient: effects of position on tolerance to apnea. *Br J Anaesth.* 2005;95(5):706–709.
22. **Stacpoole PW, Wright EC, Baumgartner TG, et al.** Natural history and course of acquired lactic acidosis in adults. DCA-Lactic Acidosis Study Group. *Am J Med.* 1994;97(1):47–54.
23. **Dellinger RP, Levy MM, Rhodes A, et al.** Surviving Sepsis Campaign: international guidelines for management of severe sepsis and septic shock, 2012. *Intensive Care Med.* 2013;39(2):165–228.
24. **Rockwood K, Song X, MacKnight C, et al.** A global clinical measure of fitness and frailty in elderly people. *CMAJ.* 2005;173(5):489–495.
25. **McDermid RC, Stelfox HT, Bagshaw SM.** Frailty in the critically ill: a novel concept. *Crit Care.* 2011;15(1):301.

SECTION II

General Endocrine and Metabolic Aspects of Acute Medical and Critical Illness

SECTION INTRODUCTION

Endocrine Responses and Testing in Acute Medical and Critical Illness

David B Sacks

The clinical laboratory has an integral role in the management of patients with acute medical and critical illness. This group of patients has diverse presentations, multi-organ dysfunction is frequent, and some life-threatening pathophysiological disruptions may be occult. The laboratory is necessary to detect many of these conditions and is essential for both monitoring responses to treatment and detecting or avoiding deleterious consequences of therapy. For example, during treatment of hyperglycemia with insulin, blood glucose concentrations need to be measured frequently to avoid hypoglycemia and serum potassium must be monitored to prevent hypokalemia, which may occur due to stimulation of potassium uptake into cells by insulin.

Critically ill patients are prone to metabolic derangements and alterations to endocrine systems. Several factors contribute to this (1). The stress of acute illness may augment (eg, hypothalamic-pituitary-adrenal) or attenuate (eg, hypothalamic-pituitary-gonadal) the activity of hormone axes. In addition to changes in hormone secretion, hormone metabolism and clearance can be altered by reduced circulation, inflammation, hypoxia, or other insults. The normal diurnal variation that occurs with a number of hormones is also disrupted. Moreover, critically ill patients usually receive numerous therapeutic agents, some of which may alter endocrine homeostasis. Thus, endocrine evaluation of an acutely ill patient requires consideration of numerous elements.

Hormone binding proteins are another aspect that needs to be contemplated. Several hormones, including thyroid hormones (T_3 and T_4), cortisol, and testosterone, are transported in the circulation by carrier proteins. During acute illness the amount of binding protein may change considerably, and the direction of the change (increase or decrease) is dependent on the underlying condition(s). In addition, the binding of hormone to carrier protein may be altered by medication, renal failure, pH change, or other conditions common to critical illness. It is generally believed that only the free hormone is biologically active. Importantly, the free hormone comprises a small fraction (eg, ~0.1% and 5% for T_3 and cortisol, respectively) of the total circulating hormone. Most assays measure the total hormone concentration, which may not correlate with the biologically active moiety, especially when amounts or binding affinities of carrier proteins are altered. Attempts to overcome this limitation with equations to calculate the free hormone have met with limited success. Several techniques, including equilibrium dialysis and ultrafiltration, have been used to separate free from bound hormone, followed by measurement of the free fraction. These approaches require rigorous attention to detail, because temperature, pH, leakage, or adsorption can substantially influence the results. The overwhelming majority of endocrine analyses are performed using antibodies (termed immunoassays). These assays frequently have inadequate sensitivity to quantify the low concentrations of free hormone accurately. Moreover, immunoassays suffer from inaccuracy, lack specificity, and often are not standardized so the results can vary widely among different laboratories and different instruments. The implementation in clinical laboratories of mass spectrometry has the potential to address many of these problems. A considerable advantage of mass spectrometry is the exquisite sensitivity, which enables measurement of very low concentrations of substances, yielding accurate results for free hormones.

Although a lack of standardization limits most hormone assays, this problem has essentially been resolved for hemoglobin A1c (HbA1c or AIC), a ubiquitous test in patients with diabetes. Although early methods to measure HbA1c were not standardized, the establishment in 1995 of the NGSP (previously known as the National Glycohemoglobin Standardization Program) has resulted in significantly reduced variability among methods and laboratories (2). This improvement led to the adoption over the last few years of HbA1c as a criterion for diagnosis of diabetes. HbA1c, which reflects long-term blood glucose concentration, is not altered by stress, food ingestion, diurnal variation, or other factors that modulate glucose in critically ill patients (3). Nevertheless, it may be influenced by certain conditions in the critically ill, such as blood loss, hemolysis, or blood transfusion.

Until recently, HbA1c was reported throughout the world as a percentage of total hemoglobin. The development by the International Federation of Clinical Chemistry (IFCC) of a reference method employing mass spectrometry yields values lower than NGSP standardized results by 1.5%–2.0% HbA1c (4). To avoid confusion, a decision was reached to report IFCC values in Systeme International (SI) units as mmol HbA1c per mol Hb. For example, HbA1c of 6.5% and 7% correspond to 48 and 53 mmol/mol, respectively. (A linear equation is required to convert between the 2 sets of units (5).) Several countries, predominantly in Europe, have elected to report HbA1c exclusively in SI units (5). Many journals now require that both sets of HbA1c units be used in publications.

Measuring patient samples at the bedside (termed point-of-care [POC]), usually performed on a blood or urine sample using a small handheld device, has several appealing features. Advantages include eliminating transport of the sample to the central laboratory, no or minimal sample processing (analysis is usually conducted with whole blood, obviating the need for centrifugation), simple analytical process, minimal sample requirement (eg, only a drop of blood), and very rapid availability of results (1–2 min). By contrast, POC test results are generally less accurate than those obtained from laboratory analyzers, usually cost substantially more, and, in general, are more prone to interference from drugs and other substances. Although several different analytes can be measured with POC devices, glucose is by far the most common substance measured in patients' blood at the bedside.

A highly contentious subject is the use of POC glucose meters in critically ill patients. Several published studies document increased mortality in hospitalized patients who have hyperglycemia or hypoglycemia. Compelling evidence revealed that intensive insulin therapy to maintain blood glucose concentrations at 80–110 mg/dL (4.4–6.1 mmol/L) significantly reduced the morbidity and mortality of patients in a surgical intensive care unit (ICU) (6). This approach, termed "tight glucose control," was rapidly and widely adopted in hospital ICUs. The publication 8 years later of the Normoglycemia in Intensive Care Evaluation-Survival Using Glucose Algorithm Regulation (NICE-SUGAR) trial (7) considerably dampened enthusiasm for tight glucose control protocols. The latter study observed that the intensive-control group had significantly higher mortality than the conventional-control group. Multiple other studies have been performed, and these have variably reported that tight glucose control protocols in ICU patients result in better, equivalent, or worse outcomes than standard glucose control. Reasons for the discrepancies in the published literature include variations in insulin protocols, patient populations, mortality rates, glucose targets, and parenteral nutrition. The methods and samples used for glucose analysis are likely to contribute substantially (8). The initial study by Van den Berge et al (6) measured glucose in arterial blood using an accurate arterial blood gas analyzer. Many of the subsequent studies used capillary blood and measured glucose with POC meters (the sample and/or method of analysis is not mentioned in many publications). The different glucose results that are produced by the diverse methods and samples will lead to different insulin doses, with potentially wide variations in the true glucose concentrations among patients.

In the United States, the Food and Drug Administration (FDA) has not approved the use of glucose meters for tight glucose control protocols in ICUs. Glucose meters are considerably less accurate than blood gas or central laboratory analyzers. For many years, the most widely accepted criteria for meter performance were that 95% of the time the result should be ±20% of the "true" glucose value at ≥75 mg/dL (4.2 mmol/L) and ±15 mg/dL (0.83 mmol/L) at glucose concentrations <75 mg/dL (4.2 mmol/L). Guidelines published in 2013 advocate tighter acceptance criteria requiring 95% of results to be within ±12.5% of the "true" glucose value at ≥100 mg/dL (5.55 mmol/L) and ±12 mg/dL (0.67 mmol/L) at glucose concentrations <100 mg/dL (5.55 mmol/L). Note that virtually all glucose meters available at the time of writing were evaluated using the old criteria. In addition, patient factors, especially in critically ill subjects, contribute to inaccurate results with meters. Some glucose meters are affected by pO_2, pH, hypothermia, drugs, or hematocrit (9). The reduced tissue perfusion in hypotensive patients creates large differences between glucose concentrations in capillary and arterial blood samples. It is important to be aware that postprandial capillary glucose values are 20–25 mg/dL (1.1 to 1.4 mmol/L) higher than those in venous blood.

As mentioned above, critically ill patients pose multiple challenges for laboratory analysis. These range from alteration of circulating concentrations of hormones and electrolytes to interferences in the assays. The myriad underlying conditions can exert diverse effects on hormone secretion, elimination, and function. Thus, the "normal" concentration of many hormones in acutely ill patients differs from what is found in other patient populations. Interference in laboratory analysis is also common in critical illness. For example, parenteral nutrition can markedly increase serum lipids, which can artefactually alter several measurement procedures. The severe nature of the condition often requires frequent and rapid modifications of therapy. The need for virtually immediate availability of laboratory results (short turnaround time) creates problems. POC testing is a solution that provides rapid results, but the compromise is often considerably reduced accuracy.

Notwithstanding these issues, advances in technology are likely to alleviate or even resolve many of these concerns in the future. A number of approaches can reduce turnaround time for critically ill patients. Some can be adopted now; for example, using whole blood in the central laboratory to measure glucose and electrolytes, shortening turnaround time to minutes (analogous to current blood gas analysis). Alternatively, small, tabletop analyzers can be set up in ICUs and operating rooms with assays performed by trained medical technologists. Improvements in indwelling devices with continuous—and accurate—measurement of glucose and electrolytes have the promise to improve tight glucose control protocols substantially. Considerable effort is being invested in developing closed-loop systems with automated, accurate, continuous blood measurement and computer-controlled insulin delivery. The successful development of such a system should improve tight glucose control in ICUs. Current mass spectrometers are expensive as well as labor-intensive and require considerable technical expertise to operate. Therefore, they are predominantly confined to large-scale reference laboratories and university-based medical centers. In the future, user-friendly, relatively inexpensive, high-throughput, automated mass spectrometers are likely to become available and be widely adopted by clinical laboratories. In addition, analysis by mass spectrometry of panels of multiple different steroids for endocrine evaluation using only a few microliters of blood should become widespread. In the longer term, the introduction into the clinical laboratory of metabolomics, although challenging in many respects, may yield considerable insight into both our comprehension and management of acutely ill patients.

ACKNOWLEDGMENTS

Work in the author's laboratory is funded by the Intramural Research Program of the National Institutes of Health.

REFERENCES

1. **Hassan-Smith Z, Cooper MS.** Overview of the endocrine response to critical illness: how to measure it and when to treat. *Best Pract Res Clin Endocrinol Metab.* 2011;25:705–717.
2. **Little RR, Rohlfing CL, Sacks DB.** Status of hemoglobin A1c measurement and goals for improvement: from chaos to order for improving diabetes care. *Clin Chem.* 2011;57:205–214.
3. **Sacks DB.** A1C versus glucose testing: a comparison. *Diabetes Care.* 2011;34:518–523.
4. **Hoelzel W, Weykamp C, Jeppsson JO, et al.** IFCC reference system for measurement of hemoglobin A1c in human blood and the national standardization schemes in the United States, Japan, and Sweden: a method-comparison study. *Clin Chem.* 2004;50:166–174.
5. **Sacks DB.** Measurement of hemoglobin A(1c): a new twist on the path to harmony. *Diabetes Care.* 2012;35:2674–2680.
6. **van den Berghe G, Wouters P, Weekers F, et al.** Intensive insulin therapy in critically ill patients. *N Engl J Med.* 2001;345:1359–1367.
7. **Finfer S, Chittock DR, Su SY, et al.** Intensive versus conventional glucose control in critically ill patients. *N Engl J Med.* 2009;360:1283–1297.
8. **Scott MG, Bruns DE, Boyd JC, Sacks DB.** Tight glucose control in the intensive care unit: are glucose meters up to the task? *Clin Chem.* 2009;55:18–20.
9. **Dungan K, Chapman J, Braithwaite SS, Buse J.** Glucose measurement: confounding issues in setting targets for inpatient management. *Diabetes Care.* 2007;30:403–409.

CHAPTER 2

Endocrine Testing in Acute and Critical Illness

Penny M Clark and Julian H Barth

ABSTRACT

Many factors combine to increase the complexity of endocrine testing in the acute and critically ill, not only in terms of laboratory service provision but particularly in the interpretation of results. This chapter aims to highlight some of the pitfalls to be avoided by both the clinician and the laboratory. The endocrine changes in the critically ill patient involve most systems and vary with primary pathology and with time. The changes are further complicated by changes in hormone-binding proteins and by drug therapy. Interference in hormone assays can be difficult to identify, and differences in assay bias and difficulties with standardization determine that assay-specific reference ranges must be applied. It cannot be overemphasized that laboratory results should be reviewed critically and any discordance with the patient's condition or with previous results be considered with suspicion and discussed with the laboratory.

INTRODUCTION

Many factors combine to increase the complexity of endocrine testing in the acute and critically ill, not only in terms of laboratory service provision but particularly in the interpretation of results. The aim of this chapter is to highlight some of the pitfalls to be avoided by both the clinician and the laboratory.

PHYSIOLOGICAL CHANGES IN THE CRITICALLY ILL

Throughout the endocrine system, common changes found in acute illness impact investigations and their interpretation (Table 2-1). Examples will be given in later sections, but key effects are listed below:

- The stress response that overrides the normal biological rhythms (eg, loss of diurnal rhythm and menstrual cycle).
- Changes in hormone-binding proteins—concentrations of and affinity for binding (influenced by drugs, acid-base status).
- The definition of "normal" in the critically ill may not be relevant and thus the commonly reported reference intervals may be inappropriate.
- The use of dynamic function tests in the critically ill—these may well be contraindicated and in practice, other than the short adrenocorticotropic hormone (ACTH) stimulation test, are rarely performed in the critically ill patient. It should be noted that the effect of pharmacological stimulation in addition to the physiological stimulation of the stress response may be difficult to assess and may not accurately reflect endocrine status.
- The metabolic response to stress results in major changes in fat distribution and protein catabolism. This may have an

Table 2-1. Effects of Acute/Critical Illness on Specific Hormones

Hormone	Effect of Acute Illness	Explanation
Thyroid hormones	Acute phase ↓ T_3, ↑ rT_3	↓ activity of type 1 deiodinase, +/− ↑ activity of type 3 deiodinase
	Chronic phase ↓ T_4, ↓ or normal TSH	Central suppression
Cortisol	Acute ↑↑ Chronic ↑	Stress response, complex mechanisms
Prolactin	↑	Stress response
ACTH	Acute ↔ ↑ Chronic ↔↓	Stress response
Catecholamines	Acute ↑↑ Chronic ↑	Stress response
LH and FSH	↓	Prolactin suppression
Androgens	↓	↓ LH, FSH, Leydig cell function
Growth hormone	↑ loss of pulsatility	GH resistance
IGF-1	↓	Nutritional effect; also ↑ binding protein and ↑ protease activity
PTH	↑	In vitamin D-deficient patients
Vitamin D	↓	In at-risk groups
Insulin	↑ relative insulin insufficiency	↑ counter-regulatory hormones lead to hyperglycemia and insulin resistance

Abbreviations: ACTH = adrenocorticotropic hormone; FSH = follicle-stimulating hormone; IGF-1 = insulin-like growth factor 1; LH = luteinizing hormone; PTH = parathyroid hormone; T_3 = triiodothyronine; rT_3 = reverse T_3; T_4 = thyroxine; TSH = thyroid-stimulating hormone.

important influence on hormone secretion and action, which is dynamic and will vary throughout the course of the disease.

PHARMACOLOGICAL INFLUENCES

Pharmacological effects on endocrine systems may be due to either direct effects on hormone secretion and metabolism (Table 2-2) or to interferences in the hormone assays (Table 2-3) (1–6). There are limitations in our understanding of these effects in the acutely ill, where many drugs are given simultaneously and where drug pharmacokinetics and metabolite concentrations are more variable.

PATHOLOGICAL CHANGES

Hypothalamic-Pituitary Disease

Patients in the intensive care unit (ICU) have been documented to have significant abnormalities of pituitary hormone secretion. In addition, the cause of admission to the ICU (eg, traumatic brain injury [TBI] or subarachnoid hemorrhage) may result in damage to the hypothalamic-pituitary axis. In terms of laboratory investigations, two illustrative examples highlight this complexity: (a) the investigation of prolactinomas; and (b) the temporal development of endocrine changes following TBI.

In the first case, measurement of serum prolactin, along with other pituitary hormones at baseline is required. However, the interpretation of the prolactin result is complicated by the fact that there will be a significant overlap in serum prolactin concentrations found due to stress of acute illness and those due to a prolactinoma. In addition, the presence of macroprolactin (immunoglobulin-bound prolactin, which is biologically inactive) as a cause of elevated serum prolactin must be excluded. This can be detected with polyethylene glycol (PEG) precipitation followed by analysis of the supernatant for monomeric prolactin. Reference intervals for PEG-treated samples should be used (7,8).

Table 2-2. Physiological Drug Effects on Circulating Concentrations of Specific Hormones (1–6)

Hormone	Drugs That Cause Physiological Increase	Drugs That Cause Physiological Decrease
Prolactin	SSRI antidepressants, antipsychotic agents (phenothiazines, benzodiazepines, and butyrophenones), bezafibrate, tricyclic antidepressants (rare), MAO inhibitors, metoclopramide, omeprazole and H2 antagonists, sulpiride, trimethoprim, verapamil, opiates, cimetidine, methyldopa, high-dose estrogens	Bromocriptine and other dopamine agonists, lisuride, pergolide, L-dopa, clonidine, carbamazepine, phenytoin, morphine
Growth hormone	Fenfluramine, clonidine, glucagon, indomethacin	Alpha blockers, serotonin antagonists, chlorpromazine, glucocorticoids, pyridostigmine, pirenzepine
ACTH	Amphetamines, metyrapone	Glucocorticoids, cyproterone acetate, clonidine
Gonadotropins	Phenytoin, primidone, phenobarbitone	Sex hormones, opioids
Vasopressin and oxytocin	Potentially any drug, but commonly: sulfonylureas, carbamazepine, MAO inhibitors, thiazide diuretics, lithium and demeclocycline secondary to the development of nephrogenic diabetes insipidus	Ethanol, phenytoin, some opioids
TSH	Sertraline (question only with thyroxine replacement)	Thyroxine, glucocorticoids
Thyroxine (T_4) and triiodothyronine (T_3)	1. T_4 increased (and T_3 lowered) by amiodarone and propranolol (dose-dependent) 2. Rare cases of lithium-induced hyperthyroidism have occurred	1. T_3 and T_4 are lowered by displacement from binding proteins by salicylates, NSAIDs, and anticonvulsants (but not valproate) 2. Thyroid hormones may be cleared faster and lowered by hepatic enzyme-inducing drugs such as rifampin 3. Lithium may reduce T_4 and T_3 secretion by the thyroid gland and cause primary hypothyroidism
TBG	Estrogens, heroin and methadone, clofibrate	Androgens
Parathyroid hormone	Lithium	Diltiazem, vinblastine, colchicine, furosemide
Catecholamines	All alpha-adrenergic stimulants, methyldopa, small increase in norepinephrine with beta blockers, increase in metanephrines with MAO inhibitors	Alpha and beta blockers
5-HIAA	Increased secretion due to serotonin-containing foods (eg, aubergines/eggplants, avocados, bananas, pineapples, plums, walnuts) or the effects of some drugs (eg, acetaminophen [paracetamol], caffeine, fluorouracil, melphalan, or reserpine)	Chlorpromazine, imipramine, isoniazid, MAO inhibitors, L-dopa, methyldopa, phenothiazines, promethazine
Cortisol	ACTH analogs (cosyntropin and synacthen), glucagon	Metyrapone, aminoglutethimide, ketoconazole, etomidate
CBG	Estrogens, anticonvulsants	
Aldosterone	Primary: Mimicked by licorice and carbenoxolone Secondary: Oral contraceptives, thiazides, minoxidil	Heparin, beta blockers, ACE inhibitors, calcium channel antagonists
Plasma renin activity	Diuretics, ACE inhibitors, minoxidil, calcium channel antagonists	Beta blockers, clonidine, reserpine
Estradiol	Anabolic steroids, carbamazepine, cimetidine, clomiphene, DHEA, tamoxifen	Gonadotropin-releasing hormone agonists, danazol

(Continued)

Table 2-2. Physiological Drug Effects on Circulating Concentrations of Specific Hormones (1–6) (Continued)

Hormone	Drugs That Cause Physiological Increase	Drugs That Cause Physiological Decrease
Testosterone	Anabolic steroids, bromocriptine, cimetidine, finasteride (>50 mg/day), flutamide, tamoxifen	Gonadotropin-releasing hormone agonists, carbamazepine, digoxin, tetracycline (20%), sulfasalazine (oligospermia), cyproterone acetate Females: danazol, dexamethasone, spironolactone
SHBG	Oral estrogens, hyperthyroidism, diazoxide, metformin, tamoxifen	Oral androgens, anticonvulsants, hypothyroidism, anabolic steroids, danazol
Urine and plasma catecholamines, metanephrines	Alpha and beta blockers, calcium channel blockers, tricyclic antidepressants, phenoxybenzamine, monoamine oxidase inhibitors, phenothiazines, dopamine agonists, amphetamines	

Abbreviations: 5-HIAA = 5-hydroxyindoleacetic acid; ACE = angiotensin-converting enzyme; ACTH = adrenocorticotropic hormone; CBG, cortisol-binding globulin; DHEA = dihydroepiandrosterone; H2 = histamine H2; MAO = monoamine oxidase; SHBG, sex hormone-binding globulin; SSRI = selective serotonin reuptake inhibitors; TBG = thyroid-binding globulin; TSH = thyroid-stimulating hormone.

Table 2-3. Drug Interferences in Hormone Assays[a]

Hormone	Analytical Interference
GH	GH assays may give different values following stimulation tests because there is differential clearance of the GH isoforms. The specific GH assays (eg, DELFIA) may give slightly raised values due to the delayed clearance of the 22kDa isoform.
Gonadotropins	hCG; effect rare with immunometric assays
Thyroxine and triiodothyronine (free)	Displacement from protein-binding sites by anticonvulsants, aspirin, NSAIDs, and furosemide
Catecholamines	Alpha-methyldopa, labetalol
Cortisol	Prednisone (prednisolone)
Estradiol	Nonhuman estrogens in hormone replacement therapy preparations
Testosterone	Norethisterone, DHEAS

Abbreviations: DHEAS = dihydroepiandrosterone sulfate; GH = growth hormone; hCG = human chorionic gonadotropin; NSAIDs = nonsteroidal anti-inflammatory drugs.

[a] Effects are often assay-dependent, and the laboratory should be consulted (1–6).

In the case of TBI, permanent pituitary hormone insufficiency is well recognized and guidelines for screening after the acute phase have been proposed (9). However, for the critically ill patient, in the acute phase the case for investigation is not proven other than for life-threatening cortisol deficiency. Profound changes in pituitary hormones in the first week after TBI have been described, including low concentrations of thyroid-stimulating hormone (TSH), suppression of the pituitary gonadotropins, and increased prolactin (10).

Growth Hormone

Derangements in the growth hormone (GH)/insulin-like growth factor 1 (IGF-1) axis in the critically ill patient, whether attributable to GH resistance or GH insufficiency/suppression, have profound effects on metabolism. These changes result in skeletal muscle loss and delayed wound healing with important clinical consequences. Other than for research purposes, the measurement of GH and IGF-1 is not likely to be required in the critically ill patient.

GH assays have recently been restandardized to a new International Standard with a fixed relationship between the 2 prevalent reporting units (mU/L and μg/L). Moreover, there has been a recommendation to use μg/L, which will change numerical values of GH (11). IGF-1 assays are also in the process of restandardization to a purer form of the peptide (12). The changes in both assays will be important when using historical research data to determine relative changes.

Hypothalamic-Pituitary-Thyroid Axis

Changes in thyroid physiology occur in severe illness, which may be instrumental in the regulation of metabolic changes. These are generally described as nonthyroidal illness (NTI) or the euthyroid sick syndrome. The syndrome is characterized by a decrease in triiodothyronine (T_3) with an accompanying increase in reverse T_3 (rT_3), most probably due to changes in the activity of the Type 1 and Type 3 deiodinase, respectively. With severe and prolonged illness there is a fall in thyroxine (T_4) with no accompanying rise in serum TSH, reflecting hypothalamic downregulation of the hypothalamic-pituitary-thyroid (HPT) set point. Earlier studies of attempts to restore serum concentrations of thyroid hormones therapeutically and improve prognosis were unsuccessful and have served to highlight the discordance between serum concentrations and tissue effects (13). Indeed the effects are known to be time-dependent and dependent on tissue type and also affected by nutrition, drug therapy, and associated organ failure (14).

Assessment of the thyroid axis in the critically ill patient is one of the most common endocrine investigations, whether it is for monitoring of previously diagnosed disease or for de novo investigation. Interpretation of results may seem straightforward, but it is important to recognize those factors that can cause significantly abnormal results. Drug effects are well described (eg, glucocorticoids suppress serum TSH (6); furosemide can cause a false elevation of serum free T_4) (Table 2-3). Administration of heparin causes an in vivo activation of lipoprotein lipase and hepatic lipase, which results in the release of free fatty acids (FFAs). These interfere with the binding of thyroxine to thyroxine-binding globulin (TBG), resulting in an increase in serum free T_4.

Laboratory protocols for the investigation of the HPT axis are likely to vary worldwide. Individual laboratories have different practices with first-line profiles of either one or both T_4 and TSH and may use either free or total T_4. The critically ill patient is likely to need both TSH and (free) T_4 as the use of only one hormone may mislead. The choice of free or total T_4 is debated. The use of total T_4 is complicated by changes in circulating TBG concentration, which is elevated by pregnancy and oral estrogen therapy but lowered by acute illness. The use of free T_4 is complicated by T_4 displacement from binding sites by FFAs and various medications (see Table 2-3) and by lowered circulating albumin concentrations. Historically, free thyroxine measurement by the older analog immunoassays has been shown to be compromised because of the effect of hypoalbuminemia on the measurement. Although the newer free T_4 assays have been improved in this regard, there remain a few assays for which this analytical approach is not robust. Methods based on equilibrium dialysis (ED) might circumvent these problems but are not yet suited for routine use because these procedures are lengthy and not completely standardized. Furthermore, the temperature and pH at which the ED step is performed are critical and currently subject to international debate as to the standard conditions. Standardization of thyroid function test (TFT) assays is proving difficult, and the lack of it is reflected in the range of reference ranges quoted.

Hypothalamic-Pituitary-Adrenal Axis

Adrenal cortex. It is well recognized that hypercortisolemia is found in critical illness as part of the stress response. However, this response may not be sufficient to lead to a good prognosis and has led to the concept of "relative" or "functional" adrenal insufficiency (15), although the concept has not been endorsed by all (16). The changes in both cortisol synthesis and release and cortisol clearance are complex in critical illness and lead to difficulty in diagnosis and indeed on the need and degree of glucocorticoid therapy (17). Clearly, a random serum/plasma cortisol is too variable to allow adequate assessment of adrenal reserve, and the short ACTH stimulation test (eg, cosyntropin or synacthen tests) has been the most widely used test.

- The definition of a "normal" response to the 250 μg short ACTH stimulation test in the noncritically ill has been shown to be assay-dependent (18) and most reliable when the absolute value of the 30-minute post-ACTH cortisol value is used rather than the 60-minute cortisol value or the incremental value. However, this may not be the case in the critically ill patient. Indeed the nature of the response may depend on the nature of the acute illness. Thus the definition of a normal response might be different in a brain injured patient as compared with a patient in septic shock. It has also been noted that the distribution of cortisol responses to the short ACTH stimulation test does not always follow a Gaussian distribution when cortisol is measured by immunoassay (19). In such cases log transformation of the data or use of nonparametric statistics is required. This has not always been the case in the published literature, which should thus be interpreted with caution.
- Pharmaceutical inhibition of cortisol synthesis may invalidate the usual criteria used for the interpretation of the short ACTH stimulation test. A common example would be use of the drug etomidate, an inhibitor of the enzyme 11-beta-hydroxylase (20).
- Circulating concentrations of cortisol-binding globulin (CBG) have been shown to fall in ill health (negative acute phase reactant) in parallel with the fall in serum albumin. Thus total serum cortisol concentrations may not represent the biologically active form. However, CBG assays are not widely available and techniques for measuring free cortisol are laborious and technically demanding (21). Salivary cortisol (an ultrafiltrate of serum) is an alternative measure of free cortisol and is now measured in many laboratories (22). Saliva samples are usually collected into special containers avoiding contamination with blood, which containing higher concentrations of cortisol will cause a false elevation.
- Comparison of cortisol results obtained with different assays (immunoassays and liquid chromatographic-mass spectrometric [LC-MS] assays) are poor, especially in samples collected after short ACTH stimulation testing both in health and in patients with septic shock. Interpretation of results thus requires method-specific cut-off values (18,23,24).
- The results of short ACTH stimulation are not repeatable in patients with septic shock (25); however, this requires confirmation in critically ill patients not in septic shock.
- Patients with a normal hypothalamic-pituitary-adrenal (HPA) axis undergoing the severe stress of cardiac surgery have been shown to mount a further increase in serum cortisol after stimulation with low-dose (1 μg) short ACTH stimulation test. In this context an absence of response in the stressed patient is most likely to be pathological (26).
- Despite the poor repeatability of the short ACTH stimulation test, a "poor" response (a peak value at 30 or 60 minutes minus the baseline cortisol value of ≤9 ug/dL [248 nmol/L]) to the short ACTH stimulation test has been shown to be associated with a poor chance of survival in patients with septic shock (27). However, consideration needs to be given to the bias of the cortisol assay used, whether the 30- or 60-minute response or the incremental value was used. Further prospective studies are required.

Adrenal medulla. Pheochromocytomas are catecholamine-secreting tumors arising from chromaffin cells in the adrenal medulla and while the clinical presentation is variable, they may present "in crisis" as an endocrine emergency and are associated with significant mortality. Extra-adrenal chromaffin tumors (paragangliomas) may also secrete catecholamines and present in a similar crisis (28).

The cornerstone of biochemical investigation is the measurement of urine and plasma catecholamines and metanephrines. It is now clear that catecholamines are metabolized within the chromaffin cells (ie, norepinephrine to normetanephrine; epinephrine to metanephrine) independently of catecholamine release. Thus it is now recommended that the first line of investigation be the measurement of these catecholamine metabolites (ie, fractionated metanephrines) with methoxytyramine individually (29). Sample-collection conditions and requirements vary among laboratories and the assays may not be available urgently, with a turnaround time of days. The effects of patient posture (supine vs seated) and fasting status on plasma/urine metanephrines have been documented and shown to affect diagnostic sensitivity (best diagnostic sensitivity with supine fasting conditions [30]), although whether these are applicable to the critically ill patient is not known. Challenges associated with biochemical testing include the collection of a complete 24h urine specimen, avoidance of drug interference in the test, and interpretation of the results in a critically ill patient where there is an appropriate increase in catecholamine secretion. Drugs causing physiological interferences (Table 2-2) vary in whether the effect is found in plasma and/or urine and which catecholamine/metadrenaline is affected. Generally the effect is to increase the marker leading to a false-positive test result (4,5). Scholten et al (31) in a retrospective study of 25 pheochromocytoma patients in crisis as compared with noncrisis patients (n = 112) found 24 urine catecholamine and metabolites (expressed as a ratio to the upper limit of the reference range) to be 3.5–645.6 (catecholamines, range) and 1.9–511.0 (catecholamine metabolites) versus 0.0–54.0 and 0.0–90.1, respectively. Thus while extreme elevations were found, it is noteworthy that there was overlap in results between the 2 groups. Absolute values will be method-dependent, and assay details were not available in this publication.

Hypothalamic-Pituitary-Gonadal Axis

Suppression of the hypothalamic-pituitary-gonadal (HPG) axis occurs in critical illness. The reduction in sex steroids in both males and females is a complex process involving reduced gonadotropin secretion, inhibition of Leydig cell function in the male, and increased peripheral aromatization (32). Despite this effect, there is no clear difference between genders in relation to survival (33,34). Both testosterone and estradiol circulate bound to albumin and sex hormone-binding globulin (SHBG) with about 1% of testosterone in women and 2% in men being unbound. Critically ill men have low bioavailable testosterone (the free fraction of testosterone plus that loosely bound to albumin) (35), and serum concentrations of both total testosterone and bioavailable testosterone may fall to within the female reference range. Acute falls in the circulating concentrations of the adrenal androgen dehydroepiandrosterone sulfate (DHEAS) have also been described. However, treatment with testosterone or analogs has not been supported for the critically ill male patient (36).

Changes in the HPG axis in females are difficult to assess because status with regard to oral contraceptive therapy, menopausal status, or day of menstrual cycle may be impossible to ascertain. If clinically indicated, investigation would be best performed on recovery.

Vitamin D

Vitamin D deficiency and insufficiency have a high prevalence in many populations, and this is likely to be exacerbated in the critically ill. Given the range of beneficial biological actions of vitamin D there is growing awareness of the potential need for identification and treatment of deficiency in the critically ill patient (37). Vitamin D deficiency has been demonstrated in patients prior to admission to the ICU and may be exacerbated after admission for prolonged periods. However, it is not clear whether the fall in vitamin D merely reflects an acute phase reaction (38) or not (39). Secondary hyperparathyroidism has been demonstrated. Whether there is a relationship to mortality remains controversial, and analytical problems have probably complicated the literature.

25-Hydroxy vitamin D (either as the endogenously derived cholecalciferol, vitamin D_3, or plant/fish derived ergocalciferol, vitamin D_2) accounts for 95% of the total circulating pool unless vitamin D_2 containing supplements are being taken. In addition, vitamin D exists in the circulation in a number of further hydroxylated forms and as a 3 epimer. The main analytical issues for the laboratory revolve around the lack of specificity of immunoassays as compared with high-performance liquid chromatography (HPLC) and LC-MS/MS in quantitating 1,25 and 25 hydroxy vitamin D_2 and D_3 (and not the 3 epimers); the problems of standardization of assays; and the need to displace the hormone from the high-affinity vitamin D-binding protein (VDBP). Much of the recent literature is complicated by the use of nonspecific and poorly standardized assays. More recently, Reference Method Procedures and a Standard Reference Material 972 have become available and their use may lead to better agreement among assays but may not help the varying and conflicting views about the definition of vitamin D adequacy.

PITFALLS IN LABORATORY MEASUREMENTS

Two basic techniques are used for the measurement of hormones: immunoassay and chromatographic-mass spectrometric assays. However, hormone assays are subject to a number of limitations detailed below.

Immunoassay

These assays are based on the use of antibodies as reagents that react with the analyte of interest. Generally they are highly automated with a small sample size and short assay time. The assays may be of the competitive format used for small molecules such as cortisol and thyroxine or of immunometric format for larger molecules such as TSH and GH. The reagent antibodies can be raised and selected to achieve high degrees of specificity. There are, nevertheless, limitations to their use, namely cross-reactivity and antibody interferences (40).

Chromatographic Techniques

A number of chromatographic separation techniques can be coupled to detection systems to provide assays that can achieve great analytical sensitivity and specificity (eg, LC-MS/MS). In this technique there is often a prior purification step (solvent or solid phase extraction) followed by chromatography. Compounds are eluted off the column and analyzed by mass spectrometry. The technique has been applied to the steroids (eg, testosterone, cortisol, cortisone, and vitamin D) and in some instances to thyroxine. The assays require sophisticated instrumentation and technical skill. Rigorous assay validation should minimize the chances of interference, but given the variability among sample matrix, patient, and drug therapy interference cannot always be excluded. The interferences may be endogenous metabolites, drugs, and even preservatives and plasticizers leached from blood collection tubes (41,42). Generally the assays would be considered as "in-house assays" or "laboratory-developed tests" and in some countries subject to separate regulatory oversight.

Analytical Challenges

- *Multiple molecular weight forms.* Many hormones exist in multiple molecular weight forms, the proportions of which vary in healthy subjects and in disease (eg, human chorionic gonadotropin [hCG], GH). In addition, the hormone metabolites may have very similar structures. However measured, these different forms may react differently or not at all in the hormone assay.
- *Cross-reactivity.* Cross-reactivity is a characteristic of the antibody and assay system such that molecules of similar structure are detected. This can be determined experimentally to a limited extent. For example, the cross-reactivity of synthetic steroids in cortisol assays has been quoted as between 0.0% and 0.2% for dexamethasone, 12.3%–171% for prednisolone, and 0.2%–31.1% for cortisone. However, the pace of drug development is such that not all drugs will have been tested in all assay systems for all analytes and the clinician should be aware of the potential for false results due to exogenous drug interference. In addition, many of the drug metabolites will not have been tested for cross-reactivity (23,24).

- *Endogenous antibodies.* These may interfere in assays for hormones and indeed may form circulating complexes with the hormone with long half-lives (eg, macroprolactin). Some patients may develop antibodies that react with the reagent antibodies used in immunoassays and therapeutic antibodies may also interfere in assays, leading to inaccurate results (43,44).
- *Hook effect.* Very high concentrations of a hormone may "swamp" the reagent antibodies used in an immunoassay, leading to falsely low results (eg, severe hyperprolactinemia). Laboratories should have procedures in place to identify this effect (eg, samples for prolactin measurement should be run at 1:100 v/v dilution in patients with large (>3 cm) macroincidentalomas. However, this may be more difficult for point-of-care (POC) devices, and false-negative results on POC qualitative hCG devices ("pregnancy test") due to excess hCG beta core fragments have been identified (45).
- *Standardization of methods.* A key concept in laboratory medicine is the traceability of a result (the measurand in a given system, eg, serum collected under standard conditions and expressed in defined units) to a Reference Material Procedure and a Reference Method that have been certified by an international authority. For many hormones this is not yet possible, and results from different assays, from different laboratories, and from different countries vary widely. With regard to units of reporting, for analytes of known molecular weight (eg, T_4, cortisol, and testosterone) it should be possible to report results in molar terms (Systeme International), although some countries continue to report in mass terms. The clinician should always check the unit of reporting and take care when implementing electronic reporting systems so that the impact on the numerical result is noted. For hormones of variable or unknown molecular weight, standardization is more problematic. Initially, such hormones were often reported in terms of their biological activity; for example, the International Unit of insulin is defined in terms of its hypoglycemic actions. This approach still impacts on assays today, such that assays for renin may be reported either in mass terms (pg/mL) or if measured by enzyme activity as plasma renin activity (ng/mL/h at 37° C). These differences in units result in different numerical results and different reference ranges, but few guidelines refer to this heterogeneity. Thus for any assay result, it is important to note the units of reporting and the assay-specific reference ranges.
- *Point-of-care testing.* Although point-of-care testing (POCT) is well established in the ICU for blood gases, electrolytes, and hemoglobin, its potential has yet to be established for hormone assays. Consideration has to be given as to whether an immediate result is required (with the potential for inaccuracy and imprecision) or whether a laboratory result within hours would be more effective. Urgent endocrine tests might include, for example, prolactin for macroprolactinomas or cortisol for adrenal crisis, and where inappropriate treatment might be harmful. Differences between POC and central laboratory assays have been demonstrated (eg, for glycated hemoglobin), although their performance is not adequate for diagnosis and should not be used in sick patients to assess acute glycemic deterioration due to the time delay in hemoglobin glycation in relation to disease course. Pregnancy test devices may be used for the investigation of ectopic pregnancy and diagnosis of pregnancy in the critically ill patient. There are significant limitations to their use in the ICU and confirmation using a serum hCG assay is suggested.

Laboratory Errors

Any method of measurement is subject to error and laboratories are required to have in place procedures for the selection of appropriate assays, for their continuing evaluation and for quality assessment and control. This can be determined by external accreditation of the laboratory and the use of internal and external quality assurance. However, the errors described above due to pharmacological and immunological interference are due to within-patient factors and will not be identified by laboratory quality control systems. They are difficult to identify without good liaison between clinicians and laboratories.

Most studies of laboratory errors are clear that the majority of errors are due to either preanalytical factors such as incorrect sample identification, sample timing, or collection tube, or to postanalytical factors such as misinterpretation.

CONCLUSIONS

The endocrine changes in the critically ill patient involve most systems and vary with primary pathology and with time. The changes are further complicated by changes in hormone-binding proteins and by drug therapy. Interference in hormone assays can be difficult to identify, and differences in assay bias and difficulties with standardization determine that assay-specific reference ranges must be applied. It cannot be overemphasized that laboratory results should be reviewed critically and any discordance with the patient's condition or with previous results be considered with suspicion and discussed with the laboratory.

ACKNOWLEDGMENTS

The authors have nothing to disclose.

REFERENCES

1. **Baylis PH.** Drug-induced endocrine disorders. *Adverse Drug Reaction Bulletin.* 1986;116:432–435.
2. **Vanderpump MPJ, Tunbridge WMG.** The effect of drugs on endocrine function. *Clin Endocrinol (Oxf).* 1993;39:389–397.
3. **Young DS.** *Effects of Drugs on Clinical Laboratory Tests.* 4th ed. Washington DC: American Association of Clinical Chemistry Press; 1995.
4. **Eisenhofer G, Goldstein DS, Walther MM, et al.** Biochemical diagnosis of pheochromocytoma: How to distinguish true- from false-positive test results. *J Clin Endocrinol Metab.* 2003;88:2656–2666.
5. **Barron J.** Phaeochromocytoma: diagnostic challenges for biochemical screening and diagnosis. *J Clin Pathol.* 2010;63:669–674.
6. **Haugen BR.** Drugs that suppress TSH or cause central hypothyroidism. *Best Pract Res Clin Endocrinol Metab.* 2009;23:793–800.
7. **Jassam NF, Paterson A, Lippiatt C, Barth JH.** Macroprolactin on the Advia Centaur: experience with 409 patients over a three-year period. *Ann Clin Biochem.* 2009;46:501–504.
8. **Fahie-Wilson M, Smith TP.** Determination of prolactin: The macroprolactin problem. *Best Pract Res Clin Endocrinol Metab.* 2013;27:725–742.
9. **Ghigo E, Masel B, Aimaretti G, et al.** Consensus guidelines on screening for hypopituitarism following traumatic brain injury. *Brain Inj.* 2005;19:711–724.
10. **Olivecrona Z, Dahlqvist P, Koskinen L-O D.** Acute neuro-endocrine profile and prediction of outcome after severe brain injury. *Scand J Trauma Resus Emergency Med.* 2013;21:33–45.
11. **Wieringa GE, Barth JH, Trainer PJ.** Growth hormone assay standardization: a biased view? *Clin Endocrinol (Oxf).* 2004;60:538–539.
12. **Burns C, Rigsby P, Moore M, Rafferty B.** The First International Standard For Insulin-like Growth Factor-1 (IGF-1) for immunoassay: preparation and calibration in an international collaborative study. *Growth Horm IGF Res.* 2009;19:457–462.
13. **Boelen A, Kwakkei J, Fliers E.** Beyond low plasma T_3: local thyroid hormone metabolism during inflammation and infection. *Endocrine Rev.* 2011;32: 670–693.
14. **Langouche L, Perre SV, Marques M, et al.** Impact of early nutrient restriction during critical illness on the nonthyroidal illness syndrome and its relation with outcome: a randomized, controlled clinical study. *J Clin Endocrinol Metab.* 2013;98:1006–1013.
15. **Cooper MS, Stewart PM.** Corticosteroid insufficiency in acutely ill patients. *N Engl J Med.* 2003;348:727–734.
16. **Marik PE, Pastores SM, Annane D, et al.** Recommendations for the diagnosis and management of corticosteroid insufficiency in critically ill adult patients: consensus statements from an international task force by the American College of Critical Care Medicine. *Crit Care Med.* 2008;36:1937–1949.
17. **Boonen E, Vervenne H, Meersseman P, et al.** Reduced cortisol metabolism during critical illness. *N Engl J Med.* 2013; 368:1477–1488.
18. **El-Farhan N, Pickett A, Ducroq D, et al.** Method-specific serum cortisol responses to the adrenocorticotrophin test: comparison of gas chromatography-mass spectrometry and five automated immunoassays. *Clin Endocrinol (Oxf).* 2013;78:673–680.
19. **Clark PM, Neylon I, Raggatt PR, Sheppard MC, Stewart PM.** Defining the normal cortisol response to the short Synacthen test: implications for the investigation of hypothalamic-pituitary disorders. *Clin Endocrinol (Oxf).* 1998;49:287–292.
20. **Albert SG, Ariyan S, Rather A.** The effect of etomidate on adrenal function in critical illness: a systematic review. *Intensive Care Med.* 2011;37: 901–910.
21. **Hamrahian AH, Oseni TS, Arafah BM.** Measurements of serum free cortisol in critically ill patients. *N Engl J Med.* 2004;350;1629–1638.

22. **Arafah BM, Nishiyama FJ, Tlaygeh H, Hejal R.** Measurement of salivary cortisol concentration in the assessment of adrenal function in critically ill subjects: a surrogate marker of the circulating free cortisol. *J Clin Endocrinol Metab.* 2007;92: 2965–2971.
23. **Cohen J, Ward G, Prins J, Jones M, Venkatesh B.** Variability of cortisol assays can confound the diagnosis of adrenal insufficiency in the critically ill population. *Intensive Care Med.* 2006;32:1901–1905.
24. **Briegel J, Sprung CL, Annane D, et al for the CORTICUS Study Group.** Multicenter comparison of cortisol as measured by different methods in samples of patients with septic shock. *Intensive Care Med.* 2009;35:2151–2156.
25. **Loisa P, Uusaro A, Ruokonen E.** A single adrenocorticotropic hormone stimulation test does not reveal adrenal insufficiency in septic shock. *Anesth Analg.* 2005;101:1792–1798.
26. **Henzen C, Kobza R, Schwaller-Protzmann B, Stulz P, Briner VA.** Adrenal function during coronary artery bypass grafting. *Eur J Endocrinol.* 2003;148: 663–668.
27. **Annane D, SébilleV, Troché G, Raphaël JC, Gajdos P, Bellissant E.** A 3-level prognostic classification in septic shock based on cortisol levels and cortisol response to corticotrophin. *JAMA.* 2000;283: 1038–1045.
28. **Whitelaw BC, Prague JK, Mustafa OG, et al.** Pheochromocytoma crisis. *Clin Endocrinol (Oxf).* 2013;80:13–22.
29. **Pacak K, Eisenhofer G, Ahlman H, et al.** Pheochromocytoma: recommendations for clinical practice from the First International Symposium. October 2005. *Nat Clin Pract Endocrinol Metab.* 2007;3:92–102.
30. **Därr R, Pamporaki C, Peitzsch M, et al.** Biochemical diagnosis of phaeochromocytoma using plasma free normetanephrine, metanephrine and methoxytyramine: importance of supine sampling under fasting conditions. *Clin Endocrinol (Oxf).* 2014;80:478–486.
31. **Scholten A, Cisco RM, Vriens MR, et al.** Pheochromocytoma crisis is not a surgical emergency. *J Clin Endocrinol Metab.* 2013;98:581–591.
32. **Mechanick, JI, Nierman DM.** Gonadal steroids in critical illness. *Crit Care Clin.* 2006;22;87–103
33. **Adrie C, Azoulay E, Francais A, et al.** for the OutcomeRea Study Group. Influence of gender on the outcome of severe sepsis. A reappraisal. *Chest.* 2007;132; 1786–1793.
34. **Heffernan DS, Dossett LA, Lightfoot MA, et al.** Gender and ARDS in critically injured adults: a prospective study. *J Trauma.* 2011;71;878–885.
35. **Nierman DM, Mechanick JI.** Hypotestosteronemia in chronically critically ill men. *Crit Care Med.* 1999;27;2418–2421.
36. **Weitzel L-R, Sandoval PA, Mayles J, Wischmeyer PE.** Performance-enhancing sports supplements: role in critical care. *Crit Care Med.* 2009;37;S400–S409.
37. **Krishnan A, Venkatesh B.** Vitamin D measurement in the intensive care unit: methodology, clinical relevance and interpretation of a random value. *Inflamm Allergy Drug Targets.* 2013;12:230–238.
38. **Reid D, Toole BJ, Knox S, et al.** The relation between acute changes in the systemic inflammatory response and plasma 25-hydroxyvitamin D concentrations after elective knee arthroplasty. *Am J Clin Nutr.* 2011;93:1006–1011.
39. **Barth JH, Field HP, Mather AN, Plein S.** Serum 25 hydroxy-vitamin D does not exhibit an acute phase reaction after acute myocardial infarction. *Ann Clin Biochem.* 2012;49:399–401.
40. **Wild D, ed.** *The Immunoassay Handbook.* 4th ed. London: Elsevier Ltd; 2013.
41. **Keller Bo, Sui J, Young AB, Whittal RM.** Interference and contaminants encountered in modern mass spectrometry. *Anal Chim Acta.* 2008;627:71–81.
42. **Vogeser M, Seger C.** Pitfalls associated with the use of liquid chromatography-tandem mass spectrometry in the clinical laboratory. *Clin Chem.* 2010;56:1234–1244.
43. **Halsall DJ.** Antibody interference in immunoassays: know your enemy. *Ann Clin Biochem.* 2013;50:397–399.
44. **Ismail AAA, Walker PL, Cawood M, Barth JH.** Interference in immunoassay is an underestimated problem. *Ann Clin Biochem.* 2002;39:366–373.
45. **Nerenz RD, Gronowski AM.** Point-of-care and over-the-counter qualitative human chorionic gonadotropin (hCG) devices remain susceptible to false-negative results caused by excess hCG beta core. *Clin Chem.* 2013;59:1672–1674.

CHAPTER 3

Endocrine Responses to Critical Illness

Novel Insights and Therapeutic Implications

Eva Boonen and Greet Van den Berghe

ABSTRACT

Critical illness, an extreme form of severe physical stress, is characterized by important endocrine and metabolic changes. Due to critical care medicine, survival from previously lethal conditions has become possible, but many patients now enter a chronic phase of critical illness. The role of the endocrine and metabolic responses to acute and prolonged critical illness in mediating or hampering recovery remains highly debated. In recent years, important novel insights in the pathophysiology and the consequences of these endocrine responses to critical illness were generated. This chapter summarizes these insights with a specific focus on the hypothalamic-pituitary-thyroid axis, the hypothalamic-pituitary-adrenal axis, and the impact of the hyperglycemic response on recovery from critical illness. Any therapeutic implications of these novel insights are critically analyzed.

INTRODUCTION

Critical illness is defined as any life-threatening condition requiring support of vital organ functions to prevent imminent death. This condition can be evoked by a variety of insults such as multiple trauma, complicated surgery, and severe medical illnesses. Without modern critical care medicine, critically ill patients would not survive. Critical illness is thus the ultimate form of severe physical stress, and all the immediate biological responses that are evoked are expected to be of greater magnitude in critically ill patients. These immediate stress responses comprise many orchestrated endocrine adaptations that are presumably directed toward providing the required energy for the "fight or flight" response in a context of exogenous substrate deprivation. Indeed, alterations within the different hypothalamic-pituitary axes bring about lipolysis and proteolysis, as well as gluconeogenesis, and redirect energy consumption toward those processes that mediate acute survival, while anabolism is postponed to more prosperous times.

Although survival from previously lethal conditions is nowadays possible, often recovery does not swiftly follow and patients enter a chronic phase of critical illness during which they continue to depend upon vital organ support for weeks, while the original trigger of the critical illness has long been resolved. This stage is characterized by distinct endocrine and metabolic alterations that may no longer be solely beneficial because they may hamper recovery. An example is the relative maintenance of fat stores while large amounts of proteins continue to be wasted from skeletal muscle and organs (1). This response may impair recovery of vital organ functions, extend weakness, and hamper rehabilitation (2), as well as expose patients to severe, often infectious, complications (3). The understanding of the mechanisms determining why certain patients recover and others do not remains very limited, but recent studies point to variable abilities to remove cell damage as playing a key role (4,5). When patients remain dependent upon critical care support, it is ultimately decided to withdraw care because of futility. Hence, further understanding the underlying pathways of recovery and investigating whether these pathways can be beneficially affected by treatment is of high clinical relevance.

In recent years, important novel insights into the pathophysiology and the consequences of these endocrine responses to critical illness were generated. This chapter summarizes these insights with a specific focus on the hypothalamic-pituitary-thyroid axis, the hypothalamic-pituitary-adrenal axis, and on the impact of the hyperglycemic response on recovery from critical illness. Any therapeutic implications of these novel insights are critically analyzed.

HYPOTHALAMIC-PITUITARY-THYROID AXIS

Responses Within the Hypothalamic-Pituitary-Thyroid Axis During Acute Critical Illness

It has long been known that both fasting and acute illness immediately affect circulating levels of thyroid hormones. Most typically, plasma concentrations of triiodothyronine (T_3) decrease and plasma concentrations of reverse T_3 (rT_3) rise, suggesting an immediate inactivation of thyroid hormone in peripheral tissues such as the liver, likely mediated by a suppressed activity of the type-1 deiodinase (D_1) and/or an activated type-3 deiodinase (D_3) (6,7). Concentrations of thyroxine (T_4) and thyroid-stimulating hormone (TSH) have shown to be briefly increased immediately after surgery (7). Thereafter, plasma TSH and T_4 concentrations often return to "normal," although a normal nocturnal TSH surge is absent (8,9). This constellation of low plasma T_3 concentrations and elevated rT_3 is generally referred to as the *acute low T_3 syndrome, the euthyroid-sick syndrome, or the nonthyroidal illness syndrome* (Figure 3-1).

Several possible mediators of the acute fall in plasma T_3 concentrations in critically ill patients include the lack of nutrients, the release of cytokines, or hypoxia (10–12). Tumor necrosis factor-alpha, interleukin-1, and interleukin-6 are capable of mimicking the acute stress–induced alterations within the thyroid axis. However, neutralizing antibodies to these cytokines in a human experiment of LPS-induced inflammation failed to restore normal thyroid hormone concentrations (13). Acute decreases in plasma concentrations of thyroid hormone-binding proteins and the inhibition of hormone binding, transport, and metabolism by elevated levels of free fatty acids and bilirubin may also play a role (14).

The low T_3 concentrations that occur with fasting have shown to be adaptive, because they appear to protect the organism against the deleterious catabolic consequences of lack of macronutrients (15,16). In critical illness, it was suggested that the low T_3 concentrations could be maladaptive, because the magnitude of the acute T_3 decrease was associated with the severity of illness and with the risk of death (17,18). However, the acute fall in circulating levels of thyroid hormone in response to illness could also be an adaptive attempt to reduce energy expenditure, as happens with fasting in healthy subjects, in which case it should be left untreated (15). Improved postoperative cardiac function was observed after short-term intravenous (IV) administration of T_3 to patients during elective cardiac surgery (19,20). However, supranormal plasma T_3 concentrations were evoked, and thus it is uncertain whether these findings were merely due to a pharmacological effect. Recently, the results of a large randomized controlled trial (RCT), investigating the impact of early parenteral nutrition as compared with tolerating pronounced caloric deficit in critically ill patients, provided indirect evidence for an adaptive nature of the low T_3 levels (21,22). This study revealed that providing nutrition in the acute phase of critical illness impaired rather than improved

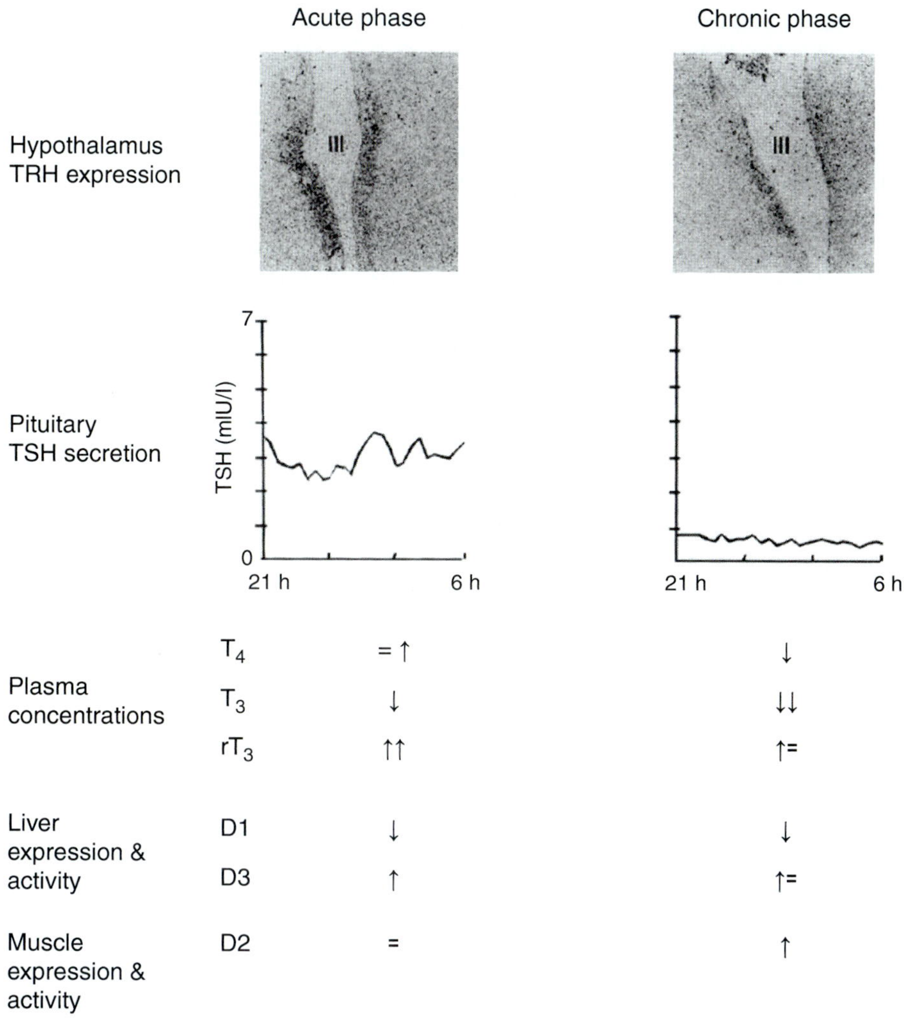

Figure 3-1. Changes in the central and peripheral thyroid axis in acute versus prolonged critical illness. The top panel shows reduced TRH gene expression in the hypothalamus of patients with prolonged illness. The central panel illustrates adaptations in nocturnal TSH secretion with a loss of pulsatility during prolonged critical illness. The bottom panel schematically summarizes the changes in circulating thyroid hormone concentrations and changes in peripheral deiodinase enzyme activity levels. D1 = type-1 deiodinase; D2 = type-2 deiodinase; D3 = type-3 deiodinase. *Drafted from original data in Fliers et al (26), Vanhorebeek et al (122), Mebis et al (123), and Debaveye et al (46).*

outcome. The provision of macronutrients prevented partially the acute thyroid hormone changes, which was recently also observed in a rabbit model of critical illness (23). In the clinical study, specifically the rise in T_3 and in the ratio of T_3 over rT_3 with early forceful feeding statistically explained the worsening of the outcome (22). These data, therefore, suggest that at least part of the acute fall in T_3 concentrations during critical illness is related to the concomitant fasting and that this part of the response is likely adaptive. Benefits include the expected reduction in energy expenditure with low T_3 levels, or a direct effect of increased D_3 activity locally in granulocytes, which could optimize bacterial killing capacity (12,24).

Responses Within the Hypothalamic-Pituitary-Thyroid Axis During Prolonged Critical Illness

When patients receiving full enteral and/or parenteral nutrition are treated in intensive care units (ICUs) for several weeks, the alterations within the thyroid axis appear different. In this phase of critical illness, low plasma T_3 concentrations now coincide with low T_4

concentrations and low-normal TSH concentrations in a single morning sample (25). Moreover, overnight repeated sampling revealed that the pulsatility of TSH secretion is virtually lost, which relates to low plasma thyroid hormone levels, a presentation resembling central hypothyroidism (Figure 3-1) (25). In line with this interpretation, Fliers and colleagues (26) demonstrated in postmortem brain samples of chronic critically ill patients that the gene expression of thyrotropin-releasing hormone (TRH) in the hypothalamic paraventricular nuclei was much lower than in patients who died after acute insults (Figure 3-1). Furthermore, a positive correlation was observed between the TRH mRNA expression and the plasma concentrations of TSH and T_3. Together, these data indicate that production and/or release of thyroid hormones is reduced in prolonged critical illness due to reduced hypothalamic stimulation of the thyrotropes, in turn leading to reduced stimulation of the thyroid gland. The observation that a rise in TSH levels precedes the onset of recovery from severe illness further supports this interpretation (27).

The factors triggering hypothalamic suppression during prolonged critical illness are unknown. Because plasma cytokine concentrations are usually much lower in the prolonged phase of critical illness (28) other mechanisms likely play a role, like endogenous dopamine or elevated cortisol levels in the hypothalamus, given that exogenous dopamine and hydrocortisone are known to provoke or aggravate hypothyroidism in critical illness (29–31). A local increase in type-2 deiodinase (D_2) activity in the hypothalamus could elevate local thyroid hormone levels, whereby the set point for feedback inhibition could be altered (32). Indeed, in a rabbit model of prolonged critical illness and low thyroid hormone plasma concentrations, hypothalamic TRH mRNA was low and D_2 mRNA was high. However, the hypothalamic T_4 and T_3 concentrations were not increased (33). Increased pituitary D_2 could also play a role in suppressing local TSH mRNA (34), although this was not confirmed in an animal model of prolonged critical illness (35).

During prolonged critical illness, peripheral tissues seem to respond to low T_3 levels to increase local hormone availability and effects. For example, in skeletal muscle and liver biopsies from prolonged critically ill patients, the monocarboxylate transporter, MCT-8, was overexpressed (Figure 3-2) (36). This was confirmed in an animal model, where the upregulation of the monocarboxylate transporters in liver and kidney was reversible by treatment with thyroid hormones (36,37). Also, in skeletal muscle biopsies from prolonged critically ill patients, D_2 expression and activity was upregulated as compared with healthy controls and with acutely ill patients (Figure 3-1) (37). Upregulation of D_2 in lungs was recently found to be adaptive in sepsis and acute lung injury, further accentuated by the observation that a D_2 polymorphism was associated with less sepsis susceptability (38). At the level of the thyroid hormone receptor (TR), an inverse correlation was observed between the active TR-1/inactive TR-2 ratio, a surrogate marker of thyroid hormone sensitivity, and the ratio of T_3/rT_3 in liver biopsies of prolonged critically ill patients (39). Together, the data suggest that when the production of thyroid hormones falls in prolonged critical illness, peripheral tissues adapt by increasing thyroid hormone transporters, local activation of thyroid hormone, and gene expression of the active receptor isoform.

In protracted critical illness, low T_3 levels were found to correlate inversely with markers of muscle breakdown and of bone loss, which could indicate either an adaptive and protective response against catabolism or a causal maladaptive relationship (40). Given that the cause of the low thyroid hormone levels during prolonged critical illness appears to be a suppressed TRH expression, whereby thyroid hormone production is reduced, the question could be addressed by assessing the effect of TRH treatment. When patients were given a TRH infusion, plasma T_3 and T_4 could be increased, but rT_3 concentrations also rose (41). However, when TRH was combined with a growth hormone (GH)-secretagogue, this rise in rT_3 was prevented, explained by a GH-mediated effect on the inactivating D_3 (42). This treatment also induced an anabolic response, which suggested a causal relationship between low thyroid hormone levels and the impaired anabolism during prolonged critical illness (40). Furthermore, the negative feedback

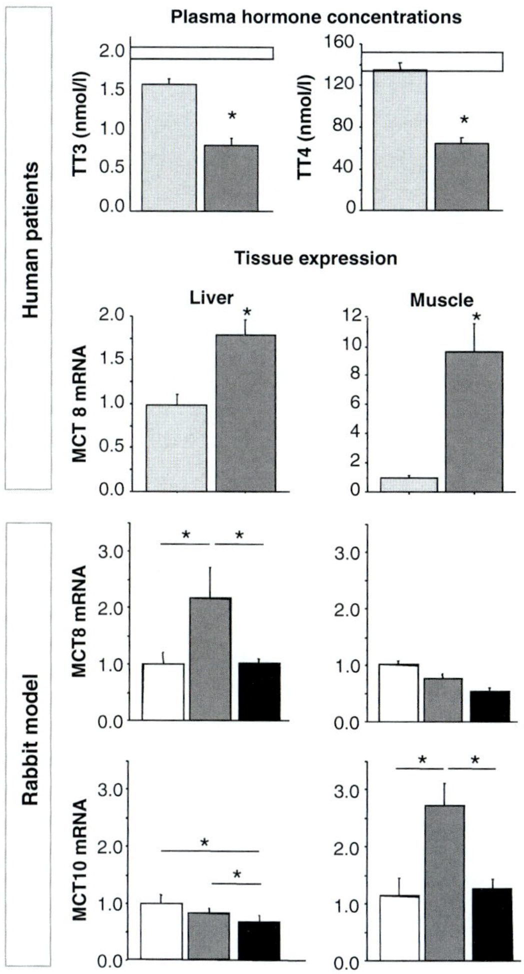

Figure 3-2. The top panel represents the circulating thyroid hormone parameters in acutely stressed (light gray bars, n = 22) and chronically ill patients (dark gray bars, n = 64). The white bars designate the normal ranges. The central panel shows the relative *MCT8* mRNA expression levels measured in liver and skeletal muscle of acutely stressed (light gray) and chronically ill (dark gray) patients. The lower panels represent the relative expression levels of *MCT8* and *MCT10* in the liver and muscle of healthy control rabbits (white bar), saline-treated rabbits with prolonged illness (dark gray), and T3- + T4-treated (black bar) ill rabbits. Data expressed as mean ± SEM; $*P < 0.05$ versus acute values. *Drafted from original data in Mebis et al (36).*

exerted by thyroid hormones on the thyrotropes was found to be maintained during TRH infusion, a self-limitation that precludes overstimulation of the thyroid axis (41,43).

Diagnostic Implications

Given the nature of the changes within the thyroid axis evoked by critical illness, the diagnosis of preexisting thyroid disease during critical illness is very difficult. Patients with preexisting primary hypothyroidism are expected to reveal low serum levels of T_4 and T_3 in combination with high TSH concentrations. However, when primary hypothyroidism and severe nonthyroidal critical illness coincide, TSH levels may be lower than anticipated. Moreover, serum TSH may be paradoxically low because of iatrogenic factors such as iodine wound dressings, iodine-containing contrast agents, and drugs such as high-dose corticosteroids, dopamine, somatostatin ana-logs, and amiodarone (30,44). So, a normal or low TSH during critical illness does not exclude primary hypothyroidism. Also, the low T_4 and T_3 levels in patients with severe hypothyroidism can be indistinguishable from those values observed in prolonged nonthyroidal critical illness. A high ratio of T_3/T_4 in serum, a low thyroid hormone-binding ratio, and a low serum rT_3 may favor the presence of primary hypothyroidism. However, the diagnostic accuracy is limited. In these patients, history, physical examination, and the possible presence of thyroid autoantibodies may give further clues to the presence of thyroid disease. Repeated thyroid function tests after improvement of the nonthyroidal illness are required to confirm the diagnosis.

Elevated plasma T_4 and T_3 concentrations are so unusual during critical illness that they should always raise concern of preexisting hyperthyroidism. However, undetectable TSH has no diagnostic value for hyperthyroidism during critical illness.

Therapeutic Implications

Given that the available evidence now indicates that the acute "low T_3 syndrome" appears to be an adaptive response partially explained by fasting, treatment likely is not indicated (22,23). In contrast, the low T_4 and T_3 levels during the prolonged phase of critical illness could be maladaptive. Experimental studies showed that in animal models of prolonged critical illness and in prolonged critically ill patients who are receiving nutrition, the syndrome can be reversed via hypothalamic releasing factors, with an anabolic response at the tissue level (40). However, the effect on clinical outcome of such a treatment remains to be investigated, so therapeutic implications are currently lacking.

An alternative option for treatment could be the administration of thyroid hormones T_4 or T_3 or the combination to normalize the plasma concentrations. In animal studies, substitution doses of T_4, T_3 or their combination were unable to alter circulating levels of thyroid hormones, likely explained by the increased metabolism of thyroid hormones during critical illness, perhaps in part mediated by sulfoconjugation, as was also shown in patients (45–48). Three times, the substitution dose of T_4 normalized plasma T_3 concentrations in this model but resulted in supranormal T_4 levels and a rise in rT_3. A dose of T_3 that was able to normalize the plasma T_3 concentrations, 5 times the substitution dose, suppressed TSH and T_4 to subnormal levels via negative feedback inhibition. A combination of these doses of T_4 and T_3 resulted in dramatic overtreatment. Similar dosing issues were present in the few available small RCTs in critically ill patients, which also did not show outcome benefits (49–52).

Controversy also remains regarding when and how to treat primary hypothyroidism during critical illness. When patients were receiving active treatment for hypothyroidism before critical illness, it seems wise to continue their usual dose of thyroid hormone. For myxedema coma it is generally accepted that patients should be treated with parenteral infusion of thyroid hormones. However, the proper initiation of replacement therapy during other types of critical illness remains controversial. There is no consensus on the type of thyroid hormone or on the optimal initial dose for replacement therapy. Many clinicians prefer a high IV loading dose of 300–500 μg of T_4 to reach quickly 50% of the euthyroid value of T_4 (53–55), followed by 50–100 μg of IV T_4 daily until oral medication can be given. Some authors have suggested the use of a co-infusion of the biologically active form of T_3 and T_4. Morreale de Escobar and colleagues (56) showed in an animal study that T_4 alone did not ensure euthyroidism in all tissues, which was achieved by combined treatment with T_4 and T_3. An experimental protocol for thyroid hormone therapy during prolonged intensive care of presumed hypothyroidism advises administering a 100–200 μg bolus of T_4 IV per 24 hours alone or, when required to also increase plasma T_3, combined with T_3 at 0.6 μg/kg ideal body weight per 24 hours in a continuous IV infusion, targeting serum thyroid hormone levels in the low-normal range (57). When the patient starts to recover, a prompt tapering of this dose may be required.

The treatment for primary hyperthyroidism is less affected by concomitant critical illness, except that treatment requirements could be lower in the presence of increased thyroid hormone metabolism. Furthermore, when patients are receiving active treatment for hyperthyroidism, they should be monitored because of potential toxicity of the medication and the impact of other frequently used medication on thyroid hormone levels.

HYPOTHALAMIC-PITUITARY-ADRENAL AXIS

Responses Within the Hypothalamic-Pituitary-Adrenal Axis During Acute and Prolonged Critical Illness

The stress hormone cortisol is an essential component of the fight or flight reaction to the stress of illness and trauma, and both very high and low cortisol levels have been associated with risk of death in such patients (58). Whenever the brain senses a stressful event, activation of the hypothalamic-pituitary-adrenal (HPA) axis initiates the release of the corticotropin-releasing hormone (CRH) and arginine vasopressin (AVP) from the hypothalamus, which stimulates the anterior pituitary corticotrophs to secrete adrenocorticotropic hormone (ACTH). High cortisol levels during critical illness likely contribute to the provision of extra energy to vital organs by acutely shifting carbohydrate, fat, and protein metabolism and by delaying anabolism. Moreover, cortisol likely affects the hemodynamic system by intravascular fluid retention and by enhancing inotropic and vasopressor responses to catecholamines and angiotensin II, respectively. In addition, the anti-inflammatory effects of cortisol can be interpreted as an attempt to prevent overactivation of the inflammatory cascade (59,60).

During critical illness, plasma cortisol concentrations are substantially elevated, traditionally explained by several-fold elevated cortisol production in the adrenal cortex driven by ACTH. However, Vermes et al reported only transiently elevated ACTH concentrations in patients with multiple trauma or sepsis, whereas cortisol concentrations remained high (61). This was recently confirmed in a more heterogeneous critically ill patient population. In this study, plasma ACTH concentrations were found to be suppressed already from ICU admission onward and stayed below the lower limit of normality throughout the first week of critical illness (62). Whether the expected initial ACTH rise in response to stress was missed in this study and had already occurred before ICU admission, for example, in the operating room or emergency department, remains unknown.

Low plasma ACTH in the presence of high plasma cortisol concentrations has been interpreted as non-ACTH driven cortisol production (61,63). Alternatively, this constellation could be caused by reduced cortisol breakdown suppressing the production of adrenocortical hormones via feedback inhibition. In fact, direct evidence of increased cortisol production during critical illness has been lacking. Recent work that used a state of the art cortisol-tracer technique showed that daytime cortisol production during critical illness was only slightly higher than in healthy subjects. Furthermore, cortisol production was only increased in patients with excessive inflammation while it was unaltered in other critically ill patients (Figure 3-3) (62). Cortisol breakdown on the other hand was substantially reduced, irrespective of the inflammatory status, attributable to suppressed expression and activity of A-ring reductases in the liver and by suppressed activity 11β-hydroxysteroid dehydrogenase type 2 in the kidneys (62). It remains unclear, however, what is driving the suppression of these enzymes, but an inverse correlation between elevated plasma concentrations of bile acids and the expression level of the A-ring reductases could point to bile acids playing a role (Figure 3-3) (62,64). Indeed, bile acids are potent inhibitors of the cortisol metabolizing enzymes, both via competitive inhibition and by suppression of gene and protein expression (65–67).

The concept of increasing the bioavailability of cortisol levels primarily in tissues that produce these enzymes and to a lesser extent in the circulation could be interpreted as a highly economic way to keep cortisol levels high without spending too much energy producing it. This concept is further supported by low plasma cortisol-binding globulin (CBG) levels in critical illness, causing increased levels of free cortisol, the biologically active form. Furthermore, such cortisol is elevated locally in the liver and kidneys, where it is needed for an optimal "fight or flight" response, without an undue exposure of immune cells and vulnerable target tissues such as skeletal muscle or brain to the deleterious side effects of hypercortisolism. The local effects of cortisol appear to be further regulated at the level of glucocorticoid receptor (GR) expression. Previous work indeed showed suppressed expression of GR in white blood cells of critically ill children, which could be a way to allow the innate immune response to effectively protect the host against infections in the presence of hypercortisolism (68). Clearly this novel concept of tissue-specific regulation of glucocorticoid activity during critical illness requires further investigation.

The new insight that during critical illness cortisol metabolism is suppressed, contributing to hypercortisolism, could theoretically explain the concomitantly low plasma ACTH concentrations via negative feedback inhibition at the level of the pituitary gland and/or the hypothalamus, but studies assessing this at the tissue level are currently lacking. It remains unclear whether such a sustained suppressed ACTH secretion could cause adrenal atrophy in the prolonged phase of critical illness. However, this could explain the reported 20-fold higher incidence of symptomatic adrenal insufficiency in critically ill patients being treated in the ICU for more than 14 days (69). Other factors contributing to adrenal failure are also possible, such as endothelial dysfunction (70,71), although conformational human studies are lacking.

Diagnostic Implications

Since the last decade, reference is made to "relative adrenal insufficiency" in the context of critical illness (72–74). This refers to the condition in which, despite a maximally ACTH-activated adrenal cortex in response to critical illness, cortisol production is still insufficient to generate enough glucocorticoid and mineralocorticoid receptor activation to maintain hemodynamic stability. From large association studies, such a condition is thought to be identifiable by an insufficient rise (<9 μg/dL [250 nmol/L]) in plasma cortisol in response to a 250 μg ACTH bolus, irrespective of the baseline plasma cortisol concentration, which is usually much higher than in healthy humans (72). In such a condition of insufficiently increased cortisol production, a very high plasma ACTH concentration would be expected. However, the recent robust findings that ACTH plasma concentrations are suppressed, that cortisol production is not much elevated, if at all, and that instead reduced cortisol breakdown plays a major role during critical illness, further complicate the issue of diagnostic criteria for adrenal failure in that setting. Moreover, it was recently shown that cortisol responses to ACTH stimulation in critically ill patients correlated positively with both cortisol production rate and cortisol plasma clearance, but patients who revealed the lowest response to ACTH, to the extent of absolute adrenal failure, were the ones with the most suppressed cortisol breakdown, while their cortisol production was similar to healthy subjects (65). These findings hint that a low cortisol response to an ACTH injection reflect the degree of negative feedback inhibition exerted by the high levels of circulating cortisol, a situation similar to patients treated with exogenous glucocorticoids for an extended time, who also reveal a suppressed response to ACTH injection. Whether this low response during critical illness indicates that cortisol availability would be "insufficient" to cope with the stress of illness remains unclear.

Alternatively, a random total cortisol of <10 μg/dL (276 nmol/L) during critical illness has been suggested for the diagnosis of "relative adrenal insufficiency" (75). However, total plasma cortisol concentration is the net effect of adrenal production and secretion, distribution, binding, and elimination of cortisol. Judging the adequacy of the adrenal cortisol production in response to critical illness based on a single measurement of total plasma cortisol is merely indicative. Furthermore, circulation total cortisol concentrations do not reveal the glucocorticoid effect. Given that only free cortisol can pass the cell membrane to bind to GR and suppressed circulating levels of the binding proteins, CBG and albumin, as well as decreased CBG binding affinity via increased cleavage from CBG at inflammatory loci or by increased temperature was established (76–79), plasma free cortisol may be more appropriate to assess HPA-axis function. However, more research is needed because plasma free cortisol assays are not readily available and normal ranges for plasma free cortisol during critical illness have not been defined. Additionally, increasing evidence from both animal and human experiments suggests altered GR regulation during critical illness (68,80–84), precluding conclusions about "adequacy" of cortisol availability and function during illness. Finally, assays to quantify plasma cortisol concentrations are often inaccurate and vary substantially (85) making it impossible to identify one cut-off value for clinical practice.

Recently, measuring interstitial cortisol levels was introduced to assess the amount of active tissue cortisol levels in critically ill patients (86,87). Therefore, a microdialysis catheter is inserted into the subcutaneous adipose tissue. However, critical illness frequently presents with edema and regional blood flow is variable. Furthermore, the subcutaneous adipose tissue is not the main target tissue for cortisol nor is it the main cortisol-metabolizing organ during critical illness (62). Hence, the benefit of this invasive technique could be questioned.

Therapeutic Implications

It is generally accepted that patients with an established diagnosis of primary or central adrenal failure or patients on chronic treatment with systemic glucocorticoids prior to critical illness, should receive additional coverage to cope with the acute stress (53,88). Also, patients who are diagnosed with an acute addisonian crisis in the ICU are typically treated with high doses of glucocorticoids. This therapeutic strategy is based on the assumption that cortisol production is increased several-fold in critical illness. The conventional treatment proposes the administration of a bolus of 100 mg of hydrocortisone followed by 50 to 100 mg every 6 hours on the first day, 50 mg every 6 hours on the second day, and 25 mg every 6 hours on the third day, tapering to a maintenance dose by the fourth to fifth day (53,88).

The doses of hydrocortisone advised for treatment of "relative adrenal failure" is another controversial issue. The proposed dose of 300 mg of hydrocortisone per day, referred to as "low dose" in the literature, is, in fact, approximately 10 times higher than the normal amount of daily cortisol production in healthy humans (89–92) and between 3- and 6-fold higher than the production that now has been quantified in critically ill patients (Figure 3-3). In view of the substantially reduced cortisol breakdown during critical illness, the currently proposed doses for adrenal failure during critical illness may be too high. This may further explain why the multicenter RCT that assessed the effect of hydrocortisone treatment could not confirm the benefit that was originally observed in the pilot trial (89,92).

Also the duration of treatment is under debate. Treating critically ill patients with glucocorticoids in an excessively high dose for too long a time could inferentially aggravate the loss of lean tissue, increase the risk of myopathy, and prolong ICU dependence, which could increase the susceptibility to potentially lethal complications (93,94).

Finally, given that glucocorticoid sensitivity likely varies among individuals (95) and among cell types in critically ill patients (68,81,83), and given that glucocorticoid treatment may downregulate GR-α via induction of miR-124, the dosing issue is further complicated (96). Moreover, single nucleotide polymorphisms in the GR gene, with an altered response to glucocorticoids, have been identified (97). However, it remains a challenge to identify specific clinical biomarkers of GR activation to guide optimal glucocorticoid therapy for individual patients and illnesses.

Based on the results of stable isotope studies (62), a dose of +/−60 mg of hydrocortisone,

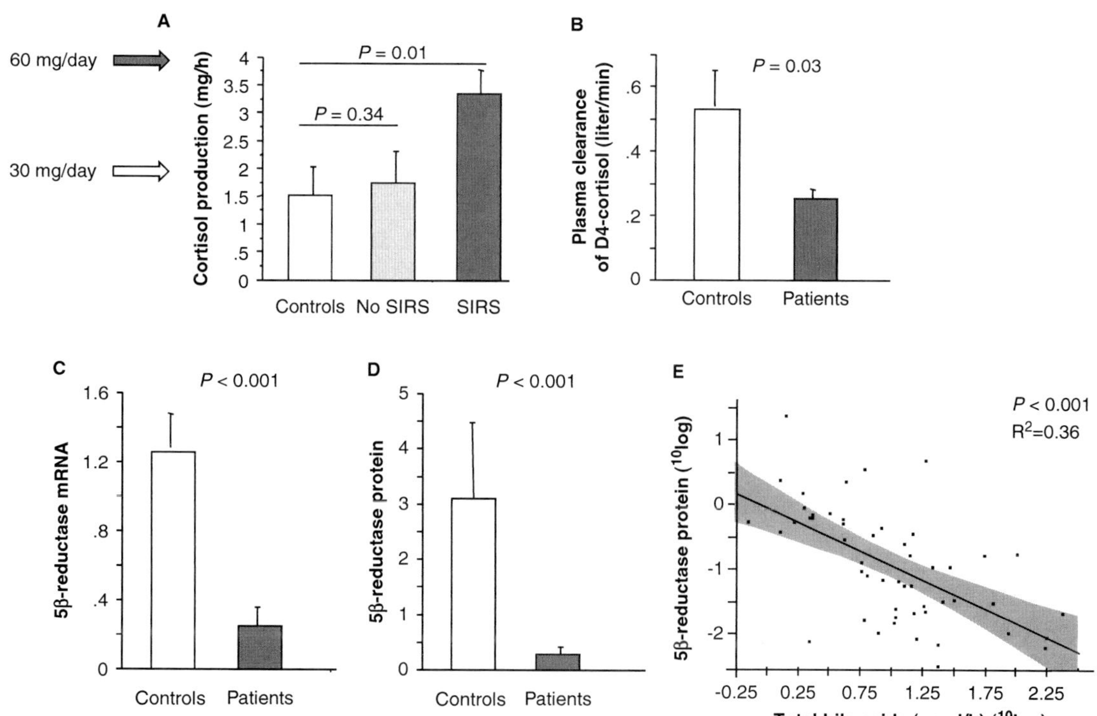

Figure 3-3. Panel A depicts cortisol production in critically ill patients with the systemic inflammatory response syndrome (SIRS) (dark gray bar, n = 7) and no systemic inflammatory response syndrome (light gray bar, n = 4) compared to controls (white bar, n = 9). Based on these results, 24-h cortisol production was estimated and depicted with the arrows.

Panel B depicts cortisol plasma clearance as assessed with a small dose of deuterated-cortisol tracer. Bar charts represent means and standard errors. Panels C–E show mRNA and protein expression of 5β-reductase in the liver of 20 controls (white bar) and 44 patients (gray bar) and the relation to plasma total bile acid concentrations. Bar charts represent means and standard errors. The mRNA data are expressed, normalized to GAPDH, as a -fold difference from the mean of the controls. Protein data are expressed normalized for CK-18 protein expression as a -fold difference from the mean of the controls. *Drafted from original data in Boonen et al (62).*

equivalent to about a doubling of the normal daily cortisol production, may be interesting to further investigate when patients at risk can be identified. A fast tapering down to the lowest effective dose should limit the adverse effects of excessive amounts of glucocorticoids during critical illness.

THE HYPERGLYCEMIC RESPONSE TO CRITICAL ILLNESS: TO TREAT OR NOT TO TREAT?

Blood Glucose and Critical Illness: Robust Associative Data

In humans, the natural endocrine and immunological responses to stress ensure adequate availability of glucose by activating gluconeogenesis and by reducing the sensitivity to insulin for those organs and tissues that predominantly rely upon glucose as metabolic substrate, such as the brain and the blood cells. In young and lean patients not receiving macronutrients, this stress response will maintain normoglycemia. However, when patients are older, overweight, suffer from chronic comorbidity, receive drugs that affect insulin sensitivity, or enteral/parenteral nutrition, the circulating glucose concentrations usually rise quickly above the upper limit of normality (98–102), which could be adaptive or maladaptive. In the condition of prolonged critical illness, stress-induced hyperglycemia may be quite severe and persist for a long period of time. Hyperglycemia in critically ill patients repeatedly has been shown to be associated with risk of mortality, an association that appears to have a J-shape with the lowest risk in the normoglycemic zone (Figure 3-4) (103). In critically ill patients with established diabetes mellitus the J-shaped curve is significantly blunted in the hyperglycemic zone and the nadir is shifted to higher blood glucose levels (103,104).

Hyperglycemia and Adverse Outcome: Cause or Consequence?

The first RCT on blood glucose management was the 2001 Leuven surgical ICU (SICU) study (105). In this study, a "strictly normal level for fasting blood glucose," namely, 80–110 mg/dL (4.4–6.0 mmol/L) was targeted in the intervention group, as compared to the "usual care" of adult surgical ICU patients in the year 2000, which was to tolerate hyperglycemia

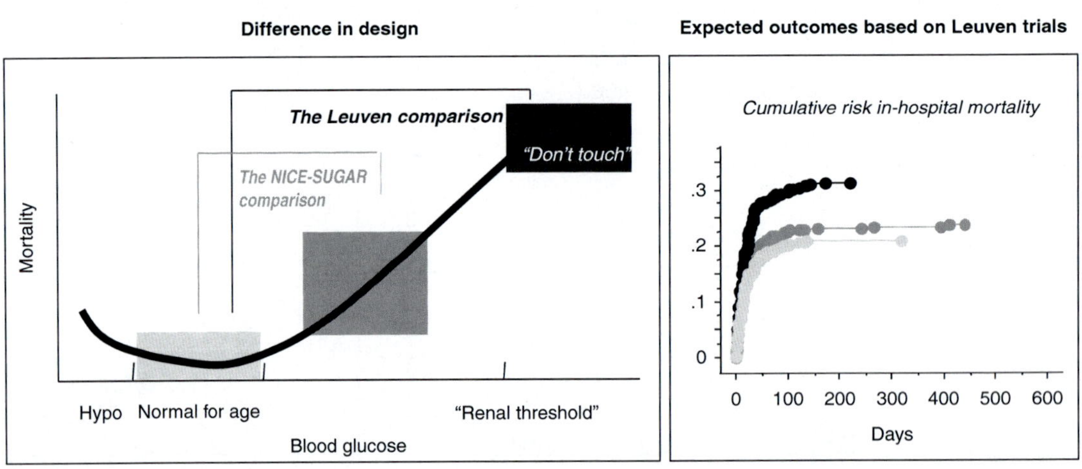

Figure 3-4. Different designs of key intervention trials and expected outcome benefits. The left panel shows J-shaped association curve between blood glucose and risk of death. The NICE–SUGAR trial was executed in the flatter part of the J-shaped curve. A very small benefit from aiming at lowering blood glucose further down from an intermediate level to strict normoglycemia was hereby traded off against a similar risk of harm by hypoglycemia, particularly when using inaccurate tools. The right panel shows the dose response in the 2 adult Leuven Trials compared to the NICE-SUGAR trial. Black circles represent blood glucose >150 mg/dL, dark gray circles represent blood glucose 110–150 mg/dL, and light gray circles represent blood glucose > 110 mg/dL. The maximal benefit that could be expected from lowering blood glucose from an intermediate level to normoglycemia is <1%, provided that blood glucose could be perfectly separated between the 2 study arms. In order to conclude confidently that such a small benefit is not present, 70,000 patients should have been included. Hence, NICE-SUGAR, with 6,100 patients, was, in fact, underpowered to address this hypothesis. *Reproduced from Van den Berghe (124) with permission.*

up to 215 mg/dL (11.9 mmol/L). The study was highly standardized, resulting in a strong internal validity. For example, frequent blood glucose measurements (interval 0.5h–4h) on whole arterial blood by an accurate blood gas analyzer were done by well-trained nurses, and insulin was continuously infused exclusively via a dedicated lumen of a central venous line with an accurate syringe pump. Maintaining strict normoglycemia lowered ICU and in-hospital mortality and reduced morbidity by preventing organ failure, reflected in a shorter duration of mechanical ventilation, along with a decreased incidence of acute kidney failure, severe infections, and critical illness polyneuropathy. In a second study performed in patients admitted to a medical ICU in Leuven, these morbidity benefits were confirmed (106). A subsequent randomized controlled study was performed in critically ill children, in which the intervention group was targeted to normal fasting glucose levels for the age groups (50–80 mg/dL for infants and 70–100 mg/dL for children) as compared with tolerating hyperglycemia up to 215 mg/dL (107). Also in this young patient population, the intervention reduced ICU morbidity and mortality and also had long-term beneficial effects on neurocognitive development up to 4 years after inclusion in the study (107,108). In a subsequent study, targeting the much higher adult range for normal fasting blood glucose levels in such young infants in the ICU did not alter the level of blood glucose concentration nor the outcome (109), suggesting that the normal fasting level is key in preventing toxicity of hyperglycemia in each age group. The underlying mechanisms of hyperglycemia-induced toxicity were identified to involve cellular damage occurring in those cells that do not require insulin for glucose uptake, such as hepatocytes, renal tubular cells, the endothelium, immune cells, and neurons (93,107–110). Soon after the first Leuven study was published, the intervention was swiftly implemented in clinical practice worldwide (111,112). After several smaller studies, the NICE-SUGAR multi-center trial (Normoglycemia in Intensive Care Evaluation and Survival Using Glucose Algorithm Regulation) was designed to be the definitive study to answer this question. The study compared tight blood glucose control to a normoglycemic target (80–100 mg/dL [4.4–6.0 mmol/L]) in the intervention group with an intermediate target of 140–180 mg/dL (8–10 mmol/L) in the control group (113). The study revealed that blood glucose control to a normoglycemic target increased mortality as compared with the intermediate level in the control group (113), subsequently explained by a 13-fold increase in hypoglycemia (114). As this study was designed for a high external validity, the first conclusion is that very tight blood glucose control is not readily applicable in general daily clinical practice. However, the usual care had already evolved significantly between the first Leuven study and the start of NICE-SUGAR: tolerating excessive hyperglycemia was now the new no-go zone, compared with the 215 mg/dL (11.9 mmol/L) tolerance threshold 5 years earlier. Second, due to its pragmatic nature, there was no emphasis on standardization in NICE-SUGAR. All sorts of glucose measurement methodologies were allowed, and practitioners were not specifically trained to perform the complex treatment. Now it has become clear that tight blood glucose control requires accurate blood gas analyzers, like those used in the Leuven studies, to target a narrow range of blood glucose (115). It is also clear that extensive experience is crucial to avoid undetected episodes of hypoglycemia and to treat hypoglycemia when it occurs. Certainly profound, prolonged/undetected hypoglycemia can have grave consequences and may even result in death. Hence, hypoglycemia should be avoided as much as possible. Nevertheless, recent data show that in cardiac patients and in critically ill children iatrogenic hypoglycemia may not by itself affect outcome (108,116,117). Spontaneous hypoglycemia is in contrast a strong predictor of poor outcome. For example, patients with liver failure, acute kidney injury requiring renal replacement therapy, diabetes mellitus, and septic shock have higher risk to develop spontaneous hypoglycemia. Furthermore, adequate treatment of hypoglycemia is essential to avoid rebound hyperglycemia, which causes cerebral neuronal damage (118). Detailed protocols for prompt and gentle correction of hypoglycemia are often not in place, which again contrasts with the Leuven studies (113).

Table 3-1. Novel Insights into Endocrine Changes in Critical Illness

- Part of the acute fall in T_3 plasma concentrations during critical illness is related to the concomitant fasting and this part of the response seems adaptive.
- Cortisol production during critical illness is only moderately increased during critical illness and only in patients suffering from the systemic inflammatory response syndrome (SIRS), while unaltered in patients without SIRS, in the face of several-fold higher plasma cortisol in all patients.
- Cortisol plasma clearance is substantially reduced in all critically ill patients and contributes substantially to hypercortisolism during critical illness, irrespective of type and severity of illness and irrespective of the inflammation status.
- The largest benefit of blood glucose control may be brought about by preventing overt hyperglycemia, hence targeting blood glucose to intermediate ranges during critical illness seems a reasonable compromise.

Therapeutic implications: How to Translate This into General Clinical Practice?

What could then be a sensible approach for daily practice? Tight blood glucose control with current technologies and experience is not yet ready to be broadly implemented in every ICU as clearly demonstrated by NICE-SUGAR. Post-hoc analyses of the Leuven clinical trials revealed that the bulk of the beneficial effects of blood glucose control lay in bringing overt hyperglycemia to moderate levels (Figure 3-4) (119,120). More can be gained by further tightening the glycemic control, but this requires a substantial investment in training and technology to do safely. Hence, targeting blood glucose below 145 mg/dL (8.1 mmol/L) seems a reasonable compromise (112). Critically ill patients with diabetes may benefit from treatment to somewhat higher glycemic targets, depending on their premorbid levels (102,103). However, irrespective of the chosen target level, several methodological aspects ought to be taken into account to ensure patient safety whenever insulin treatment is used. These include frequent blood glucose measurements, the use of on-site blood gas analyzers as the preferred measurement tool, the avoidance of capillary blood samples, and the continuous infusion of insulin with accurate syringe pumps through a dedicated lumen of a central venous catheter. Finally, insulin dosing decisions should not be based on a sliding scale system but rather on a (computerized) algorithm, which has been clinically validated for critically ill patients (121).

CONCLUSIONS

Recent studies generated important novel insights into the endocrine and metabolic responses to critical illness (Table 3-1). Although many aspects remain unresolved, an important recent insight with therapeutic implications is that most acute endocrine responses are likely adaptive and thus should probably not be treated. Nevertheless, many patients who survived the initial phase of critical illness still remain in the ICU for long periods and face a risk of death that increases steadily with every day that recovery does not set in. Hence, more work is required to find better treatments to further prevent protracted critical illness, to enhance recovery from multi-organ failure, and to optimize rehabilitation.

ACKNOWLEDGMENTS

The work summarized in this chapter has been supported by research grants from the Fund for Scientific Research Flanders Belgium, the Methusalem Program funded by the Flemish Government, and the European Research Council under the European Union's Seventh Framework Program (FP7/2007-2013 ERC Advanced Grant Agreement n° 307523).

REFERENCES

1. **Casaer MP, Langouche L, Coudyzer W, et al.** Impact of early parenteral nutrition on muscle and adipose tissue compartments during critical illness. *Crit Care Med.* 2013;41:2298–2309.
2. **Puthucheary ZA, Rawal J, McPhail M, et al.** Acute skeletal muscle wasting in critical illness. *JAMA.* 2013;310:1591–1600.
3. **Villet S, Chiolero RL, Bollmann MD, et al.** Negative impact of hypocaloric feeding and energy balance on clinical outcome in ICU patients. *Clin Nutr.* 2005;24:502–509.
4. **Hermans G, Casaer MP, Clerckx B, et al.** Effect of tolerating macronutrient deficit on the development of intensive-care unit acquired weakness: a subanalysis of the EPaNIC trial. *Lancet Respir Med.* 2013;1:621–629.
5. **Vanhorebeek I, Gunst J, Derde S, et al.** Insufficient activation of autophagy allows cellular damage to accumulate in critically ill patients. *J Clin Endocrinol Metab.* 2011;96:E633–E645.

6. **Chopra IJ, Huang TS, Beredo A, Solomon DH, Chua Teco GN, Mead JF.** Evidence for an inhibitor of extrathyroidal conversion of thyroxine to 3,5,3′-triiodothyronine in sera of patients with nonthyroidal illnesses. *J Clin Endocrinol Metab.* 1985;60:666–672.
7. **Michalaki M, Vagenakis AG, Makri M, Kalfarentzos F, Kyriazopoulou V.** Dissociation of the early decline in serum T(3) concentration and serum IL-6 rise and TNFalpha in nonthyroidal illness syndrome induced by abdominal surgery. *J Clin Endocrinol Metab.* 2001;86:4198–4205.
8. **Bartalena L, Martino E, Brandi LS, et al.** Lack of nocturnal serum thyrotropin surge after surgery. *J Clin Endocrinol Metab.* 1990;70:293–296.
9. **Romijn JA, Wiersinga WM.** Decreased nocturnal surge of thyrotropin in nonthyroidal illness. *J Clin Endocrinol Metab.* 1990;70:35–42.
10. **Redout EM, van der Toorn A, Zuidwijk MJ, et al.** Antioxidant treatment attenuates pulmonary arterial hypertension-induced heart failure. *Am J Physiol Heart Circ Physiol.* 2010;298:H1038–H1047.
11. **Wajner SM, Goemann IM, Bueno AL, Larsen PR, Maia AL.** IL-6 promotes nonthyroidal illness syndrome by blocking thyroxine activation while promoting thyroid hormone inactivation in human cells. *J Clin Invest.* 2011;121:1834–1845.
12. **Boelen A, Kwakkel J, Fliers E.** Beyond low plasma T3: local thyroid hormone metabolism during inflammation and infection. *Endocr Rev.* 2011;32:670–693.
13. **van der Poll T, Van Zee KJ, Endert E, et al.** Interleukin-1 receptor blockade does not affect endotoxin-induced changes in plasma thyroid hormone and thyrotropin concentrations in man. *J Clin Endocrinol Metab.* 1995;80:1341–1346.
14. **Lim CF, Docter R, Visser TJ, et al.** Inhibition of thyroxine transport into cultured rat hepatocytes by serum of nonuremic critically ill patients: effects of bilirubin and nonesterified fatty acids. *J Clin Endocrinol Metab.* 1993;76:1165–1172.
15. **Gardner DF, Kaplan MM, Stanley CA, Utiger RD.** Effect of tri-iodothyronine replacement on the metabolic and pituitary responses to starvation. *N Engl J Med.* 1979;300:579–584.
16. **Moshang T, Jr, Parks JS, Baker L, et al.** Low serum triiodothyronine in patients with anorexia nervosa. *J Clin Endocrinol Metab.* 1975;40:470–473.
17. **Peeters RP, Wouters PJ, van Toor H, Kaptein E, Visser TJ, Van den Berghe G.** Serum 3,3′,5′-triiodothyronine (rT3) and 3,5,3′-triiodothyronine/rT3 are prognostic markers in critically ill patients and are associated with postmortem tissue deiodinase activities. *J Clin Endocrinol Metab.* 2005;90:4559–4565.
18. **Rothwell PM, Lawler PG.** Prediction of outcome in intensive care patients using endocrine parameters. *Crit Care Med.* 1995;23:78–83.
19. **Klemperer JD, Klein I, Gomez M, et al.** Thyroid hormone treatment after coronary-artery bypass surgery. *N Engl J Med.* 1995;333:1522–1527.
20. **Mullis-Jansson SL, Argenziano M, Corwin S, et al.** A randomized double-blind study of the effect of triiodothyronine on cardiac function and morbidity after coronary bypass surgery. *J Thorac Cardiovasc Surg.* 1999;117:1128–1134.
21. **Casaer MP, Mesotten D, Hermans G, et al.** Early versus late parenteral nutrition in critically ill adults. *N Engl J Med.* 2011;365:506–517.
22. **Langouche L, Vander Perre S, Marques M, et al.** Impact of early nutrient restriction during critical illness on the nonthyroidal illness syndrome and its relation with outcome: a randomized, controlled clinical study. *J Clin Endocrinol Metab.* 2013;98:1006–1013.
23. **Mebis L, Eerdekens A, Guiza F, et al.** Contribution of nutritional deficit to the pathogenesis of the nonthyroidal illness syndrome in critical illness: a rabbit model study. *Endocrinology.* 2012;153:973–984.
24. **Boelen A, Boorsma J, Kwakkel J, et al.** Type 3 deiodinase is highly expressed in infiltrating neutrophilic granulocytes in response to acute bacterial infection. *Thyroid.* 2008;18:1095–1103.
25. **Van den Berghe G, de Zegher F, Veldhuis JD, et al.** Thyrotrophin and prolactin release in prolonged critical illness: dynamics of spontaneous secretion and effects of growth hormone-secretagogues. *Clin Endocrinol (Oxf).* 1997;47:599–612.
26. **Fliers E, Guldenaar SE, Wiersinga WM, Swaab DF.** Decreased hypothalamic thyrotropin-releasing hormone gene expression in patients with nonthyroidal illness. *J Clin Endocrinol Metab.* 1997;82:4032–4036.
27. **Bacci V, Schussler GC, Kaplan TB.** The relationship between serum triiodothyronine and thyrotropin during systemic illness. *J Clin Endocrinol Metab.* 1982;54:1229–1235.
28. **Damas P, Reuter A, Gysen P, Demonty J, Lamy M, Franchimont P.** Tumor necrosis factor and interleukin-1 serum levels during severe sepsis in humans. *Crit Care Med.* 1989;17:975–978.
29. **Faglia G, Ferrari C, Beck-Peccoz P, Spada A, Travaglini P, Ambrosi B.** Reduced plasma thyrotropin response to thyrotropin releasing hormone after dexamethasone administration in normal subjects. *Horm Metab Res.* 1973;5:289–292.
30. **Van den Berghe G, de Zegher F, Lauwers P.** Dopamine and the sick euthyroid syndrome in critical illness. *Clin Endocrinol (Oxf).* 1994;41:731–737.
31. **Van den Berghe G, de Zegher F, Lauwers P.** Dopamine suppresses pituitary function in infants and children. *Crit Care Med.* 1994;22:1747–1753.
32. **Boelen A, Kwakkel J, Thijssen-Timmer DC, Alkemade A, Fliers E, Wiersinga WM.** Simultaneous changes in central and peripheral components of the hypothalamus-pituitary-thyroid axis in lipopolysaccharide-induced acute illness in mice. *J Endocrinol.* 2004;182:315–323.
33. **Mebis L, Debaveye Y, Ellger B, et al.** Changes in the central component of the hypothalamus-pituitary-thyroid axis in a rabbit model of prolonged critical illness. *Crit Care.* 2009;13:R147.
34. **Alkemade A, Friesema EC, Kuiper GG, et al.** Novel neuroanatomical pathways for thyroid hormone action in the human anterior pituitary. *Eur J Endocrinol.* 2006;154:491–500.
35. **Langouche L, Princen L, Gunst J, Guiza F, Derde S, Van den Berghe G.** Anterior pituitary morphology and hormone production during sustained critical illness in a rabbit model. *Horm Metab Res.* 2013;45:277–282.

36. **Mebis L, Paletta D, Debaveye Y, et al.** Expression of thyroid hormone transporters during critical illness. *Eur J Endocrinol.* 2009;161:243–250.
37. **Mebis L, Langouche L, Visser TJ, Van den Berghe G.** The type II iodothyronine deiodinase is up-regulated in skeletal muscle during prolonged critical illness. *J Clin Endocrinol Metab.* 2007;92:3330–3333.
38. **Ma SF, Xie L, Pino-Yanes M, et al.** Type 2 deiodinase and host responses of sepsis and acute lung injury. *Am J Respir Cell Mol Biol.* 2011;45:1203–1211.
39. **Thijssen-Timmer DC, Peeters RP, Wouters P, et al.** Thyroid hormone receptor isoform expression in livers of critically ill patients. *Thyroid.* 2007;17: 105–112.
40. **Van den Berghe G, Wouters P, Weekers F, et al.** Reactivation of pituitary hormone release and metabolic improvement by infusion of growth hormone-releasing peptide and thyrotropin-releasing hormone in patients with protracted critical illness. *J Clin Endocrinol Metab.* 1999;84:1311–1323.
41. **Van den Berghe G, de Zegher F, Baxter RC, et al.** Neuroendocrinology of prolonged critical illness: effects of exogenous thyrotropin-releasing hormone and its combination with growth hormone secretagogues. *J Clin Endocrinol Metab.* 1998;83: 309–319.
42. **Weekers F, Michalaki M, Coopmans W, et al.** Endocrine and metabolic effects of growth hormone (GH) compared with GH-releasing peptide, thyrotropin-releasing hormone, and insulin infusion in a rabbit model of prolonged critical illness. *Endocrinology.* 2004;145:205–213.
43. **Van den Berghe G, Baxter RC, Weekers F, et al.** The combined administration of GH-releasing peptide-2 (GHRP-2), TRH and GnRH to men with prolonged critical illness evokes superior endocrine and metabolic effects compared to treatment with GHRP-2 alone. *Clin Endocrinol (Oxf).* 2002;56: 655–669.
44. **Mebis L, Van den Berghe G.** The hypothalamus-pituitary-thyroid axis in critical illness. *Neth J Med.* 2009;67:332–340.
45. **Debaveye Y, Ellger B, Mebis L, et al.** Tissue deiodinase activity during prolonged critical illness: effects of exogenous thyrotropin-releasing hormone and its combination with growth hormone-releasing peptide-2. *Endocrinology.* 2005;146:5604–5611.
46. **Debaveye Y, Ellger B, Mebis L, Darras VM, Van den Berghe G.** Regulation of tissue iodothyronine deiodinase activity in a model of prolonged critical illness. *Thyroid.* 2008;18:551–560.
47. **Debaveye Y, Ellger B, Mebis L, Visser TJ, Darras VM, Van den Berghe G.** Effects of substitution and high-dose thyroid hormone therapy on deiodination, sulfoconjugation, and tissue thyroid hormone levels in prolonged critically ill rabbits. *Endocrinology.* 2008;149:4218–4228.
48. **Peeters RP, van der Geyten S, Wouters PJ, et al.** Tissue thyroid hormone levels in critical illness. *J Clin Endocrinol Metab.* 2005;90:6498–6507.
49. **Acker CG, Singh AR, Flick RP, Bernardini J, Greenberg A, Johnson JP.** A trial of thyroxine in acute renal failure. *Kidney Int.* 2000;57:293–298.
50. **Becker RA, Vaughan GM, Ziegler MG, et al.** Hypermetabolic low triiodothyronine syndrome of burn injury. *Crit Care Med.* 1982;10:870–875.
51. **Brent GA, Hershman JM.** Thyroxine therapy in patients with severe nonthyroidal illnesses and low serum thyroxine concentration. *J Clin Endocrinol Metab.* 1986;63:1–8.
52. **Sirlak M, Yazicioglu L, Inan MB, et al.** Oral thyroid hormone pretreatment in left ventricular dysfunction. *Eur J Cardiothorac Surg.* 2004;26:720–725.
53. **Debaveye Y, Vandenbrande J, Van den Berghe G.** Endocrine emergencies. In: Tubaro M, Danchin N, Filippatos G, Goldstein P, Vranckx P, Zahger D, eds. *The ESC Textbook of Intensive and Acute Cardiac Care.* New York: Oxford University Press; 2011: 709–717.
54. **Nicoloff JT.** Thyroid storm and myxedema coma. *Med Clin North Am.* 1985;69:1005–1017.
55. **Ringel MD.** Management of hypothyroidism and hyperthyroidism in the intensive care unit. *Crit Care Clin.* 2001;17:59–74.
56. **Escobar-Morreale HF, Obregon MJ, Escobar del RF, Morreale de Escobar G.** Replacement therapy for hypothyroidism with thyroxine alone does not ensure euthyroidism in all tissues, as studied in thyroidectomized rats. *J Clin Invest.* 1995;96:2828–2838.
57. **Van den Berghe G 2010** Endocrine aspects of critical care medicine. In: Jameson JL, De Groot LJ, eds. *Endocrinology: Adult and Pediatric.* St Louis, MO: WB Saunders; 2010: 2084–2085.
58. **Finlay WE, McKee JI.** Serum cortisol levels in severely stressed patients. *Lancet.* 1982;1:1414–1415.
59. **Munck A, Guyre PM, Holbrook NJ.** Physiological functions of glucocorticoids in stress and their relation to pharmacological actions. *Endocr Rev.* 1984;5:25–44.
60. **Starling EH.** The wisdom of the body: The Harveian Oration, delivered before The Royal College of Physicians of London on St. Luke's Day, 1923. *Br Med J.* 1923;2:685–690.
61. **Vermes I, Beishuizen A, Hampsink RM, Haanen C.** Dissociation of plasma adrenocorticotropin and cortisol levels in critically ill patients: possible role of endothelin and atrial natriuretic hormone. *J Clin Endocrinol Metab.* 1995;80:1238–1242.
62. **Boonen E, Vervenne H, Meersseman P, et al.** Reduced cortisol metabolism during critical illness. *N Engl J Med.* 2013;368:1477–1488.
63. **Bornstein SR, Engeland WC, Ehrhart-Bornstein M, Herman JP.** Dissociation of ACTH and glucocorticoids. *Trends Endocrinol Metab.* 2008;19:175–180.
64. **Vanwijngaerden YM, Wauters J, Langouche L, et al.** Critical illness evokes elevated circulating bile acids related to altered hepatic transporter and nuclear receptor expression. *Hepatology.* 2011;54:1741–1752.
65. **Ackermann D, Vogt B, Escher G, et al.** Inhibition of 11beta-hydroxysteroid dehydrogenase by bile acids in rats with cirrhosis. *Hepatology.* 1999;30:623–629.
66. **McNeilly AD, Macfarlane DP, O'Flaherty E, et al.** Bile acids modulate glucocorticoid metabolism and the hypothalamic-pituitary-adrenal axis in obstructive jaundice. *J Hepatol.* 2010;52:705–711.
67. **Stauffer AT, Rochat MK, Dick B, Frey FJ, Odermatt A.** Chenodeoxycholic acid and deoxycholic acid

inhibit 11 beta-hydroxysteroid dehydrogenase type 2 and cause cortisol-induced transcriptional activation of the mineralocorticoid receptor. *J Biol Chem.* 2002;277:26286–26292.

68. **van den Akker EL, Koper JW, Joosten K, et al.** Glucocorticoid receptor mRNA levels are selectively decreased in neutrophils of children with sepsis. *Intensive Care Med.* 2009;35:1247–1254.
69. **Barquist E, Kirton O.** Adrenal insufficiency in the surgical intensive care unit patient. *J Trauma.* 1997;42:27–31.
70. **Kanczkowski W, Chatzigeorgiou A, Grossklaus S, Sprott D, Bornstein SR, Chavakis T.** Role of the endothelial-derived endogenous anti-inflammatory factor Del-1 in inflammation-mediated adrenal gland dysfunction. *Endocrinology.* 2013;154:1181–1189.
71. **Prigent H, Maxime V, Annane D.** Science review: mechanisms of impaired adrenal function in sepsis and molecular actions of glucocorticoids. *Crit Care.* 2004;8:243–252.
72. **Annane D, Sebille V, Troche G, Raphael JC, Gajdos P, Bellissant E.** A 3-level prognostic classification in septic shock based on cortisol levels and cortisol response to corticotropin. *JAMA.* 2000;283: 1038–1045.
73. **Beishuizen A, Vermes I, Hylkema BS, Haanen C.** Relative eosinophilia and functional adrenal insufficiency in critically ill patients. *Lancet.* 1999;353:1675–1676.
74. **Richards ML, Caplan RH, Wickus GG, Lambert PJ, Kisken WA.** The rapid low-dose (1 microgram) cosyntropin test in the immediate postoperative period: results in elderly subjects after major abdominal surgery. *Surgery.* 1999;125:431–440.
75. **Marik PE, Pastores SM, Annane D, et al.** Recommendations for the diagnosis and management of corticosteroid insufficiency in critically ill adult patients: consensus statements from an international task force by the American College of Critical Care Medicine. *Crit Care Med.* 2008;36:1937–1949.
76. **Chan WL, Carrell RW, Zhou A, Read RJ.** How changes in affinity of corticosteroid-binding globulin modulate free cortisol concentration. *J Clin Endocrinol Metab.* 2013;98:3315–3322.
77. **Hamrahian AH, Oseni TS, Arafah BM.** Measurements of serum free cortisol in critically ill patients. *N Engl J Med.* 2004;350:1629–1638.
78. **Holland PC, Hancock SW, Hodge D, Thompson D, Shires S, Evans S.** Degradation of albumin in meningococcal sepsis. *Lancet.* 2001;357:2102–2104.
79. **Pugeat M, Bonneton A, Perrot D, et al.** Decreased immunoreactivity and binding activity of corticosteroid-binding globulin in serum in septic shock. *Clin Chem.* 1989;35:1675–1679.
80. **Bergquist M, Nurkkala M, Rylander C, Kristiansson E, Hedenstierna G, Lindholm C.** Expression of the glucocorticoid receptor is decreased in experimental *Staphylococcus aureus* sepsis. *J Infect.* 2013;67: 574–583.
81. **Guerrero J, Gatica HA, Rodriguez M, Estay R, Goecke IA.** Septic serum induces glucocorticoid resistance and modifies the expression of glucocorticoid isoforms receptors: a prospective cohort study and in vitro experimental assay. *Crit Care.* 2013;17:R107.
82. **Indyk JA, Candido-Vitto C, Wolf IM, et al.** Reduced glucocorticoid receptor protein expression in children with critical illness. *Horm Res Paediatr.* 2013;79: 169–178.
83. **Peeters RP, Hagendorf A, Vanhorebeek I, et al.** Tissue mRNA expression of the glucocorticoid receptor and its splice variants in fatal critical illness. *Clin Endocrinol (Oxf).* 2009;71:145–153.
84. **Siebig S, Meinel A, Rogler G, et al.** Decreased cytosolic glucocorticoid receptor levels in critically ill patients. *Anaesth Intensive Care.* 2010;38:133–140.
85. **Cohen J, Ward G, Prins J, Jones M, Venkatesh B.** Variability of cortisol assays can confound the diagnosis of adrenal insufficiency in the critically ill population. *Intensive Care Med.* 2006;32:1901–1905.
86. **Vassiliadi DA, Ilias I, Tzanela M, et al.** Interstitial cortisol obtained by microdialysis in mechanically ventilated septic patients: correlations with total and free serum cortisol. *J Crit Care.* 2013;28:158–165.
87. **Venkatesh B, Morgan TJ, Cohen J.** Interstitium: the next diagnostic and therapeutic platform in critical illness. *Crit Care Med.* 2010;38:S630–S636.
88. **Chung TT, Grossman A, Clark AJL.** Adrenal Insufficiency. In: Jameson JL, De Groot LJ, eds. *Endocrinology: Adult and Pediatric.* 2010: 1853–1863.
89. **Annane D, Sebille V, Charpentier C, et al.** Effect of treatment with low doses of hydrocortisone and fludrocortisone on mortality in patients with septic shock. *JAMA.* 2002;288:862–871.
90. **Bollaert PE, Charpentier C, Levy B, Debouverie M, Audibert G, Larcan A.** Reversal of late septic shock with supraphysiologic doses of hydrocortisone. *Crit Care Med.* 1998;26:645–650.
91. **Briegel J, Forst H, Haller M, et al.** Stress doses of hydrocortisone reverse hyperdynamic septic shock: a prospective, randomized, double-blind, single-center study. *Crit Care Med.* 1999;27:723–732.
92. **Sprung CL, Annane D, Keh D, et al.** Hydrocortisone therapy for patients with septic shock. *N Engl J Med.* 2008;358:111–124.
93. **Hermans G, Wilmer A, Meersseman W, et al.** Impact of intensive insulin therapy on neuromuscular complications and ventilator dependency in the medical intensive care unit. *Am J Respir Crit Care Med.* 2007;175:480–489.
94. **Hermans G, De Jonghe B.,** Bruyninckx F, Van den Berghe G. Clinical review: critical illness polyneuropathy and myopathy. *Crit Care.* 2008;12:238.
95. **Hauer D, Weis F, Papassotiropoulos A, et al.** Relationship of a common polymorphism of the glucocorticoid receptor gene to traumatic memories and posttraumatic stress disorder in patients after intensive care therapy. *Crit Care Med.* 2011;39:643–650.
96. **Ledderose C, Mohnle P, Limbeck E, et al.** Corticosteroid resistance in sepsis is influenced by microRNA-124–induced downregulation of glucocorticoid receptor-alpha. *Crit Care Med.* 2012;40:2745–2753.
97. **Baker AC, Chew VW, Green TL, et al.** Single nucleotide polymorphisms and type of steroid impact the functional response of the human glucocorticoid receptor. *J Surg Res.* 2013;180:27–34.

98. **Ahrens CL, Barletta JF, Kanji S, et al.** Effect of low-calorie parenteral nutrition on the incidence and severity of hyperglycemia in surgical patients: a randomized, controlled trial. *Crit Care Med.* 2005;33:2507–2512.
99. **Olveira G, Tapia MJ, Ocon J, et al.** Parenteral nutrition-associated hyperglycemia in non-critically ill inpatients increases the risk of in-hospital mortality (multicenter study). *Diabetes Care.* 2013;36:1061–1066.
100. **Pasquel FJ, Smiley D, Spiegelman R, Lin E, Peng L, Umpierrez GE.** Hyperglycemia is associated with increased hospital complications and mortality during parenteral nutrition. *Hosp Pract (1995).* 2011;39:81–88.
101. **Pieracci F, Hydo L, Eachempati S, Pomp A, Shou J, Barie PS.** Higher body mass index predicts need for insulin but not hyperglycemia, nosocomial infection, or death in critically ill surgical patients. *Surg Infect (Larchmt).* 2008;9:121–130.
102. **Weiss M, Kron M, Hay B, Taenzer M, Radermacher P, Georgieff M.** Which variables are associated with blood glucose levels outside the target range in surgical critically ill patients? A retrospective observational study. *Patient Saf Surg.* 2011;5:5.
103. **Krinsley JS.** Glycemic control in the critically ill—3 domains and diabetic status means one size does not fit all! *Crit Care.* 2013;17:131.
104. **Falciglia M, Freyberg RW, Almenoff PL, D'Alessio DA, Render ML.** Hyperglycemia-related mortality in critically ill patients varies with admission diagnosis. *Crit Care Med.* 2009;37:3001–3009.
105. **Van den Berghe G, Wouters P, Weekers F, et al.** Intensive insulin therapy in the critically ill patients. *N Engl J Med.* 2001;345:1359–1367.
106. **Van den Berghe G, Wilmer A, Hermans G, et al.** Intensive insulin therapy in the medical ICU. *N Engl J Med.* 2006;354:449–461.
107. **Gunst J, Derese I, Aertgeerts A, et al.** Insufficient autophagy contributes to mitochondrial dysfunction, organ failure, and adverse outcome in an animal model of critical illness. *Crit Care Med.* 2013;41:182–194.
108. **Langouche L, Vanhorebeek I, Vlasselaers D, et al.** Intensive insulin therapy protects the endothelium of critically ill patients. *J Clin Invest.* 2005;115:2277–2286.
109. **Vanhorebeek I, De Vos R, Mesotten D, Wouters PJ, De Wolf-Peeters C, Van den Berghe G.** Protection of hepatocyte mitochondrial ultrastructure and function by strict blood glucose control with insulin in critically ill patients. *Lancet.* 2005;365:53–59.
110. **Vanhorebeek I, Gunst J, Ellger B, et al.** Hyperglycemic kidney damage in an animal model of prolonged critical illness. *Kidney Int.* 2009;76:512–520.
111. **Garber AJ, Moghissi ES, Bransome ED, Jr, et al.** American College of Endocrinology position statement on inpatient diabetes and metabolic control. *Endocr Pract.* 2004;10:77–82.
112. **Umpierrez GE, Hellman R, Korytkowski MT, et al.** Management of hyperglycemia in hospitalized patients in non-critical care setting: an endocrine society clinical practice guideline. *J Clin Endocrinol Metab.* 2012;97:16–38.
113. **Finfer S, Chittock DR, Su SY, et al.** Intensive versus conventional glucose control in critically ill patients. *N Engl J Med.* 2009;360:1283–1297.
114. **Finfer S, Liu B, Chittock DR, et al.** Hypoglycemia and risk of death in critically ill patients. *N Engl J Med.* 2012;367:1108–1118.
115. **Finfer S, Billot L.** Managing blood glucose in critically ill patients with or without diabetes. *Crit Care.* 2013;17:134.
116. **Kosiborod M, Inzucchi SE, Goyal A, et al.** Relationship between spontaneous and iatrogenic hypoglycemia and mortality in patients hospitalized with acute myocardial infarction. *JAMA.* 2009;301:1556–1564.
117. **Tin W, Brunskill G, Kelly T, Fritz S.** 15-year follow-up of recurrent "hypoglycemia" in preterm infants. *Pediatrics.* 2012;130:e1497–e1503.
118. **Suh SW, Gum ET, Hamby AM, Chan PH, Swanson RA.** Hypoglycemic neuronal death is triggered by glucose reperfusion and activation of neuronal NADPH oxidase. *J Clin Invest.* 2007;117:910–918.
119. **Van den Berghe G, Wouters PJ, Bouillon R, et al.** Outcome benefit of intensive insulin therapy in the critically ill: insulin dose versus glycemic control. *Crit Care Med.* 2003;31:359–366.
120. **Van den Berghe G, Wilmer A, Milants I, et al.** Intensive insulin therapy in mixed medical/surgical intensive care units: benefit versus harm. *Diabetes.* 2006;55:3151–3159.
121. **Kavanagh BP, McCowen KC.** Clinical practice. Glycemic control in the ICU. *N Engl J Med.* 2010;363:2540–2546.
122. **Vanhorebeek I, Langouche L, Van den Berghe G.** Endocrine aspects of acute and prolonged critical illness. *Nat Clin Pract Endocrinol Metab.* 2006;2:20–31.
123. **Mebis L, Van den Berghe G.** Thyroid axis function and dysfunction in critical illness. *Best Pract Res Clin Endocrinol Metab.* 2011;25:745–757.
124. **Van den Berghe G.** Intensive insulin therapy in the ICU–reconciling the evidence. *Nat Rev Endocrinol.* 2012;8:374–378.

SECTION III

Special Populations

CHAPTER 4

Endocrine and Metabolic Changes with Aging

Physiology or Pathophysiology

Johannes D Veldhuis

ABSTRACT

We are all living in increasingly "graying" societies due to growth in the older population. In the United States alone, this population (defined as persons 65 years or older) number 41.4 million in 2011 or 1 in every 8 Americans. This has important implications for health care. The frail elderly in particular make up a large proportion of patients presenting for acute medical care, including endocrine and metabolic emergencies. Aging is marked by initially subtle but eventually overt erosion of endocrine and metabolic physiological control mechanisms. For example, these changes in the pituitary result in depressed hormone secretory-burst amplitude and disrupted secretory-pattern regularity of growth hormone (GH), luteinizing and follicle-stimulating hormone (LH and FSH), adrenocorticotropic hormone (ACTH), prolactin, and thyroid-stimulating hormone (TSH) release. Concomitantly, 24-hour rhythmic (circadian and nycthemeral) concentrations of GH and TSH (and possibly nocturnal antidiuretic hormone [ADH]) decrease, whereas the diurnal ACTH nadir and maximum occur earlier. However, major confounding variables exist in aging, including gender, body composition, medication use, physical frailty, caloric intake, exercise, and neurocognitive decline. This chapter will briefly discuss some of the endocrine (predominantly pituitary) and metabolic changes that occur with aging and how this may impact endocrine evaluation and treatment in this population.

INTRODUCTION

Within the theme of endocrine changes in the elderly, a central issue is how anterior and posterior pituitary reserve (maximal secretory capacity) changes with age. Table 4-1 summarizes current knowledge on this point. An important insight is that hormone, type of stimulus (secretagogue), and gender together determine estimates of pituitary reserve. GH is a prototypical example, wherein all known single secretagogues, except insulin-induced hypoglycemia, predict a decrease in GH reserve with age. The decrease in GH secretion with age is more rapid in men than women before age 50, but similar thereafter (1).

Other endocrine and metabolic systems also undergo important changes with aging (eg, glucose metabolism, calcium and metabolic bone diseases) and are discussed in the relevant chapters.

HYPOTHALAMIC-PITUITARY-THYROID AXIS

A tendency for baseline (unstimulated) TSH concentrations and thyroid autoantibodies to rise with age is more evident in women

Table 4-1. Overall Hypothalamo-Pituitary Reserve in Aging

Hormone	Effect of Age	Secretagogue Used
ACTH	No change[a]	Hypoglycemia, surgery, metyrapone, naloxone
GH	No change[a]	Hypoglycemia, triple secretagogue stimulus
GH	Decreased (both sexes)[a]	Exercise, fasting, deep sleep, L-arginine, GHRP, L-dopa, GHRH, and any pair of stimuli
LH	Decreased burst size (both sexes)[a]	Antiandrogen, antiestrogen
LH and FSH	Mean and basal increased (both sexes)[a]	Gonadoprivation, antiestrogen, GnRH
Prolactin	Decreased[a] (especially women)	Nighttime (during sleep)
TSH	Unchanged[a]; increased (women) or decreased (men >50)	Hypothyroidism; TRH stimulation
ADH	Normal to increased	Hypertonic saline infusion, dehydration

[a]*24-h hormone secretion (10-min sampling).*

(2,3), whereas a decrease in baseline, overnight, and thyrotropin-releasing hormone (TRH)-stimulated TSH release with age is better demonstrated in men (4,5). Lower serum triiodothyronine (T_3) concentrations occur in older adults of both sexes, especially in the presence of organ-level failure, systemic inflammation, or debilitating illness. Reductions in mean and 24-hour rhythmic (nycthemeral) TSH concentrations become prominent after the 8th decade of life (4,6). Typically, total thyroxine (T_4) levels are preserved in older healthy adults while free T_3 and TSH levels fall, yielding lower free T_3/free T_4 and TSH/T_4 ratios. Postulated mechanisms for the ensemble changes observed in aging include augmented inhibition by T_3 of or diminished central drive to TSH output, and increased thyrotrope but decreased systemic and thyroidal T_3 activation from T_4.

Confounding issues in TSH regulation in elderly adults are decreased exercise; reduced caloric intake; muted symptoms and signs of deficient or excessive T_3/T_4; exposure to glucocorticoids, iodine, or L-dopa (2); supervening systemic illness, including traumatic brain injury; inanition, and psychiatric depression, all of which can inhibit TSH secretion. Conversely, chronic fatigue syndrome, morbid obesity, type 2 diabetes mellitus, certain drugs, and autoimmune thyroid disease (3) can all potentiate TSH secretion. At any age, ethnic differences in TSH concentrations (7) and the existence of single-nucleotide polymorphisms (eg, PDE8B) further expand intersubject variability.

HYPOTHALAMIC-PITUITARY-ADRENAL AXIS

The stress-responsive hypothalamic-pituitary-adrenal (HPA; corticotropic) axis is a vital neuroendocrine system regulating cognition, well-being, memory, behavior, appetite, work capacity, inflammation, glucose metabolism, fat, muscle and skeletal mass, blood pressure, insulin sensitivity, immune responses, and water and electrolyte balance. The inferred effects of age are complex, involving adaptations in feedback (inhibition) and feedforward (stimulation) in a gender-modulated and stressor-selective manner. Certain potent amplifiers of ACTH/cortisol secretion appear to be more effective in older than young adults; ie, cholinergic agonists, corticotropin-releasing hormone (CRH) and/or injection arginine vasopressin (AVP) and hypertonic saline infusion (8). Feedback disinhibition using a mineralocorticoid-receptor (MR) antagonist also augments ACTH release more in older than young subjects (9). Other ACTH secretagogues are equally effective in young and older volunteers, namely major surgery, insulin-induced hypoglycemia, feedback disinhibition via metyrapone-induced hypocortisolemia (10), and opiate-receptor antagonism (10,11). In contrast, feedback suppression via hydrocortisone or dexamethasone (glucocorticoid agonists) or via 9 alpha-fludrocortisone (MR agonist) is less effective in older volunteers (12).

The 24-hour (circadian) rhythm of ACTH/cortisol concentrations is consistently blunted in absolute amplitude (algebraic difference between peak and nadir) due to a higher late-day cortisol minimum (13,14). Additionally, the times of the nycthemeral cortisol peak and nadir are consistently advanced (earlier in the day by about 2 h) in elderly volunteers.

Clinical implications of altered ACTH regulation with age are (a) valid comparisons must match study subjects for age, gender, mental-health status, obesity, medication exposure, systemic illness, and stress or depressive history; (b) stress-dose glucocorticoid coverage is not required in aging per se, because adrenal responses to ACTH and pituitary ACTH responses to induced hypocortisolemia, surgery, and critical illness are largely age-invariant (10,11,15); (c) obesity can elevate urinary but not usually plasma free cortisol (16,17); (d) glucocorticoid-receptor (GR) polymorphisms may be relevant markers of tissue cortisol activity; and (e) ACTH deficiency is not the basis for low adrenal dehydroepiandrosterone (DHEA) in older men and women. Significant unresolved questions include whether and how age and comorbidities affect CRH and AVP receptors, endocannabinoid signaling, and 11 beta-hydroxysteroid dehydrogenase activity in brain and pituitary. Because this enzyme can both activate cortisone (type I activity) and inactivate cortisol (type II activity), its regulation might play a role in age-related modulation of gluco- and mineralocorticoid feedback, neurodegeneration, cognitive function, and/or memory (18,19).

ADH AND WATER BALANCE

In animals and humans, water deprivation, hypertonic saline infusion, heart failure, low renal perfusion, plasma hyperosmolarity, nausea and vomiting, certain medications (especially thiazides, anesthetics, antidepressants, and analgesics), intracranial lesions, and various pulmonary diseases drive ADH secretion (20). Aging may be associated with reduced nighttime ADH secretion, but normal or exaggerated ADH (and possibly atrial natriuretic peptide [ANP]) release during experimental hypertonicity, water deprivation, ethanol exposure, or volume contraction has also been demonstrated (21): Table 4-2. However, ADH release in response to upright posture (orthostasis) and baroreceptor activation is reduced in aging. Hypodipsia may also pertain, increasing the potential for life-threatening hypernatremia (21). Maximal urine-concentrating capability is reduced in older adults after ADH secretion or injection. Renal defects in both AVP-receptor and aquaporin-channel expression (22) accentuate the risks of severe dehydration when access to water is restricted during anesthesia, postoperatively or in coma, after acute myocardial infarction (MI) or stroke, and in the face of fever, glycosuria, diarrhea, diuresis, emesis, burn injury, or blood loss (23). Age-associated decreases in renin and aldosterone levels and measurable (7%–21%) contraction of total body water and plasma volume potentiate the adverse effects of salt and water deprivation (24). Moreover, dehydration and hypernatremia in older patients may be exacerbated by cerebral salt wasting, and medication-induced or ischemia-related renal tubulopathies (20). Clinical literature suggests that neurological sequelae of hypernatremia may be more frequent in older patients. Hypernatremia also predicts greater in-hospital mortality in aged individuals.

Table 4-2. Aging and Water Balance

• ↓ Plasma volume (and ECF)
• ↑ ANF (↑ Na^+ loss in urine)
• ↓ Renal-tubular response to ADH
• Exaggerated ADH release
• Hypodipsia
• ↓ Free water clearance (↓ GFR)

The syndrome of inappropriate ADH release (SIADH) may be exacerbated in the elderly by decreases in renin activity, aldosterone secretion and renal glomerular filtration rate (GFR) (24,25), an increase in ANP secretion, and use of multiple medications (20,26).

Chronic hyponatremia in humans and animals seems to accompany and aggravate frailty. Mechanisms include a neoplasia (associated with autonomous ectopic ADH secretion), cardiopulmonary and hepatic disease, antidepressant medications, and impairment of renal perfusion and tubular diluting capacity (25).

In aggregate, elderly individuals have less robust homeostatic adjustments to both under- and overhydration, thereby worsening the clinical severity and frequency of hyper- and hypo-osmolar states. Rapid or overcorrection of hypo- and hypernatremia carries the risk of iatrogenic neurological injury putatively due to strong osmotic shifts (20). Thus, repeated assessment of water and electrolyte balance and frequently titrated fluid adjustments constitute good medical practice in the elderly (20). These precepts are especially pertinent in older persons with diabetes, and in febrile, frail, and postoperative patients with reduced cardiopulmonary and renal function.

Table 4-3. GH-IGF-I Axis in Aging

- ↓ GH response to all single secretagogues, except insulin-induced hypoglycemia
- ↓ Before age 50 yr is more rapid in men than women
- ↑ Abdominal visceral fat and hyperinsulinemia force further ↓ GH in aging
- ↓ Pulsatile GH secretion via ↓ burst mass
- ↓ IGF-I, ↓ IGFBP-1
- Preserved hepatic IGF-I response to exogenous GH
- ? Accompanies and/or causes metabolic syndrome
- ↓ Lean body mass and bone mineral density

GH/INSULIN-LIKE GROWTH FACTOR-1 AXIS

Clinical features of organic/structural GH deficiency are less vivid in older subjects, who already often have low insulin-like growth factor-I (IGF-I), high waist/hip ratios, and perceived reduction in quality of life (27). Specifically, aging per se is accompanied by adverse changes in body composition, glucose metabolism, lipid profiles, muscle and bone mass, physical endurance, and well-being. These features are mimicked by organic GH deficiency in younger adults. Older adults have lower GH secretion during fasting, exercise, or sleep, and in response to nearly all pharmaceutical secretagogues (28) (eg, one exception is insulin-induced hypoglycemia): Table 4-3 (29). Gender and sex steroids also determine GH secretion. In particular, mean 24-hour GH concentrations decline more rapidly with age in young men than premenopausal women (1). A less vivid gender difference pertains after oophorectomy or menopause, consistent with an interaction between body composition and withdrawal of gonadal sex steroids. In particular, abdominal visceral adiposity and hyperinsulinemia are strongly negative, whereas estrogen and testosterone (acting via estrogen) are strongly positive, determinants of 24-hour pulsatile GH secretion (30,31). The age-related decrement in pulsatile GH secretion, and thereby IGF-I production, is due to smaller GH pulses (diminished secretory-burst mass) with no change in pulse frequency (32).

The clinical impact of age-related hyposomatotropism (decreased GH and IGF-I availability) as well as of organic GH deficiency in older individuals has been explored indirectly by assessing the effects of short-term GH supplementation. The most consistent effects are 2–3 kg loss of total-body (but especially visceral) fat, 1–2 kg gain of lean body mass (water, bone, and muscle), reduction of low-density lipoprotein (LDL), and elevation of IGF-I levels, with modestly improved physical endurance. Balance, muscle strength, coordination, and other functional measures often remain unaffected (33,34). Fluid-retention side effects (edema, hypertension, congestive heart failure, carpal tunnel syndrome, intracranial hypertension, and arthralgias or gynecomastia) and glucose intolerance particularly emerge at higher GH doses, prompting IGF-I-targeted GH dosing. The possibility of an increased incidence of neoplasia with long-term GH IGF-I supplementation in the elderly is raised from animal models of genetic GH/IGF-I deficiency (35). Moreover, no studies have assessed GH treatment after the eighth decade of life. Thus, GH supplementation in healthy elderly adults without hypopituitarism whether directly (via injections of biosynthetic GH) or indirectly (via administration of growth hormone-releasing hormone [GHRH] and/or growth hormone-releasing peptide [GHRP]) cannot be recommended at present outside of research contexts (36).

PROLACTIN

Mean and peak prolactin levels during the nighttime fall by about 40% after menopause, but decline less markedly in aging men (37). The young-adult gender difference (women > men) is lost in older subjects (38). Overall, age (negatively especially in women) and estrogen or adiposity/BMI (positively in both sexes) jointly determine physiological prolactin production (39). Thus, combined decrements in prolactin burst size and basal (nonpulsatile) prolactin secretion with age could reflect withdrawal of estrogen, accentuation of dopamine, and inhibition or attenuation of putative prolactin-releasing factor stimulation (37). Whether cytokines or adipokines modulate these 3 mechanisms to explain mild hyperprolactinemia in obesity is not known.

HYPOTHALAMIC-PITUITARY-GONADAL AXIS

The principal known function of the gonadotropic hormones is maintenance of gonadal steroidogenesis (estrogen and testosterone secretion) and gametogenesis (sperm and egg maturation). LH and FSH gradually rise in aging men, putatively reflecting reduced Leydig-cell androgen (and estrogen) secretion and decreased Sertoli-cell inhibin B secretion (40–42). Spermatogenesis, however, is relatively preserved. FSH concentrations subtly increase in midlife in premenopausal women due to decreased ovarian follicle reserve inferable by ultrasonography and falling concentrations of antimüllerian hormone and inhibin B (43). The initial elevation of FSH may precede clinical menopause by 5–10 years. After menopause, LH (by 2–3-fold) and FSH (by 3–20-fold) in women markedly exceed corresponding levels in age-matched men. A significant confounding factor is obesity, which decreases LH (but not FSH) pulse size in both sexes (44). Serum free (dissociated) and beta subunit levels also increase with age in both sexes (45).

Pituitary gonadotropic responses to an injected pulse of GnRH are usually normal or enhanced in older men and women (46–48). Protracted critical illness can reversibly suppress gonadotropin output at all ages in both men and women (49). Thus, measurements of ACTH/cortisol, prolactin, GH/IGF-I, and TSH/T_4 may be required to evaluate pituitary function in this setting (50). Higher glycoprotein alpha-subunit levels in aged versus young adults might falsely suggest a clinically silent gonadotropic tumor when accompanied by a pituitary incidentaloma (51), which are more common in the elderly.

HEAD TRAUMA

Severe head injuries at any age can damage the hypothalamus, infundibular stalk, and/or pituitary gland, often via hemorrhage or contusion. Deficiencies include ADH, GH, LH, ACTH, TSH, and less evidently FSH or prolactin (52). The exact risk of pituitary deficits is not known. The emergence of endocrine deficits may be either acute or delayed and either transient or permanent. There is a possible increase in pituitary injury in older individuals, and concomitant decrease in quality of life (53). Two important clinical challenges in evaluating possible hypopituitarism in elderly patients are (a) possibly increased medical risks of pituitary stimulation tests, such as insulin-induced hypoglycemia, and (b) less vivid clinical signs and symptoms of hypopituitarism.

CONCLUSIONS

Confounding issues in evaluating pituitary function (and potentially other endocrine systems) include increased comorbidities with age, gender-by-age interactions, sex-hormone deficiency or replacement in menopausal individuals, disruption of sleep, altered body composition, reduced physical activity, elevated inflammatory mediators, greater medication use (ie, polypharmacy) and risk of misdiagnosis (54), and interstudy methodological inconsistencies. These factors restrict the rigor of evidence-based decisions, which require longitudinal, double-blind, randomized, placebo-controlled interventional data replicated across multiple centers.

ACKNOWLEDGMENTS

We thank Jill Smith for support of manuscript preparation. Supported in part via AG019695, DK073148, AG029362, AG031763, and DK050456 (Metabolic Studies Core of the Minnesota Obesity Center) from the National Institutes of Health (Bethesda, Maryland). The content is solely the responsibility of the author and does not necessarily represent the official views of the National Institute on

Aging or the National Institutes of Health. The project described was supported by the National Center for Research Resources and by Grant Number UL1 TR000135 from the National Center for Advancing Translational Sciences (NCATS).

REFERENCES

1. **Weltman A, Weltman JY, Hartman ML, et al.** Relationship between age, percentage body fat, fitness, and 24-hour growth hormone release in healthy young adults: effects of gender. *J Clin Endocrinol Metab.* 1994;78:543–548.
2. **Fisher DA.** Physiological variations in thyroid hormones: physiological and pathophysiological considerations. *Clin Chem.* 1996;42:135–139.
3. **Tietz NW, Shuey DF, Wekstein DR.** Laboratory values in fit aging individuals—sexagenarians through centenarians. *Clin Chem.* 1992;38:1167–1185.
4. **van Coevorden A, Laurent E, Decoster C, et al.** Decreased basal and stimulated thyrotropin secretion in healthy elderly men. *J Clin Endocrinol Metab.* 1989;69:177–185.
5. **Roelfsema F, Pereira AM, Veldhuis JD, et al.** Thyrotropin secretion profiles are not different in men and women. *J Clin Endocrinol Metab.* 2009;94: 3964–3967.
6. **Magri F, Muzzoni B, Cravello L, et al.** Thyroid function in physiological aging and in centenarians: possible relationships with some nutritional markers. *Metabolism.* 2002;51:105–109.
7. **Surks MI, Boucai L.** Age- and race-based serum thyrotropin reference limits. *J Clin Endocrinol Metab.* 2010;95:496–502.
8. **Heuser IJ, Gotthardt U, Schweiger U, et al.** Age-associated changes of pituitary-adrenocortical hormone regulation in humans: importance of gender. *Neurobiol Aging.* 1994;15:227–231.
9. **Giordano R, Bo M, Pellegrino M, et al.** Hypothalamus-pituitary-adrenal hyperactivity in human aging is partially refractory to stimulation by mineralocorticoid receptor blockade. *J Clin Endocrinol Metab.* 2005;90:5656–5662.
10. **Blicher-Toft M, Hummer L.** Immunoreactive corticotrophin reserve in old age in man during and after surgical stress. *J Gerontol.* 1976;31:539–545.
11. **Beale E, Zhu J, Belzberg H.** Changes in serum cortisol with age in critically ill patients. *Gerontology.* 2002;48:84–92.
12. **Wilkinson CW, Petrie EC, Murray SR, Colasurdo EA, Raskind MA, Peskind ER.** Human glucocorticoid feedback inhibition is reduced in older individuals: evening study. *J Clin Endocrinol Metab.* 2001;86:545–550.
13. **Van Cauter E, Leproult R, Kupfer DJ.** Effects of gender and age on the levels and circadian rhythmicity of plasma cortisol. *J Clin Endocrinol Metab.* 1996;81:2468–2473.
14. **Deuschle M, Weber B, Colla M, Depner M, Heuser I.** Effects of major depression, aging and gender upon calculated diurnal free plasma cortisol concentrations: a re-evaluation study. *Stress.* 1998;2:281–287.
15. **Impallomeni M, Yeo T, Rudd A, Carr D, Aber V.** Investigation of anterior pituitary function in elderly in-patients over the age of 75. *Q J Med.* 1987;63:505–515.
16. **Andrew R, Phillips DI, Walker BR.** Obesity and gender influence cortisol secretion and metabolism in man. *J Clin Endocrinol Metab.* 1998;83:1806–1809.
17. **Purnell JQ, Brandon DD, Isabelle LM, Loriaux DL, Samuels MH.** Association of 24-hour cortisol production rates, cortisol-binding globulin, and plasma-free cortisol levels with body composition, leptin levels, and aging in adult men and women. *J Clin Endocrinol Metab.* 2004;89:281–287.
18. **Swaab DF, Bao AM.** (Re-)activation of neurons in aging and dementia: Lessons from the hypothalamus. *Exp Gerontol.* 2010;46:178–184.
19. **Holmes MC, Carter RN, Noble J, et al.** 11beta-hydroxysteroid dehydrogenase type 1 expression is increased in the aged mouse hippocampus and parietal cortex and causes memory impairments. *J Neurosci.* 2010;30:6916–6920.
20. **Andreucci VE, Russo D, Cianciaruso B, Andreucci M.** Some sodium, potassium and water changes in the elderly and their treatment. *Nephrol Dial Transplant.* 1996;11(suppl 9):9–17.
21. **Phillips PA, Rolls BJ, Ledingham JG, et al.** Reduced thirst after water deprivation in healthy elderly men. *N Engl J Med.* 1984;311:753–759.
22. **Tian Y, Serino R, Verbalis JG.** Downregulation of renal vasopressin V2 receptor and aquaporin-2 expression parallels age-associated defects in urine concentration. *Am J Physiol Renal Physiol.* 2004;287: F797–F805.
23. **Hawkins RC.** Age and gender as risk factors for hyponatremia and hypernatremia. *Clin Chim Acta.* 2003;337:169–172.
24. **Weidmann P, De Myttenaere-Bursztein S, Maxwell MH, de Lima J.** Effect on aging on plasma renin and aldosterone in normal man. *Kidney Int.* 1975;8: 325–333.
25. **Davis PJ, Davis FB.** Water excretion in the elderly. *Endocrinol Metab Clin North Am.* 1987;16:867–875.
26. **Miller M, Hecker MS, Friedlander DA, Carter JM.** Apparent idiopathic hyponatremia in an ambulatory geriatric population. *J Am Geriatr Soc.* 1996;44: 404–408.
27. **van der Lely AJ, Janssen JM, Lamberts SW.** Adult vs childhood onset GHD: is there a real clinical difference? *Growth Horm IGF Res.* 1998;8(suppl A): 21–23.
28. **Broglio F, Benso A, Castiglioni C, et al.** The endocrine response to ghrelin as a function of gender in humans in young and elderly subjects. *J Clin Endocrinol Metab.* 2003;88:1537–1542.
29. **Greenwood FC, Landon J, Stamp TCB.** The plasma sugar, free fatty acid, cortisol, and growth hormone response to insulin. I. In control subjects. *J Clin Invest.* 1966;45:429–436.
30. **Iranmanesh A, Lizarralde G, Veldhuis JD.** Age and relative adiposity are specific negative determinants of the frequency and amplitude of growth hormone (GH) secretory bursts and the half-life of

endogenous GH in healthy men. *J Clin Endocrinol Metab.* 1991;73:1081–1088.

31. **Veldhuis JD, Roelfsema F, Keenan DM, Pincus SM.** Gender, age, body mass index and IGF-I individually and jointly determine distinct GH dynamics: analyses in one hundred healthy adults. *J Clin Endocrinol Metab.* 2011;96:115–121.
32. **Aimaretti G, Corneli G, Baldelli R, et al.** Diagnostic reliability of a single IGF-I measurement in 237 adults with total anterior hypopituitarism and severe GH deficiency. *Clin Endocrinol (Oxf).* 2003;59: 56–61.
33. **Giannoulis MG, Sonksen PH, Umpleby M, et al.** The effects of growth hormone and/or testosterone in healthy elderly men: a randomized controlled trial. *J Clin Endocrinol Metab.* 2006;91:477–484.
34. **Brill KT, Weltman AL, Gentili A, et al.** Single and combined effects of growth hormone and testosterone administration on measures of body composition, physical performance, mood, sexual function, bone turnover, and muscle gene expression in healthy older men. *J Clin Endocrinol Metab.* 2002;87: 5649–5657.
35. **Barzilai N, Huffman DM, Muzumdar RH, Bartke A.** The critical role of metabolic pathways in aging. *Diabetes.* 2012;61:1315–1322.
36. **Bowers CY, Granda R, Mohan S, Kuipers J, Baylink D, Veldhuis JD.** Sustained elevation of pulsatile growth hormone (GH) secretion and insulin-like growth factor I (IGF-I), IGF-binding protein-3 (IGFBP-3), and IGFBP-5 concentrations during 30-day continuous subcutaneous infusion of GH-releasing peptide-2 in older men and women. *J Clin Endocrinol Metab.* 2004;89:2290–2300.
37. **Iranmanesh A, Mulligan T, Veldhuis JD.** Mechanisms subserving the physiological nocturnal relative hypoprolactinemia of healthy older men: dual decline in prolactin secretory burst mass and basal release with preservation of pulse duration, frequency, and interpulse interval. *J Clin Endocrinol Metab.* 1999;84:1083–1090.
38. **Yamaji T, Shimamoto K, Ishibashi M, Kosaka K, Orimo H.** Effect of age and sex on circulating and pituitary prolactin levels in human. *Acta Endocrinol (Copenh).* 1976;83:711–719.
39. **Kok P, Roelfsema F, Langendonk JG, et al.** Increased circadian prolactin release is blunted after body weight loss in obese premenopausal women. *Am J Physiol Endocrinol Metab.* 2006;290:E218–E224.
40. **Vermeulen A, Kaufman JM.** Ageing of the hypothalamo-pituitary-testicular axis in men. *Horm Res.* 1995;43:25–28.
41. **Veldhuis JD, Keenan DM, Iranmanesh A, Takahashi PY, Nehra AX.** The ensemble male hypothalamo-pituitary-gonadal axis. In: Timiras PS, ed. *Physiological Basis of Aging and Geriatrics.* New York: Taylor & Francis Group, LLC, Health Science Division; 2007:185–203.
42. **Tenover JS, McLachlan RI, Dahl KD, Burger HG, de Kretser DM, Bremner WJ.** Decreased serum inhibin levels in normal elderly men: evidence for a decline in Sertoli cell function with aging. *J Clin Endocrinol Metab.* 1988;67:455–461.
43. **Sowers MR, Eyvazzadeh AD, McConnell D, et al.** Anti-mullerian hormone and inhibin B in the definition of ovarian aging and the menopause transition. *J Clin Endocrinol Metab.* 2008;93:3478–3483.
44. **Veldhuis JD, Urban RJ, Lizarralde G, Johnson ML, Iranmanesh A.** Attenuation of luteinizing hormone secretory burst amplitude is a proximate basis for the hypoandrogenism of healthy aging in men. *J Clin Endocrinol Metab.* 1992;75:707–713.
45. **Madersbacher S, Stulnig T, Huber LA, et al.** Serum glycoprotein hormones and their free alpha-subunit in a healthy elderly population selected according to the SENIEUR protocol. Analyses with ultrasensitive time resolved fluoroimmunoassays. *Mech Aging & Devel.* 1993;71:223–233.
46. **Keenan DM, Takahashi PY, Liu PY, et al.** An ensemble model of the male gonadal axis: illustrative application in aging men. *Endocrinol.* 2006;147:2817–2828.
47. **Mulligan T, Iranmanesh A, Kerzner R, Demers LW, Veldhuis JD.** Two-week pulsatile gonadotropin releasing hormone infusion unmasks dual (hypothalamic and Leydig-cell) defects in the healthy aging male gonadotropic axis. *Eur J Endocrinol.* 1999;141:257–266.
48. **Pincus SM, Mulligan T, Iranmanesh A, Gheorghiu S, Godschalk M, Veldhuis JD.** Older males secrete luteinizing hormone and testosterone more irregularly, and jointly more asynchronously, than younger males. *Proc Natl Acad Sci U S A.* 1996;93:14100–14105.
49. **Van den Berghe G, Wouters P, Weekers F, et al.** Five-day pulsatile gonadotropin-releasing hormone administration unveils combined hypothalamic-pituitary-gonadal defects underlying profound hypoandrogenism in men with prolonged critical illness. *J Clin Endocrinol Metab.* 2001;86:3217–3226.
50. **Langouche L, Van den Berghe G.** The dynamic neuroendocrine response to critical illness. *Endocrinol Metab Clin North Am.* 2006;35:777–791, ix.
51. **Kastelan D, Korsic M.** High prevalence rate of pituitary incidentaloma: is it associated with the age-related decline of the sex hormones levels? *Med Hypotheses.* 2007;69:307–309.
52. **Tandon A, Suri A, Kasliwal MK, et al.** Assessment of endocrine abnormalities in severe traumatic brain injury: a prospective study. *Acta Neurochir (Wien).* 2009;151:1411–1417.
53. **van der Klaauw AA, Kars M, Biermasz NR, et al.** Disease-specific impairments in quality of life during long-term follow-up of patients with different pituitary adenomas. *Clin Endocrinol (Oxf).* 2008;69:775–784.
54. **Naing KK, Dewar JA, Leese GP.** Megestrol acetate therapy and secondary adrenal suppression. *Cancer.* 1999;86:1044–1049.

CHAPTER 5

Endocrine and Metabolic Emergencies in Pregnancy

Anita Banerjee and Catherine Williamson

ABSTRACT

Endocrine disease may present for the first time as an emergency during pregnancy, or endocrine emergencies can occur in pregnant women with preexisting endocrine conditions.

Diabetes mellitus is the most common endocrine disorder in pregnant women and can be complicated by diabetic ketoacidosis and hypoglycemia. In women with pituitary tumors, pressure effects from symptomatic expansion of the tumor or normal adjacent pituitary tissue may cause problems. Hypothalamic or posterior pituitary disorders are more commonly complicated by emergencies as a consequence of inadequate treatment or overtreatment (eg, resulting in electrolyte imbalance in diabetes insipidus or development of hypoadrenalism in women with adrenocorticotropic hormone [ACTH] deficiency). The maternal consequences of uncontrolled secretion of a hormone (eg, ACTH in Cushing's disease or growth hormone in acromegaly) may cause severe hypertension or superimposed preeclampsia. Sheehan's syndrome is possible after postpartum hemorrhage. However, pituitary apoplexy is a rare complication. Most adrenal adenomas are preexisting during pregnancy, but the first presentation of a pheochromocytoma may occur and requires a multidisciplinary approach. Thyroid diseases are common in pregnancy but, if adequately treated, hypothyroidism and hyperthyroidism are rarely complicated by medical emergencies. However, thyroid storm may occur and it is important to distinguish between gestational thyrotoxicosis and thyrotoxicosis. Severe hypercalcemia can occur during pregnancy and may be a consequence of hyperparathyroidism. As with other disorders of excessive hormone secretion, pregnant women with hyperparathyroidism may present with preeclampsia.

This chapter will discuss the endocrine and metabolic changes that occur in normal pregnancy and the current management of common endocrine and metabolic emergencies during pregnancy.

INTRODUCTION

Most endocrine disorders have a good prognosis if diagnosed and treated prior to pregnancy. Emergencies may be the consequence of a new diagnosis in pregnancy or due to women avoiding treatment when they conceive, often due to an incorrect assumption that drugs used to treat an endocrine disorder will harm the fetus. It may be difficult to establish the underlying etiology in women presenting with gestational endocrine emergencies, given that the normal ranges for many endocrine tests change in normal pregnancy. The influence of pregnancy on hormones that are used for diagnostic tests in endocrinology is summarized in Table 5-1.

DIABETES MELLITUS

Carbohydrate metabolism is adapted during pregnancy, to maintain glucose homeostasis and ensure that energy is available to the fetus during the maternal fasting state. The management of diabetes during pregnancy is described in detail in the recent 2013 Endocrine Society Clinical Practice Guidelines (1). In addition, diabetes emergencies occurring during pregnancy are discussed more comprehensively in the associated commentary.

Diabetic Ketoacidosis

Diabetic ketoacidosis (DKA) is a medical emergency during pregnancy and can be complicated by fetal loss rates as high as 10%–25% (2). The incidence is 1%–3%. During pregnancy there is an accelerated maternal response to starvation and this predisposes women with diabetes mellitus to DKA. Common precipitants during pregnancy include urinary infections, hyperemesis gravidarum, and insulin "pump failure" in women using continuous subcutaneous

Table 5-1. Effects of Pregnancy on Specific Hormones

Hormone	Effect of Pregnancy	Explanation
LH and FSH	• Undetectable during pregnancy	• Suppressed by high circulating levels of estrogen and progesterone
GH	• Total GH concentration increases	• Placental GH production (assays cannot distinguish this from pituitary GH)
ACTH	• Total ACTH level increases approximately 2-fold after the first trimester	• Placental production of cortisol releasing factor and ACTH; pituitary ACTH secretion, however, is unchanged
IGF-1	• Increases in normal pregnancy	• IGF-1 production stimulated by human placental lactogen
ADH	• Reduction in circulating ADH	• Placental vasopressinase production
Prolactin	• Progressive increase throughout pregnancy	• Increased estrogen stimulates pituitary prolactin release • Prolactin synthesized by decidual tissue but only small amounts enter fetal or maternal circulation
Renin	• Increase up to 4-fold by 20 weeks of gestation then plateaus	• Renin aldosterone system activation results from the fall in total peripheral resistance and resulting afterload reduction, and therefore allows the expansion of plasma volume
Aldosterone	• Levels increase up to 3-fold in the first trimester and 10-fold in the third trimester	• Response to increased renin and angiotensin II
Angiotensin II	• Increased 3-fold	• Increased renin and angiotensinogen
Thyroid hormones	• 50% more thyroid hormone required • Increased iodine requirement • Increased T_4 production and subsequent TSH suppression, particularly in first trimester • Upper end of normal range for free T_3 and T_4 reduced in later pregnancy • Higher levels of total T_3 and T_4	• De-iodination in placenta and increase in TBG • Increased renal iodine clearance and fetal iodine uptake • Structural similarity of TSH and hCG leading to hCG mediated stimulation of TSH receptors in thyroid tissue • Hemodilution • Increase in TBG
Cortisol	• Serum cortisol (reflecting total cortisol) increases up to 3-fold • Urinary 24-hour free cortisol (reflecting free cortisol only) increases • Suppression by exogenous corticosteroid is blunted	• Increase in CBG, corticotropin releasing hormone and progesterone
PTH	• No known change in reference range	
Vitamin D	• Reference ranges for normal pregnancy not established	
Catecholamines	• No known change in reference range	

Abbreviations: ACTH = adrenocorticotropic hormone; ADH = antidiuretic hormone; CBG = cortisol-binding globulin; FSH = follicle-stimulating hormone; GH = growth hormone; hCG = human chorionic gonadotropin; IGF-1 = insulin growth factor-1; LH = Luteinizing hormone; PTH = parathyroid hormone; T_3 = triiodothyronine; T_4 = thyroxine; TBG = thyroid-binding globulin; TSH = thyroid-stimulating hormone.

Reproduced from Frise CJ, Williamson C. Endocrine disease in pregnancy. Clin Med. *2013;13:176–181. Copyright © 2013 Royal College of Physicians. With permission.*

insulin infusion (CSII). The diagnosis and treatment algorithm of DKA in pregnancy is similar to nonpregnant cases. The management of DKA requires close maternal and fetal monitoring. Prompt management and adherence to standard guidelines are essential (3).

Hypoglycemia During Pregnancy

Hypoglycemia is common during pregnancy (4). Insulin sensitivity increases during the first trimester, and insulin requirements may fall at this stage of pregnancy. Therefore, it is not surprising that women with type 1 diabetes mellitus are reported to have severe hypoglycemia (ie, requiring third-party assistance) occurring 3–5 times more frequently in the first trimester (5). Associated risk factors for severe hypoglycemia in pregnancy include duration of pregnancy, a long history of severe hypoglycemia in the preceding year, impaired hypoglycemia awareness, and tight glycemic control in early pregnancy. Insulin doses should be reduced within the first trimester of pregnancy, and women encouraged to increase the frequency of self-monitoring of blood glucose (SMBG). If hypoglycemia awareness is blunted, patients are encouraged to use continuous glucose monitoring (CGM) if the resources are available. The Confidential Enquiries into Maternal and Child Health (CEMACH) study in the United Kingdom described recurrent hypoglycemia in 61% of type 1 diabetes patients, and 25% experienced severe hypoglycemia (6). Reassuringly, there has been no evidence of teratogenicity associated with hypoglycemia.

Nondiabetic Starvation Ketoacidosis

In the third trimester of pregnancy, ketoacidosis develops more rapidly than in nonpregnant individuals following episodes of starvation or protracted vomiting. This can result in metabolic acidosis that has similar risks of fetal mortality to DKA (7). This condition responds well to infusion of 10% dextrose and it is possible to avoid emergency delivery with rapid diagnosis and treatment.

PITUITARY DISEASE

Pregnant women with pituitary disease most commonly have tumors of the anterior pituitary gland. Nonfunctioning tumors are likely to be the most common pituitary tumor, given that they have been reported in approximately 10% of individuals at autopsy. However, prolactinoma is the most common pituitary tumor in women of reproductive age, followed by growth hormone (GH) and adrenocorticotropic hormone (ACTH)-secreting tumors. Pituitary tumors may cause an acute presentation due to pressure effects or excessive secretion of a specific hormone. Pituitary apoplexy is rarely reported in pregnancy.

Prolactinomas

The management of hyperprolactinemia in the nonpregnant and pregnant state is described in detail in the 2011 Endocrine Society Clinical Practice Guidelines (8). Hyperprolactinemia is a common cause of infertility in women because it inhibits pulsatile gonadotropin-releasing hormone release from the hypothalamus; treatment with a dopamine agonist can result in rapid return of fertility, and therefore conception. If a pregnant woman has a microprolactinoma, it is unlikely to enlarge in a clinically relevant manner in pregnancy. In contrast, women with macroprolactinomas have a 28%–46% chance of symptomatic expansion in pregnancy (9,10). Formal visual field testing should be performed every 6–8 weeks in women with macroprolactinoma. Pituitary imaging is required if tumor enlargement is suspected due to changes in visual fields or if there are new symptoms of headache, nausea, or diabetes insipidus (DI). Figure 5-1 demonstrates a pituitary macroadenoma with suprasellar extension but no chiasmal compression. As the pregnancy progresses, the figure demonstrates the macroadenoma with chiasmal compression causing a bilateral superior temporal field defect. Magnetic resonance imaging (MRI) with contrast is safe in pregnancy and can be performed in the first trimester if required (11).

Dopamine receptor agonists are usually discontinued in early pregnancy, but can be continued in cases of macroprolactinoma at risk of symptomatic tumor expansion. If there is confirmed evidence of tumor enlargement they should be restarted. Bromocriptine and cabergoline are not associated with increased rates of congenital malformation, or with

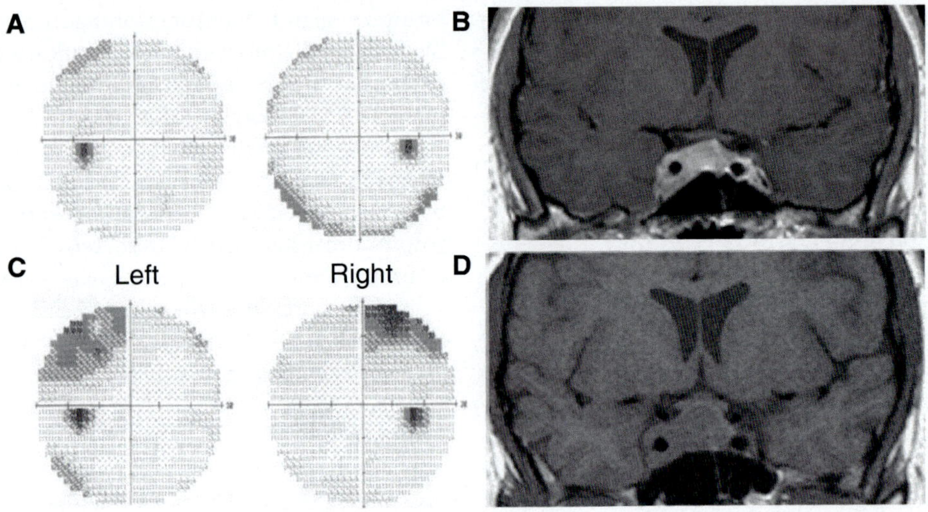

Figure 5-1. (A) Normal visual fields assessed using Humphrey's perimetry; (B) T_1-weighted MRI (coronal view) showing a pituitary macroadenoma with suprasellar extension but no chiasmal compression; (C) perimetry demonstrating a bilateral superior temporal field defect; (D) T_1-weighted MRI (coronal view) showing a pituitary macroadenoma with chiasmal compression. Reproduced from Banerjee A, Wynne K, Tan T, et al. High dose cabergoline therapy for a resistant macroprolactinoma during pregnancy. *Clin Endocrinol (Oxf)*. 2009;70:812–813. Copyright © John Wiley & Sons Ltd. With permission.

adverse pregnancy outcome (eg, preterm labor, intrauterine growth restriction [IUGR], or preeclampsia) (10,12). It is important to be aware that the UK Medicine and Healthcare Products Regulatory Authority has advised that pregnancy should be excluded before using ergot derivatives (cabergoline and bromocriptine) due to a theoretical risk of maternal or fetal cardiac valve fibrosis. However, at present there are no studies that report these complications in women treated with dopamine agonists in pregnancy, and bromocriptine or cabergoline should be used if a pregnant woman has symptomatic enlargement of a pituitary tumor.

Nonfunctioning Pituitary Tumors

There is a paucity of information regarding the course of nonfunctioning pituitary tumors in pregnancy. However, there are isolated case reports of symptomatic enlargement, although this is likely to relate to enlargement of adjacent pituitary tissue. Nonfunctioning tumors may be complicated by pituitary apoplexy.

Acromegaly

Pregnancy in patients with acromegaly is uncommon, because the majority of affected women have reduced fertility due to hyperprolactinemia from pituitary stalk compression. They also have increased rates of polycystic ovary syndrome and may have reduced secretion of gonadotropins. Most diagnostic assays cannot distinguish between pituitary and placental GH (Table 5-1) so confirmation of the diagnosis may have to wait until after delivery when the placental GH falls rapidly. Macroadenomas are relatively common in acromegaly and enlargement of normal adjacent pituitary tissue can cause an emergency presentation with visual symptoms, as with nonfunctioning pituitary tumors. Acromegaly can increase the risk of gestational diabetes, pregnancy-induced hypertension, and preeclampsia, and these complications occur more commonly in women with high levels of GH and insulin growth factor-1 (IGF-1) before pregnancy (13,14). Acromegaly-associated cardiac disease, including coronary artery disease and cardiomyopathy, can manifest for the first time in pregnancy as cardiac emergencies.

Medical treatment is usually interrupted at the time of pregnancy. Dopamine receptor agonists are normally stopped early in pregnancy and somatostatin analogs withheld due to a lack of clear safety data surrounding their use (and there are some data implicating them in IUGR) (13,14). Interruption for the duration of pregnancy will not usually affect the course of the condition but should be decided on a case-by-case basis. If the clinical team believes it is appropriate to continue both classes of drugs, this is a reasonable approach if the benefits of treatment are thought to outweigh the potential risks. Only a small number of women with acromegaly have been reported to have deteriorated in pregnancy, with tumor growth and one case of pituitary apoplexy. Therefore, the same advice as for prolactinomas should be followed with respect to tumor size and monitoring.

Pituitary Apoplexy

Pituitary apoplexy has been reported in association with prolactinoma and ACTH-secreting and nonfunctioning pituitary tumors. In a series of 7 cases, all presented with severe headache and visual symptoms, and some had coexisting vomiting or altered consciousness (15). Investigation and treatment should be the same as for nonpregnant women. Computed tomography (CT) and MRI scans can be used, and there is no contraindication to treatment with glucocorticoids.

Pituitary Insufficiency

This can result from previous pituitary surgery or radiotherapy, lesions such as adenomas, infarction, or lymphocytic hypophysitis and may lead to subfertility because the gonadotropin stimulus to ovulation may be absent. Hence ovulation induction therapies may be required. If adequate hormonal replacement has been achieved prior to pregnancy, there is no effect of this condition on maternal or fetal outcome. If the condition is not diagnosed or is inadequately treated, it can be associated with miscarriage and stillbirth (16). The principal emergencies associated with pituitary insufficiency are hypoadrenalism and severe DI.

Lymphocytic Hypophysitis

Lymphocytic hypophysitis occurs with increased frequency in late pregnancy and postpartum, and it can cause isolated ACTH deficiency. Diagnosis in the acute setting is challenging because the hormone levels used to diagnose pituitary insufficiency are affected by pregnancy. Luteinizing hormone (LH) and follicle-stimulating hormone (FSH) are suppressed, so the diagnosis is limited to assessment of the thyroid and hypothalamic-pituitary-adrenal (HPA) axis. Thyroid function may be normal initially due to the long half-life of thyroxine (T_4) so repeated measurements are important. HPA axis assessment relies on ACTH and cortisol levels. The adrenal response to ACTH will remain normal in acute pituitary insufficiency, so a short ACTH stimulation test is not diagnostically useful initially. Prolactin can be useful as the level may be abnormally low. Plasma sodium levels do not usually change significantly in pregnancy, although there is a slight reduction in the normal reference range due to a "reset osmostat" mechanism (see section SIADH and Hyponatremia below). However, in most cases hyponatremia can be diagnosed using normal laboratory reference ranges. Hormone replacement should be given in the same way as for nonpregnant individuals. There is no evidence that replacement levels of glucocorticoids cause risks for the mother or fetus.

Diabetes Insipidus

The symptoms of DI can worsen in pregnancy as a result of placental vasopressinase production and an associated reduction in antidiuretic hormone (ADH) levels. ADH analogs such as desmopressin can be continued and no adverse effects have been reported, but a higher dose may be required. It is important to reduce the dose rapidly to prepregnancy levels after delivery because otherwise hyponatremia may occur. Transient DI can occur in pregnancy secondary to placental vasopressinase production. This may be a feature of significant hepatic pathology (eg, acute fatty liver of pregnancy). In this condition the hepatic breakdown of placental vasopressinase is reduced. It is, therefore, important to exclude liver disease in addition to other pituitary disorders that may cause de novo DI in pregnancy. Polyuria and polydipsia are included in the "Swansea criteria" that are valuable in the diagnosis of acute fatty liver of pregnancy (17).

Because DI is a disorder of the posterior pituitary, it can be associated with reduced oxytocin production. This can have important consequences at delivery, because labor may not progress and there is an increased rate of uterine atony.

SIADH and Hyponatremia

In normal pregnancy there is altered sensitivity to ADH, resulting in a "reset osmostat" phenomenon. This correlates to raised levels of human chorionic gonadotropin (hCG), although the underlying mechanism is not fully understood. Pregnant women typically develop thirst at a plasma osmolality that is 5–10 mOsm/kg lower than nonpregnant individuals, and the sodium concentration is 5 mEq/L (5 mmol/L) lower (18). It is important to be aware of this when women present with hyponatremia in pregnancy. Conditions that may be complicated by maternal hyponatremia include hyperemesis gravidarum, hypoadrenalism, drug reactions (eg, carbamazepine), fluid overload, aggressive oxytocin therapy, and syndrome of inappropriate ADH (SIADH).

Hyponatremia rarely occurs as a result of SIADH in pregnant women. Approximately 50% of cases have preeclampsia, and most other cases have recognized associated disorders (19). It is important to be aware of the normal gestational alterations in ADH secretion and plasma osmolality when assessing these cases. If clinicians attempt to raise the plasma sodium inappropriately in women with hyponatremia that is not due to SIADH, they will cause thirst and polydipsia.

ADRENAL DISEASE

Pregnant women may present with endocrine emergencies as a result of adrenal tumors or insufficiency.

Pheochromocytoma

The incidence of pheochromocytoma in pregnancy is estimated to be 1 in 50,000 (20). Maternal and fetal mortality rates have fallen considerably over the years, declining to 17% and 20%, respectively, in the 1980s and to 4% and 11% from 1988 to 1997. More recent studies have reported low maternal mortality if the diagnosis is made during the antenatal period,

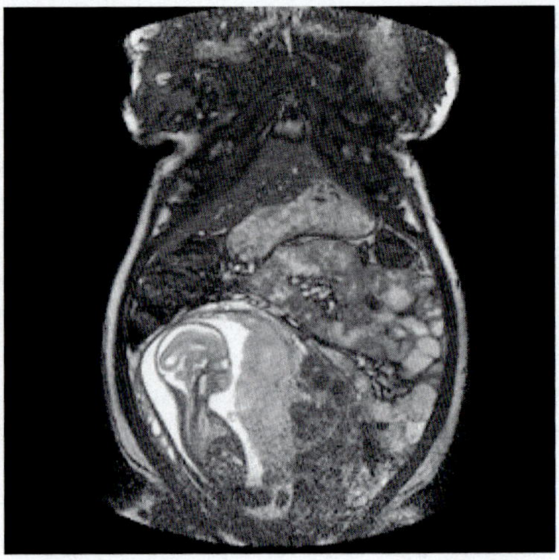

Figure 5-2. T_1-weighted MRI (coronal view) showing a pheochromocytoma and fetus in utero.

but the risk of fetal death remains relatively high at 15%. A high mortality rate is associated with the presence of an unanticipated pheochromocytoma. A low threshold for investigation of hypertension presenting in the first half of pregnancy is likely to explain the increasing number of cases that are diagnosed in the antenatal period. Management should be undertaken through a multidisciplinary approach. Figure 5-2 depicts a left adrenal mass (pheochromocytoma) and a fetus in utero. The aim should be to treat blood pressure appropriately with initial use of an alpha blocker and review for hyperglycemia. Phenoxybenzamine should be used during pregnancy as the safety data are reassuring (21,22). If pheochromocytoma is diagnosed in the first half of pregnancy, it is reasonable to consider laparoscopic removal during the second trimester.

Conn's Syndrome

This is uncommon during pregnancy and there are very few cases described in the literature. There is a rise in aldosterone levels and plasma renin activity during pregnancy, and this can pose challenges for diagnosis of the condition (Table 5-1). Conn's syndrome may present with hypokalemia and hypertension in pregnancy, and when this occurs it is important to correct blood pressure and the electrolyte imbalance. Spironolactone is the treatment of choice outside of pregnancy, but it is rarely used to treat Conn's syndrome in pregnant women due to theoretical concerns about antiandrogenic effects causing ambiguous genitalia in a male fetus. Alternative antihypertensive drugs include eplerenone and amiloride, both of which have been reported in single cases (23,24). Reported maternal and fetal complications of Conn's syndrome include placental abruption, intrauterine death, and fetal distress (25,26).

Adrenal Insufficiency

In the developed world Addison's disease is the most common cause of hypoadrenalism in fertile women. Newly diagnosed Addison's disease is very uncommon during pregnancy. It may be challenging to recognize the symptoms during pregnancy. Nonspecific symptoms include nausea, fatigue, and anorexia, all of which are common in pregnant women. During pregnancy there is a rise in total plasma cortisol, cortisol-binding globulin, and 24-hour urinary cortisol. During the third trimester there is a 3–10-fold rise in cortisol levels (27). There is also a rise in aldosterone levels and plasma renin activity during pregnancy (Table 5-1). A morning cortisol test and short ACTH stimulation test are safe during pregnancy. Trimester specific cortisol test levels should be used to interpret these results. A morning cortisol level of less than 11 mcg/dL (300 nmol/L), 16.3 mcg/dL (450 nmol/L), and 21.7 mcg/dL (600 nmol/L) in the first, second, and third trimester, respectively, raises the suspicion of hypocortisolism. The optimal cut-off for the 60-minute cortisol level as part of the short ACTH stimulation test should be greater than 25.3 mcg/dL (700 nmol/L), 29 mcg/dL (800 nmol/L), and 32.6 mcg/dL (900 nmol/L) in the first, second, and third trimester, respectively (28). Maternal and fetal risks of inadequately treated adrenal insufficiency include preterm delivery, IUGR, and adrenal crisis. An acute adrenal crisis may occur due to hyperemesis gravidarum or intercurrent illness. Most women with preexisting Addison's disease require a 30%–40% rise in their hydrocortisone dose during the third trimester. Fludrocortisone doses are not usually affected during pregnancy due to the antimineralocorticoid effects of progesterone. Hydrocortisone is the drug of choice for this condition. All women require intrapartum hydrocortisone regardless of mode of delivery. Hydrocortisone doses of 50 mg–100 mg three to four times a day are usually administered. Immediately, postpartum women should remain on twice their predelivery dose for the first 24–48 hours and then be rapidly tapered back to maintenance dose.

THYROID DISEASE IN PREGNANCY

Thyroid disease is common during pregnancy, and if treated appropriately medical emergencies are rare. Trimester specific thyroid-stimulating hormone (TSH) and T_4 ranges are important to account for the pregnancy effects on the hypothalamic-pituitary-thyroid axis (Table 5-2). An underactive thyroid is more common during pregnancy with a prevalence of 2%–5%, while overt hypothyroidism is seen in 0.3%–0.5% of pregnancies. An overactive thyroid during pregnancy has a prevalence of 0.1%–0.4%, and Graves' disease accounts for 85% of all cases. Distinguishing between hyperthyroidism and gestational thyrotoxicosis is important and can be challenging.

Hypothyroidism

Hypothyroidism is common in women of childbearing age (29). It is recognized either by the clinical presentation of classic symptoms or incidentally during the work-up of infertility. If inadequately treated there is an increased risk of gestational hypertension, placental abruption, and postpartum hemorrhage. If untreated there is a risk of low birth weight, preterm delivery, and neonatal respiratory distress. Ideally thyroid disease should be stable prior to conception. The TSH value prior to conception should ideally be <2.5 mIU/L (30). During pregnancy some women with known hypothyroidism require an increase in their thyroxine dose (31,32). This may be due to increased levels of thyroid-binding globulin,

Table 5-2. Trimester-Specific Thyroid-Stimulating Hormone

Trimester	TSH (IU/L)
First	0.1–2.5
Second	0.2–3.0
Third	0.3–3.5

or because they were inadequately treated prior to conception. Once the thyroid function tests are stable, pregnant women only require surveillance each trimester and at 6–8 weeks postpartum, unless they become symptomatic. If symptomatic or first diagnosed during pregnancy the thyroid function tests may be measured more frequently until stable. Hypothyroidism is rarely associated with medical emergencies in pregnancy.

Hyperthyroidism

The symptoms of hyperthyroidism usually predate pregnancy. If inadequately treated there is a risk of IUGR, low birth weight, preeclampsia, preterm delivery, stillbirth, and miscarriage (30). The symptoms of Graves' disease tend to worsen in the first trimester and improve in the latter half of pregnancy. When diagnosed before pregnancy the disease should be stabilized prior to conception. Definitive treatments such as radioactive iodine (RAI) are contraindicated during pregnancy and women considering pregnancy are counselled to wait at least 6 months after RAI treatment to conceive. Surgical interventions should only be considered during pregnancy if medical treatment cannot be tolerated. The optimal time to perform surgery is the second trimester.

During pregnancy, antithyroid medication is the first-line treatment for thyrotoxicosis (33). Options include methimazole (MMI), carbimazole (CBM), and propylthiouracil (PTU). All have similar transplacental transfer kinetics. Antithyroid medication is associated with a 0.3%–0.5% risk of agranulocytosis. PTU in adults can lead to hepatotoxicity in 1 in 10,000. Both MMI and CBM are associated with increased risk of congenital anomalies. The congenital anomalies seen include aplasia cutis, choanal atresia, and intestinal anomalies (30,34,35). Due to these effects current guidelines advocate the use of PTU in the first trimester and MMI/CBM in the second and third trimester. However, a recent Danish cohort study of 817,093 children, including 1,820 exposed to PTU or MMI/CBM demonstrated congenital malformations in 8% of children exposed to PTU, 9% of those taking MMI/CBM, and 10% of children treated with both drugs (36). Thus, clinicians should individualize decisions about treatment with antithyroid drugs in pregnancy, with cognizance of the need to maintain good maternal control while minimizing the risk to the fetus. Consensus statements have proposed that "practitioners should use their clinical judgment in choosing the antithyroid medication, including the potential difficulties in switching from one drug to another" (37). Thyroid function tests should be measured every 4–6 weeks with the aim of maintaining the T_4 in the upper limits of the nonpregnant normal range. If the TSH becomes detectable, the antithyroid medication should be reduced further. MMI, CBM, and PTU are all safe during breast-feeding, although in the context of high maternal doses it is advisable to ensure the neonate remains euthyroid. Antenatal management of thyrotoxicosis may include symptomatic treatment with beta blockers. They are safe during pregnancy, and short-acting beta blockers such as propranolol and metoprolol are effective. After delivery hyperthyroidism may relapse or worsen.

TSH receptor antibodies should be measured at 22–26 weeks gestation. These antibodies cross the placenta. If raised more than 2–3-fold, there is an increased risk of fetal thyrotoxicosis. Management includes fetal surveillance and treatment with antithyroid drugs in utero.

Gestational Thyrotoxicosis

Gestational thyrotoxicosis is usually limited to the first half of pregnancy and associated with hyperemesis gravidarum in 5–10 cases per 1,000 pregnancies. Biochemically there is a raised T_4 and suppressed TSH. The condition is thought to be caused by elevated hCG in the first trimester, and the homology with TSH leads to these biochemical findings. It occurs in the absence of thyroid antibodies. Other causes of this clinical picture include multiple gestation, hydatidiform mole, hyperreactio luteinalis, and hyperplacentosis.

It is important to distinguish between gestational thyrotoxicosis and Graves' disease because the conditions are managed differently. With gestational thyrotoxicosis the symptoms only occur during pregnancy; nausea and vomiting are profound and usually the main symptoms. Rehydration, appropriate antiemetic medication, and reassurance are necessary. With Graves' disease the symptoms often predate the pregnancy and can be associated with the usual clinical features (eg, Graves' ophthalmopathy).

Thyroid Storm

This is an uncommon event in pregnancy, but may be life-threatening. It can be precipitated by infection or preeclampsia, and during the intrapartum period by labor or cesarean-section (38). It can also occur in women with severe hyperemesis gravidarum in whom severe vomiting prevents ingestion of antithyroid medication. Symptoms are similar to nonpregnant individuals. The management is supportive in an intensive care unit setting with a multidisciplinary approach. Antithyroid medication should be commenced immediately. PTU is preferred due to its ability to block conversion of T_4 to triiodothyronine (T_3) (39). Tachyarrhythmias may be managed with beta-blocking medication. Other additional medications include high-dose glucocorticoids and oral potassium iodide (40).

PARATHYROID DISEASE IN PREGNANCY

Primary hyperparathyroidism in pregnancy is rare, with a reported annual incidence of 8 cases per 100,000 women of childbearing age. The actual incidence in pregnancy is unknown due to likely under-reporting; there are fewer than 250 cases in the peer-reviewed literature to date. Primary hyperparathyroidism causes hypercalcemia as a consequence of excessive secretion of parathyroid hormone (PTH), usually due to an adenoma of the parathyroid gland. Maternal complications are reported in approximately 65% of cases. These include hyperemesis gravidarum, nephrolithiasis, peptic ulcer disease, and pancreatitis. Hypertension or preeclampsia occurs in up to 25% of cases (41). Primary hyperparathyroidism can occasionally precipitate a life-threatening hypercalcemic crisis. The incidence of fetal complications is approximately 50%, and these include miscarriage, IUGR, stillbirth, neonatal tetany, and neonatal death (42).

Hyperparathyroidism is diagnosed by identifying a high plasma calcium concentration with a corresponding high or inappropriately normal PTH concentration and high urinary calcium levels. Identification of hypercalcemia in pregnancy can be difficult because the total calcium concentration can appear normal as a result of the lower albumin concentration. Isotope studies are contraindicated in pregnancy, but ultrasound or arterial phase CT scan can be used to identify adenomas. Most pregnant women with hypercalcemia respond well to admission and hydration. However, many cannot maintain normocalcemia without ongoing administration of intravenous fluids. Furthermore, the increased risk of adverse pregnancy outcome, including stillbirth, is of concern in women with hypercalcemia secondary to hyperparathyroidism; therefore, parathyroidectomy is the treatment of choice in the majority of cases. Ideally, parathyroidectomy should be performed at the end of the first trimester or in the second trimester, but it can be performed in pregnancy at most gestational ages. If surgery is not performed, management involves maintaining hydration and administering oral phosphates. In addition to the increased risk of preeclampsia in women with primary hyperparathyroidism in pregnancy, those with a history of parathyroidectomy more than 2 years prior to pregnancy also have increased rates of hypertensive disease in pregnancy (43).

CONCLUSIONS

Endocrine and metabolic emergencies in pregnancy should be managed by a multidisciplinary team that includes endocrinologists, obstetricians, obstetrical anesthetists, and neonatologists. Prepregnancy counselling should be offered to all women with preexisting endocrine disease to ensure stability of the disease prior to conception and to discuss the safety profile of medication(s) during pregnancy.

ACKNOWLEDGMENTS

The authors have nothing to disclose.

REFERENCES

1. **Blumer I, Hader E, Hadden DR, et al.** Diabetes and pregnancy: an Endocrine Society clinical practice guideline. *J Clin Endocrinol Metab.* 2013;98:4227–4249.
2. **de Veciana M.** Diabetes ketoacidosis in pregnancy. *Semin Perinatol.* 2013; 37:267–273.

3. **Dhatariya K, Savage M, Claydon A, et al.** Joint British Diabetes Societies Inpatient Care Group. *The Management of Diabetic Ketoacidosis in Adults.* second ed. Update: September 2013. http://www.diabetologistsabcd.org.uk/JBDS/JBDS_IP_DKA_Adults_Revised.pdf. 2013.
4. **Seaquist ER, Anderson J, Childs B, et al.** Hypoglycemia and diabetes: a report of a workgroup of the American Diabetes Association and the Endocrine Society. *J Clin Endocrinol Metab.* 2013;98:1845–1859.
5. **Ringholm L, Pedersen-Bjergaard U, Thorsteinsson B, Damm P, Mathiesen ER.** Hypoglycaemia during pregnancy in women with Type 1 diabetes. *Diabet Med.* 2012;29:558–566.
6. **Modder J, ed.** *Confidential Enquiry into Maternal and Child Health: Diabetes in Pregnancy in Women with Type 1 and Type 2 Diabetes in 2002–03, England, Wales and Northern Ireland.* London: CEMACH; 2010.
7. **Frise CJ, Mackillop L, Joash K, Williamson C.** Starvation ketoacidosis in pregnancy. *Eur J Obstet Gynecol Reprod Biol.* 2013;167:1–7.
8. **Melmed S, Casaneuva FF, Hoffman AR, et al.** Diagnosis and treatment of hyperprolactinemia. An Endocrine Society Clinical Practice Guideline. *J Clin Endocrinol Metab.* 2011;96:273–288.
9. **Bronstein MD, Paraiba DB, Jallad RS.** Management of pituitary tumors in pregnancy. *Nat Rev Endocrinol.* 2011;7:301–310.
10. **Lebbe M, Hubinont C, Bernard P, Maiter D.** Outcome of 100 pregnancies initiated under treatment with cabergoline in hyperprolactinaemic women. *Clin Endocrinol (Oxf).* 2010;73:236–242.
11. **Kanal E, Barkovich AJ, Bell C, et al.** ACR guidance document for safe MR practices: 2007. *AJR Am J Roentgenol.* 2007;188:1447–1474.
12. **Raymond JP, Goldstein E, Konopka P, Leleu MF, Merceron RE, Loria Y.** Follow-up of children born of bromocriptine-treated mothers. *Horm Res.* 1985;22:239–246.
13. **Caron P, Broussaud S, Bertherat J, et al.** Acromegaly and pregnancy: a retrospective multicenter study of 59 pregnancies in 46 women. *J Clin Endocrinol Metab.* 2010;95:4680–4687.
14. **Cheng S, Grasso L, Martinez-Orozco JA, et al.** Pregnancy in acromegaly: experience from two referral centers and systematic review of the literature. *Clin Endocrinol (Oxf).* 2012;76:264–271.
15. **de Heide LJ, van Tol KM, Doorenbos B.** Pituitary apoplexy presenting during pregnancy. *Neth J Med.* 2004;62:393–396.
16. **Overton CE, Davis CJ, West C, Davies MC, Conway GS.** High risk pregnancies in hypopituitary women. *Hum Reprod.* 2002;17:1464–1467.
17. **Ch'ng CL, Morgan M, Hainsworth I, Kingham JG.** Prospective study of liver dysfunction in pregnancy in Southwest Wales. *Gut.* 2002;51:876–880.
18. **Harris K, Shankar R, Black K, Rochelson B.** Reset osmostat in pregnancy: a case report. *J Matern Fetal Neonatal Med.* 2013. PMID:23859494.
19. **Nawathe A, Govind A.** Pregnancy with known syndrome of inappropriate antidiuretic hormone. *J Obstet Gynaecol.* 2013;33:9–13.
20. **Ahlawat SK, Jain S, Kumari S, Varma S, Sharma BK.** Pheochromocytoma associated with pregnancy: case report and review of the literature. *Obstet Gynecol Surv.* 1999;54:728–737.
21. **Darr R, Lenders JW, Hofbauer LC, Naumann B, Bornstein SR, Eisenhofer G.** Pheochromocytoma—update on disease management. *Ther Adv Endocrinol Metab.* 2012;3:11–26.
22. **Oliva R, Angelos P, Kaplan E, Bakris G.** Pheochromocytoma in pregnancy: a case series and review. *Hypertension.* 2010;55:600–606.
23. **Al-Ali NA, El-Sandabesee D, Steel SA, Roland JM.** Conn's syndrome in pregnancy successfully treated with amiloride. *J Obstet Gynaecol.* 2007;27:730–731.
24. **Cabassi A, Rocco R, Berretta R, Regolisti G, Bacchi-Modena A.** Eplerenone use in primary aldosteronism during pregnancy. *Hypertension.* 2012;59:e18–e19.
25. **Lu W, Zheng F, Li H, Ruan L.** Primary aldosteronism and pregnancy: a case report. *Aust N Z J Obstet Gynaecol.* 2009;49:558.
26. **Ronconi V, Turchi F, Zennaro MC, Boscaro M, Giacchetti G.** Progesterone increase counteracts aldosterone action in a pregnant woman with primary aldosteronism. *Clin Endocrinol (Oxf).* 2011;74:278–279.
27. **Jung C, Ho JT, Torpy DJ, et al.** A longitudinal study of plasma and urinary cortisol in pregnancy and postpartum. *J Clin Endocrinol Metab.* 2011;96:1533–1540.
28. **Lebbe M, Arlt W.** What is the best diagnostic and therapeutic management strategy for an Addison patient during pregnancy? *Clin Endocrinol (Oxf).* 2013;78:497–502.
29. **Teng W, Shan Z, Patil K, et al.** Hypothyroidism in pregnancy. *Lancet Diabetes Endocrinol.* 2013;1:228–237.
30. **De GL, Abalovich M, Alexander EK, et al.** Management of thyroid dysfunction during pregnancy and postpartum: an Endocrine Society clinical practice guideline. *J Clin Endocrinol Metab.* 2012;97:2543–2565.
31. **Alexander EK, Marqusee E, Lawrence J, Jarolim P, Fischer GA, Larsen PR.** Timing and magnitude of increases in levothyroxine requirements during pregnancy in women with hypothyroidism. *N Engl J Med.* 2004;351:241–249.
32. **Reid SM, Middleton P, Cossich MC, Crowther CA, Bain E.** Interventions for clinical and subclinical hypothyroidism pre-pregnancy and during pregnancy. *Cochrane Database Syst Rev.* 2013;5:CD007752.
33. **Cooper DS, Laurberg P.** Hyperthyroidism in pregnancy. *Lancet Diabetes Endocrinol.* 2013;1:238–249.
34. **Clementi M, Di GE, Cassina M, Leoncini E, Botto LD, Mastroiacovo P.** Treatment of hyperthyroidism in pregnancy and birth defects. *J Clin Endocrinol Metab.* 2010;95:E337–E341.
35. **Yoshihara A, Noh J, Yamaguchi T, et al.** Treatment of Graves' disease with antithyroid drugs in the first trimester of pregnancy and the prevalence of congenital malformation. *J Clin Endocrinol Metab.* 2012;97:2396–2403.
36. **Andersen SL, Olsen J, Wu CS, Laurberg P.** Birth defects after early pregnancy use of antithyroid drugs: a Danish nationwide study. *J Clin Endocrinol Metab.* 2013;98:4373–4381.

37. **Rivkees SA.** Propylthiouracil versus methimazole during pregnancy: an evolving tale of difficult choices. *J Clin Endocrinol Metab.* 2013;98:4332–4335.
38. **Chan GW, Mandel SJ.** Therapy insight: management of Graves' disease during pregnancy. *Nat Clin Pract Endocrinol Metab.* 2007;3:470–478.
39. **Cooper DS.** Antithyroid drugs. *N Engl J Med.* 2005;352:905–917.
40. **Mestman JH.** Hyperthyroidism in pregnancy. *Best Pract Res Clin Endocrinol Metab.* 2004;18:267–288.
41. **Schnatz PF, Thaxton S.** Parathyroidectomy in the third trimester of pregnancy. *Obstet Gynecol Surv.* 2005;60:672–682.
42. **Norman J, Politz D, Politz L.** Hyperparathyroidism during pregnancy and the effect of rising calcium on pregnancy loss: a call for earlier intervention. *Clin Endocrinol (Oxf).* 2009;71:104–109.
43. **Hultin H, Hellman P, Lundgren E, et al.** Association of parathyroid adenoma and pregnancy with preeclampsia. *J Clin Endocrinol Metab.* 2009;94:3394–3399.

CHAPTER 6

Endocrine and Metabolic Emergencies in HIV and AIDS

Chelsea McMahon and Katherine Samaras

ABSTRACT

The widespread use of combined antiretroviral therapy (cART) has dramatically improved the life expectancy of people living with HIV. Both treated and untreated HIV infection can be associated with a spectrum of endocrine and metabolic disorders. Some of these can present as potentially life-threatening emergencies. This review focuses on the endocrine and metabolic emergencies that can occur in people with HIV and acquired immunodeficiency syndrome (AIDS), including adrenal crisis, lactic acidosis, diabetic ketoacidosis (DKA), hyperglycemic hyperosmolar state (HHS), hypertriglyceridemia, thyrotoxicosis, and hypercalcemia. The HIV- and cART-specific contributions to the development of these emergencies are reviewed.

INTRODUCTION

HIV infection currently affects 39.5 million people worldwide (http://www.unaids.org/globalreports). The natural history of HIV infection has been transformed into a chronic disease, since widespread combined antiretroviral therapy (cART) availability has substantially reduced HIV- and acquired immunodeficiency syndrome (AIDS)-related morbidity and mortality and dramatically improved the life expectancy of people living with HIV infection. Table 6-1 lists drugs by drug class that are in current use in combination regimens. AIDS is no longer the dominant health issue in countries where cART is available to treat HIV infection.

The priorities of HIV care are now focused primarily on suppression of viral replication and immune system restoration and managing the chronic health issues associated with treated HIV infection, including cART toxicities. Increasingly, endocrine dysfunction is a recognized accompaniment in people with HIV infection and can occur as a result of (i) opportunistic infections and infiltration processes associated with untreated infection or disease progression; (ii) immune reconstitution in treated infection; and/or (iii) as a complication of cART. Table 6-2 summarizes the numerous endocrine emergencies that can occur in HIV infection, treated and untreated. Endocrinologists play an integral role in managing hormonal and metabolic diseases in HIV and its treatment. In this chapter, we will focus on the endocrine emergencies that can occur in people with HIV/AIDs.

HYPOADRENALISM

Adrenal dysfunction is common in both treated and untreated HIV infection with a pluripotent etiology (1). If unrecognized, it is associated with significant morbidity and mortality risk. Clinical attention to the heightened risk of adrenal dysfunction in HIV infection is essential, with evaluation of the hypothalamic-pituitary-adrenal (HPA) axis necessary in all symptomatic patients.

Table 6-1. Drug Classes Used in the Treatment of HIV Infection

Protease Inhibitors	NRTIs	NNRTIs	Entry Inhibitors	Integrase Inhibitors
Atazanavir	Abacavir	Efavirenz	Fusion inhibitors	Dolutegravir
Darunavir	Didanosine	Etravirine	Enfuvirtide	Raltegravir
Fosamprenavir	Emtricitabine	Nevirapine	CCR 5 inhibitors	
Indinavir	Lamivudine	Rilpivirine	Maraviroc	
Lopinavir	Stavudine			
Nelfinavir	Tenofovir			
Ritonavir	Zidovudine			
Saquinavir				
Tipranavir				

Abbreviations: NRTI = nucleoside reverse transcription inhibitor; NNRTI = non-nucleoside reverse transcription inhibitor.

Table 6-2. Endocrine and Metabolic Emergencies in HIV Infection

	Cause	Explanation
Lactic acidosis	NRTIs	Treatment-associated: mitochondrial toxicity
DKA	Insulin deficiency	Immune reconstitution Drug-associated: • pentamidine (beta-cell toxic) • protease inhibitors (acute)
HHS	Relative insulin deficiency	Drug-associated: • pentamidine (beta-cell toxic) • protease inhibitor (acute)
Hypertriglyceridemia		Drug-induced: • protease inhibitor (especially tipranavir, lopinavir, fosamprenavir, and ritonavir) • NRTI (stavudine, didanosine, zidovudine) • NNRTI (efavirenz)
Hypercalcemia		Drug-induced Immune reconstitution Lymphoma Granulomatous disorders Parathyroid disorders
Adrenal failure/Addisonian crisis	Primary	Adrenalitis (infectious) Iatrogenic suppression: • azole antifungals • protease inhibitor and P450 3A4 interactions - inhaled glucocorticoids and other synthetic glucocorticoids (eg, intra-articular triamcinolone) - megestrol - rifampicin
	Secondary	Hypophysitis: • autoimmune • HIV-associated
Thyrotoxicosis	Autoimmune	Graves' disease: • immune reconstitution • interferon therapy Hashimoto's thyroiditis: • immune reconstitution

Abbreviations: DKA = diabetic ketoacidosis; HHS = hyperglycemic hyperosmolar state; NRTI = nucleoside reverse transcription inhibitor; NNRTI = non-nucleoside reverse transcription inhibitor; P450 3A4 = cytochrome P450 3A4.

Prior to the introduction of cART, infection and infiltration were the most common causes of adrenal abnormalities. However, with the widespread use of cART and less opportunistic infection, iatrogenic adrenal suppression is the more prevalent cause.

Cytomegalovirus (CMV) infection is the most common infective cause of adrenal failure and is known to affect both the adrenal medulla and cortex. There is often bilateral adrenal gland involvement and the spectrum of severity is wide ranging, from mild adrenalitis to necrosis and overwhelming infection (2). Other infectious agents causing adrenalitis include *Mycobacterium tuberculosis* (3), cryptococcal infection (4), *Nocardia* (5), *Mycobacterium avium* complex (4), and *Histoplasma capsulatum* (6). In addition, the HIV virus itself may cause adrenalitis (7). Infiltrative processes can also result in primary adrenal insufficiency with lymphoma, malignancy, and Kaposi sarcoma reported in advanced HIV infection or AIDS (8,9).

Since the advent of cART, there has been an increased incidence of medication-induced iatrogenic adrenal suppression, steroid interactions, and cytokine-induced complications known to affect the function of the HPA axis. These include the azole anti-fungal agents (ketoconazole and itraconazole), which impair steroidogenesis in the adrenal gland; rifampicin, which increases hepatic cortisol metabolism; and megestrol acetate, which nonspecifically binds the glucocorticoid receptor and may suppress the HPA axis. Protease inhibitors inhibit hepatic cytochrome P450 3A4 drug metabolism, potentiating the half-life of drugs that can affect adrenal steroidogenesis, including synthetic steroids. This can result in iatrogenic Cushing's syndrome and HPA suppression. Iatrogenic Cushing's syndrome in HIV-infected patients receiving ritonavir and inhaled fluticasone has been reported (10). The concomitant use of other synthetic glucocorticoids such as triamcinolone, budesonide, dexamethasone, and prednisolone, and additional HIV agents such as atazanavir has also resulted in exaggerated serum concentrations of glucocorticoids. The degree of adrenal suppression in these cases can be substantial, leading to adrenal failure and addisonian crisis if the steroids are ceased without glucocorticoid support (10).

The HPA axis requires evaluation in HIV-infected individuals symptomatic of fatigue, weight loss, nausea, postural presyncope, or with hypoglycemia or hyponatremia, especially those with risk factors mentioned previously. The approach is the same as in seronegative patients, with the appropriate first step being a short adrenocorticotropic hormone (ACTH) stimulation test. If insufficiency is demonstrated, the clinician should proceed to ACTH levels and imaging to locate the cause of insufficiency. Care should be taken in abruptly ceasing any steroid-containing medications (even if inhaled or administered by different routes) in a patient who is on one of the previously mentioned medications due to the risk of precipitating an addisonian crisis, as has been described (10). Patients with evidence of hypocortisolism, regardless of the etiology, should be treated with physiological replacement doses of glucocorticoids (with fludrocortisone if there is evidence of mineralocorticoid deficiency) and have appropriate clinical and biochemical monitoring.

LACTIC ACIDOSIS AND MITOCHONDRIAL TOXICITY

Hyperlactinemia is the most significant manifestation arising from nucleoside reverse transcriptase inhibitor (NRTI)-associated mitochondrial toxicity, although it is becoming less common as older NRTIs are less frequently prescribed. NRTIs inhibit HIV reverse transcriptase (an enzyme critical to viral replication), but also inhibit mitochondrial DNA polymerase γ (an enzyme responsible for DNA replication) (11). Inhibition results in the production of dysfunctional mitochondria proteins, which accumulate and impair crucial aspects of mitochondrial metabolic function, such as oxidative phosphorylation. With insufficient oxidative phosphorylation pyruvate is metabolized to lactate rather than acetyl CoA, and lactate accumulates. The propensity for lactate accumulation is further exacerbated by concomitant impaired hepatic dysfunction with reduced lactate clearance (12).

The clinical manifestations of hyperlactinemia are broad and nonspecific and diagnosis may be delayed by the unpredictability of the onset of mitochondrial toxicity. Signs and symptoms may include abdominal pain, nausea, vomiting, weight loss, fatigue, tachypnea, dyspnea, seizures, impaired cognition, arrhythmias, and heart failure. Blood investigations may reveal anemia and leukopenia, as well as elevation in aminotransferases, lipase, and creatine phosphokinase. Hepatic steatosis may be evident on abdominal imaging. All NRTIs may cause hyperlactinemia. Some drugs, however, are more problematic than others. Zidovudine, lamivudine, stavudine, and didanosine have been most often reported (12).

In a patient who develops lactic acidosis, the NRTI medication should be immediately ceased. Supportive care is the mainstay of treatment, aiming to optimize tissue oxygen delivery by cardiopulmonary support. This includes fluid resuscitation and mechanical ventilation, if required. The use of alkali therapy is controversial and may actually worsen the intracellular acidosis. There is limited evidence for the use of metabolic cofactors such as riboflavin, carnitine, and thiamine, although some authors support their use (13). Resolution of hyperlactinemia requires replenishment of mitochondrial DNA, which may take 4–28 weeks (14). After normalization of lactate levels a new antiretroviral regimen should be considered, with non-nucleoside reverse-transcriptase inhibitors (NNRTIs) and protease inhibitors being a safer regimen for these patients.

HYPERGLYCEMIA

Diabetes in HIV infection was uncommon in the era prior to cART, with early studies suggesting diabetes rates of around 2.0% in treatment-naïve HIV-infected subjects (15,16). Since cART became the treatment standard in HIV infection the prevalence of diabetes has increased substantially due to the impact on adipocyte and lipid metabolism (17–19). Initially, the development of insulin resistance and diabetes was considered a consequence of protease inhibitors, but certain NRTIs are also implicated (20), and it has become apparent that individual genetic susceptibility to antiretroviral medications exists (21). Duration of antiretroviral medication exposure is also associated with an increased risk of incident diabetes (22) with the Data Collection on Adverse Events of Anti-HIV Drugs study showing cumulative antiretroviral exposure was independently associated with incident diabetes (23). In addition the HIV-infected population are also affected by the traditional risk factors, including family history, abdominal obesity, increasing age, and gender (24).

The exact prevalence and incidence of diabetes in treated HIV infection is difficult to establish due to multiple confounders, not limited to diverse ethnic susceptibilities and medication regimens. Prevalence has been quoted to range from 7%–13% in individuals treated with protease inhibitors (18,25,26).

The recognition of hyperglycemia is important because of the long-term consequence of diabetes mellitus (DM) (multi-organ macro- and microvascular disease) and also the potentially severe adverse effects of rapid-onset hyperglycemia, as has been described with some protease inhibitors. Diabetic ketoacidosis (DKA), a potentially fatal metabolic complication of diabetes, has been reported in patients commencing protease inhibitor therapy with no other diabetes risk factors (27–29). Patients present with the biochemical triad of hyperglycemia, ketonemia, and anion gap metabolic acidosis, which often develops rapidly following the precipitating event. Hyperglycemic hyperosmolar state (HHS), the prototype of hyperglycemic crises in type 2 diabetes mellitus, often has a more insidious onset over days or weeks with the final symptoms including clouding of the sensorium, which may progress to seizure, focal neurology, and coma. The common clinical picture of both conditions includes symptoms of hyperglycemia (eg, polyuria, polydipsia, polyphagia, and weight loss), in addition to physical signs of dehydration. Treatment involves fluid resuscitation, correction of electrolyte disturbances, and a gradual reduction in serum glucose and plasma osmolality. The underlying precipitating cause requires identification and treatment.

HYPERTRIGLYCERIDEMIA

Lipid disorders are highly prevalent in both treated and untreated HIV infection (30). With the introduction of cART and the subsequent improvement in long-term survival, individuals with HIV infection face the same causes of major morbidity and mortality as the uninfected population, increasing the importance of appropriate intervention for lipid disorders and cardiovascular risk reduction.

In untreated HIV infection multiple lipid disorders are reported, including increased serum triglycerides and reduced total, low-density lipoprotein (LDL) and high-density lipoprotein (HDL) cholesterol. Hypertriglyceridemia is associated with greater immune system activation (31). In addition, some antiretroviral medications can also cause lipid abnormalities and each medication can have its own unique effect, making it difficult to assign a "class effect" to any particular drug class (30). Hypertriglyceridemia is common with certain protease inhibitors, in particular those where ritonavir is used to boost other protease inhibitors, such as tipranavir (32), lopinavir, and fosamprenavir (33). In these regimens, ritonavir is used at a low dose to boost circulating levels of these other protease inhibitors, due to its efficiency in blocking cytochrome p450 metabolism of these other medications. The incidence of hypertriglyceridemia-associated pancreatitis is higher in cohorts of patients with HIV infection, compared with seronegative populations (34). The pathophysiology is not understood, however, and there is no overall clear evidence supporting an increased risk of pancreatitis associated with protease inhibitor use (34–36).

The management of hypertriglyceridemia should follow established general guidelines. Careful consideration must be given to the potential for adverse drug interactions between lipid-lowering drugs and the agents used to treat HIV infection (30). In cases of hypertriglyceridemia-associated pancreatitis, the severity should be determined (using various scoring systems), and, if severe, intensive care admission is warranted. Decreasing the serum triglyceride concentration is a priority. If hyperglycemia is present, an insulin infusion can reduce free fatty acid release from tissues, decrease the glucose substrate for hepatic triglyceride synthesis, and enhance lipoprotein lipase (LPL) activity. Initial management is identical to that for other causes of acute pancreatitis (ie, analgesia, intravenous [IV] fluids, nothing by mouth [NPO]). However, as the patient begins oral intake (usually after pain is controlled), hypertriglyceridemia-associated pancreatitis patients need to avoid oral fat intake. In addition, IV hyperalimentation with fat emulsions is also contraindicated. Secondary causes of hypertriglyceridemia should be addressed, and precipitating drugs should be reviewed and ideally discontinued.

THYROTOXICOSIS

Prior to the introduction of cART overt thyroid dysfunction occurred at similar rates to the seronegative population (37). The use of antiretroviral medications, however, can result in thyrotoxicosis through drug interactions or the immune reconstitution inflammatory syndrome (IRIS).

Graves' disease in HIV-infected individuals may be seen as a late complication after initiation of cART and is thought to occur as part of IRIS (38). It may also occur in HIV infection with hepatitis C coinfection as a result of interferon-alpha therapy (39,40).

The therapeutic options include antithyroid medications (methimazole, carbimazole, and propylthiouracil) or definitive treatment with radioactive iodine or total thyroidectomy. Interferon therapy may need to be ceased if the thyrotoxicosis is severe. Beta blockers may be used for symptomatic relief of the associated adrenergic symptoms and may be stopped once thyroid function has normalized, as would be standard treatment.

HYPERCALCEMIA

Hypercalcemic crisis carries a high risk of mortality and may be complicated by metabolic encephalopathy, renal failure, and cardiac arrhythmias. Successful management of hypercalcemia depends on identifying and treating its cause. The causes of hypercalcemia are numerous, including abnormal parathyroid function, malignancy, granulomatous disorders, multiple myeloma, iatrogenic causes, and renal failure.

In HIV-infected individuals, hypercalcemia may occur as a result of IRIS. Cases of hypercalcemia associated with immune reconstitution-related sarcoidosis (41) and tuberculosis (42) have been reported.

CONCLUSIONS

Disorders of endocrine and metabolic function are well-recognized complications or accompaniments of HIV infection. With the introduction of cART to treat HIV infection there has been a paradigm shift from infectious and infiltrative causes to complications associated with cART and IRIS. Endocrine and metabolic disorders contribute to increased morbidity in this population, highlighting the importance of the endocrinologist in supporting the overall care in people living with HIV infection and its complications. Awareness of the endocrine and metabolic emergencies that can occur and their unique pathophysiology in HIV infection is critical.

ACKNOWLEDGMENTS

The authors were supported by the Gilead Grant.

REFERENCES

1. **Lo J, Grinspoon SK.** Adrenal function in HIV infection. *Curr Opin Endocrinol Diabetes Obes.* 2010;17(3):205–209.
2. **Marks JB.** Endocrine manifestations of human immunodeficiency virus (HIV) infection. *Am J Med Sci.* 1991;302(2):110–117.
3. **Baker R, Rook GA, Zumla A.** Adrenal function and the hypothalamo-pituitary adrenal axis in immunodeficiency virus-associated tuberculosis. *Int J Tuberc Lung Dis.* 1997;1(3): 289–290.
4. **Glasgow BJ, Steinsapir KD, Anders K, Layfield LJ.** Adrenal pathology in the acquired immune deficiency syndrome. *Am J Clin Pathol.* 1985;84(5):594–597.
5. **Arabi Y, Fairfax MR, Szuba MJ, Crane L, Schuman P.** Adrenal insufficiency, recurrent bacteremia, and disseminated abscesses caused by Nocardia asteroides in a patient with acquired immunodeficiency syndrome. *Diagn Microbiol Infect Dis.* 1996;24(1):47–51.
6. **Baraia-Etxaburu Artetxe J, Astigarraga Aguirre B, Elorza Olabegova R, et al.** [Primary adrenal failure and AIDS: report of 11 cases and review of the literature]. *Rev Clin Esp.* 1998;198(2):74–79.
7. **Freda PU, Wardlaw SL, Brudney K, Goland RS.** Primary adrenal insufficiency in patients with the acquired immunodeficiency syndrome: a report of five cases. *J Clin Endocrinol Metab.* 1994;79(6):1540–1545.
8. **Radin DR, Esplin JA, Levine AM, Ralls PW.** AIDS-related non-Hodgkin's lymphoma: abdominal CT findings in 112 patients. *AJR Am J Roentgenol.* 1993;160(5):1133–1139.
9. **Tappero JW, Conant MA, Wolfe SF, Berger TG.** Kaposi's sarcoma. Epidemiology, pathogenesis, histology, clinical spectrum, staging criteria and therapy. *J Am Acad Dermatol.* 1993;28(3):371–395.
10. **Samaras K, Pett S, Gowers A, McMurchie M, Cooper DA.** Iatrogenic Cushing's syndrome with osteoporosis and secondary adrenal failure in human immunodeficiency virus-infected patients receiving inhaled corticosteroids and ritonavir-boosted protease inhibitors: six cases. *J Clin Endocrinol Metab.* 2005;90(7):4394–4398.
11. **Kakuda TN.** Pharmacology of nucleoside and nucleotide reverse transcriptase inhibitor-induced mitochondrial toxicity. *Clin Ther.* 2000;22(6):685–708.
12. **Margolis AM, Heverling H, Pham PA, Stolbach A.** A review of the toxicity of HIV medications. *J Med Toxicol.* [Published online ahead of print August 21, 2013]. PMID:23963694.
13. **Falcó V, Rodríguez D, Ribera E, et al.** Severe nucleoside-associated lactic acidosis in human immunodeficiency virus-infected patients: report of 12 cases and review of the literature. *Clin Infect Dis.* 2002;34(6):838–846.
14. **Côté HC, Brumme ZL, Craib KJ, et al.** Changes in mitochondrial DNA as a marker of nucleoside toxicity in HIV-infected patients. *N Engl J Med.* 2002;346(11):811–820.
15. **Kilby JM, Tabereaux PB.** Severe hyperglycemia in an HIV clinic: preexisting versus drug-associated diabetes mellitus. *J Acquir Immune Defic Syndr Hum Retrovirol.* 1998;17(1):46–50.
16. **El-Sadr WM, Mullin CM, Carr A, et al.** Effects of HIV disease on lipid, glucose and insulin levels: results from a large antiretroviral-naive cohort. *HIV Med.* 2005;6(2):114–121.
17. **Bradbury RA, Samaras K.** Antiretroviral therapy and the human immunodeficiency virus–improved survival but at what cost? *Diabetes Obes Metab.* 2008;10(6):441–450.
18. **Eastone JA, Decker CF.** New-onset diabetes mellitus associated with use of protease inhibitor. *Ann Intern Med.* 1997;127(10):948.
19. **Dubé MP, Johnson DL, Currier JS, Leedom JM.** Protease inhibitor-associated hyperglycaemia. *Lancet.* 1997;350(9079):713–714.
20. **Brinkman K, Smeitink JA, Romijn JA, Reiss P.** Mitochondrial toxicity induced by nucleoside-analogue reverse-transcriptase inhibitors is a key factor in the pathogenesis of antiretroviral-therapy-related lipodystrophy. *Lancet.* 1999;354(9184):1112–1115.
21. **Ranade K, Geese WJ, Noor M, et al.** Genetic analysis implicates resistin in HIV lipodystrophy. *AIDS.* 2008;22(13):1561–1568.
22. **Samaras K.** The burden of diabetes and hyperlipidemia in treated HIV infection and approaches for cardiometabolic care. *Curr HIV/AIDS Rep.* 2012;9(3): 206–217.
23. **De Wit S, Sabin CA, Weber R, et al.** Incidence and risk factors for new-onset diabetes in HIV-infected patients: the Data Collection on Adverse Events of Anti-HIV Drugs (D:A:D) study. *Diabetes Care.* 2008;31(6):1224–1229.
24. **Wohl DA, McComsey G, Tebas P, et al.** Current concepts in the diagnosis and management of metabolic complications of HIV infection and its therapy. *Clin Infect Dis.* 2006;43(5):645–653.
25. **Carr A, Samaras K, Thorisdottir A, Kaufmann GR, Chisholm DJ, Cooper DA.** Diagnosis, prediction, and natural course of HIV-1 protease-inhibitor-associated lipodystrophy, hyperlipidaemia, and diabetes mellitus: a cohort study. *Lancet.* 1999;353(9170):2093–2099.
26. **Gelato MC.** Insulin and carbohydrate dysregulation. *Clin Infect Dis.* 2003;36(suppl 2):S91–S95.

27. **Besson C, Jubault V, Viard JP, Pialoux, G.** Ketoacidosis associated with protease inhibitor therapy. *AIDS.* 1998;12(11):1399–1400.
28. **Kan VL, Nylen ES.** Diabetic ketoacidosis in an HIV patient: a new mechanism of HIV protease inhibitor-induced glucose intolerance. *AIDS.* 1999; 13(14):1987–1989.
29. **Hughes CA, Taylor GD.** Metformin in an HIV-infected patient with protease inhibitor-induced diabetic ketoacidosis. *Ann Pharmacother.* 2001;35(7–8): 877–880.
30. **Dube MP, Cadden JJ.** Lipid metabolism in treated HIV infection. *Best Pract Res Clin Endocrinol Metab.* 2011;25(3):429–442.
31. **Grunfeld C, Pang M, Doerrler W, Shigenaga JK, Jensen P, Feingold KR.** Lipids, lipoproteins, triglyceride clearance, and cytokines in human immunodeficiency virus infection and the acquired immunodeficiency syndrome. *J Clin Endocrinol Metab.* 1992;74(5):1045–1052.
32. **Hicks CB, Cahn P, Cooper DA, et al.** Durable efficacy of tipranavir-ritonavir in combination with an optimised background regimen of antiretroviral drugs for treatment-experienced HIV-1-infected patients at 48 weeks in the Randomized Evaluation of Strategic Intervention in multi-drug resistant patients with Tipranavir (RESIST) studies: an analysis of combined data from two randomised open-label trials. *Lancet.* 2006;368(9534):466–475.
33. **Eron J Jr, Yeni P, Gathe J Jr, et al.** The KLEAN study of fosamprenavir-ritonavir versus lopinavir-ritonavir, each in combination with abacavir-lamivudine, for initial treatment of HIV infection over 48 weeks: a randomised non-inferiority trial. *Lancet.* 2006;368(9534):476–482.
34. **Riedel DJ, Gebo KA, Moore RD, Lucas GM.** A ten-year analysis of the incidence and risk factors for acute pancreatitis requiring hospitalization in an urban HIV clinical cohort. *AIDS Patient Care STDS.* 2008;22(2):113–121.
35. **Reisler RB, Murphy RL, Redfield RR, Parker RA.** Incidence of pancreatitis in HIV-1-infected individuals enrolled in 20 adult AIDS clinical trials group studies: lessons learned. *J Acquir Immune Defic Syndr.* 2005;39(2):159–166.
36. **Bush ZM, Kosmiski LA.** Acute pancreatitis in HIV-infected patients: are etiologies changing since the introduction of protease inhibitor therapy? *Pancreas.* 2003;27(1):e1–e5.
37. **Parsa AA, Bhangoo A.** HIV and thyroid dysfunction. *Rev Endocr Metab Disord.* **2013;14**(2):127–131.
38. **Rasul S, Delapenha R, Farhat F, Gajjala J, Zahra SM.** Graves' disease as a manifestation of immune reconstitution in HIV-infected individuals after initiation of highly active antiretroviral therapy. *AIDS Res Treat.* 2011;743597.
39. **Prummel MF, Laurberg P.** Interferon-alpha and autoimmune thyroid disease. *Thyroid.* 2003;13(6): 547–551.
40. **Koh LK, Greenspan FS, Yeo PP.** Interferon-alpha induced thyroid dysfunction: three clinical presentations and a review of the literature. *Thyroid.* 1997;7(6):891–896.
41. **Ferrand RA, Cartledge JD, Connolly J, Standish RA, Miller RF.** Immune reconstitution sarcoidosis presenting with hypercalcaemia and renal failure in HIV infection. *Int J STD AIDS.* 2007;18(2):138–139.
42. **Tsao YT, Wu CC, Chu P.** Immune reconstitution syndrome-induced hypercalcemic crisis. *Am J Emerg Med.* 2010;29(2):244 e3–e6.

SECTION IV

Pituitary Disorders

SECTION INTRODUCTION

Emergent Management of Pituitary Disorders

Edward R Laws and Ursula B Kaiser

Because of its complex control mechanisms over vital hormonal functions and its strategic location at the base of the brain, endocrine emergencies related to the pituitary are important clinical problems, and they are regularly encountered. Both the blood supply of the pituitary and the hypothalamic stimulatory and inhibitory factors that control its physiology are related to the pituitary stalk (infundibulum) that connects the pituitary gland to the hypothalamus. Lodged within the confines of the bony sella turcica, the pituitary is directly related to the optic chiasm superiorly and to the cranial nerves of the cavernous sinus laterally. These nerves control pupillary action, extraocular muscle function, and trigeminal nerve sensation.

The pituitary gland can be affected by both primary and metastatic tumors; trauma to the head; hemorrhage; vasospasm and vascular insufficiency; infection; inflammatory and autoimmune processes; the influence of drugs; and the reaction to radiation therapy.

Pituitary insufficiency can lead to profound fatigue and loss of support for vital endocrine and metabolic functions. This can occur as a result of enlarging pituitary tumors and pituitary tumor apoplexy (hemorrhage or infarction of a preexisting pituitary adenoma). Acute and subacute hypopituitarism can also occur following head trauma with damage to the pituitary stalk and the blood supply of the pituitary, during or after pregnancy from Sheehan's syndrome (infarction of the normal pituitary), and as a result of metastatic cancers involving the pituitary gland, its infundibulum, or the hypothalamus. Other primary inflammatory and infectious processes can also result in the abrupt onset of hypopituitarism. These include lymphocytic hypophysitis, granulomatous disease, sarcoidosis, tuberculosis, and sellar abscesses.

Afflictions of the pituitary, either sudden or chronic, can cause secondary (central) adrenal insufficiency—a true endocrine emergency. Considering this possibility is of crucial importance in critically ill patients. Patients with acute adrenal insufficiency (or adrenal crisis) often present with shock but may also present with anorexia, weight loss, nausea, vomiting, abdominal pain, weakness, fatigue, lethargy, confusion, and coma frequently accompanied by fever. An adrenal crisis may be precipitated in a patient with chronic adrenal insufficiency by a concurrent infection. If hypopituitarism is suspected, stress doses of intravenous (IV) hydrocortisone should be administered empirically even before hormonal test results are available, together with IV fluids. Central hypothyroidism also needs to be considered, and patients may present in myxedema coma or with bradycardia, shock, hypothermia, hypoventilation, and altered mental status.

Patients with acute pituitary insults can be affected by fluid and electrolyte disturbances manifested as either central diabetes insipidus (DI) or, occasionally, syndrome of inappropriate antidiuretic hormone production (SIADH). DI occurs rarely in patients with pituitary adenomas but can manifest in patients with inflammatory or infiltrative pituitary lesions or after surgery or radiation, typically as a result of hypothalamic or infundibular involvement. Tumors metastatic to the pituitary area may often present clinically with fluid and electrolyte disturbances from DI, the theory being that the network of portal vessels feeding the neurohypophysis may trap circulating tumor cells that then proliferate into a mass lesion. Careful management of fluid and electrolyte balance is essential, together with desmopressin administration as needed. Management of these afflictions can be particularly challenging if thirst regulation is also disordered.

Enlargement of the pituitary, acute or chronic, can lead to visual loss from compression or distortion of the optic nerves and chiasm. Sudden visual loss from pituitary tumor apoplexy can be a true endocrine emergency, prompting emergent surgical management. Progressive failure of visual acuity and visual field deficits can occur with a variety of sellar and parasellar lesions, including not only pituitary adenomas but also Rathke cleft cysts, craniopharyngiomas, arachnoid cysts, meningiomas, and other problems in this area, making the differential diagnosis broad and often difficult.

Occasionally, cystic pituitary lesions such as Rathke cleft cysts and craniopharyngiomas can rupture, leaking caustic fluid contents into the subarachnoid space. This can produce an acute meningitis-like clinical picture, and the inflammatory response to the cyst contents can contribute to visual loss and hypopituitarism.

Head injury, intracranial hemorrhage, and aneurysmal rupture may be accompanied by vasospasm, which may compromise the blood supply to the pituitary and damage the infundibulum and the hypothalamus. These phenomena can lead to DI or SIADH with severe acute electrolyte disturbances. Cerebral salt wasting can also occur under these circumstances. The differential diagnosis and correct management can be challenging. In addition to DI and SIADH, head trauma may produce differing degrees of deficiency of anterior pituitary hormones, subsequent to the injury.

A variety of medications can alter or interfere with normal pituitary function. These include psychoactive drugs, therapeutic medications to correct pituitary disorders, some forms of cancer chemotherapy, and a variety of hormones that can be toxic or poorly tolerated. One uncommon emergency is the development of cerebrospinal rhinorrhea (CSF leak) from dramatic shrinkage of an invasive prolactin-secreting macroadenoma treated successfully by dopamine agonists.

The thoughtful clinician in the office, the emergency department, the hospital, or the operating room should keep in mind the many functions of the pituitary and the consequences to the patient when it malfunctions or is injured. A thorough differential diagnosis and the appropriate gathering of information from laboratory testing and imaging can save lives and remain a challenge in effective patient care.

ACKNOWLEDGMENTS

The authors have nothing to disclose.

CHAPTER 7

Hypopituitarism

Nicholas A Tritos and Anne Klibanski

ABSTRACT

Hypopituitarism may be caused by a variety of conditions, including pituitary adenomas and other sellar masses, pituitary surgery or radiation therapy, traumatic brain injury, medications, hemorrhage (pituitary apoplexy or subarachnoid hemorrhage), postpartum pituitary infarction (Sheehan's syndrome), inflammation, infection, iron overload, and deleterious mutations of genes involved in pituitary development and function. In a few cases, hypopituitarism can also be idiopathic.

Potentially life-threatening manifestations of hypopituitarism include central hypoadrenalism, diabetes insipidus, or, rarely, central hypothyroidism. In contrast, although gonadotropin deficiency and growth hormone deficiency are not life-threatening, they are nevertheless associated with significant morbidity, impaired quality of life, and possibly increased mortality.

In acutely ill patients at risk for hypopituitarism, glucocorticoid replacement should be administered without awaiting the results of confirmatory diagnostic testing; this can be subsequently performed. Judicious administration of desmopressin, as well as monitoring of fluid balance and serum sodium, are essential in the management of diabetes insipidus. Levothyroxine replacement should only be administered after glucocorticoid replacement in order to avoid precipitating adrenal crisis. Further studies are needed to optimize the long-term management of hypopituitary patients and minimize associated morbidity and excess mortality.

INTRODUCTION

Hypopituitarism may occur as a result of diverse etiologies and lead to substantial morbidity and mortality. Acute manifestations of hypopituitarism may include central hypoadrenalism (due to deficiency of corticotropin [adrenocorticotropic hormone, ACTH]), diabetes insipidus or, rarely, central hypothyroidism. In contrast, deficiencies of other pituitary hormones, including gonadotropins, growth hormone (GH), and prolactin, are not immediately life-threatening. Despite advances in the diagnosis and management of pituitary disorders, hypopituitarism is still associated with increased long-term cardiovascular mortality (1,2).

The aims of the present chapter include a review of the causes, pathophysiology, clinical features, diagnosis, and management of hypopituitarism in adults, with emphasis placed on the evaluation and management of acutely ill patients.

ETIOLOGY

Pituitary adenomas are the most common cause of hypopituitarism in adult patients seen at pituitary centers. Patients with macroadenomas (defined as lesions 10 mm or larger in greatest diameter) are clearly at risk for anterior hypopituitarism. However, it has been suggested that some patients with smaller pituitary adenomas (microadenomas) may also be at risk (3). It should be noted that central diabetes insipidus (CDI) is extremely unlikely to occur in patients with pituitary adenomas before pituitary surgery. As a corollary, the presence of CDI in patients with a sellar mass, who have not had pituitary surgery, strongly suggests that the underlying lesion is not a pituitary adenoma.

In addition, patients with larger (>10 mm) sellar masses other than adenomas (Table 7-1) are at risk of anterior hypopituitarism and in some cases, including those with craniopharyngiomas and metastases, CDI (4). In particular, infiltrating or inflammatory lesions and/or those involving the pituitary stalk may lead to hypopituitarism regardless of size. A minority of patients with primary empty sellae may also have anterior hypopituitarism.

Pituitary surgery leads to CDI in ~15% of patients early postoperatively (5). However, persistent CDI only occurs in ~5% of postoperative patients. In addition, new deficits of anterior pituitary hormone secretion may occur in ~10% of patients postoperatively. It is unknown whether some of these patients had marginal anterior pituitary function prior to surgery. Conversely, improvement in preexisting pituitary function deficits occurs in ~40% of patients undergoing pituitary surgery, presumably due to decompression of the normal anterior pituitary gland.

Radiation therapy to the sella is associated with a lifelong risk of anterior hypopituitarism that becomes more prevalent over time, affecting ~40% of patients at 5 years and ~60% at 10 years after therapy (6). In these patients, GH and gonadotropin deficits tend to occur before the development of thyrotropin or corticotropin deficiency. In addition to gonadotroph failure, radiation-induced hyperprolactinemia may lead to hypogonadism in some cases (7). It may be noted that conventional radiation therapy of brain tumors distant from the sella is also associated with a substantial risk of hypopituitarism. Whether stereotactic radiosurgery, used to treat brain lesions remote from the hypothalamus and pituitary, is safer with regard to pituitary function has not been established.

Traumatic brain injury (TBI) has recently emerged as an important, yet likely underappreciated, cause of hypopituitarism (8,9). It has been estimated that ~25% of patients with TBI severe enough to require hospitalization develop one or more pituitary hormone deficiencies. Of note, at least partial recovery of pituitary function may occur in some of these patients.

A variety of nontraumatic vascular insults have been associated with hypopituitarism, including aneurysmal subarachnoid hemorrhage, pituitary apoplexy (hemorrhage and/or infarction of a pituitary adenoma), and postpartum pituitary infarction in women with severe obstetric hemorrhage, resulting in hypovolemic shock (Sheehan's syndrome) (10). It may be noted that Sheehan's syndrome

Table 7-1. Differential Diagnosis of Sellar Masses[a]

Pituitary adenomas (~91%)	Prolactinoma; clinically nonfunctioning pituitary adenoma; growth hormone-secreting adenoma (acromegaly and gigantism); corticotropinoma (Cushing's disease); thyrotropinoma; gonadotroph cell adenoma
Nonadenomatous lesions (~9%)	
Neoplastic	Craniopharyngioma; pituicytoma; meningioma; germ cell tumor; glioma; chordoma; chondrosarcoma; metastases; lymphoma
Cystic	Rathke's cleft cyst; arachnoid cyst; epidermoid cyst; dermoid cyst
Vascular	Aneurysm; cavernous malformation
Inflammatory	Primary hypophysitis (lymphocytic, granulomatous, xanthomatous, necrotizing); secondary hypophysitis (associated with sarcoidosis, Langerhans cell histiocytosis, granulomatosis with polyangiitis [GPA, formerly known as Wegener's granulomatosis]); drug-induced (ipilimumab, interferon alpha)
Infectious	Pituitary abscess; Whipple's disease; fungal infection; cysticercosis
Pituitary hyperplasia	Associated with pregnancy, target gland hypofunction (including severe primary hypothyroidism), or ectopic-releasing hormone secretion

[a] *The list includes most pituitary pathologies but is not exhaustive.*

has become rare in western countries as a result of global improvements in obstetric care.

Medications associated with hypopituitarism include agents that may result in hypophysitis, namely alpha interferon and ipilimumab (the latter in routine clinical use in patients with metastatic melanoma). In addition, some medications may selectively suppress aspects of pituitary function, including pharmacological doses of glucocorticoids, which inhibit corticotropin, thyrotropin, GH, and gonadotropins. Opioids suppress corticotropin and gonadotropins, and bexarotene (retinoic acid receptor agonist) inhibits thyrotropin secretion.

In addition to drug-related hypophysitis, pituitary inflammation may occur as a primary pituitary pathology (classified as lymphocytic, granulomatous, xanthomatous, or necrotizing) or can be associated with systemic inflammatory/autoimmune conditions (eg, sarcoidosis, Langerhans cell histiocytosis, granulomatosis with polyangiitis [GPA, formerly known as Wegener's granulomatosis], and immunoglobulin G4-related disease [IgG4-RD]). Infiltrative conditions, including hemochromatosis, may also result in hypopituitarism with a predilection for central hypogonadism. Infectious conditions associated with hypopituitarism include meningitis, pituitary abscess, Whipple's disease, tuberculosis, fungal infection, and cysticercosis.

Genetic causes of hypopituitarism have been identified in some patients with congenital or childhood onset and/or familial hypopituitarism, and may involve inactivating mutations of genes encoding transcription factors having a role in pituitary development (such as *POU1F1 [Pit1], PROP1, LHX3, LHX4, HESX1, OTX2, PITX2, SOX2, SOX3, TPIT*) or inactivating mutations of genes encoding hypothalamic or pituitary hormones or their respective receptors (11).

PATHOPHYSIOLOGY

In patients with nonfunctioning sellar masses, hypopituitarism may occur as a result of mass effect upon the normal secretory cells in the pars distalis or interference with the hypothalamo-hypophyseal portal system. At diagnosis, central hypogonadism and GH deficiency are the most frequent deficits in patients with clinically nonfunctioning pituitary macroadenomas, followed in prevalence by central hypoadrenalism and hypothyroidism. Stalk transection is associated with multiple pituitary hormone deficits (12). Suprasellar lesions may additionally impinge upon hypothalamic nuclei involved in the secretion of releasing hormones with a critical role in the regulation of pituitary function. Hemorrhage, ischemia, the chronic effects of radiation therapy, inflammation, and infection may all disrupt pituitary function by means of incompletely characterized mechanisms. Secretory pituitary adenomas may selectively inhibit the function of specific anterior pituitary cell populations (including inhibition of gonadotropin secretion by hyperprolactinemia and suppression of GH, gonadotropin, and thyrotropin secretion by cortisol excess).

Hypopituitary patients may become acutely ill as a result of severe pituitary hormone deficits (including lack of corticotropin, thyrotropin, or vasopressin) or as a consequence of partial pituitary deficiencies when faced with intercurrent homeostatic stressors, such as injury, surgery, or infection. Central hypoadrenalism may lead to dehydration, hyponatremia, and shock unresponsive to fluid resuscitation and vasopressor therapy before glucocorticoid replacement is administered. Central hypothyroidism may rarely lead to myxedema coma. Vasopressin deficiency causes CDI, which may become clinically apparent only after the initiation of glucocorticoid and thyroid hormone replacement therapies as a result of improvements in renal hemodynamics, glomerular filtration rate, and free water clearance.

CLINICAL FEATURES AND FINDINGS

Patients with central hypoadrenalism may present with prostration, headache, nausea, vomiting, orthostatic dizziness, joint aches, dehydration, confusion, shock, and hyponatremia (1). Patients with disease of long duration may additionally report fatigue and unexplained weight loss. Notably absent are skin and mucosal hyperpigmentation as well as hyperkalemia (in contrast to patients with Addison's disease).

Patients with central hypothyroidism may rarely present in myxedema coma, characterized by bradycardia, shock, bradypnea, hypoventilation, hypothermia, abnormal mental status, jaundice, hyponatremia, and abnormal liver function tests. If history can be obtained, information elicited may include chronic fatigue, weight gain, constipation, muscle cramps, irregular menses, dry skin, edema, hair loss, and cold intolerance.

In patients with acute pituitary insults affecting the posterior pituitary, including TBI and pituitary surgery, CDI typically presents within 24 to 48 hours and is characterized by polyuria (urine output exceeding 200 mL/hr for >2 hr) and hyposthenuria (in general, urine specific gravity <1.005 or osmolality <300 mOsm/kg [300 mmol/kg]) (13). Serum sodium levels are generally high normal or mildly elevated. However, severe hypernatremic dehydration may occur if patients are unable to compensate for aquaresis by increasing their water intake. Such a scenario is possible in patients with impaired sensorium, deficient thirst, or restricted access to water. Transient CDI may be followed by hyponatremia as a result of the syndrome of inappropriate antidiuretic hormone secretion (SIADH), which generally resolves within 2 weeks and can be succeeded by recurrent CDI (a sequence of events termed the "triple phase response").

Deficiencies of gonadotropins, prolactin, or GH are not likely to be immediately relevant in an acute setting. However, the presence of symptoms and findings suggestive of deficiencies in these hormones should raise suspicion for the presence of hypopituitarism in patients at risk. Women with gonadotropin deficiency generally note oligomenorrhea or secondary amenorrhea, whereas men may note low libido, erectile dysfunction, fatigue, or increased central adiposity. Patients of both genders may also experience hot flashes, involution of secondary sex characteristics, or infertility and are at risk for bone loss. Women with prolactin deficiency may report failure to lactate in the postpartum state, as is frequently the case in women with Sheehan's syndrome. There are no established consequences of prolactin deficiency in men. In children and adolescents, GH deficiency leads to delays in growth and may also impair the normal accrual of bone mineral and muscle mass. In adults of both genders, GH deficiency is associated with abnormal body composition (increased visceral adiposity, decreased muscle mass and bone mineral density), decreased exercise capacity, dyslipidemia, insulin resistance, and impaired quality of life.

In addition to symptoms and signs of pituitary hormone deficiencies, patients may note evidence of local mass effect, including headache, vision loss (as a result of compression of the optic apparatus by a sellar mass, most commonly bitemporal hemianopsia), or, less commonly, other cranial neuropathies (involving the III, IV, V, and VI cranial nerves). Pituitary apoplexy presents with acute, very severe headache, vision loss, and ophthalmoplegia, and constitutes an endocrine and neurosurgical emergency.

DIAGNOSIS

Evaluation of the hypothalamic-pituitary-adrenal (HPA) axis is the highest diagnostic (as well as therapeutic) priority in patients at risk of hypopituitarism (Table 7-2) (1). Morning (or random) serum cortisol levels exceeding 18 mcg/dL (~500 nmol/L) assure sufficient adrenocortical function with high specificity but low sensitivity. Conversely, morning serum cortisol levels below 3 mcg/dL (~80 nmol/L) are diagnostic of adrenal insufficiency. Intermediate morning cortisol levels are considered nondiagnostic and require additional testing. Measuring plasma corticotropin levels in a concurrent specimen helps to distinguish between central hypoadrenalism (characterized by low or "normal" plasma corticotropin) and primary adrenal insufficiency (characterized by elevated plasma corticotropin). It should be emphasized that acutely ill patients at risk for central hypoadrenalism should be presumed to be adrenally insufficient and treated with stress doses of glucocorticoids (preferably after drawing a blood specimen to assay cortisol and corticotropin) without awaiting the results of diagnostic testing.

Stimulation testing is helpful in assessing the integrity of the HPA axis in stable patients, but is not informative or practical in the acute setting. The insulin tolerance test (ITT) is considered the gold standard test in the evaluation of pituitary adrenal function and additionally helps to evaluate GH secretion. However, the test requires the induction of severe hypoglycemia (<45 mg/dL [~2.2 mmol/L]) in order

Table 7-2. Diagnostic Evaluation of Adult Patients with Suspected Hypopituitarism

Pituitary Function	Test Name	Procedure	Test Interpretation	Comments
Pituitary adrenal axis	Morning serum cortisol and plasma corticotropin	Draw specimens at 8 am	Serum cortisol >18 mcg/dL (~500 nmol/L) assures sufficiency; cortisol <3 mcg/dL (~80 nmol/L) is diagnostic of hypoadrenalism Plasma corticotropin levels that are not elevated in patients with untreated hypoadrenalism are diagnostic of a central etiology	Serum cortisol between 3 and 18 mcg/dL (~80–500 nmol/L) is indeterminate and requires stimulation testing
	Insulin tolerance test	Short-acting insulin 0.1–0.15 units/kg IV Serum cortisol at 0, 30, 60, 90, and 120 min	Peak serum cortisol >18 mcg/dL (~500 nmol/L) assures sufficiency	Diagnostic gold standard; nadir plasma glucose <45 mg/dL (~2.2 mmol/L) needed to assure sufficient corticotroph stimulation Requires physician in attendance; avoid test in the elderly and patients with cardiovascular disease or seizures
	Metyrapone test	Metyrapone (30 mg/kg) po × 1 at 11 pm Serum cortisol, ACTH, 11-DOC at 8 am (next morning)	Serum 11-DOC >7 mcg/dL (~200 nmol/L) assures sufficiency (ACTH >50 pg/mL [11 pmol/L] is normal; however, ACTH response is less reliable than 11-DOC response) Serum cortisol <5 mcg/dL (~140 nmol/L) needed to assure sufficient enzymatic blockade	Avoid test in patients with abnormal cosyntropin stimulation test Risk of precipitating acute adrenal insufficiency
	Short-ACTH stimulation test	Cosyntropin (Cortrosyn or Synacthen) 250 mcg IV or IM x 1[a] Serum cortisol at 0, 30, and 60 min	Peak serum cortisol >18 mcg/dL (~500 nmol/L) assures sufficient adrenal function	Test often falsely normal in patients with corticotroph failure of recent onset (within several weeks)
Pituitary thyroid axis	Serum thyrotropin and free T_4	Random serum specimens are drawn to measure thyrotropin and free T_4	Serum free T_4 is low in patients with central hypothyroidism "Normal" serum thyrotropin levels are common in central hypothyroidism	Similar biochemical findings may occur in patients with euthyroid sick syndrome
Posterior pituitary (vasopressin)	Serum sodium and osmolality; urine osmolality (or specific gravity)	Specimens obtained in patients with polyuria; early morning specimens preferred	Urine osmolality >700 mOsm/kg (700 mmol/kg) excludes DI	Exclude hypokalemia, hypercalcemia, and hyperglycemia Consider performing a water deprivation test in stable patients with normal serum sodium/osmolality and insufficiently concentrated urine

(Continued)

Table 7-2. Diagnostic Evaluation of Adult Patients with Suspected Hypopituitarism (Continued)

Pituitary Function	Test Name	Procedure	Test Interpretation	Comments
	Water deprivation test	All fluid intake withheld with careful monitoring of blood pressure, pulse, urine output, and weight Specimens for serum sodium and osmolality and urine osmolality are obtained every 2 hr until urine osmolality plateaus or evidence of significant dehydration is noted Desmopressin (1–2 mcg SC) is given at the end of the test and urine specimens are obtained in 1 and 2 hr	Urine osmolality >700 mOsm/kg (700 mmol/kg) assures sufficient vasopressin secretion and action Patients with severe DI have peak urine osmolality <300 mOsm/kg (300 mmol/kg) Serum sodium >145 mEq/L (145 mmol/L) (or serum osmolality >300 mOsm/kg [300 mmol/kg]) needed to assure sufficient stimulus for vasopressin stimulation Normalization of urine osmolality (>700 mOsm/kg [700 mmol/kg]) after desmopressin administration is consistent with central DI; absence of an increase in urine osmolality after desmopressin is consistent with nephrogenic DI	This test is performed under close supervision in stable patients; serum potassium, calcium, and glucose should be normal; thyroid and adrenal function known to be normal or replaced before test Terminate test if loss of weight >3% over baseline occurs or if clinical evidence of dehydration or hyperosmolality (>300 mOsm/kg [300 mmol/kg]) occurs
Gonadotropin gonadal axis	Serum gonadotropins (FSH and LH) Estradiol and menstrual history in women; testosterone and SHBG (or free testosterone) in men	In menstruating women, specimens are preferably drawn on day 3 after onset of menses Morning serum specimens are drawn in men	Regular spontaneous menses suggest that hypogonadism is unlikely; amenorrhea in women and low gonadal steroid levels (in both genders) are consistent with hypogonadism Serum gonadotropin levels that are not elevated in patients with hypogonadism are diagnostic of a central etiology	Avoid testing in hospitalized patients; abnormal results should be confirmed with repeated testing
GH	Insulin tolerance test[b]	Short-acting insulin 0.1–0.15 units/kg IV Serum GH at 0, 30, 60, 90, and 120 min	Peak GH >3 ng/mL (3 mcg/L) is considered a normal response	Diagnostic gold standard; nadir plasma glucose <45 mg/dL (~2.2 mmol/L) needed to assure sufficient somatotroph stimulation Requires physician in attendance; avoid in the elderly and patients with cardiovascular disease or seizures
	Glucagon stimulation test[b]	Glucagon 1 mg IM x 1 (1.5 mg in patients >90 kg) Serum GH at 0, 30, 60, 90, 120, 150, and 180 min	Peak GH >3 ng/mL (3 mcg/L) considered a normal response	Good diagnostic accuracy in adults

(Continued)

Table 7-2. Diagnostic Evaluation of Adult Patients with Suspected Hypopituitarism (Continued)

Pituitary Function	Test Name	Procedure	Test Interpretation	Comments
	GHRH arginine stimulation test[b]	GHRH = 1 mcg/kg IV bolus plus arginine 0.5 g/kg (up to 30 g) IV infused over 30 min Serum GH at 0, 30, 60, 90, and 120 min	BMI-dependent diagnostic cut-points recommended as follows: • If BMI <25 kg/m^2, then peak GH >11.5 ng/mL (11.5 mcg/L) is a normal response • If BMI 25–30 kg/m^2, then peak GH >8 ng/mL (8 mcg/L) is a normal response • If BMI >30 kg/m^2, then peak GH >4.2 ng/mL (4.2 mcg/L) is a normal response	Good diagnostic accuracy (except in patients with recent brain irradiation)
	Arginine stimulation test[b]	Arginine 0.5 g/kg (up to 30 g) IV infused over 30 min Serum GH at 0, 30, 60, 90, and 120 min	Peak GH >0.4 ng/mL (0.4 mcg/L) considered a normal response	Lower diagnostic accuracy than other tests in adults
	IGF-1	Randomly obtained serum specimens are assayed for IGF-1	Normal serum IGF-1 levels occur in ~50% of adults with GH deficiency (low sensitivity) Low serum IGF-1 levels in the presence of 3 or more additional pituitary deficiencies and known pituitary pathology are highly specific for GH deficiency	Low serum IGF-1 levels may also occur in patients with severe liver disease, uncontrolled diabetes mellitus, or on oral estrogen
Prolactin	Serum prolactin	Specimen for serum prolactin drawn (after overnight fast) Domperidone administration can be used to stimulate prolactin secretion (used in research)	Undetectable serum prolactin levels are diagnostic	Prolactin deficiency generally occurs in patients with multiple additional pituitary hormone deficiencies

Abbreviations: ACTH = corticotropin; DI = diabetes insipidus; 11-DOC = 11 deoxycortisol; FSH = follicle-stimulating hormone; GH = growth hormone; GHRH = growth hormone-releasing hormone; IGF-1 = insulin-like growth factor 1; IM = intramuscularly; IV = intravenously; LH = luteinizing hormone; PO = by mouth; T_4 = thyroxine.

[a] A low-dose (1-mcg) short-ACTH stimulation test has been suggested in some studies to be more sensitive than the 250-mcg short-ACTH in the diagnosis of central hypoadrenalism.

[b] GH stimulation testing is performed after other pituitary hormone deficits are replaced. An overnight fast is required.

to achieve adequate diagnostic accuracy. As a result, it is often perceived as unpleasant by patients, carries some risk associated with severe hypoglycemia, and is contraindicated in the elderly, patients with seizures, or those with cardiovascular disease. The metyrapone test is also reliable in the assessment of the HPA axis. However, the currently limited availability of metyrapone and the potential of precipitating acute adrenal insufficiency, particularly in an unmonitored outpatient setting, have limited use of this test in the United States. The short-ACTH (cosyntropin [Synacthen]) stimulation test directly evaluates adrenocortical responsiveness and is quite accurate in the diagnosis of primary adrenal insufficiency. However, the diagnostic accuracy of this test in patients with central hypoadrenalism of recent onset is lower, because it takes 4 to 6 weeks or longer after endogenous corticotropin secretion is blunted for the adrenals to become atrophic and lose responsiveness to exogenous ACTH administration.

Evaluation of the pituitary thyroid axis requires assays for both thyrotropin and free thyroxine (T_4) levels, because serum thyrotropin is often inappropriately "normal" in the presence of low free T_4 levels in patients with central hypothyroidism (1). Similar biochemical findings may be present in acutely ill patients with the "euthyroid sick" syndrome. The latter condition may not be reliably distinguished from central hypothyroidism in the critically ill. Unless myxedema coma is suspected, cautious observation with serial laboratory assessments of the pituitary thyroid axis may be appropriate and can help to distinguish between the 2 diagnostic possibilities, given that the biochemical abnormalities in euthyroid sick syndrome improve and eventually resolve in parallel with overall improvement in patients' clinical status.

Evaluation of posterior pituitary function includes careful assessment of urine output, fluid balance, serum sodium and osmolality, and urine specific gravity or osmolality (14). Patients with DI have polyuria with inappropriately dilute urine despite the presence of hypernatremia/hyperosmolality. If needed, a water deprivation test can be performed in stable patients under monitored conditions in order to exclude the presence of primary polydipsia, establish the diagnosis of DI, and identify the cause. However, a water deprivation test is not appropriate in acutely ill patients. In patients with DI, a substantial increase in urine osmolality in response to desmopressin administration is consistent with CDI. In contrast, lack of such a response is most consistent with nephrogenic DI. In these patients, the history may also provide important clues, including use of medications, such as lithium, associated with resistance to vasopressin.

Patients with SIADH are euvolemic and have hypotonic hyponatremia with inappropriately concentrated urine (urine osmolality >100–150 mOsm/kg [100–150 mmol/kg]). Hypoadrenalism and hypothyroidism should be excluded before the diagnosis of SIADH can be established, because both conditions decrease free water clearance. Review of the medical record helps to exclude medications (such as carbamazepine, opioids, or selective serotonin reuptake inhibitors) as potential contributing factors resulting in SIADH.

Assays for vasopressin often lack sufficient accuracy to be clinically useful in the diagnosis of DI and SIADH. An assay for copeptin, which is the C-terminal portion of the vasopressin precursor and is secreted in an equimolar ratio to vasopressin, is being evaluated and appears to hold promise in the differential diagnosis of DI and SIADH (15).

Evaluation of the remaining anterior pituitary hormones (gonadotropins, GH, prolactin) may often be confounded by acute illness and is best deferred until patients are medically stable and assessed in the outpatient setting. Obtaining a menstrual history is critical in women, in addition to tests for serum gonadotropins and estradiol. In men, measuring serum testosterone (including total testosterone and sex hormone-binding globulin, or free testosterone) and gonadotropins in the morning is advised.

Fasting serum prolactin levels (either at baseline or after stimulation by thyrotropin releasing hormone or domperidone; both stimulation tests being used primarily in research settings) are very low or undetectable in patients with prolactin deficiency. Evaluation of GH secretion generally requires stimulation testing in adults, as serum insulin-like growth factor levels are below normal in only 50% of adults with GH deficiency (16). Several GH stimulation tests are of diagnostic utility in adults, using insulin, glucagon, growth hormone-releasing hormone (GHRH), and arginine, or arginine alone as provocative stimuli (1,17).

MANAGEMENT

Glucocorticoid replacement is a high priority in patients with known or suspected central hypoadrenalism (Table 7-3) (1). Acutely ill, hospitalized patients with central hypoadrenalism should be given stress dose glucocorticoid coverage, including hydrocortisone 50–100 mg intravenously (IV) every 8 hours (or equivalent). Patients with pituitary apoplexy should receive stress dose glucocorticoid replacement, given that they are at high

Table 7-3. Management of Adult Patients with Hypopituitarism

Pituitary Function	Acute Management	Maintenance Therapy	Comments
Pituitary adrenal axis	Hydrocortisone 50–100 mg IV every 8 hr (acutely ill hospitalized patients) In outpatients with minor illness: Hydrocortisone or prednisone at 2–3 times maintenance should be advised	Hydrocortisone 15–25 mg PO daily (in 2–3 divided doses with the largest dose in the morning) or prednisone 2.5–5 mg PO daily in a single morning dose	Dose adjustment based on clinical criteria (well-being, weight, blood pressure, glycemia, etc) Patients are advised to wear a medical identification tag
Pituitary thyroid axis[a]	Suspected myxedema coma: Levothyroxine 300–500 mcg IV x 1 followed by levothyroxine 50–100 mcg IV daily	Levothyroxine 1.6 mcg/kg PO daily	Lower starting doses are advised in the elderly, patients with cardiovascular disease, or those with mild hypothyroidism Monitor free T_4 levels
Posterior pituitary (vasopressin)	Desmopressin 1–2 mcg SC or IV every 8–24 hr as needed	Desmopressin 10–20 mcg intranasally daily or twice daily or desmopressin 100–400 mcg PO daily or twice daily	Allowing the effect of the medication to wear off between doses may avoid hyponatremia Patients with intact thirst should drink water only when thirsty; patients with impaired thirst need to drink water on schedule Monitor fluid balance and serum sodium levels
Gonadotropin gonadal axis	Not recommended	In women: Combination oral contraceptive or oral/topical estrogen (with progesterone in women with intact uterus) In men: Testosterone in transdermal, intramuscular, or subcutaneous implant form	Gonadotropin therapy (rFSH and hCG) advised to restore fertility in women; hCG alone may be sufficient in men Monitor serum testosterone levels, prostate health, and hematocrit in men
GH	Not recommended	Recombinant human GH: 0.2–0.3 mg SC daily (starting dose)	Higher starting doses are appropriate in younger patients or women on oral contraceptives; lower starting doses appropriate in the elderly Monitor serum IGF-1 levels, body composition and mineral density, serum lipids, and quality of life
Prolactin	Not applicable	Not routinely available (used in clinical research)	

Abbreviations: GH = growth hormone; hCG = human chorionic gonadotropin; IGF-1 = insulin-like growth factor 1; IV = intravenously; PO = by mouth; rFSH = recombinant follicle-stimulating hormone; SC = subcutaneously; T_4 = thyroxine.

[a] *Thyroid hormone should only be administered after glucocorticoid replacement is given (or sufficient cortisol secretion assured).*

risk for hypopituitarism, including central hypoadrenalism (10,18). Of note, neurosurgeons generally recommend pharmacological doses of glucocorticoids (including dexamethasone 4 mg IV every 6 hr) in patients with pituitary apoplexy and cranial neuropathies before surgical decompression is undertaken.

In the outpatient setting, patients with central hypoadrenalism and acute intercurrent illness should be taught to increase their glucocorticoid replacement to 2–3 times their usual maintenance dose until recovery, and then resume taking their usual glucocorticoid replacement (prednisone 2.5–5 mg by mouth daily in a single morning dose or hydrocortisone 15–25 mg by mouth daily in divided doses). Use of a modified release hydrocortisone tablet has been associated with improvements in metabolic profile, including lower body weight, blood pressure, and glycemia (19). This medication has been approved for use in Europe but is not currently FDA approved. Patients with central hypoadrenalism are also advised to wear a medical identification tag.

Levothyroxine replacement should always be deferred until after glucocorticoid replacement has been administered (or hypoadrenalism excluded); failure to do so may precipitate acute adrenal crisis. In acutely ill patients with suspected myxedema coma, 300–500 mcg of levothyroxine is administered IV (after stress dose glucocorticoid replacement is given), followed by 50–100 mcg of IV levothyroxine daily. In the outpatient setting, levothyroxine replacement is given as a single daily dose. Usual levothyroxine replacement doses are ~1.6 mcg/kg. However, patients with mild central hypothyroidism, the elderly, and those with cardiovascular disease are generally advised to begin therapy with a lower levothyroxine dose (25–50 mcg/daily) and careful monitoring of free thyroxine levels in 6 weeks after dose adjustment. In these patients, serum thyrotropin levels must not be relied upon as an index of the adequacy of thyroid hormone replacement.

In hospitalized patients, CDI requires careful monitoring of fluid balance, sodium levels, and judicious administration of desmopressin as needed (20). Patients with intact thirst are advised to drink to thirst. In contrast, patients with impaired thirst sensation need to drink on schedule, guided by changes in fluid balance, body weight, and serum sodium levels. Desmopressin administration is given only on demand in the hospital (desmopressin dose = 1–2 mcg subcutaneously or intravenously every 8–24 hr as needed), with careful monitoring of sodium levels because CDI can be transient or can be followed by SIADH. Stable outpatients with persistent CDI generally experience good symptomatic relief from polyuria and excessive thirst on once or twice daily desmopressin therapy, administered either nasally or orally. Patients are advised to drink to thirst and allow for the medication effect to wear off before taking the next desmopressin dose in order to minimize the possibility of hyponatremia. Frequent monitoring of serum sodium levels is important to do, particularly at the start of therapy.

Replacement therapies for other hormone deficiencies (eg, gonadotropins, GH) are not administered in the acute setting because of unclear efficacy and safety in severely ill patients. An overview of sex steroid and GH replacement is outlined in Table 7-3. However, a detailed review of these therapies is outside the scope of this manuscript. Prolactin replacement is not available. However, a recombinant human prolactin preparation has been successfully administered (within the scope of a clinical trial) in women who failed to lactate postpartum and have very low prolactin levels.

Supportive care, including ventilation, correction of volume and electrolyte or temperature abnormalities, and treatment of the underlying cause of hypopituitarism are obviously important. Pituitary adenomectomy may improve pituitary function in 30%–40% of patients. However, pituitary function rarely, if ever, improves in patients with craniopharyngioma after tumor resection.

CONCLUSIONS

Hypopituitarism is caused by a wide variety of pathologies affecting the hypothalamic pituitary unit. Prompt institution of glucocorticoid replacement and careful attention to fluid and electrolyte balance can be life-saving in acutely ill patients.

Despite substantial advances in the diagnosis and management of pituitary disorders, hypopituitarism remains a serious condition and has been associated with excess mortality, as a result of inadequately treated hypoadrenalism, long-term excess risk of cardiovascular and cerebrovascular disease, and possibly increased risk of malignancy in irradiated patients (2,21). Possible factors contributing to increased cardiovascular risk may include excessive glucocorticoid replacement, lack of appropriate sex steroid and/or GH replacement therapies, and radiation therapy (22,23).

Further improvements in the accuracy of diagnostic testing and replacement therapies are needed in order to improve the long-term outlook of these patients.

ACKNOWLEDGMENTS

The authors have nothing to disclose.

REFERENCES

1. **Toogood AA, Stewart PM.** Hypopituitarism: clinical features, diagnosis, and management. *Endocrinol Metab Clin North Am.* 2008;37(1):235–261, x.
2. **Stewart PM, Sherlock M.** Mortality and pituitary disease. *Ann Endocrinol (Paris).* 2012;73(2):81–82.
3. **Yuen KC, Cook DM, Sahasranam P, et al.** Prevalence of GH and other anterior pituitary hormone deficiencies in adults with nonsecreting pituitary microadenomas and normal serum IGF-1 levels. *Clin Endocrinol (Oxf).* 2008;69(2):292–298.
4. **Crowley RK, Hamnvik OP, O'Sullivan EP, et al.** Morbidity and mortality in patients with craniopharyngioma after surgery. *Clin Endocrinol (Oxf).* 2010;73(4):516–521.
5. **Hannon MJ, Finucane FM, Sherlock M, Agha A, Thompson CJ.** Clinical review: disorders of water homeostasis in neurosurgical patients. *J Clin Endocrinol Metab.* 2012;97(5):1423–1433.
6. **Darzy KH.** Radiation-induced hypopituitarism. *Curr Opin Endocrinol Diabetes Obes.* 2013;20(4): 342–353.
7. **Pai HH, Thornton A, Katznelson L, et al.** Hypothalamic/pituitary function following high-dose conformal radiotherapy to the base of skull: demonstration of a dose-effect relationship using dose-volume histogram analysis. *Int J Radiat Oncol Biol Phys.* 2001;49(4):1079–1092.
8. **Hannon MJ, Sherlock M, Thompson CJ.** Pituitary dysfunction following traumatic brain injury or subarachnoid haemorrhage. In: "Endocrine Management in the Intensive Care Unit". *Best Pract Res Clin Endocrinol Metab.* 2011;25(5):783–798.
9. **Hannon MJ, Crowley RK, Behan LA, et al.** Acute glucocorticoid deficiency and diabetes insipidus are common after acute traumatic brain injury and predict mortality. *J Clin Endocrinol Metab.* 2013;98(8): 3229–3237.
10. **Nawar RN, AbdelMannan D, Selman WR, Arafah BM.** Pituitary tumor apoplexy: a review. *J Intensive Care Med.* 2008;23(2):75–90.
11. **Romero CJ, Nesi-Franca S, Radovick S.** The molecular basis of hypopituitarism. *Trends Endocrinol Metab.* 2009;20(10):506–516.
12. **Ioachimescu AG, Hamrahian AH, Stevens M, Zimmerman RS.** The pituitary stalk transection syndrome: multifaceted presentation in adulthood. *Pituitary.* 2012;15(3):405–411.
13. **Devin JK.** Hypopituitarism and central diabetes insipidus: perioperative diagnosis and management. *Neurosurg Clin N Am.* 2012;23(4):679–689.
14. **Jahangiri A, Wagner J, Tran MT, et al.** Factors predicting postoperative hyponatremia and efficacy of hyponatremia management strategies after more than 1000 pituitary operations. *J Neurosurg.* 2013; 119:1478–1483.
15. **Fenske W, Allolio B.** Clinical review: Current state and future perspectives in the diagnosis of diabetes insipidus: a clinical review. *J Clin Endocrinol Metab.* 2012;97(10):3426–3437.
16. **Molitch ME, Clemmons DR, Malozowski S, Merriam GR, Vance ML.** Evaluation and treatment of adult growth hormone deficiency: an Endocrine Society clinical practice guideline. *J Clin Endocrinol Metab.* 2011;96(6):1587–1609.
17. **Biller BM, Samuels MH, Zagar A, et al.** Sensitivity and specificity of six tests for the diagnosis of adult GH deficiency. *J Clin Endocrinol Metab.* 2002;87(5): 2067–2079.
18. **Chanson P, Lepeintre JF, Ducreux D.** Management of pituitary apoplexy. *Expert Opin Pharmacother.* 2004;5(6):1287–1298.
19. **Johannsson G, Nilsson AG, Bergthorsdottir R, et al.** Improved cortisol exposure-time profile and outcome in patients with adrenal insufficiency: a prospective randomized trial of a novel hydrocortisone dual-release formulation. *J Clin Endocrinol Metab.* 2012;97(2):473–481.
20. **Oiso Y, Robertson GL, Norgard JP, Juul KV.** Clinical review: treatment of neurophyseal diabetes insipidus. *J Clin Endocrinol Metab.* 2013;98:3958–3967.
21. **Burman P, Mattsson AF, Johannsson G, et al.** Deaths among adult patients with hypopituitarism: hypocortisolism during acute stress, and de novo malignant brain tumors contribute to an increased mortality. *J Clin Endocrinol Metab.* 2013;98(4):1466–1475.
22. **Sherlock M, Reulen RC, Alonso AA, et al.** ACTH deficiency, higher doses of hydrocortisone replacement, and radiotherapy are independent predictors of mortality in patients with acromegaly. *J Clin Endocrinol Metab.* 2009;94(11):4216–4223.
23. **Sherlock M, Stewart PM.** Updates in growth hormone treatment and mortality. *Curr Opin Endocrinol Diabetes Obes.* 2013;20(4):314–320.

CHAPTER 8

Pituitary Apoplexy

Aikaterini Theodoraki and Mark Vanderpump

ABSTRACT

Pituitary apoplexy is an endocrine emergency resulting from catastrophic hemorrhage or infarct of the pituitary gland that typically manifests with headache, nausea and vomiting, visual impairment, and reduced consciousness. In most cases, apoplexy occurs in an undiagnosed, preexisting pituitary adenoma. Patients with suspected pituitary apoplexy require detailed visual field, visual acuity, and oculomotor nerve examination, pituitary hormone profile assessment, and emergency glucocorticoid treatment. Extensive or deteriorating visual field or visual acuity deficits, or reduced consciousness, necessitate urgent surgical intervention. In patients with mild visual impairment, conservative management results in similar visual and endocrine outcomes compared to early surgical intervention. No evidence from randomized studies exists in the management of pituitary apoplexy. The recently introduced pituitary apoplexy score (PAS) is a scoring system that aims to assess the clinical severity of patients objectively and serve as a management and audit tool for randomized studies.

INTRODUCTION

Classic pituitary apoplexy is a clinical syndrome caused by hemorrhage or infarction of the pituitary gland. It is characterized by sudden headache, vomiting, visual impairment, and reduced consciousness. It has to be differentiated from asymptomatic pituitary hemorrhage (or subclinical pituitary apoplexy), in which pituitary hemorrhage is found on routine imaging or during histopathologic examination. It is a rare condition with an annual incidence of 1.2 in 10,000,000 (1). Apoplexy usually occurs in preexisting pituitary tumors and often in patients with undiagnosed pituitary adenomas, with an incidence of 2%–7% in pituitary adenomas. It usually occurs between the fifth and the sixth decade and is more prevalent in men (2). It may evolve within hours or days.

PATHOPHYSIOLOGY

It has been suggested that tumor ischemia usually occurs as a result of the pituitary tumor outgrowing its blood supply. The abnormal vasculature in tumors may also contribute to the apoplectic event. Kinking of the superior hypophyseal artery against the diaphragma sellae is another mechanism that can lead to ischemia, although others support that pituitary adenomas derive their blood supply from the inferior and not the superior hypophyseal arteries, which get compressed with the impaction of the enlarging tumor against the diaphragmatic notch (3,4).

During hemorrhage of the pituitary gland there is increase of the intrasellar contents with an increase in the intrasellar pressure (5). This can explain the earliest and most common symptom, namely, the headache that can be retro-orbital, bifrontal, or diffuse and associated with nausea and vomiting. If pressure is exerted laterally to the sella, the contents of the cavernous sinus can be affected with ocular palsies resulting in 70% of patients. The most common cranial nerve affected in more than 50% of the patients is the third cranial nerve. Enlargement of the intrasellar contents can cause optic chiasmal compression with resulting visual field defects and a reduction in the visual acuity. The most common visual field defect is bitemporal hemianopia. Further pressure upon the hypothalamus and midbrain might account for the disturbance of consciousness and vital functions. Extravasation of blood or necrotic tissue in the subarachnoid space can cause meningism with resultant fever, photophobia, and reduction in the level of consciousness. Mechanical compression of the carotid artery against the anterior clinoid and vasospasm secondary to subarachnoid hemorrhage can cause cerebral ischemia. Hypocortisolemia renders the vasculature less responsive to the pressor effects of catecholamines, and hemodynamic instability results. Low serum cortisol additionally increases the release of vasopressin and decreases free water clearance, resulting in hyponatremia (4,6).

ETIOLOGY

Precipitating factors for pituitary apoplexy have been found in up to 40% of patients (7,8) and include major surgery, especially coronary artery bypass grafting (CABG), dynamic endocrine testing of the pituitary gland, anticoagulation treatment, coagulopathies, initiation or withdrawal of dopamine agonists, estrogen treatment, radiation therapy, pregnancy, head trauma, and acute systemic illness (4,9). Dynamic testing of the pituitary gland associated with pituitary apoplexy has been observed in thyrotropin-releasing hormone (TRH) testing, gonadotropin-releasing hormone (GnRH) testing, insulin tolerance testing (ITT), and corticotropin-releasing hormone (CRH) testing, and in the majority of patients (83%) pituitary apoplexy occurs within 2 hours (10). Although hypertension is commonly present in patients with apoplexy (6,11), a controlled study has not suggested it is a risk factor for pituitary apoplexy (12). The precipitating factors for pituitary apoplexy are summarized in Table 8-1.

DIAGNOSTIC CONSIDERATIONS

The clinical symptoms and signs of pituitary apoplexy coincide with those of more common medical emergencies. Subarachnoid hemorrhage, internal carotid artery aneurysm, meningitis, migraine, cluster headache, temporal arteritis, stroke, encephalitis, and cavernous sinus thrombosis are conditions from which pituitary apoplexy must be differentiated. Patients with pituitary apoplexy present to various clinical specialities, which may result in delays in diagnosis (4,13).

CLINICAL SIGNS AND FEATURES

Initial assessment of patients presenting with symptoms consistent with pituitary apoplexy should include a detailed history focusing on symptoms of pituitary dysfunction followed by a thorough physical examination including cranial nerves and visual fields to confrontation (Figure 8-1). Sudden headache is the most common presenting symptom and can be retro-orbital, bifrontal, or diffuse (6,13,14). It can be associated with nausea and vomiting. Oculomotor nerve palsies occur in up to 70% of cases, and the most common is third cranial nerve palsy. Visual field defects and a reduction in visual acuity are commonly present (75%). Meningism with fever and photophobia, reduction of the level of consciousness, and cerebral ischemia occur less often (4,7).

Table 8-1. Precipitating Factors for Pituitary Apoplexy

Major surgery, in particular coronary artery bypass surgery
Dynamic pituitary function tests with GnRH, TRH, and CRH
Anticoagulation therapy
Coagulopathies
Estrogen therapy
Initiation or withdrawal of dopamine receptor agonist
Radiation therapy
Pregnancy
Head trauma
Acute systemic illness
Systemic hypertension (common, but debatable whether it contributes)

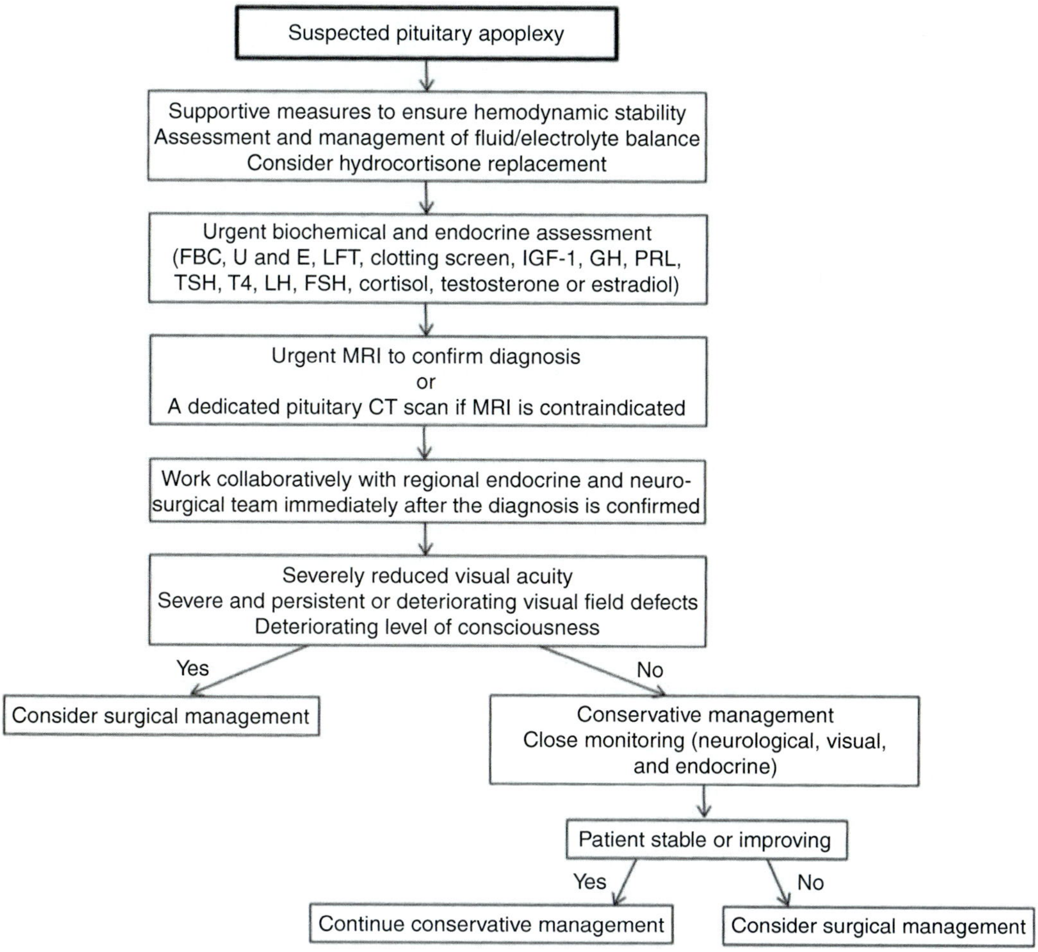

Figure 8-1. Algorithm for the management of pituitary apoplexy (13). FBC = full (complete) blood count; U and E = urea and electrolytes; LFT = liver function tests; IGF-1 = insulin-like growth factor 1; GH = growth hormone; TSH = thyroid-stimulating hormone; T4 = thyroxine; LH = luteinizing hormone; FSH = follicle-stimulating hormone; MRI = magnetic resonance imaging; CT = computed tomography.

In the event of a functioning pituitary adenoma, clinical features suggestive of hormone hypersecretion are usually present. Galactorrhea, oligomenorrhea, and infertility in women, and erectile dysfunction (ED) and infertility in men are common in prolactinomas. Obesity, proximal myopathy, skin bruising, colored abdominal striae, supraclavicular fat pads, and buffalo hump are seen in Cushing's disease. Headache, macroglossia, prognathism, soft tissue swelling, enlargement of extremities, and gigantism (if onset prior to epiphyses closure) are seen in acromegaly. In the rare occurrence of thyrotropinomas, tachycardia, hand tremor, weight loss, anxiety, and nervousness are observed. In men, ED may have been present for years prior to the discovery of a pituitary tumor.

PITUITARY-SPECIFIC CLINICAL, LABORATORY, AND IMAGING ASSESSMENT

Visual acuity, visual fields, and oculomotor nerves need to be examined in detail. Formal visual field assessment using Humphrey's visual field analyzer or Goldmann perimeter is recommended once the patient is clinically stable. Formal visual field assessment is recommended to be organized within 48 hours of the patient's presentation (13).

At presentation with pituitary apoplexy the majority of patients have a deficiency of one or more anterior pituitary hormones. Clinically, the most crucial deficit is that of adrenocorticotropic hormone (ACTH), which has been reported in up to 70% of patients. Growth hormone (GH) deficiency is present in almost all patients after pituitary apoplexy but rarely replaced (1,15). Thyroid-stimulating hormone (TSH) deficit is found in up to 50%, gonadotropin deficit in up to 75%, and hyponatremia in up to 40% (13). In acute hypocortisolemia, hemodynamic instability may occur. Prolactin levels can be high, normal, or low. In the latter situation, a low prolactin indicates high intrasellar pressure and a gland that is less likely to recover from hypopituitarism after decompressive surgery (5).

Drawing blood samples for baseline endocrine function tests including random serum cortisol, free thyroxine (FT_4), TSH, prolactin, luteinizing hormone (LH), follicle-stimulating hormone (FSH), insulin-like growth factor 1 (IGF-1), GH, testosterone in men and estradiol in women, serum electrolytes, clotting studies, and liver function tests (LFT) is recommended at presentation and before administration of glucocorticoids.

Urgent magnetic resonance imaging (MRI) scanning confirms the diagnosis of pituitary apoplexy in more than 90% of patients. A computed tomography (CT) scan can be diagnostic in only a minority of cases (21%–28%), however, a sellar mass may be shown in up to 80% of the patients (13). Additionally, CT cannot differentiate cystic or degenerative changes from previous hemorrhage. The preoperative finding of hemorrhage or infarction on MRI scanning correlates well with the operative findings (16).

ACUTE INTERVENTION

Acute secondary adrenal insufficiency is seen in two thirds of patients with pituitary tumor apoplexy and is a major source of morbidity and, rarely, mortality associated with the condition. Indications for empirical glucocorticoid treatment in patients with pituitary apoplexy are hemodynamic instability, altered consciousness level, reduced visual acuity, or severe visual field defects. In any patient who does not fulfill at least one of the above criteria, a 9 am serum cortisol less than 20 mcg/dL (550 nmol/L) necessitates glucocorticoid treatment (13). Glucocorticoids are given most often intravenously (IV) at a stat dose of 100–200 mg of hydrocortisone followed by a hydrocortisone infusion at a rate of 2–4 mg/hr or 50–100 mg intramuscular (IM) hydrocortisone every 6 hours.

GENERAL SUPPORTIVE CARE

If the patient is hypotensive, resuscitation with IV hydration is indicated. Subsequent monitoring should include daily electrolyte measurement and fluid balance assessments. Once the patient has been medically stabilized, transfer to the local neurosurgical/endocrinology team is recommended.

PITUITARY-SPECIFIC THERAPIES

The main treatment decision that is required is whether to adopt a "watch and wait" conservative approach, or proceed to surgical decompression. Uncontrolled retrospective studies have suggested that endocrine and visual outcomes do not differ between patients managed conservatively or by early surgical intervention (2,17,18). However, studies examining the role of conservative versus surgical management of pituitary apoplexy with regard to visual loss all suffer from selection bias and a lack of appropriately matched patients; as in most series, patients in the conservative group had less visual field/acuity loss than those in the surgically treated group.

It is recommended that patients with pituitary apoplexy and severe reduction in visual acuity, severe and persistent reduction in visual fields, or a reduction in the level of consciousness undergo surgical decompression. Generally, early surgical intervention within 8 days of presentation is advised, because some evidence suggests that greater improvements in visual fields and visual acuity are achieved then (2,11,17). The improvement usually starts immediately postoperatively and continues for several weeks. Visual recovery is less likely in patients presenting with monocular or binocular blindness, and early surgical decompression again is more likely to achieve best visual outcomes (19). Oculomotor nerve paresis in the absence of any visual field defects or reduction in visual acuity is not in itself an indication for immediate surgery, and resolution will typically occur within days or weeks with conservative management (19). This can partly be explained by the fact that the oculomotor nerves are peripheral nerves, and therefore can undergo regeneration.

If surgical decompression is decided, then a transsphenoidal approach is usually used. In giant pituitary tumors a transcranial approach may be required (20). It is recommended that surgery be performed by an experienced pituitary surgeon, defined as performing at least 5 or more transsphenoidal pituitary operations per annum (13). The decision regarding conservative versus surgical treatment should be made jointly by a multidisciplinary team including neurosurgeons, endocrinologists, and ophthalmologists. Where feasible, informed consent from the patient should be sought.

It is important to emphasize that all patients with pituitary apoplexy need to have detailed cranial nerve, visual field, and visual acuity examination on presentation. The frequency of reassessment depends on the clinical severity, and whether the visual fields, visual acuity, and ocular nerve deficits are stable/improving or deteriorating. If there is a reduction in visual acuity or visual fields, formal daily assessment is indicated until a clear trend for improvement is observed. Acutely unwell patients need hourly neurological assessments and any deterioration should prompt urgent senior medical review with consideration to repeat MRI scanning if findings are unexpected, and surgery (13). In the rare occurrence of hydrocephalus in patients with pituitary apoplexy, then an external ventricular drain may be warranted.

Postoperative management of patients after surgery for pituitary apoplexy is similar to that of elective pituitary surgery for pituitary tumors. Anterior pituitary function needs to be tested postoperatively: 9 am cortisol is usually checked on day 2 and day 3 postoperatively, thyroid function (FT_4 and TSH) is done on day 3 or day 4, and then all should be repeated 4–8 weeks later. If patients are already on hydrocortisone replacement, then the evening dose the previous day before the morning measurement should be omitted for the result to be diagnostic. If there is cortisol deficiency prior to the surgical intervention, then hydrocortisone is usually continued and changed to maintenance dose when the patient is stable, with further assessment of cortisol 4–8 weeks later (13). Transient diabetes insipidus (DI) occurs postoperatively in up to 16% of patients with apoplexy during their hospital stay. Postoperative hourly reviews in order to assess fluid balance, electrolytes, paired plasma, and urine osmolalities are recommended if DI is suspected. In up to 50% of patients, partial or complete recovery of pituitary function is observed after the apoplectic event. Retrospective studies have not shown any statistically significant differences in the endocrine outcomes between patients managed medically versus those managed surgically (2,6,17).

PITUITARY APOPLEXY SCORE

It is evident that patients with pituitary apoplexy present with varying degrees of visual and oculomotor nerve involvement, and an objective tool for clinical evaluation was not available. Such a tool would allow risk-stratification at presentation and clinical monitoring of patients. Additionally, it would serve as an audit tool and would be required in order to conduct randomized controlled clinical studies. The Pituitary Apoplexy Score (PAS) is a newly designed simple scoring system, which can be used for objective clinical evaluation in patients with pituitary apoplexy. It is based on 3 neuro-ophthalmic parameters (visual acuity: 0, 1, and 2; visual field defect: 0, 1, and 2; and ocular paresis: 0, 1, and 2) and the Glasgow Coma Scale (GCS; 0, 2, and 4) (Table 8-2). This scoring system ranges from 0 to 10, with a higher score indicating extensive neuro-ophthalmic impairment (13).

The PAS score has so far been applied in 2 retrospective cohorts. In a recent review of patients with acute pituitary apoplexy treated in a single center, the mean PAS for the group treated with early surgery was 3.8 (range 1–6), and 73% of surgically treated patients had a PAS of 4 or higher, whereas the mean score for the group managed conservatively or with delayed surgery was 1.8 (range 0–5), and only 13% of the conservative management/delayed surgery group had a PAS of 4 or higher (6). In an audit from 2 UK centers of patients with pituitary apoplexy, the mean PAS in patients who had early surgery within 8 days was 3.5 (range: 1–9), the mean PAS in those who had surgery from 9 to 14 days was 3.1 (range: 0–6), and conservatively managed

Table 8-2. Pituitary Apoplexy Score (13)

Pituitary Apoplexy Score	
Variable	**Points**
Level of consciousness	
Glasgow Coma Scale 15	0
Glasgow Coma Scale <8–14	2
Glasgow Coma Scale <8	4
Visual acuity	
Normal[a] 6/6	0
Reduced—unilateral	1
Bilateral	2
Visual field defects	
Normal	0
Unilateral defect	1
Bilateral defect	2
Ocular paresis	
Absent	0
Present—unilateral	1
Bilateral	2

[a] *No change from premorbid visual acuity.*

patients had a mean PAS of 1.4 (range: 0–4) (21). In both studies, therefore, the clinical severity at the time of presentation, based on a higher PAS, appeared to influence the management toward emergency surgical intervention; this may be useful in identifying individuals who would benefit from early surgery.

TREATMENT OF PRECIPITATING CAUSE

Patients known to have a pituitary tumor must be observed for signs and symptoms of pituitary apoplexy when performing pituitary stimulation tests, commencing anticoagulation treatment, or undertaking CABG or other major surgery. Similarly, patients with a pituitary tumor should be given clear information regarding the signs and symptoms of apoplexy and the precipitating factors (13).

MAINTENANCE TREATMENT

All patients with pituitary apoplexy should be reviewed in the endocrinology clinic regarding their pituitary hormone profile 4–8 weeks after the acute event and annually thereafter. Up to 80% of patients are on one or more pituitary hormone replacement: 60%–80% on long-term glucocorticoids, 50%–60% on levothyroxine, 10%–25% on desmopressin, and 60%–80% of men on testosterone. Annual assessment should be undertaken after apoplexy. Repeat imaging with MRI scanning is advised 3–6 months after the event, followed by annual MRI imaging for 5 years (13).

Recurrent apoplexy and tumor regrowth have been documented in both surgically and conservatively managed patients, and all patients treated with apoplexy need follow-up imaging to detect recurrent growth (22). Long-term management depends on the nature of the underlying tumor. Support from endocrine nurses and patient support organizations should be provided if available (13).

CONCLUSIONS

Pituitary apoplexy is an endocrine emergency resulting from catastrophic hemorrhage or infarct involving the pituitary gland. Careful visual field, visual acuity, and oculomotor nerve assessment and a high index of suspicion are necessary for the diagnosis to be made and the condition to be managed appropriately. The majority of patients require emergency glucocorticoid replacement, and all patients need close monitoring. Surgical decompression is indicated in patients with extensive or deteriorating neuro-ophthalmic involvement or reduced consciousness. All patients need to be managed jointly under a neurosurgical and endocrine team with experience in pituitary assessment and surgery.

ACKNOWLEDGMENTS

The authors have nothing to disclose.

REFERENCES

1. **Nielsen EH, Lindholm J, Bjerre P, et al.** Frequent occurrence of pituitary apoplexy in patients with non-functioning pituitary adenoma. *Clin Endocrinol (Oxf).* 2006;64(3):319–322. PMID: 16487443.
2. **Sibal L, Ball SG, Connolly V, et al.** Pituitary apoplexy: a review of clinical presentation, management and outcome in 45 cases. *Pituitary.* 2004;7(3): 157–163. PMID: 16010459.
3. **Cardoso ER, Peterson EW.** Pituitary apoplexy: a review. *Neurosurgery.* 1984;14(3):363–373. PMID: 6369168.

4. **Watt A, Pobereskin L, Vaidya B.** Pituitary apoplexy within a macroprolactinoma. *Nat Clin Pract Endocrinol Metab.* 2008;4(11):635–641. PMID: 18797434.
5. **Zayour DH, Selman WR, Arafah BM.** Extreme elevation of intrasellar pressure in patients with pituitary tumor apoplexy: relation to pituitary function. *J Clin Endocrinol Metab.* 2004;89(11):5649–5654. PMID: 15531524.
6. **Bujawansa S, Thondam SK, Steele C, et al.** Presentation, management and outcomes in acute pituitary apoplexy: a large single-centre experience from the United Kingdom. *Clin Endocrinol (Oxf).* 2014; 80(3):419–424. PMID: 23909507.
7. **Nawar RN, AbdelMannan D, Selman WR, Arafah BM.** Pituitary tumor apoplexy: a review. *J Intensive Care Med.* 2008;23(2):75–90. PMID: 18372348.
8. **Murad-Kejbou S, Eggenberger E.** Pituitary apoplexy: evaluation, management, and prognosis. *Curr Opin Ophthalmol.* 2009;20(6):456–461. PMID: 19809320.
9. **Semple PL, Jane JA Jr, Laws ER Jr.** Clinical relevance of precipitating factors in pituitary apoplexy. *Neurosurgery.* 2007;61(5):956–961; discussion 61–62. PMID: 18091272.
10. **Yoshino A, Katayama Y, Watanabe T, et al.** Apoplexy accompanying pituitary adenoma as a complication of preoperative anterior pituitary function tests. *Acta Neurochir (Wien).* 2007;149(6):557–565; discussion 65. PMID: 17468811.
11. **Randeva HS, Schoebel J, Byrne J, Esiri M, Adams CB, Wass JA.** Classical pituitary apoplexy: clinical features, management and outcome. *Clin Endocrinol (Oxf).* 1999;51(2):181–188. PMID: 10468988.
12. **Moller-Goede DL, Brandle M, Landau K, Bernays RL, Schmid C.** Pituitary apoplexy: re-evaluation of risk factors for bleeding into pituitary adenomas and impact on outcome. *Eur J Endocrinol.* 2011;164(1):37–43. PMID: 20926593.
13. **Rajasekaran S, Vanderpump M, Baldeweg S, et al.** UK guidelines for the management of pituitary apoplexy. *Clin Endocrinol (Oxf).* 2011;74(1):9–20. PMID: 21044119.
14. **Semple PL, Webb MK, de Villiers JC, Laws ER Jr.** Pituitary apoplexy. *Neurosurgery.* 2005;56(1):65–72; discussion 72–73. PMID: 15617587.
15. **Veldhuis JD, Hammond JM.** Endocrine function after spontaneous infarction of the human pituitary: report, review, and reappraisal. *Endocr Rev.* 1980;1(1):100–107. PMID: 6785084.
16. **Semple PL, Jane JA, Lopes MB, Laws ER.** Pituitary apoplexy: correlation between magnetic resonance imaging and histopathological results. *J Neurosurg.* 2008;108(5):909–915. PMID: 18447705.
17. **Ayuk J, McGregor EJ, Mitchell RD, Gittoes NJ.** Acute management of pituitary apoplexy—surgery or conservative management? *Clin Endocrinol (Oxf).* 2004;61(6):747–752. PMID: 15579190.
18. **Gruber A, Clayton J, Kumar S, Robertson I, Howlett TA, Mansell P.** Pituitary apoplexy: retrospective review of 30 patients—is surgical intervention always necessary? *Br J Neurosurg.* 2006;20(6):379–385. PMID: 17439089.
19. **Muthukumar N, Rossette D, Soundaram M, Senthilbabu S, Badrinarayanan T.** Blindness following pituitary apoplexy: timing of surgery and neuro-ophthalmic outcome. *J Clin Neurosci.* 2008;15(8): 873–879. PMID: 18502643.
20. **Kurwale NS, Ahmad F, Suri A, et al.** Post operative pituitary apoplexy: preoperative considerations toward preventing nightmare. *Br J Neurosurg.* 2012;26(1):59–63. PMID: 22122708.
21. **Reddy NL, Rajasekaran S, Han TS, et al.** An objective scoring tool in the management of patients with pituitary apoplexy. *Clin Endocrinol (Oxf).* 2011;75(5):723. PMID: 21535071.
22. **Pal A, Capatina C, Tenreiro AP, et al.** Pituitary apoplexy in non-functioning pituitary adenomas: long term follow up is important because of significant numbers of tumour recurrences. *Clin Endocrinol (Oxf).* 2011;75(4):501–504. PMID: 21521336.

CHAPTER 9

Macroprolactinomas

Mark E Molitch

ABSTRACT

Several aspects of managing patients with macroprolactinomas may be difficult and, in some cases, can be considered emergencies. Visual field defects can be expected in about 40% of patients with macroprolactinomas. Improvement in such defects with dopamine agonist treatment appears to be at least as good as can be achieved by transsphenoidal surgery and can be accomplished with less morbidity. With both treatments, improvements can be delayed and there is no emergency in decompressing the chiasm. Cerebrospinal fluid (CSF) rhinorrhea can occur when there is a large, invasive, skull-based prolactinoma that serves as a "cork" in the base of the skull. When the tumor size is reduced substantially through dopamine agonist use, CSF can leak around the tumor into the sphenoid sinus and nasal passages, with a resultant risk of meningitis. Measurement of beta-2 transferrin in the nasal fluid is diagnostic. Surgical repair is usually required. Pituitary apoplexy is very rare, although asymptomatic hemorrhage into a pituitary adenoma is common. In patients with apoplexy, rapid assessment for hypopituitarism and treatment of deficits in ACTH with stress steroids are important. Although surgical decompression is often required, many patients may be treated conservatively. Macroprolactinoma enlargement during pregnancy occurs in about 22% of women, resulting in headaches or visual symptoms. Visual field monitoring each trimester for women with macroprolactinomas is warranted. Treatment consists of reinstitution of dopamine agonists, surgery if that is not effective, or delivery if the pregnancy is sufficiently advanced.

INTRODUCTION

Pituitary tumors account for approximately 10%–15% of all intracranial tumors (1,2). Prolactin (PRL)-secreting adenomas (prolactinomas) account for approximately 40% of all pituitary tumors (1,2). The reported population prevalence of clinically apparent prolactinomas ranges from 6 to 10 per 100,000 to approximately 50 per 100,000 (1,2). Generally, prolactinomas are diagnosed when patients present with typical findings of hyperprolactinemia, namely, galactorrhea, amenorrhea and infertility in women, erectile dysfunction and infertility in men, and lack of libido in both sexes (1). Once hyperprolactinemia is documented and other causes are excluded, magnetic resonance imaging (MRI) is done to characterize a possible tumor (1). Prolactinomas and other pituitary adenomas are divided into micro- and macroadenomas, with the cut-off being 10 mm for the greatest diameter as demonstrated on MRI or computed tomography (CT) scan (1,2). Prolactinomas are also frequently discovered as pituitary incidentalomas (previously unsuspected pituitary lesions that are discovered on an imaging study for an unrelated reason), which are present in approximately 10% of the general population and are frequently discovered in acute clinical settings (2). The management of pituitary incidentalomas is discussed in detail in an Endocrine

Society Clinical Practice Guideline on pituitary incidentalomas and is summarized in Figure 9-1 (2). It should be remembered, however, that PRL levels should be run at 1:100 dilution in patients with large (>3 cm) macroincidentalomas, to avoid missing a prolactinoma because of the "hook effect" (very high levels of PRL saturating the antibodies in some assays, giving falsely normal or mildly elevated levels) (2).

The treatment of patients with microprolactinomas and macroprolactinomas is generally very satisfying for clinicians, primarily due to the excellent efficacy of dopamine agonist therapy in reducing PRL levels, reducing adenoma size, restoring gonadal function, and improving other clinical features (1,3). The Endocrine Society guideline on treatment of hyperprolactinemia generally recommends cabergoline as the dopamine agonist of choice, due to higher efficacy in normalizing prolactin levels and pituitary tumor shrinkage (1). However, there are some aspects of treatment that are more troubling than others and some can even be considered emergencies; most of these aspects occur in patients with macroprolactinomas. Several particular aspects of management fall into this category: (1) a visual field (VF) defect at presentation; (2) the development of cerebrospinal fluid (CSF) rhinorrhea; (3) the development of pituitary apoplexy; and (4) tumor enlargement during pregnancy.

VISUAL FIELD DEFECT AT PRESENTATION

Visual field defects can be expected in about 40% of patients with macroprolactinomas (4–7). Visual field testing is only necessary, of course, in patients whose tumors are found to abut the optic chiasm on MRI. Although it is recognized that, overall, dopamine agonist treatment is more efficacious than transsphenoidal surgery for patients with prolactinomas (1,3), it is worth reviewing some of the data that would allow comparison of the efficacy of dopamine agonist treatment vs. transsphenoidal surgery with respect to improving VF defects.

In a US multicenter study, bromocriptine was found to cause VF defect improvement in 9 of 10 patients who had defects (4). Maximal improvement was found by 2 weeks in 1 patient, by 3 months in 5 patients, and by

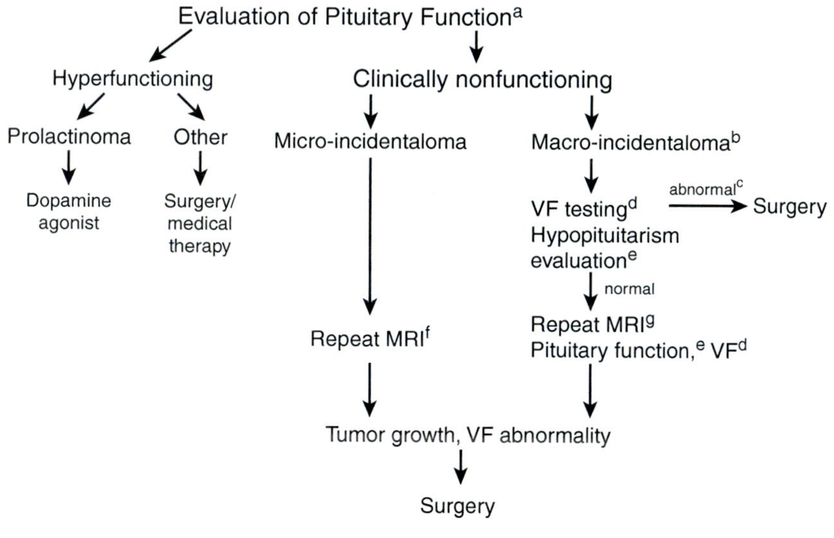

Figure 9-1. Flow diagram for the evaluation and treatment of pituitary incidentalomas. (a) Baseline evaluation in all patients should include a history and physical exam evaluating for signs and symptoms of hyperfunction and hypopituitarism and a laboratory evaluation for hypersecretion. (b) This group may also include large microlesions. (c) The recommendation for surgery includes the presence of abnormalities of VF or vision and signs of tumor compression; surgery is also suggested for other findings. (d) VF testing is recommended for patients with lesions abutting or compressing the optic nerves or chiasm at the initial evaluation and during follow-up. (e) Evaluation for hypopituitarism is recommended for the baseline evaluation and during follow-up evaluations. This is most strongly recommended for macrolesions and larger microlesions. (f) Repeat MRI in 1 year, yearly for 3 years, and then less frequently thereafter if no change in lesion size. (g) Repeat the MRI in 6 months, yearly for 3 years, and then less frequently if no change in lesion size.

6 months in the remaining 3 patients (4). In general, the improvement in VF defects parallels the change in tumor size. In their review on bromocriptine-treated macroadenomas, Bevan et al (5) found that 79% of 271 macroadenomas showed more than 25% shrinkage, and of the 102 patients with chiasmal compression, 85% showed tumor shrinkage of more than 25%. Shrinkage with VF improvement may occur as early as a few days with maximal shrinkage generally occurring by 3–6 months (4,5,8). A 75%–90% tumor shrinkage with VF improvement similarly occurs with cabergoline (1,6,7,9). Complete normalization of VF occurred in 9 of 10 patients in one series, with such normalization occurring by 3 months in 4 patients and by 6–12 months in 5 patients (6).

Because the primary treatment of most patients with prolactinomas is currently medical rather than surgical, the most appropriate comparison is with patients with clinically nonfunctioning pituitary adenomas (CNFA) who have undergone transsphenoidal surgery. In a meta-analysis that analyzed 59 series, 795 patients with CNFAs had visual field defects, and transsphenoidal surgery resulted in an improvement in VF defects in 78%, at the expense, however, of a 1% mortality and 3% worsening of VF (10). It is important to note that after surgery, the improvement in VF is not necessarily rapid. There is a rapid recovery of some function within minutes to a few days, a more delayed recovery over weeks to months, and late recovery over months to years (11).

Overall, therefore, the improvement in VF with dopamine agonist treatment appears to be at least as good as can be achieved by transsphenoidal surgery. Furthermore, medical treatment can be accomplished with less morbidity and better achievement of normal PRL levels (3). With both treatments, the improvements in VF can be quite delayed. Dekkers et al (12) performed repeat VF at a 4-week (range 1–45 weeks) interval in 34 patients with CNFAs, finding no change in VFs or visual acuity within that time period. Thus, there is no urgency to rush into surgery for the patient with a VF defect, and a trial of a dopamine agonist is indicated unless the VF defect is sudden (see section on Pituitary Apoplexy below). Consultation with an experienced pituitary surgeon can be very helpful in this setting. Given the time periods discussed above, a 3-month trial would appear to be warranted. Monitoring of PRL levels and VF every 4–6 weeks seems reasonable. A full reevaluation with PRL levels, VF, and MRI should be carried out at 3 months in such patients. If there is no change in tumor size with continued abutment of the chiasm and no improvement at all in VF and the defect is clinically significant, then surgical decompression is reasonable. If the VF defect is minimal, then perhaps surgery would not be indicated, especially if PRL levels have come down to normal or near normal. If there is substantial tumor shrinkage with relief of pressure on the chiasm, then surgery would not be expected to result in VF improvement despite persistent defects and, therefore, would not be indicated. Certainly, if there is evidence of tumor growth or a worsening of VF over the initial 3 months or later, surgical decompression of the chiasm would be indicated. One additional rare complication should be mentioned, and that is a secondary worsening of VF after successful treatment with dopamine agonists due to marked tumor shrinkage with herniation of the optic apparatus into the partially empty sella (13). Of course, the same worsening can occur after surgery as well.

CEREBROSPINAL FLUID RHINORRHEA

CSF rhinorrhea can occur when there is a large, invasive, skull-based prolactinoma that serves as a "cork" in the base of the skull. When the tumor size is reduced substantially through dopamine agonist use, CSF can leak around the tumor into the sphenoid sinus and nasal passages (14–16). Because tumor shrinkage may occur rapidly, such CSF rhinorrhea may occur within a week of starting the dopamine agonist (14,15). Although CSF rhinorrhea is relatively rare, such an occurrence has been reported in the literature in 42 patients with prolactinomas through 2012, with the CSF leak occurring following dopamine agonist therapy in 36 (86%) (16). Spontaneous CSF leaks can also occur without medical therapy, but they are much less common (16).

Typically, patients will develop excessive rhinorrhea, and then the differential diagnosis is between CSF rhinorrhea and a simple upper respiratory infection. With CSF rhinorrhea, the amount of fluid typically is increased if the patient leans forward and down. The fluid should be sent to the laboratory for measurement of β2-transferrin, which is an asialo transferrin isoform found only in CSF, ocular fluids, and perilymph and is an accepted marker of CSF leakage (17,18). The major concern with such leaks is the risk of meningitis, although pneumocephaly may also occur (14–16). The use of prophylactic antibiotics while awaiting surgery is controversial (19). Urgent consultation with an experienced pituitary neurosurgeon is important when CSF rhinorrhea is suspected, as endonasal, endoscopic surgical repair of the leak to prevent meningitis is generally recommended (15). Although such a repair is not emergent, it should be done expeditiously. Conservative approaches of reduction in dopamine agonist dose and reduction of CSF pressure through insertion of a lumbar drain are usually not successful (16).

PITUITARY APOPLEXY

Pituitary apoplexy is a clinical syndrome consisting of severe headache, stiff neck, nausea, vomiting, and often neurological symptoms such as ophthalmoplegias, cranial nerve palsies, VF defects, ptosis, or altered mental status (20,21). These symptoms are related to a rapid expansion of the contents of the sella into the parasellar and suprasellar spaces due to hemorrhage into or hemorrhagic infarction of an adenoma (20). Hemorrhage can be found in 25%–36% of pituitary adenomas removed at surgery (21,22) and was found on MRI in 16 of 79 (20.3%) macroprolactinomas and 9 of 289 (3.1%) microprolactinomas in a recent series (23). Of the surgical cases, about half are entirely asymptomatic, about one third have mild to moderate headaches, and only 10%–15% have symptoms compatible with pituitary apoplexy. In the prolactinoma series, of the 25 of 368 patients who had hemorrhage, only 3 were considered to have classic apoplexy (23). This hemorrhagic infarction is to be distinguished from the bland infarction of the normal pituitary that may be seen with hypotension, which is most commonly seen following postpartum bleeding (Sheehan's syndrome) (20). Virtually all cases of true pituitary apoplexy are due to hemorrhagic infarction of a preexisting adenoma and not to hemorrhage into normal pituitary tissue; most occur in macroadenomas rather than microadenomas (20). In general, the amount of hemorrhage correlates with the severity of symptoms (21). Although bland infarction may cause apoplexy, it usually causes less severe symptoms and a more prolonged course (20). It has been hypothesized that dopamine agonist use may precipitate apoplexy in patients with prolactinomas, but this has not been proven.

There are several factors to consider in a patient with a prolactinoma who presents with signs and symptoms compatible with pituitary apoplexy. The first issue is to distinguish apoplexy from meningitis and subarachnoid hemorrhage. The CSF may be abnormal, showing increased protein and a pleiocytosis in all three conditions, but the finding of bacteria is certainly diagnostic of meningitis (20). The finding of hemorrhage into the tumor on a noncontrast CT (hyperdensity within the tumor) is very helpful (20). With MRI (Figure 9-2), within the first 2 hours there are no specific findings, but after 3 hours an acute hemorrhage is usually isointense on T1-weighted images and very hypointense on T2-weighted images (20). Later images may show hyperintense areas on T1-weighted images and variable hypointense and hyperintense areas on T2-weighted images. The intensity changes in these images are due to the progressive breakdown of hemoglobin (20).

A second early issue is that of hypopituitarism. Varying degrees of hypopituitarism are found in up to three quarters of such patients (20,24,25). A complete hormonal profile should be obtained in all patients and hydrocortisone administered intravenously in stress doses pending return of these levels. If the cortisol level was appropriately elevated for the stress, then hydrocortisone may be discontinued. However, pituitary function may get worse over time following the apoplexy (16), so that repeated cortisol measurements are in order to detect possible later deficiencies. Thyroid hormone can be replaced as necessary.

Once the patient has been stabilized with appropriate intravenous fluids and hydrocortisone and diagnostic studies have been completed, the decision regarding operative decompression with at least removal of the hemorrhagic adenoma needs to be made.

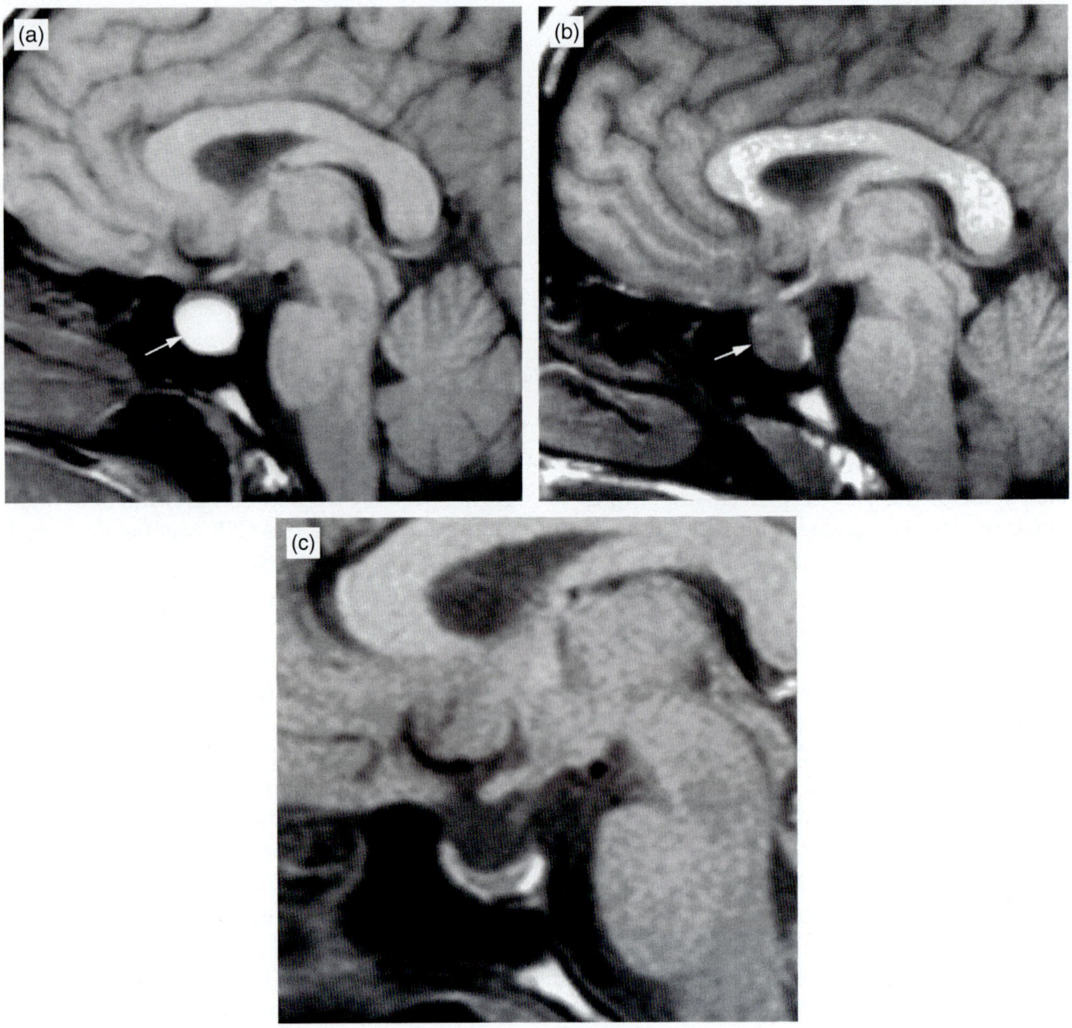

Figure 9-2. Macroadenoma with subsequent pituitary hemorrhage. (a) The macroadenoma (arrow) appears as an enlarged mass within the sella on the noncontrast T1-weighted sagittal MR image. (b) Repeat imaging obtained 2 years later shows that there is a new high signal (arrow) within the macroadenoma secondary to subacute hemorrhage. The patient had been receiving bromocriptine and was asymptomatic. (c) On the examination performed in the same patient 1 year later, the macroadenoma is no longer present and there is a partially empty sella. Presumably, there has been necrosis of the tumor following the episode of hemorrhage. (From Naidich MJ, Russell EF. Current approaches to imaging of the sellar region and pituitary. *Endocrinol Metab Clin N Amer.* 1999;28:45–70.)

Much depends upon the nature of any neurological deficits and whether or not they are progressing. A full discussion of the pros and cons of surgery versus conservative management is presented elsewhere, but suffice it to say that not all patients need surgery (20,24–27). Brisman et al (28) reported an interesting patient with an untreated macroprolactinoma who presented with pituitary apoplexy and whose tumor mass and clinical findings improved quickly and dramatically following the initiation of bromocriptine along with high-dose steroids. Starting a dopamine agonist immediately once PRL levels are found to be elevated in a patient not previously known to have a prolactinoma certainly seems like a reasonable treatment option. Following any surgery or conservative therapy, the decrease in size of the enlarged tumor mass may permit some resolution of hormonal deficits (20) and so a repeat evaluation of pituitary function should be carried out several weeks later.

TUMOR ENLARGEMENT DURING PREGNANCY

The stimulatory effect of the hormonal milieu of pregnancy and the withdrawal of the dopamine agonist may result in significant prolactinoma enlargement (Figure 9-3). Severe headaches or visual disturbances due to tumor enlargement during pregnancy have been reported in 18 of 734 (2.5%) women with microadenomas, 49 of 224 (21.9%) with macroadenomas that had not undergone prior surgery or radiotherapy, and 7 of 148 (4.7%) with macroadenomas that had undergone prior surgery or radiotherapy (29,30).

A patient with a microadenoma treated only with a dopamine agonist should be carefully followed throughout gestation. PRL levels do not always rise during pregnancy in women with prolactinomas, as they do in normal women. PRL levels may also not rise with tumor enlargement (31). Therefore, periodic checking of PRL levels is not recommended, as they are of no diagnostic benefit, and may be both misleading and the cause of unnecessary worry. Because of the low incidence of tumor enlargement, routine, periodic VF testing is not cost effective. Visual field testing and MRI scanning are performed only in patients who become symptomatic when intervention is being considered. There are no data to show that either MRI scans or the use of gadolinium is harmful to the developing fetus (29); nonetheless, many neuroradiology departments are reluctant to do any MRI scan and even more reluctant to give gadolinium to a pregnant patient. In the patient with tumor enlargement who does not respond to reinstitution of a dopamine agonist, surgery or early delivery may be required (29).

For the patient with a small intrasellar or inferiorly extending macroadenoma, dopamine agonists are also favored as the primary therapy. The likelihood that such a tumor will enlarge sufficiently to cause clinically serious

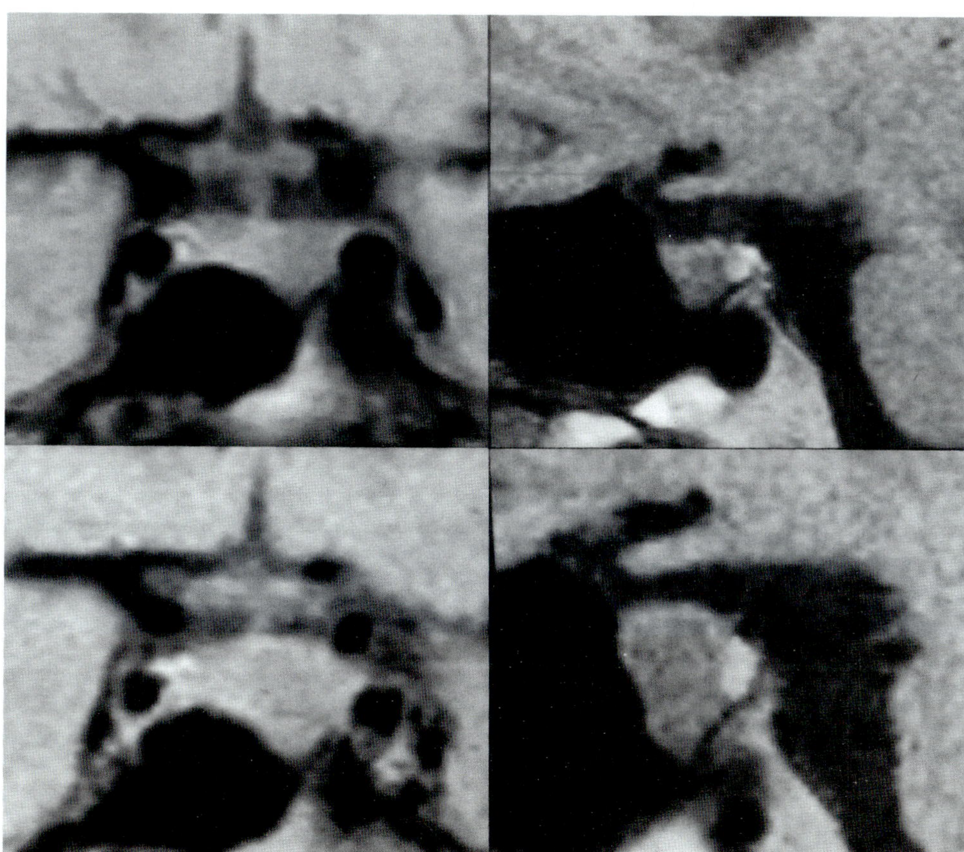

Figure 9-3. Coronal (left) and sagittal (right) MRI scans of an intrasellar prolactin secreting macroadenoma in a woman prior to conception (top) and at 7 months of gestation (below). Note the marked tumor enlargement at the latter point, at which time the patient was complaining of headaches. (From Molitch ME. Medical treatment of prolactinomas. *Endocrinol Metab Clin North Am.* 1999;28:143–170.)

complications is probably only marginally higher than the likelihood in patients with microadenomas (29).

In a woman with a larger macroadenoma that may have suprasellar extension, there is a 22% risk of clinically significant tumor enlargement during pregnancy when only dopamine agonists are used. There is no definitive answer as to the best therapeutic approach in such a patient; this has to be a highly individualized decision that the patient makes after a clear, documented discussion of the various therapeutic alternatives. One approach is to perform a prepregnancy transsphenoidal surgical debulking of the tumor. This should greatly reduce the risk of serious tumor enlargement, but cases with massive tumor expansion during pregnancy after such surgery have been reported (29). After surgical debulking, a dopamine agonist is required to restore normal PRL levels and allow ovulation. Although radiotherapy before pregnancy, followed by a dopamine agonist, also reduces the risk of tumor enlargement, it is rarely curative. It also commonly results in long-term hypopituitarism, so that this approach seems less acceptable than transsphenoidal surgery plus a dopamine agonist. A third approach, that of giving bromocriptine continuously throughout gestation, has been used but data of effects on the fetus are quite meager, and data on the effects of continuous cabergoline on the fetus are even fewer (29); therefore, such treatment cannot be recommended without reservation. Should pregnancy at an advanced stage be discovered in a woman taking bromocriptine or cabergoline, however, the data that exist are reassuring and would not justify therapeutic abortion. A fourth approach, and the one most commonly employed, is to stop the dopamine agonist after pregnancy is diagnosed, as in the patient with a microadenoma.

For patients with macroadenomas treated with a dopamine agonist alone or after surgery or irradiation, careful follow-up with 1–3 monthly formal visual field testing is warranted. Repeat MRI scanning is reserved for patients with symptoms of tumor enlargement and/or evidence of a developing visual field defect or both. Should symptomatic tumor enlargement occur with any of these approaches, reinstitution of the dopamine agonist is probably less harmful to the mother and child than surgery. There have been a number of cases reported where such reinstitution of the dopamine agonist has worked quite satisfactorily, causing rapid tumor size reduction with no adverse effects on the infant (see above). Any type of surgery during pregnancy results in a 1.5–fold increase in fetal loss in the first trimester and a 5-fold increase in fetal loss in the second trimester, although there is no risk of congenital malformations from such surgery (32). Thus, dopamine agonist reinstitution would appear to be preferable to surgical decompression. However, such medical therapy must be very closely monitored, and transsphenoidal surgery or delivery (if the pregnancy is far enough advanced) should be performed if there is no response to the dopamine agonist and vision is progressively worsening.

ACKNOWLEDGMENTS

The author has nothing to disclose.

REFERENCES

1. **Melmed S, Casaneuva FF, Hoffman AR, et al.** Diagnosis and treatment of hyperprolactinemia. An Endocrine Society Clinical Practice Guideline. *J Clin Endocrinol Metab.* 2011;96:273–288.
2. **Freda PU, Beckers AM, Katznelson L, et al.** Pituitary incidentaloma: an Endocrine Society Clinical Practice Guideline. *J Clin Endocrinol Metab.* 2011;96: 894–904.
3. **Gillam MP, Molitch MP, Lombardi G, Colao A.** Advances in the treatment of prolactinomas. *Endocrine Revs.* 2006;27:485–534.
4. **Molitch ME, Elton RL, Blackwell RE, et al.** Bromocriptine as primary therapy for prolactin-secreting macroadenomas: results of a prospective multicenter study. *J Clin Endocrinol Metab.* 1985;60:698–705.
5. **Bevan M, Webster J, Burke CW, Scanlon MF.** Dopamine agonists and pituitary tumor shrinkage. *Endocrine Revs.* 1992;13:220–240.
6. **Colao A, Di Sarno A, Landi ML, et al.** Long-term and low-dose treatment with cabergoline induces macroprolactinoma shrinkage. *J Clin Endocrinol Metab.* 1997;82:3574–3579.
7. **Colao A, Vitale G, Cappabianca P, et al.** Outcome of cabergoline treatment in men with prolactinoma: effects of a 24-month treatment on prolactin levels, tumor mass, recovery of pituitary function, and semen analysis. *J Clin Endocrinol Metab.* 2004;89:1704–1711.
8. **Lesser RL, Zheutlin JD, Boghen D, Odel JG, Robbins RJ.** Visual function improvement in patients with macroprolactinomas treated with bromocriptine. *Am J Ophthalmol.* 1990;109;535–543.

9. **Corsello SM, Libertini G, Altomara M, et al.** Giant prolactinomas in men: efficacy of cabergoline treatment. *Clin Endocrinol.* 2003;58:662–670.
10. **Murad MH, Fernández-Balsells MM, Barwise A, et al.** Outcomes of surgical treatment for nonfunctioning pituitary adenomas: a systematic review and meta-analysis. *Clin Endocrinol.* 2010;73:777–791.
11. **Kerrison JB, Lynn MJ, Baer C, Newman SA, Biousse V, Newman NJ.** Stages of improvement in visual fields after pituitary tumor resection. *Am J Ophthalmol.* 2000;130:813–820.
12. **Dekkers OM, de Keizer RJW, Roelfsema F, et al.** Progressive improvement of impaired visual acuity during the first year after transsphenoidal surgery for functioning pituitary macroadenoma. *Pituitary.* 2007;21:61–65.
13. **Raverot G, Jacob M, Jouanneau E, et al.** Secondary deterioration of visual field during cabergoline treatment for macroprolactinoma. *Clin Endocrinol.* 2009;70:588–592.
14. **Leong KS, Foy PM, Swift C, Atkin SL, Hadden DR, MacFarlane IA.** CSF rhinorrhea following treatment with dopamine agonists for massive invasive prolactinomas. *Clin Endocrinol.* 2000;52:43–49.
15. **Nadesapillai S, Balcere I, Kaye AH, Tress BM, Colman PG.** Acute complications of dopamine agonist treatment for macroprolactinoma—how uncommon? *J Clin Neurosci.* 2004;11:825–828.
16. **Lam G, Mehta V, Zada G.** Spontaneous and medically induced cerebrospinal fluid leakage in the setting of pituitary adenomas: review of the literature. *Neurosurg Focus.* 2012;32:E2. doi: 10.3171/2012.4.FOCUS1268.
17. **Rodríguez-Capote K, Turner J, Macri J.** Evaluation of a commercially available carbohydrate deficient transferrin kit to detect beta-2-transferrin in cerebrospinal fluid using capillary electrophoresis. *Clin Biochem.* 2013;46:1770–1773.
18. **Warnecke A, Averbeck T, Wurster U, Harmening M, Lenarz T, Stover T.** Diagnostic relevance of beta2-transferrin for the detection of cerebrospinal fluid fistulas. *Arch Otolaryngol Head Neck Surg.* 2004;130:1178–1184.
19. **Sherif C, Di Leva A, Gibson D, et al.** A management algorithm for cerebrospinal fluid leak associated with anterior skull base fractures: detailed clinical and radiological follow-up. *Neurosurg Rev.* 2012;35:227–237.
20. **Nawar RN, AbdlMannan D, Selman WR, Arafah BM.** Pituitary tumor apoplexy: a review. *J Intens Care Med.* 2008;23:75–90.
21. **Kim D-J, Song Y-J, Kim S-J, Park M-K, Choi S-S, Kim K-U.** Pituitary hemorrhage: classification and related factors. *J Korean Neurosurg.* 2009;46:23–30.
22. **Mohanty S, Tandon PN, Banerji AK, Prakash B.** Haemorrhage into pituitary adenomas. *J Neurol Neurosurg Psych.* 1977;40:987–991.
23. **Sarwar KN, Huda MSB, van de Velde V, et al.** The prevalence and natural history of pituitary hemorrhage in prolactinomas. *J Clin Endocrinol Metab.* 2013;98:2362–2367.
24. **Randeva HS, Schoebel J, Byrne J, Esiri M, Adams CT, Wass JAH.** Classical pituitary apoplexy: clinical features management and outcome. *Clin Endocrinol.* 1999;51:181–188.
25. **Ayuk J, McGregor EJ, Mitchell RD, Gittoes NJL.** Acute management of pituitary apoplexy—surgery or conservative management. *Clin Endocrinol.* 2004;61:747–752.
26. **Maccagnan P, Macedo CL, Kayath MJ, Nogueira RG, Abucham J.** Conservative management of pituitary apoplexy: a prospective study. *J Clin Endocrinol Metab.* 1995;80:2190–2197.
27. **Gruber A, Clayton J, Kumar S, Robertson J, Howlett TA, Mansell P.** Pituitary apoplexy: retrospective review of 30 patients—is surgical intervention always necessary? *Br J Neurosurg.* 2006;20:379–385.
28. **Brisman MH, Katz G, Post KD.** Symptoms of pituitary apoplexy rapidly reversed with bromocriptine. *J Neurosurg.* 1996;85:1153–1155.
29. **Molitch ME.** Prolactinoma in pregnancy. *Best Pract Res Clin Endocrinol Metab.* 2011;25:885–896
30. **Auriemma RS, Perone Y, DiSarno A, et al.** Results of a single-center observational 10-6314 survey study on recurrence of hyperprolactinemia after pregnancy and lactation. *J Clin Endocrinol Metab.* 2013;98:372–379.
31. **Divers WA Jr, Yen SS.** Prolactin-producing microadenomas in pregnancy. *Obstet Gynecol.* 1983;62:425–429.
32. **Cohen-Kerem R, Railton C, Oren D, Lishner M, Koren G.** Pregnancy outcome following non-obstetric surgical intervention. *Am J Surg.* 2005;190:467–473.

SECTION V

Thyroid Disorders

SECTION INTRODUCTION

Emergent Management of Thyroid Disorders

Hossein Gharib

Thyroid disorders are very common, affecting 750 million people worldwide by recent World Health Organization (WHO) estimates, being possibly even more prevalent than diabetes. Many groups, including primary care physicians and specialists, nurses, physician assistants, health educators, medical clinics, professional medical societies, and public health personnel, provide care and assistance to those with thyroid diseases. Therefore, a discussion of some of the more common, controversial, or challenging issues in thyroid practice should be of great use to those of us who provide thyroid care. This section, devoted to thyroid disorders, is developed by renowned experts and offers a state-of-the-art update on many management issues important to the care of thyroid patients.

Iodine deficiency is arguably the most common global thyroid problem. Consequences of iodine deficiency include endemic goiter, physical and mental retardation, cretinism, hypothyroidism, and poor outcomes in pregnancy, generally referred to as *iodine deficiency disorders* (IDD). Dietary iodine is essential for production of thyroid hormones, and in 1952 WHO recommended iodization of all food salts in iodine-deficient regions. Sadly, by 1980, WHO estimated that anywhere from 20% to 60% of the world population was still iodine-deficient (1). The United States has been considered iodine-sufficient in the past 100 years, although recent data suggest that pregnant women may be mildly iodine deficient. A recent review concluded that "Iodine-deficiency remains a significant health problem worldwide and affects both industrialized and developing countries" (2).

Autoimmune thyroiditis is another common thyroid problem with an approximate global prevalence of around 0.8%. It is estimated that 10% of most populations have antithyroid antibodies, and 40%–50% of women, and 20% of men, have focal thyroiditis. Hashimoto thyroiditis, which occurs mostly in women, is the most common cause of diffuse goiter and hypothyroidism in the United States. Typically, goiter is diffuse, nontender, and firm. Diagnosis is confirmed by positive antithyroid antibodies, characteristic appearance on ultrasound, and occasionally, by cytologic analysis. For patients with elevated thyroid-stimulating hormone (TSH) and/or goiter, thyroxine (T_4) therapy is prescribed.

In recent years, special attention has been paid to thyroid problems in pregnancy (3,4). Adequate iodine intake is critical in pregnancy, because it influences normal fetal development. New trimester-specific ranges are recommended for serum TSH levels in pregnancy. Subclinical hypothyroidism is common in pregnancy and diagnosed in approximately 2.5% of pregnancies. The issue of screening for thyroid function in pregnancy, however, remains a subject of debate. Current guidelines suggest "aggressive case-finding," rather than universal screening, for women planning pregnancy. Postpartum thyroiditis, another form of autoimmune thyroid disease, has a worldwide prevalence of 7.5%. It represents thyroid dysfunction within 1 year following delivery.

The typical course is one of transient hyperthyroidism, followed by hypothyroidism, with the majority of women reverting to a euthyroid state by the end of the postpartum year.

Another common and controversial clinical problem is subclinical thyroid disease, which is essentially a biochemical diagnosis. Subclinical hyperthyroidism is defined by a low TSH with normal free thyroxine (FT_4) and triiodothyronine (T_3) levels; in subclinical hypothyroidism TSH is mildly elevated with normal FT_4. Both subclinical hypo- and hyperthyroidism can be associated with morbidity, and some studies show increased mortality as well. Screening is the only effective way to diagnose these conditions early, but in the absence of controlled, randomized trials, hot debate continues on the need for screening as well as the benefits of treatment in some patients (5).

Graves' disease (GD) is the most common cause of hyperthyroidism in iodine-sufficient parts of the world; management options include antithyroid drug therapy, radioiodine, or surgical thyroidectomy. Treatment should be individualized, based on patient and physician preferences, as well as the availability of resources. Graves' ophthalmopathy is an uncommon but difficult-to-manage complication of GD. Recent reports have looked at the risk-benefit ratio for different treatment modalities, including selenium, glucocorticoids, rituximab, and surgical intervention.

Another very common clinical problem is nodular thyroid disease (NTD) with an incidence of 0.1% and a prevalence of 5%–7% by palpation, but 50%–70% by sonographic examination (6). NTD is more common in women, in the elderly, with iodine deficiency, and in populations exposed to radiation. According to a WHO report, goiter prevalence between 1993 and 2004 increased by 81% in Africa, 80% in Europe, and 63% in the eastern Mediterranean countries. Although nodules are common, they are commonly benign. Recent data show that worldwide, the incidence of thyroid cancer has increased in the past 50 years. In the United States, for example, the incidence of thyroid cancer has increased 3-fold, from 3.6 cases in 1973 to 11.6 per 100,000 in 2002 (7). It seems that this increase is most likely due to widespread use of imaging and thyroid fine-needle aspiration biopsy (FNA) in thyroid practice. Despite this significant increase in prevalence, mortality remains stable.

One should also talk about disease prevention. Disease prevention may take many forms, including public programs directed at decreasing risks for disease in healthy populations (primary prevention), early detection of disease particularly through screening programs (secondary prevention), and prevention of complications from overt disease (tertiary prevention). Primary prevention in thyroid disease includes maintaining adequate iodine intake and abstinence from tobacco use. Secondary prevention involves detection of early or mild disease, generally through screening programs. On this subject, there is considerable difference in criteria to justify screening and recommendations for screening by major professional societies. For example, an area of controversy is screening for subclinical hyper- and hypothyroidism. One form of thyroid screening that is widely accepted and practiced is screening for congenital hypothyroidism (CH), a problem that occurs in 1 out of 3,000 newborns worldwide. Screening for CH detects 6,000 cases per year, and early, adequate treatment avoids irreversible physical and mental retardation. Tertiary prevention is treatment of established disease to avoid complications. These measures are discussed in great detail in the following chapters in this section.

In summary, in order to help our patients with thyroid disorders, we should continue to improve iodine nutritional status; design studies to determine whether screening for thyroid disease, or treatment of subclinical disease, improves outcomes; develop cost-effective screening programs to detect early disease; encourage health care delivery teams to provide appropriate treatment for hypo- and hyperthyroidism; and promote public education through awareness campaigns and educational materials.

ACKNOWLEDGMENTS

The author has nothing to disclose.

REFERENCES

1. **Zimmerman MB.** Iodine deficiency and excess in children: worldwide status in 2013. *Endocr Pract.* 2013;19:839–846.
2. **Pearce EN, Andersson M, Zimmerman MB.** Global iodine nutrition: where do we stand in 2013? *Thyroid.* 2013;23:523–528.
3. **Stagnaro-Green A, Abalovich M, Alexander E, et al.** Guidelines of the American Thyroid Association for the diagnosis and management of thyroid dysfunction during pregnancy and the postpartum. *Thyroid.* 2011;21:1–45.
4. **De Groot L, Abalovich M, Alexander EK, et al.** Management of thyroid dysfunction during pregnancy and postpartum: an Endocrine Society Clinical Practice Guideline. *J Clin Endocrinol Metab.* 2012;97: 2543–2565.
5. **Cooper DS, Biondi B.** Subclinical thyroid disease. *Lancet.* 2012;379:1142–1154.
6. **Gharib H, Papini E.** Thyroid nodules: clinical importance, assessment, and treatment. *Endocrinol Metabol Clin North Am.* 2007;36:707–735.
7. **Brito JP, Morris JM, Montori VM.** Thyroid cancer: zealous imaging has increased detection and treatment of low-risk tumours. *BMJ.* 2013;347:14706.

CHAPTER 10

Myxedema Coma

Natasha Kasid and James V Hennessey

ABSTRACT

Myxedema coma is a decompensated state of hypothyroidism resulting from severe and prolonged depletion of thyroid hormones, leading to altered mental status and other clinical features related to widespread multiorgan dysfunction. Although this is a rare condition on the spectrum of thyroid disorders, myxedema coma is considered an endocrine emergency due to the danger of increased mortality, with recent rates of 20%–25% reported. Therefore, it is important to recognize and treat myxedema coma promptly in an attempt to improve outcomes.

INTRODUCTION

Myxedema coma is a decompensated state of hypothyroidism resulting from severe and prolonged depletion of thyroid hormones, leading to altered mental status and other clinical features related to widespread multiorgan dysfunction. In 1877, the term myxedema was first used by William Miller Ord after Sir William Withey Gull correlated this presentation with atrophy of the thyroid gland (1). The term myxedema coma is misleading given that most patients are merely obtunded, but not as frequently in a true state of coma. In 1953, the term myxedema coma was used in conjunction with fatal outcomes of 4 cases where coma was noted in patients in the setting of typical manifestations of myxedema (2).

Although this is a rare condition on the spectrum of thyroid disorders, with a reported incidence rate of 0.22/million/year and an estimated 300 or more reported cases in the medical literature (3,4), myxedema coma is considered an endocrine emergency due to the danger of mortality, with 60%–80% rates reported in the older literature and 20%–25% reported more recently (3,5,6). Therefore, it is important to recognize and treat myxedema coma promptly in an attempt to improve outcomes.

PATHOPHYSIOLOGY

In the setting of untreated hypothyroidism (both primary and central), after discontinuation of L-thyroxine (LT_4) therapy, or eventually following a total thyroidectomy, there will be an obligatory reduction in intracellular triiodothyronine (T_3) that will interfere with maintenance of metabolic homeostasis (7). In this situation, myxedema coma can be induced by the additional presence of common inciting factors, such as infections like urosepsis or pneumonia, or conditions such as heart failure, exposure to a cold environment, trauma, surgery, cerebrovascular accidents, or gastrointestinal bleeding (7–9). Medications that often have been implicated in precipitating myxedema coma are anesthetics, sedatives, narcotics, lithium, amiodarone, sunitinib, and phenytoin (7).

In terms of neurological dysfunction, patients can present with severe hypothermia described as core temperatures <90°F (32.2°C) or can be afebrile in the setting of an underlying infectious process (9). Altered mental status in myxedema coma is caused by underlying cerebral tissue hypothyroidism as well as multiple mechanisms such as decreased cerebral blood flow, hyponatremia, and hypoxemia. These can also lower the threshold for precipitation of seizures in the setting of myxedema coma (7,8). Besides memory impairment, dysarthria, and seizures, sensory and motor peripheral neuropathy have also been noted in this severe state of hypothyroidism (10).

Due to the innate cardiovascular-related compensatory mechanisms in the setting of reduced availability of thyroid hormone, one can develop diastolic dysfunction and peripheral vasoconstriction, which together may result in a reduction of circulating blood volume (11). Further, primary cardiac pump function is directly compromised due to the predictable onset of decreased cardiac inotropy, which may result in cardiomegaly and negative chronotropy resulting in bradycardia. Nonspecific electrocardiographic (ECG) findings are seen, which on further disruption of cardiac rhythm may also include sustained ventricular tachycardia and torsades de pointes in a severely hypothyroid state (12). Therefore, low cardiac output and hypotension can precipitate cardiogenic shock (7,8). Not only can accumulation of mucopolysaccharides and water result in pericardial effusions reducing the amplitude of electrical activity and causing electrical alternans on the ECG and obscuring ischemic findings, but they may also result in cardiac tamponade physiology (13). Other ECG findings include the presence of a J wave if hypothermia is present.

Hypoventilation occurs in the setting of altered respiratory sensitivity to hypoxia and hypercapnia, as well as in reduced respiratory drive. In addition, there is respiratory muscle dysfunction, which further impairs ventilation (7,9). It has been noted in patients with even milder forms of hypothyroidism, compared to controls, that a higher prevalence of cough, sputum production, and airway inflammation may be observed (14). In addition, an underlying anatomical process in the setting of infection or a manifestation of hypothyroidism such as pleural effusions or macroglossia can further interfere with lung volume or airway size (9,13). There is a report of neuropathic oropharyngeal dysphagia that can contribute to aspiration and further respiratory impairment (10).

In myxedema coma, the glomerular filtration rate and renal blood flow are reduced as would be expected in the hypothyroid patient (15). The occurrence of hyponatremia is based upon a diminished capacity to clear a free water load, which is a consequence of the combined effects of lower renal perfusion and the presence of elevated antidiuretic hormone levels (8,9,16,17). Due to the potential of simultaneous adrenal insufficiency and impaired gluconeogenesis, hypoglycemia can occur (7). Reduced intestinal motility has also been observed, which may result in symptoms of upper and lower gastrointestinal distress and reduced absorptive efficiency contributing to paralytic ileus with abdominal distention (8,18,19).

CLINICAL MANIFESTATIONS

One may document the typical features of hypothyroidism preceding the presentation of myxedema coma, including fatigue, weight gain, cold intolerance, and constipation, as well as cool and dry skin. In addition, brittle nails, macroglossia, hoarse voice, muscle cramps, menstrual disturbances, periorbital and nonpitting edema, or delayed deep tendon reflexes may be observed. The clinician should be especially alert to the presence of a goiter, thyroidectomy scar, or history of I^{131} treatment (7,8,20). Myxedema coma is 8-fold more common in women compared with men, and is a frequent cause of hospitalization among women over 60 years of age for a diagnosis of hypothyroidism (4,17). As a consequence of this gender difference, most cases of myxedema coma occur during the winter months in women (11).

The changes in mental status observed are along the spectrum of psychomotor slowing, deficits in impaired memory, confusion, depression, visuoperceptual skills, paranoia, hallucinations ("myxedema madness"), or dementia (8,17). One may also identify large and small fiber polyneuropathy (8). Hypothermia can be as extreme as temperatures <80°F (26.6°C) (9), or patients with obvious infections can be afebrile (11). In the setting of accumulation of pericardial and pleural effusions, patients may report progressive dyspnea. With regard to signs of hemodynamic impairment, one may note bradycardia and hypotension when cardiac function is compromised. In the setting of pericardial effusion leading to cardiac tamponade, it is important to evaluate for physical signs such as jugular venous distention, muffled heart sounds, pulsus paradoxus, low-voltage QRS complexes, electrical alternans, and tachycardia (9). Respiratory dysfunction may be frequently encountered, with up to 80% demonstrating hypoxia and over half having documented hypercapnia (21). In addition to abdominal pain, nausea, and constipation, patients with myxedema coma can develop paralytic ileus and toxic megacolon (7).

DIAGNOSIS

The diagnosis of myxedema coma is made by recognizing the clinical presentation consistent with a change in mental status, hypothermia, hypotension, and clinical signs and symptoms of hypothyroidism (7,20). In addition, the history from family members can reveal a diagnosis of hypothyroidism or past radioiodine therapy in patients with marked mental status changes. When this pattern of findings is identified, it is important to document the potential thyroid etiology biochemically and search for a nonthyroidal precipitating cause. However, treatment should not be withheld pending the results of further evaluation if this endocrine emergency is suspected.

The following laboratory studies should be obtained prior to the initiation of pharmacologic treatment: thyroid-stimulating hormone (TSH), free thyroxine (fT_4), a free thyroxine index using total T_4 (TT_4) and T_3 resin uptake, a complete (full) blood count, and chemistry panel. Evaluation of potential sources of infection with chest X-ray, urine studies, and blood cultures is also needed. In the setting of potential myocardial infarction precipitating the crisis, cardiac enzymes should be obtained (7). An elevated TSH will distinguish primary from secondary or tertiary hypothyroidism, in which TSH is normal or low (20). Moreover, TSH may not be as elevated in the setting of nonthyroidal illness (NTI) or when the patient is exposed to glucocorticoids or dopamine. However, it is important to recognize that reduced TT_3 and increased reverse T_3 levels (if obtained) may be observed in the setting of NTI without thyroid dysfunction, but both would be low in a hypothyroid patient with myxedema coma, limiting the clinical utility of these T_3 determinations. Given the risk for coexistent adrenal insufficiency in either polyendocrine failure syndrome or a central hypothyroidism, the collection of a serum cortisol level is essential with the baseline laboratory assessment (17). A short ACTH stimulation test should also be performed under these circumstances.

As mentioned previously, laboratory analysis can reveal hyponatremia, normocytic anemia, elevated lactate dehydrogenase, elevated aspartate transaminase (AST), elevated low-density lipoprotein (LDL) cholesterol, elevated creatine kinase, and hypoglycemia, which if observed should alert the clinician to potential pituitary-adrenal dysfunction (7,8,11,17). An ECG could identify bradycardia, nonspecific ST-T wave changes, and/or a prolonged QT interval (7). A baseline ECG prior to initiation of treatment is important because thyroid replacement can precipitate an acute coronary syndrome. A chest X-ray would be important to evaluate for a potential source of underlying infection as well as the presence of an enlarged cardiac silhouette. A cardiac echo should be obtained to differentiate a dilated cardiomyopathy from the presence of a pericardial effusion (9).

A lumbar puncture, if performed to evaluate the etiology of altered mental status, would note an increase in intracranial pressure and protein. Electroencephalography (EEG) may note low amplitude or a decrease of alpha wave activity with seizure activity that often is related to the presence of accompanying hyponatremia, hypoglycemia, or hypoxemia (17).

MANAGEMENT

In a critical care setting, hypoventilation and hypercapnia, as well as airway protection in the setting of a reduced Glasgow Coma Scale (GCS), are indications for immediate ventilator support (7,8,17). Given that hypotension and hemodynamic strain may be present, careful volume resuscitation with normal saline is recommended while balancing considerations for the management of concomitant hyponatremia (7,8). Dopamine should be considered if fluid resuscitation does not restore circulatory stability (22). Additionally, the presence of refractory hypotension may also be due to adrenal insufficiency, which was discussed previously. Consequently, hyponatremia management may not respond until the initiation of glucocorticoids as outlined in the next paragraph (22). For hypothermia, it is recommended to provide gentle warming with blankets, but to avoid excessive rapid external warming because this may lead to peripheral vasodilatation and potentially to cardiovascular collapse. Alternatively, careful central warming may be attempted (11,17,22).

Given the uncommon risk for coexistent adrenal insufficiency (occurs 5%–10%) in either the setting of polyendocrine failure syndrome or a secondary hypothyroidism, it is important to obtain a baseline assessment of cortisol prior to providing stress dose steroids, which should always be given before the administration of thyroid replacement. An adrenal crisis may be precipitated by the initiation of LT_4 as cortisol clearance is accelerated by the thyroid hormone. Hydrocortisone 50–100 mg intravenously (IV) every 6–8 hours should be administered for up to 7–10 days or until hemodynamically stable, followed by a taper if adrenal insufficiency is not present (7,17). Due to the frequency with which infections have been reported to result in death in the setting of myxedema coma, it has been recommended that a vigorous search for infectious precipitation of the crisis be pursued, with specific antimicrobial intervention being initiated when evidence of infection is present (9).

It is reported that the equivalent of 90 mcg of LT_4 is produced daily in healthy subjects (5). In the setting of primary hypothyroidism and myxedema coma a larger dose of LT_4 is required to make up for the deficit and saturate the excessive binding capacity that is present (5). Differences of opinion persist as to the best approach in replacing the circulating thyroid hormone levels. Some have advocated utilizing LT_4 only, emphasizing the safety of administering the prohormone, which would be activated gradually by peripheral metabolism of LT_4. When using LT_4 alone, it is suggested to initiate it quickly with an IV bolus of 300–600 mcg (4 mcg/kg lean body weight). Subsequently, 50–100 mcg (PO, nasogastric, or IV) should be given daily (8,9,11,17). Intravenous and oral routes appeared to have similar survival outcomes in a recently reported retrospective series (6).

Due to the decrease in T_3 and a potential delay in T_4 to T_3 conversion secondary to underlying NTI, a small amount of liothyronine (LT_3) can be given simultaneously. However, there are limited data demonstrating efficacy of this intervention. Suggested doses have ranged from 2.5 mcg given orally (or via nasogastric tube) at the same time that LT_4 is initiated, to doses as high as 25 mcg IV every 12 hours until stabilization of the cardiovascular system or 48 hours have passed (22). It has been suggested that the use of LT_3 would not be favored in patients with a history of coronary artery disease because it may cause increased oxygen consumption and could lead to an acute coronary syndrome (21). More recently, a middle ground has been suggested to administer 10 mcg IV of LT_3 every 8–12 hours until the patient recovers enough to adequately continue receiving monotherapy with oral LT_4 (9). Another approach is to consider LT_3 therapy if clinical status is not improved after 24–48 hours of LT_4 therapy alone (9,11). There are no prospective studies comparing outcomes with these different replacement regimens.

In the setting of severe hyponatremia (105–120 mEq/L [105–120 mmol/L]), one can administer 3% sodium chloride to achieve a modest increase in sodium level. However, it is very important to not correct sodium more than 10–12 mEq/L (10–12 mmol/L) in 24 hours and 18 mEq/L (18 mmol/L) in 48 hours to avoid precipitating central pontine myelinolysis (7,17) (Table 10-2).

PROGNOSIS

As previously noted, mortality rates as high as 25% have been reported in the contemporary literature (16,21). Smaller series have highlighted several factors associated with mortality in those diagnosed with myxedema coma (Table 10-3). Historically, coma has been cited as a poor prognostic factor, while survivors have been noted to be younger, have higher GCS scores, and lower Acute Physiology and Chronic Health Evaluation II (APACHE II) scores (3). Others have had associated higher mortality rates in myxedema coma among

Table 10-1. Aspects to Initial Evaluation

	Underlying Mechanisms	Initial Evaluation
Etiology	Primary vs. secondary vs. tertiary hypothyroidism	TSH, fT_4, total T_4, T_3 resin uptake
Precipitating causes	Infectious origin, gastrointestinal bleeding, metabolic derangements	Complete (full) blood count, blood and urine cultures, chest X-ray, cortisol, cardiac enzymes, and complete history of medications patient is taking
Downstream manifestations	Hyponatremia, hypoglycemia, elevated AST, elevated LDL, elevated creatine kinase, multiorgan failure, and neurological manifestations	Chemistry panel, liver function tests, and cardiac echo

Table 10-2. Approach to the Management of Myxedema Coma

	Evaluation	Intervention
Respiratory	• Ability to maintain airway protection in setting of altered mental status in setting of reduced Glasgow Coma Scale (GCS) • Hypoxemia and hypercapnia	Arterial blood gas
		Intubation
Cardiovascular	• Hypotension • Bradycardia • Cardiomegaly • Pericardial effusions	Volume resuscitation with normal saline
		Dopamine or other vasopressor
		ECG: bradycardia, prolonged QT interval
		Cardiac echo
		Glucocorticoids in setting of refractory hypotension
Hypothermia	• Temperature <90°F (32.2°C) • Evaluate for underlying infection	External warming with blankets
		Empiric antibiotics in setting of suspected infection
Thyroid hormone replacement	• Primary: Elevated TSH with low fT_4 • Secondary: Low or normal TSH with low fT_4 • Tertiary: Low TSH and low fT_4	Obtain baseline cortisol levels (consider short ACTH stimulation test)
		Hydrocortisone 50–100 mg IV q6–8h followed by LT_4 bolus 300–600 mcg IV
		Then, LT_4 50–100 mcg PO or IV daily
		Consider LT_3 2.5–25 mcg IV or PO daily with concomtant LT_4 initiation
Hyponatremia	• Monitor sodium closely	If <120 mEq/L (120 mmol/L), consider adminstering 3% sodium chloride, avoid increasing sodium more than 10–12 mEq/l (10–12 mmol/L) in 24 hours

those with infections, especially of the pulmonary system due to aspiration and resulting in respiratory failure (9). In the study of Dutta et al (6), 23 patients observed over a 7-year period had a 52.2% mortality rate with causes of death noted to be sepsis, respiratory failure, and upper gastrointestinal bleed. It was noted that less favorable outcomes occurred with the presence of hypotension, bradycardia, sepsis, use of mechanical ventilation, unresolved hypothermia despite intervention, and history of sedative drug use (6). With respect to the comparison of APACHE II score, GCS score, and the Sequential Organ Failure Assessment (SOFA) score in the accuracy of predicting outcome, Dutta and colleagues concluded a high SOFA score more accurately predicted a higher mortality rate (Table 10-3) (6).

CONCLUSIONS

As summarized in Table 10-1, myxedema coma is a rare but life-threatening condition. It is often seen in the elderly population and

Table 10-3. Prognostic Factors

Favorable Prognosis	Unfavorable Prognosis
Higher GCS score	Elderly
Lower APACHE II score	Associated respiratory infections
	Sepsis
	Upper gastrointestinal bleed
	Hypotension
	Bradycardia
	Use of mechanical ventilation
	Unresolved hypothermia
	History of sedative drug use
	Higher SOFA score

Compiled from Rodriguez et al (2004), Wartofsky (2013), and Dutta et al (2008).

precipitated by several factors in the setting of preexisting hypothyroidism. Over time, the mortality rate has improved from 60%–70% to 20%–25%, which has been attributed to better awareness and more aggressive interventions. Prognosis is less favorable in the elderly, and in the settings of prolonged hypothermia, bradycardia, or lower level of consciousness (17). More specifically, hypotension, bradycardia, sepsis, use of mechanical ventilation, unresolved hypothermia despite intervention, and a history of sedative drug use are factors associated with poor prognosis, and along with a high SOFA score, have correlated with a higher mortality rate (6). Treatment involves administration of hydrocortisone, LT_4, and consideration of LT_3 use, as well as general medical and cardiopulmonary support as needed.

ACKNOWLEDGMENTS

The authors have nothing to disclose.

REFERENCES

1. **Pearce JMS.** Myxoedema and Sir William Withey Gull (1816–1890). *J Neurol Neurosurg Psychiatry.* 2006;77:639.
2. **Summers VK.** Myxoedema coma. *BMJ.* 1953;2:366–368.
3. **Rodriguez I, Fluiters E, Perez-Mendez LF, Luna R, Paramo I, Garcia-Mayor RV.** Factors associated with mortality of patients with myxedema coma: prospective study in 11 cases treated in a single institution. *J Endocrinol.* 2004;180:347–350.
4. **Wartofsky L.** Myxedema coma. *Endocrinol Metab Clin N Am.* 2006;35:687–698.
5. **Arlot S, Debussche X, Lalau J-D, et al.** Myxoedema coma: response of thyroid hormones with oral and intravenous high-dose L-thyroxine treatment. *Intensive Care Med.* 1991;17:16–18.
6. **Dutta P, Bhanasali A, Masoodi SR, Bhadada S, Sharma N, Rajput R.** Predictors of outcome in myxedema coma: a study from a tertiary care centre. *Crit Care.* 2008;12:R1.
7. **Mathew V, Misgar RA, Ghosh S, et al.** Myxedema coma: a new look into an old crisis. *J Thyroid Res.* 2011:1–7.
8. **Yu CHY, Stoval R, Fox S.** Chorea—an unusual manifestation in a woman recovering from myxedema coma. *Endoc Pract.* 2012;18:e43–e48.
9. **Wartofsky L.** Myxedema coma. In: Braverman LE, Cooper CS, eds. *Werner and Ingbar's The Thyroid: A Fundamental and Clinical Text.* 10th ed. Philadelphia, PA: Wolters Kluwer Health; 2013:600–605.
10. **Urquhart AD, Rea IM, Lawson LT, Skipper M.** A new complication of hypothyroid coma: neurogenic dysphagia: presentation, diagnosis, and treatment. *Thyroid.* 2001;11:595–598.
11. **Wiersinga WM.** Myxedema coma. In: Jameson JL, DeGroot LJ, eds. *Endocrinology: Adult and Pediatric.* 6th ed. Philadelphia, PA: Saunders Elsevier; 2010: 1618–1619.
12. **Schenck JB, Rizvi AA, Lin T.** Severe primary hypothyroidism manifesting with torsades de pointes. *Am J Med Sci.* 2006;331:154–156.
13. **Parving H, Hansen JM, Nielsen SL, Rossing N, Munck O, Lassen NA.** Mechanisms of edema formation in myxedema-increased protein extravasation and relatively slow lymphatic drainage. *N Engl J Med.* 1979;301:460–465.
14. **Birring SS, Patel RB, Parker D, et al.** Airway function and markers of airway inflammation in patients with treated hypothyroidism. *Thorax.* 2005;60:249–253.
15. **Kreisman SH, Hennessey JV.** Consistent reversible elevations of serum creatinine levels in severe hypothyroidism. *Arch Intern Med.* 1999;159:79–82.
16. **Fliers E, Wiersinga WM.** Myxedema coma. *Rev Endocrin Metab Dis.* 2003;4:137–141.
17. **Klubo-Gwiezdzinska J, Wartofsky L.** Thyroid emergencies. *Med Clin N Am.* 2012;96:385–403.
18. **Ji JS, Chae HS, Cho YS, et al.** Myxedema ascites: case report and literature review. *J Korean Med Sci.* 2006;21:761–764.
19. **Chadha JS, Ashby DW, Cowan WK.** Fatal intestinal atony in myxoedema. *BMJ.* 1969;3:398.
20. **Hamburger S, Collier RE.** Myxedema coma. *Ann Emerg Med.* 1982;11:156–159.
21. **Reinhardt W, Mann K.** Incidence, clinical picture and treatment of hypothyroid coma. Results of a survey. *Med Klin (Munich).* 1997;92:521–524.
22. **Wiersinga WM.** Myxedema coma. L.J. DeGroot, ed. Thyroid Manager. http://www.thyroidmanager.org. Updated December 12, 2013.

CHAPTER 11

Life-Threatening Thyrotoxicosis

Thyroid Storm and Adverse Effects of Antithyroid Drugs

Alicia L Warnock, David S Cooper, and Henry B Burch

ABSTRACT

Thyroid storm is a dreaded, fortunately rare complication of a very common disorder. Many cases of thyroid storm occur after a precipitating event, intercurrent illness, or discontinuation of antithyroid drug therapy, frequently after the development of an adverse drug reaction. Effective management is predicated on a prompt recognition of impending thyroid storm, which is, in turn, dependent on knowledge of both the typical and atypical presentations of this disorder. An unwavering commitment to an aggressive multifaceted therapeutic intervention is critical to obtaining a satisfactory outcome. A summary of serious adverse effects associated with thionamide therapy is also included in this chapter.

INTRODUCTION

The spectrum of thyrotoxicosis ranges from asymptomatic subclinical disease to a life-threatening metabolic crisis characterized by multisystem dysfunction and high mortality. A number of factors determine where on this continuum a thyrotoxic individual presents, including patient age, the presence of comorbidities, the rapidity of onset of thyroid hormone excess, and the presence or absence of a precipitating event (1). Thyroid storm (or crisis) is triggered when the cumulative effect of these factors surpasses an individual patient's ability to maintain adequate metabolic, thermoregulatory, and cardiovascular compensatory mechanisms (1). The high morbidity and mortality associated with thyroid storm requires both early recognition and a steadfast commitment to an aggressive multifaceted therapeutic intervention. Because abrupt discontinuation of antithyroid drugs is a common precipitant of thyroid storm, and because the highest doses of antithyroid drugs (ATDs) are used to treat this disorder, a summary of adverse effects associated with thionamide therapy is included in this chapter.

CLINICAL PRESENTATION

General Features

The clinical features seen in uncomplicated thyrotoxicosis are generally present and accentuated in thyroid storm (Table 11-1). The heat intolerance and diaphoresis common in simple thyrotoxicosis are often manifested in thyroid storm as moderate-to-severe hyperpyrexia with large insensible fluid losses as temperatures frequently exceed 104°–106°F (40°–41°C) (2–4). Cardiovascular findings of sinus tachycardia in uncomplicated thyrotoxicosis become accelerated tachycardia in thyroid storm, with a high propensity for atrial

Table 11-1. Comparison of Clinical Features of Uncomplicated Thyrotoxicosis to Thyroid Storm

Clinical Feature	Uncomplicated Thyrotoxicosis	Thyroid Storm
Thermoregulatory	Heat intolerance, diaphoresis	Hyperpyrexia, large insensible fluid losses
Nervous system	Hyperkinesis, nervousness	Confusion, seizure, coma
Cardiovascular	Tachycardia (90–120 bpm)	Accelerated tachycardia (>130 bpm), atrial dysrhythmia, heart failure
Gastrointestinal	Hyperdefecation	Nausea, vomiting, diarrhea
Hepatic	Mild transaminase elevation	Hepatic dysfunction, jaundice
Psychiatric	Agitation, emotional lability	Psychosis
Precipitant history	Absent	Present
Death	Rare	Frequent (10%–20%)

dysrhythmia (3) and varying degrees of ventricular dysfunction and congestive heart failure (1). Anxiety and restlessness are extended in thyroid storm to severe agitation, delirium, or frank psychosis, progressing in some patients to stupor and coma (2,5–7). Gastrointestinal and hepatic involvement, limited to enhanced intestinal transport and mild transaminase elevation in simple thyrotoxicosis, may dominate the presentation in thyroid storm, with nausea, vomiting, frank diarrhea, and marked hepatocellular dysfunction with jaundice (1).

Although not universally present or recognized, a key clinical feature in thyroid storm is the presence of a precipitating event or intercurrent illness. Thyroid surgery, once the most common precipitant of thyroid storm, has become a relatively rare cause of this disorder (4). This is largely attributable to the current practice of rendering the thyrotoxic patient euthyroid before surgery as well as a decrease in the number of patients undergoing surgery for Graves' disease (8), owing to the popularity of radioiodine ablation therapy for hyperthyroidism (8). However, nonthyroidal surgery in patients with unrecognized thyrotoxicosis continues to act as a surgical precipitant of thyroid storm (9,10). A recent survey-based summary of thyroid storm cases in Japan found abrupt withdrawal of antithyroid drugs to be the single most commonly recognized precipitant (4). Sadly, poor access to medical care has also been implicated as a cause of thyroid storm (11). A list of known triggers or precipitants of thyroid storm is shown in Table 11-2. These can be grouped into those conditions characterized by a rapid rise in circulating thyroid hormone levels, and those associated with an underlying acute or subacute nonthyroidal illness.

Recognition of Thyroid Storm: Diagnostic Criteria

A common theme in early reported series of thyroid storm patients was a rapid downward spiral culminating in death within hours to days of onset (1,12). The most important determinants of survival in life-threatening thyrotoxicosis are early recognition and institution of appropriate therapy. Yet, diagnostic efforts are often frustrated on multiple levels. Laboratory parameters have little value in distinguishing uncomplicated thyrotoxicosis from thyroid storm owing to extensive overlap in circulating thyroid hormone levels between these two categories (4,13,14). In addition, diagnostic criteria for thyroid storm have historically been far from uniform (12,15). Based on these difficulties, a diagnostic point scale was proposed by Burch and Wartofsky in 1993 for distinguishing uncomplicated thyrotoxicosis from impending or established thyroid storm (Table 11-3). The Burch-Wartofsky Point Scale (BWPS) is an empirically derived system taking into account 3 principal observations in patients with thyroid storm, including (1) the continuum of end organ dysfunction; (2) the high variability of individual patient presentation; and (3) the high mortality associated with a missed diagnosis.

In 2012, Akamizu and colleagues reported on 356 patients with definite or possible thyroid storm over a 5-year period in Japan (4), collected from survey-elicited cases in

Table 11-2. Precipitants or Triggers of Thyroid Storm

Conditions Associated with a Rapid Rise in Thyroid Hormone Levels
Withdrawal of antithyroid drugs
Radioiodine therapy
External beam radiation therapy
Thyroid "poisoning" (overdose of thyroid hormone)
Vigorous thyroid palpation
Iodinated contrast dyes
Thyroid bed trauma
Thyroid surgery
Conditions Associated with an Acute or Subacute Nonthyroidal Illness
Nonthyroidal surgery
Infection
Cerebrovascular accident
Pulmonary thromboembolism
Parturition
Diabetic ketoacidosis
Emotional stress

large (>500 bed) hospitals, university-affiliated hospitals, and a random subset of smaller Japanese hospitals. This retrospective, questionnaire-based report provides a wealth of new clinical information pertaining to thyroid storm. Like the BWPS, the authors empirically derived diagnostic criteria for thyroid storm, based on literature review (Table 11-4). Application of these criteria to reported cases of thyroid storm in Japan led to the inclusion of 1 additional criterion, a serum of bilirubin >3 mg/dL (51 μmol/L), to signify gastrointestinal/hepatic involvement. The final criteria were referred to as the Japanese Thyroid Association (JTA) criteria for thyroid storm (4). Akamizu and colleagues provide data that allow a comparison of the JTA criteria to the BWPS for the selection of patients for treatment of impending or established thyroid storm. Assuming patients with a diagnosis of thyroid storm or impending/possible thyroid storm will receive aggressive therapy, it is apparent that among 406 patients the authors considered for a diagnosis of thyroid storm, 354 would receive therapy using both systems, 41 would receive therapy using the BWPS but not the JTA system, 2 would receive therapy based on JTA criteria but not the BWPS, and

Table 11-3. Burch-Wartofsky Point Scale for Diagnosis of Thyroid Storm

Clinical Feature	Scoring Points
Thermoregulatory dysfunction	
Temperature, °F (°C)	
<99 (37.2)	0
99–99.9 (37.2–37.7)	5
100–100.9 (37.8–38.2)	10
101–101.9 (38.3–38.8)	15
102–102.9 (38.9–39.4)	20
103–103.9 (39.5–39.9)	25
≥104 (40)	30
Cardiovascular dysfunction	
Tachycardia (beats per minute)	
<90	0
90–109	5
110–119	10
120–129	15
130–139	20
≥140	25
Congestive heart failure	
Absent	0
Mild (Pedal edema)	5
Moderate (Bibasilar rales)	10
Severe (Pulmonary edema)	15
Atrial fibrillation	
Absent	0
Present	10
Central nervous system dysfunction	
Absent	0
Mild (agitation)	10
Moderate (delirium, psychosis, extreme lethargy)	20
Severe (seizures, coma)	30
Gastrointestinal-hepatic dysfunction	
Absent	0
Moderate (diarrhea, nausea/vomiting, abdominal pain)	10
Severe (jaundice)	20
Precipitant history	
Absent	0
Present	10
Total	
≥45	Highly likely thyroid storm
25–44	Suggestive of impending storm
<25	Unlikely to represent storm

Table 11-4. Japanese Thyroid Association Diagnostic Criteria for Thyroid Storm

Thyroid Storm		Possible Thyroid Storm	
Combination-1	**Combination-2**	**Combination-1**	**Combination-2**
□ Thyrotoxicosis	□ Thyrotoxicosis	□ Thyrotoxicosis	No T_4 or T_3 levels
and	*and*	*and*	*and*
□ CNS disturbance O Restlessness *or* O Delirium *or* O Mental aberration/psychosis *or* O Somnolence/lethargy	No CNS disturbance	No CNS disturbance	Meeting other criteria for thyroid storm
*and **one** other:*	*and **three** others:*	*and **two** others:*	
□ Fever ≥100.4°F (38°C)	□ Fever ≥100.4°F (38°C)	□ Fever ≥100.4°F (38° C)	
or	*and/or*	*and/or*	
□ Tachycardia ≥130 beats per minute	□ Tachycardia ≥130 beats per minute	□ Tachycardia ≥130 beats per minute	
or	*and/or*	*and/or*	
□ Congestive heart failure	□ Congestive heart failure	□ Congestive heart failure	
or	*and/or*	*and/or*	
□ Gastrointestinal/hepatic O Nausea *or* O Vomiting *or* O Diarrhea *or* O Bilirubin ≥3 mg/dL	□ Gastrointestinal/hepatic O Nausea *or* O Vomiting *or* O Diarrhea *or* O Bilirubin ≥3 mg/dL	□ Gastrointestinal/hepatic O Nausea *or* O Vomiting *or* O Diarrhea *or* O Bilirubin ≥3 mg/dL	

Exclusions and provisos: Cases are excluded if other underlying diseases are clearly causing any of the following symptoms: fever (eg, pneumonia and malignant hyperthermia), impaired consciousness (eg, psychiatric disorders and cerebrovascular disorders), heart failure (eg, acute myocardial infarction), and liver disorders (eg, viral hepatitis and acute liver failure). However, some of these disorders trigger thyroid storm. Therefore, it is difficult to determine whether the symptom is caused by thyroid storm or is simply a symptom of an underlying disease that is possibly triggered by thyroid storm; the symptom should be regarded as being due to a thyroid storm that is caused by these precipitating factors. Clinical judgment in this matter is required (4).

Adapted from Akamizu T, et al. Diagnostic criteria, clinical features, and incidence of thyroid storm based on nationwide surveys. Thyroid. *2012;22:661–679.*

9 would not receive therapy by either system (Table 11-5). Hence, although there is overall agreement between these 2 diagnostic systems, the BWPS appears to select a higher percentage of patients for aggressive therapy than the JTA system.

It is important to note that inappropriate application of either system can lead to misdiagnosis. For example, using the JTA system, a thyrotoxic patient with hyperkinesis and a temperature of 100.4° F (38° C) would meet diagnostic criteria for thyroid storm on the basis of "restlessness" and fever alone. This same patient would have a BWPS score of 20, making thyroid storm unlikely. Likewise, using the BWPS, a thyrotoxic patient with tachycardia of 120 and a temperature of 100.0° F (37.8° C) would qualify as impending thyroid storm, while using the JTA system this same patient would not meet either possible or definite thyroid storm criteria. These cases illustrate the importance of clinical judgment in assessing each individual patient.

Atypical Presentations of Thyroid Storm

Thyrotoxic storm has occasionally been described in patients with masked or "apathetic" hyperthyroidism (16). Although most

Table 11-5. Comparison of the Decision to Treat Using the BWPS or JTA Criteria for Thyroid Storm

		Burch-Wartofsky	
		No Treatment	**Treatment**
Japanese Thyroid Association	No treatment	9	41
	Treatment[a]	2	354

[a] *Assumes that patients with either thyroid storm or impending/possible thyroid storm will receive aggressive treatment for thyroid storm.*

Based on data from Akamizu T, et al. Diagnostic criteria, clinical features, and incidence of thyroid storm based on nationwide surveys. Thyroid. *2012;22:661–679.*

classically described in the elderly, apathetic hyperthyroidism presenting with thyroid storm has been described in all age groups, including pediatric patients. A literature review reported 14 cases of apathetic thyroid storm with patients most often being in their fourth to sixth decade (17). Additional reports have described thyroid crisis presenting initially as psychosis, coma (2,5,18), status epilepticus (6), and nonembolic cerebral infarction (19). Even less common presentations have included abdominal pain and fever in young women (20,21), small bowel obstruction (22), hypercalcemia (23), and acute renal failure resulting from rhabdomyolysis (24).

PATHOPHYSIOLOGY

The pathogenetic mechanisms underlying thyroid storm remain poorly understood. The rarity of this disorder and need for immediate therapeutic intervention, as well as the diversity of precipitants and presenting features, all contribute to this knowledge gap. Modern hypotheses regarding the pathogenesis of thyroid storm should incorporate advances in our understanding of thyroid hormone action at the cellular level. Further, clues to the pathogenesis of thyroid storm lie in the known precipitants of this disorder. Specifically, precipitants associated with a rapid increase in thyroid hormone levels suggest a sudden and overwhelming intracellular availability of free thyroid hormone, while those triggers related to intercurrent illness suggest that a diminished physiological reserve plays a central role. Both mechanisms cause a failure of normal homeostatic mechanisms, and ultimately lead to life-threatening systemic decompensation.

In patients with a rapid increase in circulating thyroid hormone, a transient saturation of plasma binding capacity sufficient to increase concentrations of unbound hormone could lead to increased transporter-mediated intracellular entry of free thyroid hormone. Support for this mechanism comes from observations of a prompt clinical response in patients with refractory life-threatening thyrotoxicosis after rapid normalization of circulating hormone levels through plasmapheresis or charcoal plasmaperfusion (25–27). In addition, the development of thyroid crisis following the acute ingestion of thyroid hormone has been well-documented in case reports, although this is not a typical outcome of accidental thyroid hormone overdose (1). Although an enhanced availability of free thyroid hormone for cellular entry would intuitively seem central in the development of thyroid storm, no clear distinction from uncomplicated thyrotoxicosis can be made based on absolute levels of circulating thyroid hormones, as has been recently confirmed (4). Conversely, a 1980 report revealed a significant elevation in free T_4 concentrations in 5 thyroid storm patients compared to a larger group with simple thyrotoxicosis, despite similar levels of total T_4 (28). In some instances of thyroid storm, disproportionate elevation of free thyroid hormone levels have occurred in the setting of only modest elevations in total T_4 and normal levels of total T_3 (1).

Additional mechanisms are likely operative in patients who develop thyroid storm during an underlying acute or subacute nonthyroidal illness. A decoupling of oxidative phosphorylation, leading to an enhanced rate of lipolysis, contributes to the heightened oxygen consumption and calorigenesis characteristic of these patients. Preferential production of thermal energy over adenosine triphosphate through this mechanism could also contribute to the hyperthermia seen in thyroid storm (29). A decreased hepatic and renal clearance of thyroid hormone during systemic illness (30) as well as enhanced generation of the metabolically active T_3 congener, triiodoacetic acid (TRIAC), have each been considered to be of possible pathophysiologic significance in patients whose thyroid storm is precipitated by a nonthyroidal illness (1). Lastly, an augmented tissue response to circulating thyroid hormone during nonthyroidal illness has been proposed as a potentiator of thyroid storm. Potential mechanisms for such activity could entail enhanced intracellular transport or nuclear entry of thyroid hormone, an alteration in binding to the nuclear receptor, or altered binding of the thyroid hormone-receptor complex to thyroid hormone response elements in target genes, though experimental evidence in support of this hypothesis is lacking.

Adrenergic system activation plays an important contributory role in the pathogenesis of both uncomplicated thyrotoxicosis and thyroid storm. Many of the clinical features of severe thyrotoxicosis, including agitation, tachycardia, dysrhythmia, and hyperthermia, are related to either direct catecholamine action or an interaction between the adrenergic system and excessive circulating thyroid hormone (31). Probably the best evidence for a significant role of the adrenergic system in this disorder is the dramatic clinical improvement afforded thyroid crisis patients following the addition of specific adrenergic blockade to the therapeutic regimen (1,32). However, a supporting rather than primary role of the adrenergic system is suggested by the observation that circulating levels of catecholamines are normal or low in thyroid storm (33). Furthermore, propranolol, even at high doses, does not prevent or ameliorate thyroid storm (34,35), and propranolol has no effect on thyroid hormone synthesis or release (36). The hyperadrenergic state seen both in thyrotoxicosis and thyroid storm may result from a thyroid hormone-mediated increase in beta-adrenergic receptor density on target cells, and postreceptor mechanisms (37), although this remains speculative.

Although the mechanisms underlying thyroid storm remain incompletely understood, important inferences can be derived from the available data. A dramatic increase in free hormone levels is likely a common denominator in the precipitation of thyroid storm. Additional factors, including poor nutrition and the complicating influences of medical, surgical, and emotional stresses on thyroid hormone binding, cellular uptake, metabolic clearance, and an individual patient's physiological reserve are other likely components.

TREATMENT

General Treatment Strategy

The treatment of impending or established thyroid storm is directed at each therapeutically accessible point in the thyroid hormone's synthetic, secretory, and peripheral action pathways. Concurrently, aggressive intervention is directed at reversal of ongoing or incipient decompensation of normal homeostatic mechanisms. The rigorous level of care, including continuous monitoring and minute-to-minute titration of therapy, mandates an intensive care setting for the early management of established thyroid storm. The therapeutic approach to thyroid storm may be grouped as (1) therapy directed against the thyroid; (2) antagonism of the peripheral actions of thyroid hormone; (3) reversal or prevention of systemic decompensation; (4) therapy directed at the precipitating event or intercurrent illness; and (5) definitive therapy. These will each be considered separately as outlined in Table 11-6.

Therapy directed against the thyroid gland. A nearly complete blockade of new hormone synthesis must be established early in the treatment course through the use of the ATDs propylthiouracil (PTU) or methimazole (MMI). PTU and MMI are thionamides thought to inhibit iodine organification, which is the binding of oxidized iodine to tyrosine residues in thyroglobulin, as well as the coupling of iodotyrosine residues to form the iodothyronine thyroid hormones T_4 and T_3 (18). Carbimazole (CBM) is rapidly metabolized to MMI, and can, therefore, be considered a prodrug for MMI, and is subject to the same dosing regimen and adverse effect profile as MMI. Blockade of iodine organification is established within an hour of administration of any of the ATDs. PTU has the advantage over MMI of decreasing the conversion of T_4 to T_3 (see section "Treatment Directed Against Peripheral Effects of Thyroid Hormone"). Because of this unique property, thyroid storm continues to be one of a few conditions in which PTU is used preferentially over the more potent MMI (38).

Neither PTU nor MMI are commercially available as parenteral formulations and are, therefore, generally given orally or per

Table 11-6. Management of Thyroid Storm

Treatment Directed Against the Thyroid Gland
Inhibition of new hormone synthesis Thionamide drugs (propylthiouracil, methimazole [carbimazole])
Inhibition of thyroid hormone release Iodine Potassium iodide (SSKI), Lugol's solution, ipodate Lithium carbonate
Treatment Directed Against the Peripheral Effects of Thyroid Hormone
Inhibition of T_4 to T_3 conversion Propylthiouracil Corticosteroids Propranolol Ipodate, iopanoic acid
Beta-adrenergic blockade Propranolol, esmolol
Removal of excess thyroid hormone Plasmapheresis Charcoal plasmaperfusion Cholestyramine
Treatment Directed Against Systemic Decompensation
Treatment of hyperthermia Acetaminophen (paracetamol) Cooling
Correction of dehydration and nutritional deficit Fluids and electrolytes Glucose Vitamins
Supportive therapy Corticosteroids Vasopressors Congestive heart failure management
Treatment Directed Against the Precipitating Event
Etiology-dependent

nasogastric tube in the stuporous, comatose, or otherwise uncooperative patient. Intravenous, rectal, and even transdermal routes of administration have been utilized (see section "Non-Oral Administration of Antithyroid Drugs"). PTU should be loaded with a dose of 600 to 1,000 mg and then given at doses of 1,200 to 1,500 mg daily as 200 to 250 mg every four hours. MMI is given at a total daily dose of 120 mg in divided doses of 20 mg every 4 hours. While a history of antithyroid drug-related agranulocytosis or moderate hepatocellular dysfunction should prompt the use of alternate modes of therapy, a history of minor adverse reactions such as urticaria or rash is not sufficient cause to abandon these medications in the treatment of thyroid storm. It is important to be aware that antithyroid drug therapy, although highly effective at inhibiting new hormone synthesis, has little effect on release of preformed thyroid hormone, a role which is, therefore, relegated to inorganic iodine therapy.

Inorganic iodine directly inhibits colloid proteolysis, release of T_4 and T_3 from the thyroid gland, and has transient inhibitory effects on thyroid hormone synthesis, through the Wolff-Chaikoff effect. Recommended oral doses are either Lugol's solution (8 mg/drop [0.05 mL]) 8 drops every 6 hours, or saturated solution of potassium iodide (SSKI) (~35–50 mg/drop) 5 drops every 6 hours (1). Parenteral administration by slow intravenous infusion as sodium iodide (NaI), 0.5 to 1 g every 12 hours, has been employed, but sterile NaI for intravenous usage is not currently commercially available in the United States. Rectal administration of inorganic iodide has been described and recently summarized (39). Sublingual iodine has been used effectively as well, with 0.4 mL of a SSKI sublingually 3 times daily in a patient with bowel obstruction. By measuring urinary iodine, the authors calculated that 70% of the administered sublingual dose was absorbed (22).

It is essential that iodine therapy not be initiated until a blockade of new thyroid hormone synthesis has been established with thionamide antithyroid drugs (approximately 1 hr), as iodine alone will eventually lead to further increases of thyroid hormone stores, thereby increasing the risk of exacerbating the thyrotoxic state. Further, such "unprotected" use of iodine will complicate any planned management by delaying the effectiveness of antithyroid drug therapy, increasing surgical risk due to an enrichment of glandular hormone stores, or postponing radioiodine ablation pending clearance of the iodine load. It should be noted that oral iodine therapy has been associated with acute gastrointestinal injury (40). Lithium also reduces the release of hormone from the thyroid, and could be considered in patients unable to be treated with iodide, provided adequate patient monitoring for lithium toxicity is performed (41).

Oral cholecystographic contrast agents such as ipodate and iopanoate (no longer available in the United States) have been used to treat severe thyrotoxicosis (42). These drugs, by virtue of a large content of stable iodine (308 mg/500 mg capsule for ipodate) have beneficial effects on thyroid hormone release similar to inorganic iodide. In addition, these agents are the most potent inhibitors of peripheral conversion of T_4 to T_3, and may antagonize thyroid hormone binding to nuclear receptors. Ipodate is given at a daily dose of 1–3 g and, as with iodide, should not be used without prior blockade of new thyroid hormone synthesis with PTU or MMI. Although the utility of ipodate in thyroid storm has not been extensively examined, dramatic reductions in circulating T_4 and T_3 levels (by as much as 30%–54% within 48 hr of initiating therapy) have been reported in uncomplicated thyrotoxicosis (43).

Non-oral administration of antithyroid drugs. Oral administration of antithyroid drugs can be problematic in a patient with a poorly functioning gastrointestinal tract or who is combative or comatose. Case reports have documented the effective use of intravenous methimazole (44,45). The report by Hodak and colleagues is most informative. These authors prepared intravenous methimazole by reconstituting 500 mg of methimazole powder in 0.9% sodium chloride solution to a final volume of 50 mL. The resulting solution of 10 mg/mL was then filtered through a 0.22-mm filter and administered as a slow intravenous push over 2 minutes, followed by a saline flush (44). Standard sterile pharmacological techniques are obviously required in the preparation process for these alternate medical vehicles.

Rectal administration of antithyroid drugs also has been successful (46–49), both as enemas and suppositories, as has been recently reviewed (39). Preparation of a suppository consisting of 1,200 mg of methimazole dissolved in 12 mL of water with two drops of Span 80 (a nonionic surfactant), which was then mixed with 52 mL of cocoa butter, has been described (46). A retention enema has been tested as well, prepared by dissolving 600 mg of propylthiouracil tablets in 90 mL of sterile water, delivered to the rectum by Foley catheter with the balloon inflated to prevent leakage (50). Other authors have described the dissolution of 400 mg of propylthiouracil in 60 mL of Fleet's mineral oil or in 60 mL of Fleet's phospho soda (47), for use as a retention enema. In this report the enema preparation consisted of 400 mg of propylthiouracil dissolved in 90 mL of sterile water, and for the suppository formulation, 200 mg of propylthiouracil was dissolved in a polyethylene glycol base and put into suppository tablets. Finally, Zweig and colleagues (49) describe the use of a propylthiouracil-based suppository, prepared as follows. A total of 14.4 g of propylthiouracil tablets was solubilized in 40 mL of light mineral oil and mixed in 36 g of cocoa butter solid suppository base, melted in a hot water bath, and maintained at less than 60°C. The mixture was then distributed into thirty-six 1-g suppository molds and frozen until solid. Each suppository contained 400 mg of PTU, which was administered every 6 hours, with documentation of therapeutic drug levels (49). Suppository formulations have the benefit of ease of administration compared to retention enema preparations and appear to have similar clinical effectiveness (48).

Emergent thyroidectomy. Numerous case reports and small series have described the use of thyroidectomy in thyroid storm patients who continued to deteriorate despite the use of standard medical therapy (51). Scholz and colleagues reviewed 39 cases from the literature and 10 additional cases from their own center, in which thyroidectomy was ultimately used to treat thyroid storm. Early or late postoperative mortality was reported in 5 of 49 (10.2%) patients (51). The authors advocated early thyroidectomy to treat thyroid storm, particularly in chronically ill elderly patients with concurrent cardiopulmonary and renal failure, who fail to respond to the standard intensive multifaceted therapy for thyroid storm.

Treatment directed against peripheral effects of thyroid hormone. This category includes treatment given to diminish the adrenergic manifestations of severe hyperthyroidism, inhibition of the peripheral conversion of T_4 to T_3, and procedures designed to physically remove thyroid hormone from the circulation. The dramatic clinical response to beta blockers makes them one of the most valuable forms of therapy available for both uncomplicated thyrotoxicosis and thyroid storm. In addition to antiadrenergic effects, these agents have the added benefit of a modest inhibition of the peripheral conversion of T_4 to T_3, although studies have shown minimal changes in the serum levels, certainly not enough to fully account for the clinical response (52). The oral dose of propranolol in thyroid crisis is 60–80 mg every 4 hours, an amount notably higher than that customarily used in uncomplicated thyrotoxicosis. Plasma propranolol levels in excess of 50 ng/mL may be necessary to maintain adequate blockade in thyrotoxicosis (53,54), and it should be noted that the dose required to maintain this level may vary considerably in different thyrotoxic individuals due to the increased rate of plasma clearance (55,56). For a more rapid effect, intravenous propranolol may be given, using an initial dose of 0.5 to 1.0 mg with continuous monitoring of the patient's cardiac rhythm. Subsequent intravenous doses as high as 2–3 mg may be given over 15 minutes, to be repeated every several hours while awaiting the effects of the oral formulation (32). The alternative use of esmolol rather than propranolol is discussed under Measures Directed Against Systemic Decompensation.

Inhibition of peripheral conversion of T_4 to T_3, an important aspect of care in thyroid storm, is accomplished as an ancillary effect of other therapeutic agents used for another primary purpose in treating this disorder. These include PTU (but not MMI), propranolol, ipodate (not available in the United States), and glucocorticoids. In regard to PTU, this is achieved through inhibition of the type 1 deiodinase (T_1D) located primarily in the liver and thyroid gland. PTU is theoretically most effective in hyperthyroid states such as Graves' disease or toxic nodules where the T_1D is upregulated (57,58).

Physical removal of thyroid hormone from the circulation or gastrointestinal tract. Both plasmapheresis and charcoal plasmaperfusion techniques have been used for the physical removal of circulating hormone in thyroid storm with generally positive results (25–27, 59–67). Plasmapheresis should be considered in those patients who fail to respond rapidly to conventional therapy, those with a history of antithyroid drug-associated agranulocytosis or moderate hepatocellular dysfunction, and those who are being prepared for emergent thyroidectomy (61,66). It should be recognized, however, that the beneficial effect of plasmapheresis is transient, generally lasting only 24–48 hours (66). Cholestyramine therapy at doses of 4 grams four times daily (68) is another adjunctive measure used to physically remove thyroid hormone, in this setting from the enterohepatic circulation.

Measures directed against systemic decompensation. Combating systemic decompensation occurring in thyroid storm requires reversal of hyperthermia, dehydration, congestive heart failure, and dysrhythmia, as well as prevention of concomitant adrenal crisis. Hyperthermia should be aggressively treated with measures aimed at both thermoregulatory set point modification and peripheral cooling. Hence, acetaminophen (paracetamol) is given as antipyretic therapy, and cooling techniques such as alcohol washes, ice packs, and cooling blankets are used to enhance the dissipation of thermal energy. Salicylates are specifically avoided owing to their ability to displace thyroid hormone from serum binding sites, which could theoretically aggravate the state of thyrotoxicosis. Gastrointestinal and insensible fluid losses are potentially immense during thyroid crisis and should be aggressively replaced to prevent cardiovascular collapse and shock. Fluid requirements of 3–5 liters/day are not uncommon in thyroid storm. Elderly patients and individuals with evidence of congestive heart failure should be carefully monitored. Depletion of hepatic glycogen stores occurs readily during thyroid storm and has been cited as a characteristic histological finding at autopsy in patients dying from this disorder (9,69). As such, intravenous fluids containing 5%–10% dextrose in addition to required electrolytes should be used in patients with thyroid storm. Vitamin supplementation, particularly thiamine, should be given intravenously to replace any possible coexisting deficiency.

Cardiovascular complications including atrial dysrhythmia and congestive heart failure are treated with conventional means including antiarrhythmic agents, vasodilators, and diuretics. Congestive heart failure occurs largely as a result of impaired myocardial contractility and is aggravated by atrial dysrhythmia, particularly fibrillation. Strong consideration should be given to Swan-Ganz monitoring of central hemodynamics in these patients, because despite modern critical care advances, management of heart failure in thyroid storm continues to prove difficult. With each medication used, careful examination of its effects on thyroid hormones is required to avoid exacerbation of thyrotoxicosis. Beta blockers are a mainstay of therapy, but there are several special considerations. Propranolol is contraindicated in patients with a history of asthma or chronic obstructive pulmonary disease, who should be considered for other agents such as calcium channel blockers, β1-selective beta blockers, or reserpine. Propranolol has also been associated with cases of cardiorespiratory arrest in thyroid storm patients (70), further justifying the use of an intensive care setting.

Although propranolol has been the beta blocker of choice for many decades (because of its additional benefit of peripheral inhibition of T_4 to T_3 conversion), more recently the drug esmolol, an ultra-short-acting beta-blocking agent, has been used successfully in management of severe thyrotoxicosis as well as in thyroid storm (71–74). Esmolol has definite utility over propranolol depending on the clinical circumstance. Because it is β1-selective, it can be used in patients at risk for bronchospasm. Additionally, the half-life of esmolol's β1-selective-blockade property is 9 minutes (vs 2.5 hr with propranolol), allowing minute-to-minute titration of the medication (74). Esmolol should be loaded with a dose of 250–500 μg/kg followed by continuous infusion rates of 50–100 μg/kg per minute, facilitating a rapid titration of drug level to the desired effect (71–73).

Other pharmacological considerations include the following. Furosemide at high doses inhibits T_4 and T_3 binding to TBG, leading to increases in free thyroid hormones. Calcium-channel blockers used for atrial fibrillation can potentially lead to dramatic falls in systemic vascular resistance and consequent severe hypotension (75). In regard to digoxin, somewhat larger loading and maintenance doses may be required in thyrotoxic patients, owing, presumably, to an increased distribution space and/or rapid metabolism of this drug (75). Serum digoxin levels should be closely monitored, particularly as thyrotoxicosis improves, to prevent digitalis toxicity.

The empiric use of glucocorticoids in the treatment of thyroid storm was begun in the 1950s in an attempt to address the accelerated release and turnover of corticosteroids in thyroid storm (1). Indeed, inappropriately normal (rather than elevated) levels of serum cortisol have been observed in thyroid storm compared to other periods of significant stress (14). In addition to these effects, glucocorticoids such as dexamethasone and hydrocortisone have inhibitory effects on the peripheral conversion of T_4 to T_3. Further, the use of these agents appears to have led to improved survival in thyroid storm (7,14). Hydrocortisone is given intravenously at an initial dose of 300 mg, followed by 100 mg every 8 hours during the initial stages of thyroid storm. The dose may be subsequently reduced and discontinued as allowed by the clinical response of the individual patient.

Measures directed against precipitating events in thyroid storm. Although the event precipitating thyroid storm may be quite obvious, such as surgery, labor (76), withdrawal of thionamides (12), or recent use of radioiodine (77), this is frequently not the case. This is particularly true in the instance of an underlying infection. The fever and leukocytosis found in thyroid storm even in the absence of an infection may be difficult to distinguish from an occult infectious process (78). A careful culturing of blood, sputum, and urine is, therefore, indicated in the febrile thyrotoxic patient. The routine use of broad spectrum antibiotics is, however, not recommended in the absence of other evidence suggestive of infection. In cases of thyroid storm precipitated by hypoglycemia, diabetic ketoacidosis, stroke, or pulmonary embolism, standard therapeutic approaches apply and should be instituted simultaneously with the treatment of thyroid storm. In the stuporous or comatose patient who is unable to provide a history suggestive of a particular precipitating event, a high index of suspicion for these varied etiologies must be maintained. It should be remembered that in some individuals no precipitant will be identified, even in retrospect. In fact, in older clinical series, as many as 25%–43% of cases of thyroid storm occurred without an identified precipitating event (1,9,14,15).

After the storm: definitive treatment. For the patient successfully treated during the acute stages of thyroid storm, a key objective should be the prevention of a recurrent crisis by planning for definitive therapy with either radioactive iodine ablation or surgery. As the severely thyrotoxic patient improves clinically, a gradual withdrawal of treatment modalities is often possible. Corticosteroids should be gradually tapered and discontinued, while beta-blockade, unless contraindicated, should generally be continued during this period.

Owing to the large load of iodine used in the management of the acute stages of thyroid storm, early subsequent use of radioiodine as ablative therapy is frequently not possible until the excessive iodine has been cleared, as indicated by a return to normal levels of urinary iodine excretion. In the interim, the patient should be continued on antithyroid drug therapy. A surgical ablation with subtotal thyroidectomy is a therapeutic option with the advantage of expediency. Care must be taken, however, to ensure that the patient has adequate control of thyrotoxicosis in order to reduce the risk of another episode of thyroid crisis following anesthesia induction or the surgery itself.

PREVENTION OF THYROID STORM

In that the vast majority of cases of thyroid crisis today may be considered "medical" rather than perioperative storm, greater awareness of predisposing factors is warranted. Hence, the clinician and patient alike should be aware that the development of an intercurrent illness during the medical management of thyrotoxicosis warrants scrutiny for signs of metabolic decompensation. Likewise, elective surgical procedures should be deferred until euthyroidism has been established. Likewise, patients requiring thyroidectomy due to a poor response or inability to take antithyroid drugs require rapid preparation using all available pharmacological means to improve thyrotoxicosis preoperatively.

Selective Pretreatment with Antithyroid Drugs Before Radioiodine Therapy

The use of radioiodine ablation for thyrotoxicosis simultaneously exposes patients to 2 known precipitants of thyroid storm, namely, thionamide withdrawal (in pretreated patients) and the ablation therapy itself. Treatment of severely thyrotoxic patients with radioiodine can occasionally lead to rapid increases in thyroid hormone levels in the weeks immediately following radioiodine administration. Thyroid storm has even been described following the use of radioiodine in patients with metastatic differentiated thyroid cancer (1). Hence, patients at increased risk for developing thyroid storm, such as the elderly, patients with severe thyrotoxicosis, and those with extensive comorbidity should receive pretreatment with antithyroid drugs before radioiodine ablation therapy (38,79). In these patients, an attempt should be made to minimize the duration off antithyroid drugs to 3–5 days before radioiodine is given, as antithyroid drug discontinuation leads to rapid increases in thyroid hormone levels (79). The use of beta-adrenergic blockade in the period preceding and immediately following radioiodine provides additional protection in this circumstance. Consideration can also be given to restarting antithyroid drugs 3–7 days after radioiodine and then slowly tapering this therapy over the ensuing 4–6 weeks (38).

Rapid Preparation for Surgery in the Thyrotoxic Patient

Rapid preoperative preparation is occasionally needed for patients requiring urgent or emergent surgery (Table 11-7) (68). These patients either have insufficient time to be rendered euthyroid by thionamides before surgery or have contraindications to their use. Safe and effective oral therapy with a combination of beta blocker high-dose glucocorticoids, and cholcystographic agent (iopanoate) was effective in a small series of patients requiring urgent surgery (80). This regimen was given for 5 days with surgery performed on the sixth day. Dexamethasone and hydrocortisone decrease T_4 to T_3 conversion and have an important role in this setting. As noted previously, ipodate and iopanoic acid are no longer available in the United States.

Emergent preparation for thyroid surgery at our center in thyrotoxic patients unable to use or responding poorly to antithyroid drugs

Table 11-7. Rapid Preparation of the Thyrotoxic Patient for Surgery

Drug Class	Recommended Drug	Dose	Mechanism of Action	Continue Postoperatively?
Beta-adrenergic blockade	Propranolol	40–80 mg po tid-qid	Beta-adrenergic blockade; decreased T_4 to T_3 conversion (high dose)	Yes
	Esmolol	50–100 μg/kg/min		Change to oral propranolol
Thionamide	Propylthiouracil	200 mg po q 4 h	Inhibition of new thyroid hormone synthesis; decreased T_4 to T_3 conversion	Stop immediately after near total thyroidectomy; continue after nonthyroidal surgery
	Methimazole (carbimazole)	20 mg po q 4 h	Inhibition of new thyroid hormone synthesis	Stop immediately after near total thyroidectomy; continue after nonthyroidal surgery
Iodine[a]	SSKI	2 drops q 8 h	Inhibition of new thyroid hormone synthesis; decreased release of thyroid hormone	No
	Lugol's	3–5 drops q 8 h		No
Corticosteroid	Dexamethasone	2 mg po or IV q 6 h	Vasomotor stability; decreased T_4 to T_3	Taper over first 72 h
	Hydrocortisone	100 mg po or IV q 8 h		Taper over first 72 h
Resin agents	Cholestyramine	4 g po q 6 h	Interference with enterohepatic circulation	Stop immediately postoperatively

[a]*In countries where available, cholecystographic agents such as iopanoic acid (500 mg po bid) can be used in place of iodine, with the added benefit of inhibition of T_4 to T_3 conversion.*

Adapted from Langley RW, Burch HB. Perioperative management of the thyrotoxic patient. Endocrinol Metab Clin North Am. *2003;32:519–534.*

(68) has successfully involved the following inpatient regimen with rapid correction of thyrotoxicosis when given for 5–10 days before thyroidectomy:

- Propranolol 60 mg orally, twice daily
- Dexamethasone 2 mg intravenously, four times daily
- Cholestyramine 4 g orally, four times daily
- SSKI 2 drops orally, three times daily

ADVERSE EFFECTS OF ANTITHYROID DRUGS

Antithyroid drugs are generally well-tolerated. However, as with any drug, side effects may require cessation of therapy and the subsequent need for alternate treatment. Traditionally, the adverse reactions associated with antithyroid drugs are divided into "minor" and "major" side effects (81). The major side effects, agranulocytosis, hepatotoxicity, and vasculitis, are potentially life-threatening. A recent report has suggested that patient's with Graves' disease may be more susceptible to allergic reactions to antithyroid drugs, compared to patients with nonautoimmune etiologies of thyrotoxicosis such as toxic multinodular goiter (82).

Minor Drug Reactions

The minor side effects include skin rash, which is typically papular and pruritic, gastrointestinal (GI) distress, nausea, and arthralgias (81). In general, the minor side effects occur in about 2%–5% of patients, with skin rash being by far the most common. The development of pruritic skin rash often requires discontinuation of the drug, but some patients may be able to continue therapy along with an antihistamine with eventual resolution of the skin rash. Typically, minor reactions develop within the first few weeks of starting the medication, and while switching to the alternate drug might be possible, there is at least a 50% cross-reactivity between the 2 antithyroid drugs (81).

Major Drug Reactions

The 3 major antithyroid drug reactions are agranulocytosis, hepatotoxicity, and antineutrophil cytoplasmic antibody positive vasculitis. Each of these will be discussed individually.

Agranulocytosis. Agranulocytosis is defined as an absolute granulocyte count $<0.5 \times 10^9/L$, but most patients have granulocyte counts that are close to zero (81). Some patients also have anemia and mild thrombocytopenia. The frequency of antithyroid drug-induced agranulocytosis is in the range of 0.2%–0.6% (83), and 99% of cases occur within the first 100 days of therapy (83). The elderly may be more susceptible to agranulocytosis than younger patients (84). Also, agranulocytosis can occur after a prior innocuous first exposure to the drug many years earlier. The risk of agranulocytosis is dose-related with methimazole (85), and is extremely unusual at doses less than 5–10 mg per day. In contrast, there is no dose response relationship with PTU and the risk of agranulocytosis. Patients may have agranulocytosis and be asymptomatic, only developing typical symptoms when they become infected. The classic presentation is that of a fulminant oropharyngeal infection with severe odynophagia, lymphadenopathy, malaise, chills, and high fever (86). Pneumonia, skin infections, and anorectal infections have also been described. Bone marrow examination typically shows normal or slightly decreased cellularity but absent or markedly decreased myeloid precursors. Bone marrow examination may be helpful in predicting recovery, because the lack of myeloid precursors makes it unlikely that there will be a normal granulocyte count before 7–14 days (87). On the other hand, if there is preservation of the immature cells, recovery time will be shorter.

Treatment of agranulocytosis induced by antithyroid drugs includes the following:

- Immediate cessation of the offending drug
- Hospitalization if there is a fever, and coverage with broad-spectrum antibiotics
- Avoidance of the other antithyroid drug because of the possibility of cross-reactivity

Most patients are treated with hematopoietic growth factors (eg, G-CSF or GM-CSF). In most large cohort studies using retrospective controls and in one meta-analysis, use of these drugs reduced the fatality rate and shortened the time to hematological recovery (88). Mortality rates are in the 5%–10% range with worse outcomes in patients over age 65, patients with a neutrophil count that is $<0.1 \times 10^9/L$, and in patients who have severe underlying comorbidities such as renal failure, cardiac disease, or respiratory disease.

Hepatic involvement. Classically, liver involvement is different for the 2 antithyroid drugs (81). In the case of PTU, hepatotoxicity is typically "hepatocellular," whereas the pattern of involvement with methimazole is "cholestatic." For PTU, the frequency of mild hepatocellular dysfunction is in the 1% range, but the frequency of fulminant, life-threatening hepatic failure is more likely to be in the 1/10,000 range (89). For methimazole, there are no reliable data on the prevalence of cholestatic reactions, but it is decidedly rare. There are case reports of liver involvement developing within the first few days of treatment, but in a recent review of case reports involving PTU, the median was 120 days (90). For methimazole, the mean duration of therapy before the onset of hepatotoxicity was 36 days (91). In the case of PTU, symptoms and signs of severe hepatic involvement include lethargy, malaise, nausea and vomiting, jaundice, dark urine, and light-colored stools. Recognition of the syndrome and immediate discontinuation of PTU is essential. There then should be expectant management of hepatic involvement (coma, prolonged prothrombin time, hepatorenal syndrome, etc.) and consideration of referral to a center that can provide specialized care, including possible liver transplantation. For methimazole-induced cholestasis, liver involvement typically resolves over the course of 1–2 months once the drug is stopped. In a recent review of cases reported to the FDA using the MedWatch system, no deaths had been reported from methimazole-related hepatotoxicity (90). In patients with antithyroid drug-induced hepatotoxicity, treatment of the continuing hyperthyroidism may involve switching to the other antithyroid drug, given that the 2 drugs have different hepatotoxicity profiles.

Vasculitis. Antithyroid drug-induced vasculitis may take two forms clinically: (1) drug-induced lupus with fever, palpable purpura, splenomegaly, lymphadenopathy, and serositis involving the pleura and pericardium, or (2) drug-induced vasculitis with malaise, arthritis, myalgias, severe skin involvement, glomerulonephritis, and pulmonary hemorrhage. However, both of these forms likely represent part of a spectrum of antithyroid drug-induced vasculitis with associated antineutrophil cytoplasmic antibody (ANCA) positivity (92,93). In the case of antithyroid drug-related vasculitis, the antibodies are called *pANCA*, which stands for "perinuclear" ANCA, with the antibody directed against granulocytic myeloperoxidase (MPO). However, antibodies against other neutrophil proteins besides MPO can also be seen. Vasculitis from antithyroid drugs is far more common with PTU than with methimazole, and occurs preferentially in individuals of Asian ethnicity (94). Cross-sectional studies showed the prevalence of circulating pANCA to be in the 10%–50% range in asymptomatic individuals taking PTU, and 0%–3% in patients taking methimazole (95). Antithyroid drug-related vasculitis typically occurs 1–3 months after starting treatment, but may occur after years of treatment (94). The usual presentation includes fever, arthritis, and palpable purpura involving the extremities and often the earlobes, dermal ulceration, and, more rarely, evidence of organ dysfunction, including glomerulonephritis or pulmonary involvement (94). The syndrome generally resolves after drug cessation, but immunosuppressive therapy, including high-dose glucocorticoids and/or cyclophosphamide, has been used in more severe cases.

Birth defects. Although not classically included in the category of adverse effects, the use of methimazole in the first trimester of pregnancy has been associated with rare birth defects, including aplasia cutis, choanal atresia, esophageal atresia, and omphalocele (81). Recently, a study from Denmark noted a similar prevalence of birth defects in infants born to mothers exposed to propylthiouracil during early pregnancy, although the spectrum of defects differed between methimazole and propylthiouracil (96). These and other recent similar findings prompted a call for a greater use of definitive therapy for Graves' disease in women planning pregnancy in order to avoid exposure to antithyroid drugs during early pregnancy (97).

CONCLUSIONS

Although important strides in recognition and therapy have reduced the mortality in thyroid storm from the nearly 100% fatality rate noted by Lahey in 1928 (3), survival is by no means guaranteed (98). Most recent series have shown fatality rates between 20% and 50% (4,14,99). It is likely that these improvements are a result of early recognition of thyroid storm and the demonstration of beneficial effects of corticosteroid, antithyroid drugs, and antiadrenergic therapies for the treatment of this disorder (14,15) in the decades since Lahey's first description.

Thyroid storm is a dreaded, fortunately rare complication of a very common disorder. Many cases of thyroid storm occur after a precipitating event, intercurrent illness, or discontinuation of antithyroid drug therapy, frequently after the development of an adverse drug reaction. Effective management is predicated on a prompt recognition of impending thyroid storm, which is, in turn, dependent on knowledge of both the typical and atypical presentations of this disorder. An unwavering commitment to an aggressive multifaceted therapeutic intervention is critical to obtaining a satisfactory outcome.

ACKNOWLEDGMENTS

The views expressed in this chapter are those of the authors and do not reflect the official policy of the Department of the Army, Navy, the Department of Defense, or the U.S. government. One or more of the authors are military service members (or employees of the U.S. government). This work was prepared as part of our official duties. Title 17 U.S.C. 105 provides the "Copyright protection under this title is not available for any work of the United States Government." Title 17 U.S.C. 101 defines a U.S. government work as a work prepared by a military service member or employee of the U.S. government as part of that person's official duties. We certify that all individuals who qualify as authors have been listed; each has participated in the conception and design of this work, the analysis of data (when applicable), the writing of the document, and/or the approval of the submission of this version; that the document represents valid work; that if we used information derived from another source, we obtained all necessary approvals to use it and made appropriate acknowledgments in the document; and that each takes public responsibility for it.

REFERENCES

1. **Burch HB, Wartofsky L.** Life-threatening thyrotoxicosis. Thyroid storm. *Endocrinol Metab Clin North Am.* 1993;22:263–277.
2. **Howton JC.** Thyroid storm presenting as coma. *Ann Emerg Med.* 1988;17:343–345.
3. **Lahey FH.** The crisis of exophthalmic goiter. *N Engl J Med.* 1928;199:255–257.
4. **Akamizu T, Satoh T, Isozaki O, et al.** Diagnostic criteria, clinical features, and incidence of thyroid storm based on nationwide surveys. *Thyroid.* 2012;22:661–679.
5. **Laman DM, Berghout A, Endtz LJ, et al.** Thyroid crisis presenting as coma. *Clin Neurol Neurosurg.* 1984;86:295–298.
6. **Safe AF, Griffiths KD, Maxwell RT.** Thyrotoxic crisis presenting as status epilepticus. *Postgrad Med J.* 1990;66:150–152.
7. **Waldenstrom J.** Acute thyrotoxic encephalo- or myopathy, its cause and treatment. *Acta Med Scand.* 1945;121:251–294.
8. **Burch HB, Burman KD, Cooper DS.** A 2011 survey of clinical practice patterns in the management of Graves' disease. *J Clin Endocrinol Metab.* 2012;97:4549–4558.
9. **Nelson NC, Becker WF.** Thyroid crisis: diagnosis and treatment. *Ann Surg.* 1969;170:263–273.
10. **Bish LT, Bavaria JE, Augoustides J.** Thyroid storm after coronary artery bypass grafting. *J Thorac Cardiovasc Surg.* 2010;140:6.
11. **Sherman SI, Simonson L, Ladenson PW.** Clinical and socioeconomic predispositions to complicated thyrotoxicosis: a predictable and preventable syndrome? *Am J Med.* 1996;101:192–198.
12. **Rives JD, Shepard RM.** Thyroid crisis. *Am Surg.* 1951;17:406–418.
13. **Brooks MH, Waldstein SS, Bronsky D, Sterling K.** Serum triiodothyronine concentration in thyroid storm. *J Clin Endocrinol Metab.* 1975;40:339–341.
14. **Mazzaferri EL, Skillman TG.** Thyroid storm. A review of 22 episodes with special emphasis on the use of guanethidine. *Arch Intern Med.* 1969;124:684–690.
15. **Waldstein SS, Slodki SJ, Kaganiec GI, Bronsky D.** A clinical study of thyroid storm. *Ann Intern Med.* 1960;52:626–642.
16. **Lahey FH.** Apathetic thyroidism. *Ann Surg.* 1931;93: 1026–1030.
17. **Grossman A, Waldstein SS.** Apathetic thyroid storm in a 10-year-old child. *Pediatrics.* 1961;28:447–451.
18. **Ghobrial MW, Ruby EB.** Coma and thyroid storm in apathetic thyrotoxicosis. *South Med J.* 2002;95:552–554.
19. **Jarrett DR, Hansell DM, Zeegen R.** Thyroid crisis complicated by cerebral infarction. *Br J Clin Pract.* 1987;41:671–673.
20. **Harwood-Nuss AL, Martel TJ.** An unusual cause of abdominal pain in a young woman. *Ann Emerg Med.* 1991;20:574–582.
21. **Karanikolas M, Velissaris D, Karamouzos V, Filos KS.** Thyroid storm presenting as intra-abdominal sepsis with multi-organ failure requiring intensive care. *Anaesth Intensive Care.* 2009;37:1005–1007.
22. **Cansler CL, Latham JA, Brown PM Jr, Chapman WH, Magner JA.** Duodenal obstruction in thyroid storm. *South Med J.* 1997;90:1143–1146.
23. **Parker KI, Loftley A, Charles C, Hermayer K.** A case of apathetic thyroid storm with resultant hyperthyroidism-induced hypercalcemia. *Am J Med Sci.* 2013;19:19.
24. **Bennett WR, Huston DP.** Rhabdomyolysis in thyroid storm. *Am J Med.* 1984;77:733–735.
25. **Ashkar FS, Katims RB, Smoak WM 3rd, Gilson AJ.** Thyroid storm treatment with blood exchange and plasmapheresis. *JAMA.* 1970;214:1275–1279.
26. **Candrina R, Di Stefano O, Spandrio S, Giustina G.** Treatment of thyrotoxic storm by charcoal plasmaperfusion. *J Endocrinol Invest.* 1989;12:133–134.
27. **Tajiri J, Katsuya H, Kiyokawa T, Urata K, Okamoto K, Shimada T.** Successful treatment of thyrotoxic crisis with plasma exchange. *Crit Care Med.* 1984;12:536–537.
28. **Brooks MH, Waldstein SS.** Free thyroxine concentrations in thyroid storm. *Ann Intern Med.* 1980;93:694–697.
29. **Mackin JF, Canary JJ, Pittman CS.** Thyroid storm and its management. *N Engl J Med.* 1974;291:1396–1398.
30. **Wartofsky L, Burman KD.** Alterations in thyroid function in patients with systemic illness: the "euthyroid sick syndrome." *Endocr Rev.* 1982;3:164–217.
31. **Landsberg L.** Catecholamines and hyperthyroidism. *Clin Endocrinol Metab.* 1977;6:697–718.
32. **Das G, Krieger M.** Treatment of thyrotoxic storm with intravenous administration of propranolol. *Ann Intern Med.* 1969;70:985–988.
33. **Coulombe P, Dussault JH, Walker P.** Catecholamine metabolism in thyroid disease. II. Norepinephrine secretion rate in hyperthyroidism and hypothyroidism. *J Clin Endocrinol Metab.* 1977;44:1185–1189.
34. **Anaissie E, Tohme JF.** Reserpine in propranolol-resistant thyroid storm. *Arch Intern Med.* 1985;145:2248–2249.

35. **Jamison MH, Done HJ.** Post-operative thyrotoxic crisis in a patient prepared for thyroidectomy with propranolol. *Br J Clin Pract.* 1979;33:82–83.
36. **Wartofsky L, Dimond RC, Noel GL, Frantz AG, Earll JM.** Failure of propranolol to alter thyroid iodine release, thyroxine turnover, or the TSH and PRL responses to thyrotropin-releasing hormone in patients with thyrotoxicosis. *J Clin Endocrinol Metab.* 1975;41:485–490.
37. **Bilezikian JP, Loeb JN.** The influence of hyperthyroidism and hypothyroidism on alpha- and beta-adrenergic receptor systems and adrenergic responsiveness. *Endocr Rev.* 1983;4:378–388.
38. **Bahn RS, Burch HB, Cooper DS, et al.** Hyperthyroidism and other causes of thyrotoxicosis: management guidelines of the American Thyroid Association and American Association of Clinical Endocrinologists. *Thyroid.* 2011;21:593–646.
39. **Alfadhli E, Gianoukakis AG.** Management of severe thyrotoxicosis when the gastrointestinal tract is compromised. *Thyroid.* 2011;21:215–220.
40. **Myung Park J, Seok Lee I, Young Kang J, et al.** Acute esophageal and gastric injury: complication of Lugol's solution. *Scan J Gastroenterol.* 2007;42:135–137.
41. **Nayak B, Burman K.** Thyrotoxicosis and thyroid storm. *Endocrinol Metab Clin North Am.* 2006;35:663–686.
42. **Robuschi G, Manfredi A, Salvi M, et al.** Effect of sodium ipodate and iodide on free T4 and free T3 concentrations in patients with Graves' disease. *J Endocrinol Invest.* 1986;9:287–291.
43. **Wu SY, Chopra IJ, Solomon DH, Johnson DE.** The effect of repeated administration of ipodate (Oragrafin) in hyperthyroidism. *J Clin Endocrinol Metab.* 1978;47:1358–1362.
44. **Hodak SP, Huang C, Clarke D, Burman KD, Jonklaas J, Janicic-Kharic N.** Intravenous methimazole in the treatment of refractory hyperthyroidism. *Thyroid.* 2006;16:691–695.
45. **Thomas DJ, Hardy J, Sarwar R, et al.** Thyroid storm treated with intravenous methimazole in patients with gastrointestinal dysfunction. *Br J Hosp Med.* 2006;67:492–493.
46. **Nabil N, Miner DJ, Amatruda JM.** Methimazole: an alternative route of administration. *J Clin Endocrinol Metab.* 1982;54:180–181.
47. **Walter RM Jr, Bartle WR.** Rectal administration of propylthiouracil in the treatment of Graves' disease. *Am J Med.* 1990;88:69–70.
48. **Jongjaroenprasert W, Akarawut W, Chantasart D, Chailurkit L, Rajatanavin R.** Rectal administration of propylthiouracil in hyperthyroid patients: comparison of suspension enema and suppository form. *Thyroid.* 2002;12:627–631.
49. **Zweig SB, Schlosser JR, Thomas SA, Levy CJ, Fleckman AM.** Rectal administration of propylthiouracil in suppository form in patients with thyrotoxicosis and critical illness: case report and review of literature. *Endocr Pract.* 2006;12:43–47.
50. **Yeung SC, Go R, Balasubramanyam A.** Rectal administration of iodide and propylthiouracil in the treatment of thyroid storm. *Thyroid.* 1995;5: 403–405.
51. **Scholz GH, Hagemann E, Arkenau C, et al.** Is there a place for thyroidectomy in older patients with thyrotoxic storm and cardiorespiratory failure? *Thyroid.* 2003;13:933–940.
52. **Mintz G, Pizzarello R, Klein I.** Enhanced left ventricular diastolic function in hyperthyroidism: noninvasive assessment and response to treatment. *J Clin Endocrinol Metab.* 1991;73:146–150.
53. **Feely J, Forrest A, Gunn A, Hamilton W, Stevenson I, Crooks J.** Propranolol dosage in thyrotoxicosis. *J Clin Endocrinol Metab.* 1980;51:658–661.
54. **Hellman R, Kelly KL, Mason WD.** Propranolol for thyroid storm. *N Engl J Med.* 1977;297:671–672.
55. **Rubenfeld S, Silverman VE, Welch KM, Mallette LE, Kohler PO.** Variable plasma propranolol levels in thyrotoxicosis. *N Engl J Med.* 1979;300:353–354.
56. **Shenfield GM.** Influence of thyroid dysfunction on drug pharmacokinetics. *Clin Pharmacokinet.* 1981;6:275–297.
57. **Bianco AC, Salvatore D, Gereben B, Berry MJ, Larsen PR.** Biochemistry, cellular and molecular biology, and physiological roles of the iodothyronine selenodeiodinases. *Endocr Rev.* 2002;23:38–89.
58. **Laurberg P, Vestergaard H, Nielsen S, et al.** Sources of circulating 3,5,3'-triiodothyronine in hyperthyroidism estimated after blocking of type 1 and type 2 iodothyronine deiodinases. *J Clin Endocrinol Metab.* 2007;92:2149–2156.
59. **Horn K, Brehm G, Habermann J, Pickardt CR, Scriba PC.** [Successful treatment of thyroid storm by continuous plasmapheresis with a blood-cell separator (author's transl)]. *Klin Wochenschr.* 1976;54:983–986.
60. **Tshirch LS, Drews J, Liedtke R, Schemmel K.** [Treatment of thyroid storm with plasmapheresis (author's transl)]. *Medizinische Klinik.* 1975;70: 807–811.
61. **Ezer A, Caliskan K, Parlakgumus A, Belli S, Kozanoglu I, Yildirim S.** Preoperative therapeutic plasma exchange in patients with thyrotoxicosis. *J Clin Apher.* 2009;24:111–114.
62. **Herrmann J, Hilger P, Kruskemper HL.** Plasmapheresis in the treatment of thyrotoxic crisis (measurement of half-concentration times for free and total T3 and T4). *Acta Endocrinol.* 1973 (suppl): 173:22.
63. **Jha S, Waghdhare S, Reddi R, Bhattacharya P.** Thyroid storm due to inappropriate administration of a compounded thyroid hormone preparation successfully treated with plasmapheresis. *Thyroid.* 2012;22:1283–1286.
64. **Koball S, Hickstein H, Gloger M, et al.** Treatment of thyrotoxic crisis with plasmapheresis and single pass albumin dialysis: a case report. *Artif Organs.* 2010;34:1525–1594.
65. **Petry J, Van Schil PE, Abrams P, Jorens PG.** Plasmapheresis as effective treatment for thyrotoxic storm after sleeve pneumonectomy. *Ann Thorac Surg.* 2004;77:1839–1841.
66. **Vyas AA, Vyas P, Fillipon NL, Vijayakrishnan R, Trivedi N.** Successful treatment of thyroid storm with plasmapheresis in a patient with methimazole-induced agranulocytosis. *Endocr Pract.* 2010;16: 673–676.

67. **Pasimeni G, Caroli F, Spriano G, Antonini M, Baldelli R, Appetecchia M.** Refractory thyrotoxicosis induced by iodinated contrast agents treated with therapeutic plasma exchange. A case report. *J Clin Apher.* 2008;23:92–95.
68. **Langley RW, Burch HB.** Perioperative management of the thyrotoxic patient. *Endocrinol Metab Clin North Am.* 2003;32:519–534.
69. **Ficarra BJ.** Thyroid crisis: pathogenesis of hepatic origin. *Am J Surg.* 1945;69:325–337.
70. **Dalan R, Leow MK.** Cardiovascular collapse associated with beta blockade in thyroid storm. *Exp Clin Endocrinol Diabetes.* 2007;115:392–396.
71. **Brunette DD, Rothong C.** Emergency department management of thyrotoxic crisis with esmolol. *Am J Emerg Med.* 1991;9:232–234.
72. **Isley WL, Dahl S, Gibbs H.** Use of esmolol in managing a thyrotoxic patient needing emergency surgery. *Am J Med.* 1990;89:122–123.
73. **Thorne AC, Bedford RF.** Esmolol for perioperative management of thyrotoxic goiter. *Anesthesiology.* 1989;71:291–294.
74. **Duggal J, Singh S, Kuchinic P, Butler P, Arora R.** Utility of esmolol in thyroid crisis. *Can J Clin Pharmacol.* 2006;13:26.
75. **Fadel BM, Ellahham S, Ringel MD, Lindsay J Jr, Wartofsky L, Burman KD.** Hyperthyroid heart disease. *Clin Cardiol.* 2000;23:402–408.
76. **Kamm ML, Weaver JC, Page EP, Chappell CC.** Acute thyroid storm precipitated by labor. Report of a case. *Obstet Gynecol.* 1963;21:460–463.
77. **McDermott MT, Kidd GS, Dodson LE Jr, Hofeldt FD.** Radioiodine-induced thyroid storm. Case report and literature review. *Am J Med.* 1983;75:353–359.
78. **Urbanic RC, Mazzaferri EL.** Thyrotoxic crisis and myxedema coma. *Heart Lung.* 1978;7:435–447.
79. **Burch HB, Solomon BL, Cooper DS, Ferguson P, Walpert N, Howard R.** The effect of antithyroid drug pretreatment on acute changes in thyroid hormone levels after (131)I ablation for Graves' disease. *J Clin Endocrinol Metab.* 2001;86:3016–3021.
80. **Baeza A, Aguayo J, Barria M, Pineda G.** Rapid preoperative preparation in hyperthyroidism. *Clinical Endocrin.* 1991;35:439–442.
81. **Cooper DS.** Antithyroid drugs. *N Engl J Med.* 2005; 352:905–917.
82. **Chivu RD, Chivu LI, Ion DA, Barbu C, Fica S.** Allergic reactions to antithyroid drugs are associated with autoimmunity a retrospective case-control study. *Revista medico-chirurgicala a Societatii de Medici si Naturalisti din Iasi.* 2006;110:830–832.
83. **Watanabe N, Narimatsu H, Noh JY, et al.** Antithyroid drug-induced hematopoietic damage: a retrospective cohort study of agranulocytosis and pancytopenia involving 50,385 patients with Graves' disease. *J Clin Endocrinol Metab.* 2012;97:E49–E53.
84. **Cooper DS, Goldminz D, Levin AA, et al.** Agranulocytosis associated with antithyroid drugs. Effects of patient age and drug dose. *Ann Intern Med.* 1983;98:26–29.
85. **Takata K, Kubota S, Fukata S, et al.** Methimazole-induced agranulocytosis in patients with Graves' disease is more frequent with an initial dose of 30 mg daily than with 15 mg daily. *Thyroid.* 2009;19:559–563.
86. **Sheng WH, Hung CC, Chen YC, et al.** Antithyroid-drug-induced agranulocytosis complicated by life-threatening infections. *QJM.* 1999;92:455–461.
87. **Yang J, Zhong J, Xiao XH, et al.** The relationship between bone marrow characteristics and the clinical prognosis of antithyroid drug-induced agranulocytosis. *Endocr J.* 2013;60:185–189.
88. **Andres E, Kurtz JE, Perrin AE, Dufour P, Schlienger JL, Maloisel F.** Haematopoietic growth factor in antithyroid-drug-induced agranulocytosis. *QJM.* 2001;94:423–428.
89. **Cooper DS.** Treatment of thyrotoxicosis. In: Braverman LE, Cooper DS, eds. *The Thyroid.* 10th ed. Philadelphia, PA: Lippincott Williams and Wilkins; 2012.
90. **Cooper DS, Rivkees SA.** Putting propylthiouracil in perspective. *J Clin Endocrinol Metab.* 2009;94: 1881–1882.
91. **Woeber KA.** Methimazole-induced hepatotoxicity. *Endocr Pract.* 2002;8:222–224.
92. **Gunton JE, Stiel J, Caterson RJ, McElduff A.** Clinical case seminar: anti-thyroid drugs and antineutrophil cytoplasmic antibody positive vasculitis. A case report and review of the literature. *J Clin Endocrinol Metab.* 1999;84:13–16.
93. **Wiik A.** Drug-induced vasculitis. *Curr Opin Rheumatol.* 2008;20:35–39.
94. **Noh JY, Yasuda S, Sato S, et al.** Clinical characteristics of myeloperoxidase antineutrophil cytoplasmic antibody-associated vasculitis caused by antithyroid drugs. *J Clin Endocrinol Metab.* 2009;94:2806–2811.
95. **Wada N, Mukai M, Kohno M, Notoya A, Ito T, Yoshioka N.** Prevalence of serum anti-myeloperoxidase antineutrophil cytoplasmic antibodies (MPO-ANCA) in patients with Graves' disease treated with propylthiouracil and thiamazole. *Endocr J.* 2002;49: 329–334.
96. **Andersen SL, Olsen J, Wu CS, Laurberg P.** Birth defects after early pregnancy use of antithyroid drugs: a Danish nationwide study. *J Clin Endocrinol Metab.* 2013;98:4373–4381.
97. **Rivkees SA.** Propylthiouracil versus methimazole during pregnancy: an evolving tale of difficult choices. *J Clin Endocrinol Metab.* 2013;98:4332–4335.
98. **Parker JL, Lawson DH.** Death from thyrotoxicosis. *Lancet.* 1973;2:894–895.
99. **Ashkar FS, Miller R, Gilson AJ.** Thyroid function and serum thyroxine in thyroid storm. *South Med J.* 1972;65:372–374.

CHAPTER 12

Amiodarone-Induced Thyrotoxicosis

Fausto Bogazzi, Luca Tomisti, Luigi Bartalena, and Enio Martino

ABSTRACT

Amiodarone-induced thyrotoxicosis (AIT) occurs in patients with preexisting cardiac disease and, in some instances, can be considered an emergency because of the detrimental effects of excess thyroid hormone on underlying heart abnormalities. When AIT represents an imminent risk for cardiac function, it should be managed accordingly, without delay, because late resolution of thyrotoxicosis is associated with a high mortality rate. In these instances emergent thyroidectomy may represent the most effective and rapid way for resolving thyrotoxicosis.

INTRODUCTION

Amiodarone is a benzofuranic iodine-rich drug structurally similar to thyroid hormones (1,2). It is a class III antiarrhythmic drug, mainly inhibiting myocardial Na-K ATPase activity and eventually increasing the refractory period. However, amiodarone also has class I (decrease in conduction velocity through blockade of Na channel), class II (antiadrenergic effect reducing beta adrenergic receptor), and class IV (suppression of Ca-mediated action potentials) actions. These multiple antiarrhythmic effects of amiodarone justify its use in supraventricular and ventricular tachyarrhythmias, atrial fibrillation (when other therapies are poorly effective), and in preventing sudden cardiac death in selected patients (3–5).

Amiodarone administration is complicated in 15%–20% of patients by thyroid dysfunction, with either thyroid hormone excess (amiodarone-induced thyrotoxicosis, AIT) or deficiency (amiodarone-induced hypothyroidism, AIH). Owing to the detrimental effects of thyroid hormone excess on the heart, AIT may represent an endocrine emergency.

PATHOPHYSIOLOGY

Abnormal thyroid function tests, not indicative of thyroid disease, are found in all patients given amiodarone. A few weeks after institution of therapy serum, thyroid-stimulating hormone (TSH) concentrations transitorily increase, but usually normalize thereafter. Serum free T_4 (FT_4) and reverse T_3 (rT_3) concentrations increase, while serum free T_3 (FT_3) levels decrease because of amiodarone-induced inhibition of hepatic type 1 deiodinase. Amiodarone-induced thyroid dysfunction may result from excessive iodine load and/or the intrinsic properties of the drug (1,6).

Effects of Iodine Load

Using a standard dose of amiodarone (200 mg per day), patients are exposed to a 75-mg daily iodine load, which greatly exceeds the recommended daily iodine intake (150–200 μg). This iodine load may cause either AIH or AIT. After iodine load, the thyroid gland normally blocks thyroid hormone synthesis (Wolff-Chaikoff effect). This is associated with increased serum TSH concentrations, but is then followed by an "escape" phenomenon driven by a decrease in iodine transport and intrathyroidal concentrations to levels inadequate to maintain the block related to the Wolff-Chaikoff effect. Amiodarone inhibits iodide transport into the thyroid by either an iodine-independent mechanism or a decrease in sodium-iodide symporter mRNA expression.

Failure to escape from the Wolff-Chaikoff effect is believed to be the mechanism underpinning AIH both in patients with normal thyroid glands and in those with preexisting chronic autoimmune thyroiditis. Excessive iodine is the cause of type 1 AIT, a form of iodine-induced hyperthyroidism, in which iodine load unveils underlying thyroid autonomy or latent Graves' disease, and triggers the occurrence of hyperthyroidism (jodbasedow) (1,2,6).

Effects Intrinsic to the Molecular Structure

Amiodarone and its main metabolite, desethylamiodarone (DEA), have proapoptotic and cytotoxic effects on thyroid follicular cells. Excess iodine may directly contribute to these changes. Histopathological changes resemble those seen in other thyroid-destructive processes, such as subacute thyroiditis. Direct drug- (and/or iodine-) induced cytotoxic damage of thyroid follicular cells is considered to be the cause of type 2 AIT (destructive thyroiditis) (1,2,4,6).

AMIODARONE-INDUCED THYROID DISEASE

The overall prevalence of amiodarone-induced thyroid dysfunction, though widely variable in different series, is between 15% and 20%, but may increase to 36% or 49% in patients with congenital heart disease, with beta-thalassemia major, or under phenytoin therapy (1).

Amiodarone-Induced Thyrotoxicosis

AIT preferentially occurs in iodine-deficient areas and in men. Amiodarone therapy is not associated with de novo development of thyroid autoimmunity.

Type 1 AIT is a form of iodine-induced hyperthyroidism with the iodine load revealing preexisting, latent thyroid autonomy due to Graves' disease or nodular goiter. This explains the relative preponderance of AIT in iodine-deficient regions, where the prevalence of nodular goiter is high, and in men, given that iodine-induced thyrotoxicosis is more common in males (4,6). In iodine-replete areas the higher sensitivity of the thyroid gland to generate an iodine-induced turn-off signal for hormone biosynthesis makes it relatively resistant to the iodine load. Iodine load may rapidly trigger thyroidal hyperfunction in type 1 AIT, with a median of 3.5 months from institution of amiodarone therapy to occurrence of thyrotoxicosis (Tomisti et al, unpublished).

Type 2 AIT is a thyroid-destructive process of the thyroid gland, causing a release of preformed thyroid hormones from the damaged thyroid follicular epithelium. This may imply that a high intrathyroidal drug concentration needs to be reached before the damage to thyroid follicular cells becomes evident at a clinical level. In this regard, it is worth mentioning that in our institutional series of AIT patients, the median time interval before the occurrence of thyrotoxicosis was 30 months, much longer than in type 1 AIT (Tomisti et al, unpublished).

Differentiation of the 2 main forms of AIT is crucial, although challenging, because treatment and outcome differ. Several diagnostic procedures may be required for an accurate differentiation between type 1 and type 2 AIT, as reported in Table 12-1. Although an increased serum T_4/T_3 ratio (>4) is typical in destructive thyroiditis, it is not useful in individual amiodarone-treated patients, because serum FT_4 is relatively higher than FT_3 due to the inhibition of type 1 deiodinase (7,8).

Increased synthesis and destructive phenomena may all contribute to the pathogenesis of the challenging, indefinite forms of AIT.

Mean radioactive iodine uptake (RAIU) values are usually very low to undetectable in type 2 AIT patients, due to prevalent destructive phenomena, whereas they may be low-to-normal in type 1 AIT, owing to the underlying autonomous function (9,10).

Thyroid ultrasonography may reveal underlying nodules or goiter. However, conventional echography does not provide functional

Table 12-1. Clinical and Pathogenic Features of the Two Main Forms of AIT

	Type 1 AIT	Type 2 AIT
Preexisting thyroid disease	Yes (latent Graves' disease, single- or multinodular goiter)	No
FT_4/FT_3 ratio	Often >4	<4
Spontaneous remission	No	Possible
Thyroid ultrasound CFDS	Increased vascularity	Absent hypervascularity
Thyroidal RAIU	Low-to-normal uptake	Low-to-absent uptake
Thyroid autoantibodies	Sometimes present	Usually absent

Abbreviations: CFDS = color-flow Doppler sonography; RAIU = radioactive iodine uptake.

information, and the presence of goiter or nodules does not necessarily imply that an increased thyroid hormone synthesis is the underlying pathogenic mechanism. Color-flow Doppler echography shows an increase in thyroid vascularization in most type 1 AIT patients, whereas an absent hypervascularity, in spite of high serum thyroid hormone concentrations, is almost invariably associated with type 2 AIT (7,11).

In principle, clinical features of AIT are indistinguishable from those of the other forms of thyrotoxicosis. However, selected features may herald the occurrence of AIT in a patient under amiodarone therapy:

- Reduced appetite, absence of distal tremors, and depression may be atypical features of AIT in the elderly (apathetic hyperthyroidism).
- AIT may worsen the underlying cardiac disease; thus, difficulties in arrhythmia control in patients under chronic amiodarone therapy may reflect development of AIT.
- Thyrotoxicosis may increase degradation rate of vitamin K-dependent coagulation factors; thus, unexplained increased sensitivity to warfarin, in patients under anticoagulant and amiodarone therapy, might be related to undiagnosed AIT (12).

MEDICAL MANAGEMENT OF AIT

The choice of therapy for AIT should take into account several key points:

- The underlying thyroid disease and the consequent AIT type
- The underlying cardiac disease
- The cardiovascular conditions
- The need to continue amiodarone therapy

Type 1 AIT

Type 1 AIT is best treated by antithyroid drugs (carbimazole, methimazole, or propylthiouracil). However, the iodine-replete thyroid gland of AIT patients is less responsive to thionamides. Thus, very high daily doses of the drug (40–60 mg/d methimazole or equivalent doses of propylthiouracil) for longer than usual periods of time are needed before euthyroidism is restored (Table 12-2) (13). This is obviously not an ideal situation in patients with underlying cardiac problems, whose hyperthyroidism should be promptly controlled. To increase the sensitivity of the thyroid gland and the response to thionamides, potassium perchlorate, which decreases thyroid iodine uptake, can be usefully added, if available. To minimize the adverse effects of the drug (particularly on the kidney and blood marrow), doses not exceeding 1 g/d should be used (Table 12-2). In addition, it is recommended not to use the drug for more than 4–6 weeks. Thionamides therapy can be continued until euthyroidism is restored, if this is permitted by the underlying heart disease and cardiocirculatory compensation. After restoration of euthyroidism, definitive therapy of the hyperfunctioning thyroid gland should be considered. If amiodarone can be discontinued, radioiodine therapy can

Table 12-2. Medical Therapies of AIT

Drugs	Starting Dose	Duration
Methimazole	40–60 mg/day	To be tapered gradually to a maintenance dose
Propylthiouracil	400–600 mg/day	To be tapered gradually to a maintenance dose
Carbimazole	40–60 mg/day	To be tapered gradually to a maintenance dose
Potassium perchlorate	≤1 g/day	≤4–6 weeks
Prednisone	0.5–0.7 mg/kg/day	To be gradually tapered based on thyroid hormone levels
Methylprednisolone	0.4–0.6 mg/kg/day	To be gradually tapered based on thyroid hormone levels
Iopanoic acid	1 g/day	Usually 7–21 days before surgery[a]

[a]It may be continued for a longer period in selected cases.

be performed after iodine contamination is over, as suggested by normalized iodine urinary excretion. Otherwise total thyroidectomy should be considered.

Type 2 AIT

Type 2 AIT is currently the predominant form of AIT (89%). It is best treated by glucocorticoids. This is usually required, although mild forms may be transient and self-limiting, requiring only watchful waiting. Initial prednisone dose is about 0.5–0.7 mg/kg body weight per day (or equivalent dose of other steroids) (14), gradually tapering down the drug according to thyroid hormone reduction (Table 12-2). Although response to treatment is often dramatic, with 50% of patients being euthyroid within 4 weeks, response is sometimes delayed (Figure 12-1). Factors possibly delaying the response to glucocorticoids are thyroid volume (>25 mL) and serum FT_4 (>50 pg/mL) at diagnosis (15). Thionamides are not effective in type 2 AIT and should be avoided. Discontinuation of amiodarone therapy is advisable, if feasible, to reduce the recurrence rate of thyrotoxicosis, to allow a prompt and stable restoration of euthyroidism, and to shorten the exposure of the heart to thyroid hormone excess (16). After restoration of euthyroidism, periodical assessment of thyroid status is required, because >15% of patients will develop permanent hypothyroidism over time, requiring thyroxine replacement therapy (17).

Indefinite AIT Forms

The most difficult challenge is represented by mixed/indefinite forms of AIT because both pathogenic mechanisms described for type 1 and type 2 AIT are likely operating. The best medical treatment is a combination of thionamides (with or without potassium perchlorate) and oral glucocorticoids. However, mixed/indefinite forms of AIT, although proposed as a separate entity, have not been fully characterized so far. If the presence of underlying Graves' disease or toxic adenoma is strongly suggestive of type 1 AIT, whereas a normal thyroid gland suggests type 2 AIT, patients with multinodular goiter may potentially develop both main forms of AIT type, making it difficult to differentiate the precise etiology.

The concomitant presence of features of hyperthyroidism and destructive thyroiditis is compatible with the contribution of both pathogenetic mechanisms. If a patient initially treated with thionamides alone (because of a diagnosis of type 1 AIT) does not respond within a reasonably short period of time (3–4 weeks), most thyroidologists usually add potassium perchlorate and/or oral glucocorticoids, even though there is no evidence supporting this indication (18).

AIT and Warfarin

Particular attention should be paid to AIT patients who need to start warfarin therapy.

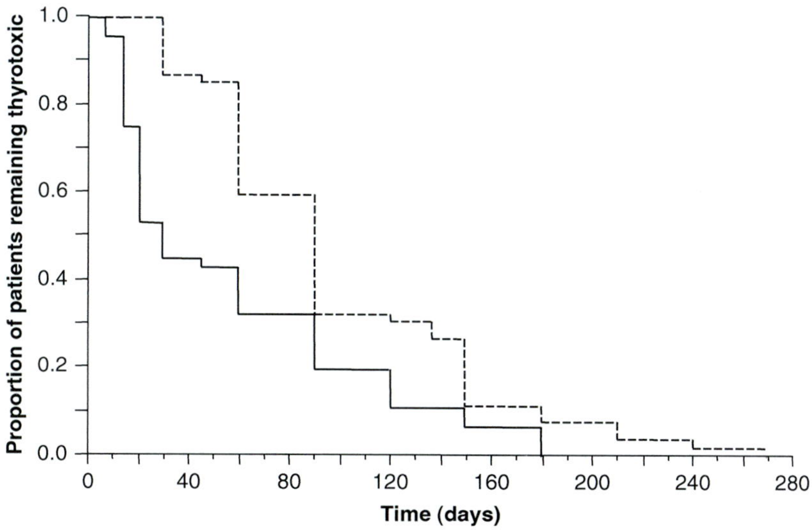

Figure 12-1. Proportion of type 2 AIT patients remaining thyrotoxic during glucocorticoid therapy, considering either the normalization of both T_4 and T_3 (continuous line) or that of TSH (dotted line). From Bogazzi F, Bartalena L, Tomisti L, et al. Glucocorticoid response in amiodarone-induced thyrotoxicosis resulting from destructive thyroiditis is predicted by thyroid volume and serum free thyroid hormone concentrations. *J Clin Endocrinol Metab.* 2007;92:556–562.

In these subjects, therapy should be instituted using a very low dose, because amiodarone per se and thyrotoxicosis increase the effect of warfarin therapy. In addition, polymorphisms in the genes involved in warfarin metabolism (*CYP2C9* and *VKORC1*), if present, can strongly increase warfarin sensitivity, exposing AIT patients to a high risk of bleeding (19).

EMERGENT THERAPY FOR AIT

AIT is a dangerous condition for the patient because of the additional risk posed by thyrotoxicosis to the underlying cardiac abnormalities. Indeed, AIT has been associated with increased morbidity and mortality (Figure 12-2), especially in older patients with impaired left ventricular function (20,21). Thus, a prompt restoration and stable maintenance of euthyroidism should be achieved as quickly as possible, particularly in some patients. Hence, in selected categories of patients, detailed in the number list that follows, emergent management of AIT should be considered in order to obtain a rapid resolution of thyrotoxicosis.

1. *Patients with deterioration of cardiac conditions.* AIT patients with stable cardiac conditions may continue medical therapy and cope with a longer exposure to thyroid hormone excess. At variance, patients with left ventricular systolic dysfunction, as assessed by the left ventricular ejection fraction (LVEF), have an increased mortality risk (Figure 12-3). AIT and left ventricular systolic dysfunction are independent factors associated with high cardiovascular morbidity and mortality. In AIT patients with low LVEF, mortality may be as high as 30%–50%. These findings suggest that in patients with severe underlying cardiac disease, prolonged exposure to high thyroid hormone levels may further deteriorate cardiac function and be responsible for the increased mortality rate (22).
2. *Patients unresponsive to medical therapy.* Patients with type 1 AIT often need large doses and a prolonged course of thionamides before achieving euthyroidism because the iodine-replete thyroid gland is less responsive to antithyroid drugs. On the other hand, approximately 20% of glucocorticoid-treated patients with type 2 AIT still are thyrotoxic after 2 months of therapy (more frequently patients with larger thyroid volume and severe thyrotoxicosis) (15).

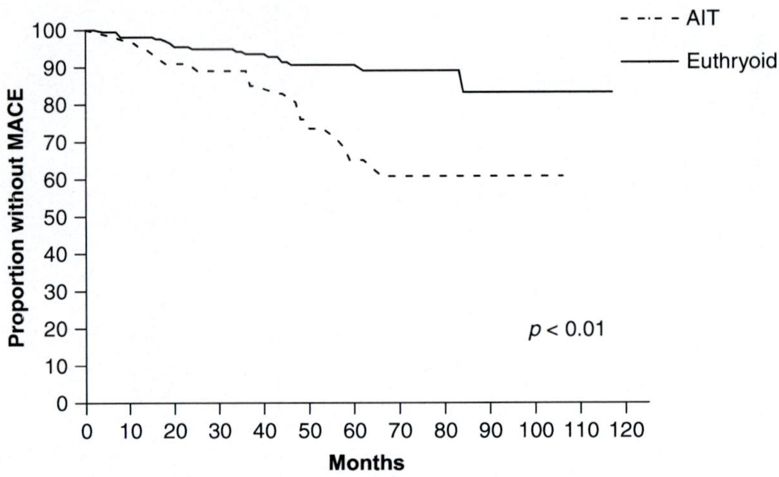

Figure 12-2. Development of major adverse cardiovascular events (MACE) in patients with AIT (dotted line) compared with euthyroid patients under amiodarone therapy (continuous line). MACE was defined as the occurrence of heart failure requiring hospitalization, cardiovascular mortality, myocardial infarction, stroke including transient ischemic attack, and ventricular arrhythmias requiring hospital admission. From Yiu KH, Jim MH, Siu CW, et al. Amiodarone-induced thyrotoxicosis is a predictor of adverse cardiovascular outcome. *J Clin Endocrinol Metab.* 2009;94:109–114.

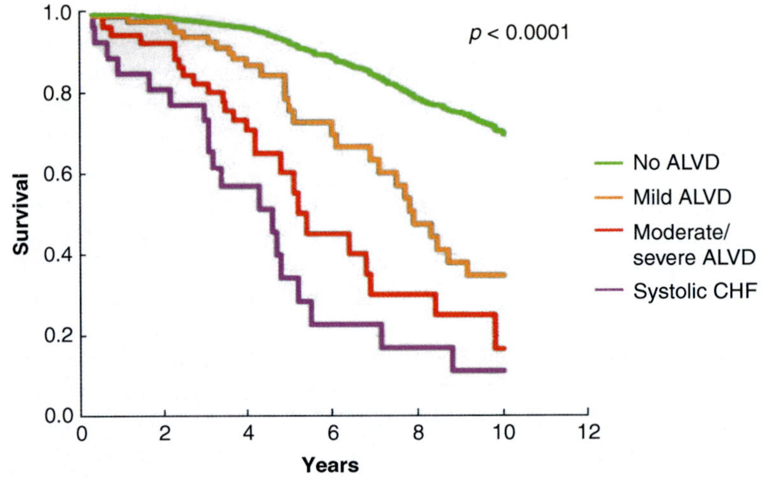

Figure 12-3. Mortality of patients with asymptomatic left ventricular systolic dysfunction (ALVD) according to ejection fraction (EF). Referent group consists of subjects with normal left ventricular systolic function (EF >50%) and no history of congestive heart failure (No ALVD). Mild ALVD: mild asymptomatic left ventricular systolic dysfunction (EF 40%–50%). Moderate/severe ALVD: moderate-to-severe asymptomatic left ventricular systolic dysfunction (EF <40%). Systolic CHF: congestive heart failure with EF ≤50%. Modified from Wang TJ, Evans JC, Benjamin EJ, et al. Natural history of asymptomatic left ventricular systolic dysfunction in the community. *Circulation.* 2003;108:977–982.

3. *Patients needing to continue amiodarone therapy.* In type 2 AIT patients treated with glucocorticoids, continuation of amiodarone does not significantly affect the first normalization of thyroid hormone. However, patients requiring continuations of amiodarone therapy show a high risk of recurrence of thyrotoxicosis during glucocorticoids therapy (about 70%), causing a delay in achieving stable restoration of euthyroidism (16).
4. *Patients with type 2 AIT showing advrse effect to glucocorticoids therapy.* These include severe hyperglycemia, hepatotoxicity, glucocorticoid-induced osteoporosis, and opportunistic infections.

In this subset of patients, total thyroidectomy can represent the only therapeutic approach to guarantee a quick resolution of thyrotoxicosis. In addition, surgery, by rapidly restoring euthyroidism, can improve cardiac function within 2 months (Figure 12-4), mainly in patients with severe left ventricular systolic dysfunction, thereby reducing the risk of death (23). Therefore, in patients with deteriorated left ventricular function, surgery should be considered without delay.

Older studies have reported frequent postoperative complications, including rehospitalization and death (24). Conversely, recent studies have shown that total thyroidectomy can be performed in AIT patients, including those with moderate-to-severe left ventricular dysfunction, without serious complications (25,26). Even though controlled studies are not available, our extensive personal experience suggests that an optimal preparation for surgery, including glucocorticoids and beta blockers, may reduce the surgical risk. Thus, in AIT patients who are candidates for total thyroidectomy, a short course with glucocorticoids is mandatory, irrespective of the AIT type. More importantly, a multidisciplinary interaction of an experienced team, including surgeon, endocrinologist, cardiologist, and anesthesiologist dedicated to the management of AIT patients, is fundamental.

We have extensively used iopanoic acid (for 7–21 days before surgery) to reduce serum FT_3 in patients unresponsive to medical therapy (Table 12-2) (27). However, in the absence of controlled studies, the real advantage of preparation with iopanoic acid for thyroidectomy in preventing surgical adverse events remains to be established. In addition, iopanoic acid is no longer available. Whether other iodinated contrast agents may replace iopanoic acid is uncertain.

Recently, radioiodine therapy with 131-1 after stimulation with recombinant human TSH (rhTSH) alone or associated with rhTSH and lithium therapy has been proposed for the treatment of AIT patients to overcome the problem of low RAIU values (28). However, owing to very limited experience in this subset of patients and to the risk of exacerbation of hyperthyroidism with consequent deleterious cardiac effects, this option should be considered with caution and is not currently recommended (29).

Plasmapheresis, aimed at removing excess thyroid hormones from the circulation, has

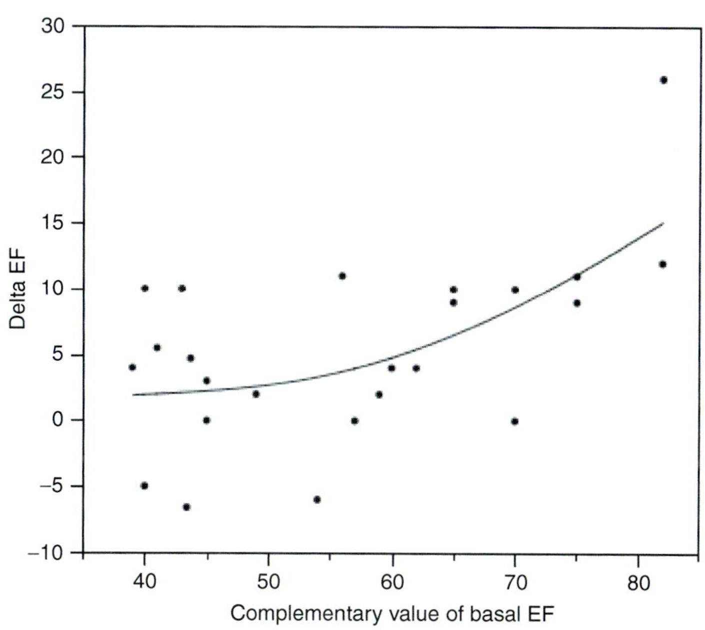

Figure 12-4. Change in ejection fraction values before and 2 months after surgery—our experience. Delta EF: difference between left ventricular ejection fraction value before and 2 months after total thyroidectomy. Complementary value of basal EF: basal left ventricular ejection fraction value expressed as complementary value of 100. For example, a patient with ejection fraction of 20% will be a complementary value of basal EF: 100–20 = 80. Based on Tomisti L, Materazzi G, Bartalena L, et al. Total thyroidectomy in patients with amiodarone-induced thyrotoxicosis and severe left ventricular systolic dysfunction. *J Clin Endocrinol Metab.* 2012;97:3515–3521.

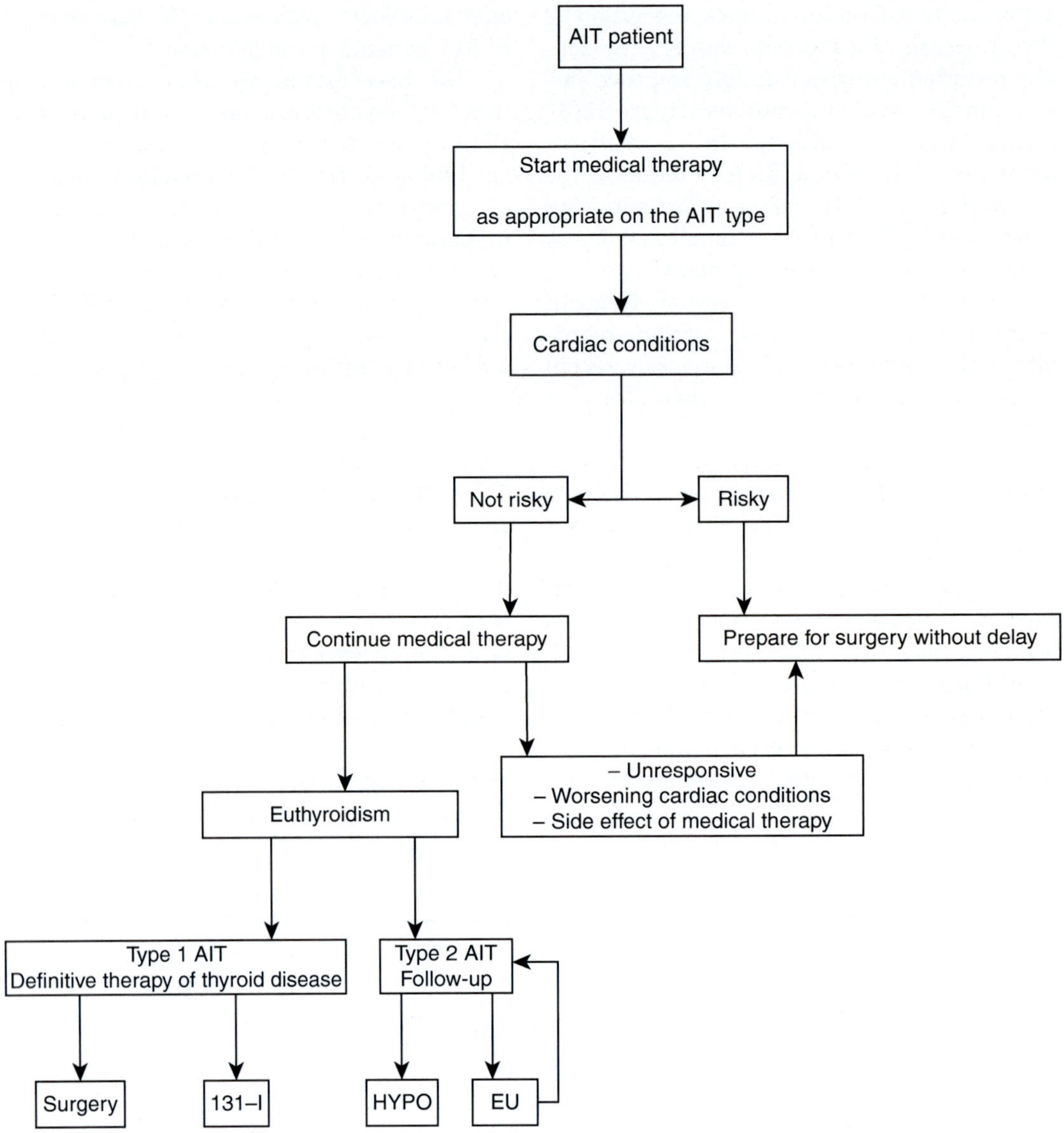

Figure 12-5. A proposed flow chart for the management of AIT patients. Patients with compromised cardiac function should be considered for total thyroidectomy shortly after diagnosis of AIT. In addition, total thyroidectomy may be considered for patients unresponsive to medical therapies, or if amiodarone should be continued during thyrotoxicosis.

been reported to be efficacious, but this is usually transient and followed by exacerbation of thyrotoxicosis. Thus, its real advantage is uncertain.

CONCLUSIONS

All patients with AIT should be considered to be at risk of requiring emergent treatment (Figure 12-5). Thyrotoxicosis may precipitate cardiac conditions even in asymptomatic patients. This is unlikely to occur in patients with subtle cardiac abnormalities and likely to be more frequent in those with severe heart disease (eg, congenital heart disease, postinfarction heart disease, or ventricular arrhythmias).

ACKNOWLEDGMENTS

The authors have nothing to disclose.

REFERENCES

1. **Martino E, Bartalena L, Bogazzi F, Braverman LE.** The effects of amiodarone on the thyroid. *Endocr Rev.* 2001;22:240–254.

2. **Bogazzi F, Bartalena L, Gasperi M, Braverman LE, Martino E.** The various effects of amiodarone on thyroid function. *Thyroid.* 2001;11:511–519.
3. **Reiffel JA, Estes NA 3rd, Waldo AL, Prystowsky EN, DiBianco R.** A consensus report on antiarrhythmic drug use. *Clin Cardiol.* 1994;17:103–116.
4. **Bogazzi F, Tomisti L, Bartalena L, Aghini-Lombardi F, Martino E.** Amiodarone and the thyroid: a 2012 update. *J Endocrinol Invest.* 2012;35:340–348.
5. **Doval HC, Nul DR, Grancelli HO, Perrone SV, Bortman GR, Curiel R.** Randomised trial of low-dose amiodarone in severe congestive heart failure. Grupo de Estudio de la Sobrevida en la Insuficiencia Cardiaca en Argentina (GESICA). *Lancet.* 1994;344:493–498.
6. **Eskes SA, Wiersinga WM.** Amiodarone and thyroid. *Best Pract Res Clin Endocrinol Metab.* 2009;23: 735–751.
7. **Eaton SE, Euinton HA, Newman CM, Weetman AP, Bennet WM.** Clinical experience of amiodarone-induced thyrotoxicosis over a 3-year period: role of colour-flow Doppler sonography. *Clin Endocrinol (Oxf).* 2002;56:33–38.
8. **Bogazzi F, Bartalena L, Dell'Unto E, et al.** Proportion of type 1 and type 2 amiodarone-induced thyrotoxicosis has changed over a 27-year period in Italy. *Clin Endocrinol (Oxf).* 2007;67:533–537.
9. **Daniels GH.** Amiodarone-induced thyrotoxicosis. *J Clin Endocrinol Metab.* 2001;86:3–8.
10. **Martino E, Aghini-Lombardi F, Lippi F.** Twenty-four hour radioactive iodine uptake in 35 patients with amiodarone associated thyrotoxicosis. *J Nucl Med.* 1985;26:1402–1407.
11. **Bogazzi F, Bartalena L, Brogioni S, et al.** Color flow Doppler sonography rapidly differentiates type I and type II amiodarone-induced thyrotoxicosis. *Thyroid.* 1997;7:541–545.
12. **Kurnik D, Loebstein R, Farfel Z, Ezra D, Halkin H, Olchovsky D.** Complex drug-drug-disease interactions between amiodarone, warfarin, and the thyroid gland. *Medicine (Baltimore).* 2004;83:107–113.
13. **Bogazzi F, Bartalena L, Martino E.** Approach to the patient with amiodarone-induced thyrotoxicosis. *J Clin Endocrinol Metab.* 2010;95:2529–2535.
14. **Bogazzi F, Tomisti L, Rossi G, et al.** Glucocorticoids are preferable to thionamides as first-line treatment for amiodarone-induced thyrotoxicosis due to destructive thyroiditis: a matched retrospective cohort study. *J Clin Endocrinol Metab.* 2009;94:3757–3762.
15. **Bogazzi F, Bartalena L, Tomisti L, et al.** Glucocorticoid response in amiodarone-induced thyrotoxicosis resulting from destructive thyroiditis is predicted by thyroid volume and serum free thyroid hormone concentrations. *J Clin Endocrinol Metab.* 2007;92: 556–562.
16. **Bogazzi F, Bartalena L, Tomisti L, et al.** Continuation of amiodarone delays restoration of euthyroidism in patients with type 2 amiodarone-induced thyrotoxicosis treated with prednisone: a pilot study. *J Clin Endocrinol Metab.* 2011;96:3374–3380.
17. **Bogazzi F, Dell'Unto E, Tanda ML, et al.** Long-term outcome of thyroid function after amiodarone-induced thyrotoxicosis, as compared to subacute thyroiditis. *J Endocrinol Invest.* 2006;29:694–699.
18. **Diehl LA, Romaldini JH, Graf H, et al.** Management of amiodarone-induced thyrotoxicosis in Latin America: an electronic survey. *Clin Endocrinol (Oxf).* 2006;65:433–438.
19. **Tomisti L, Del Re M, Bartalena L, et al.** Effects of amiodarone, thyroid hormones and CYP2C9 and VKORC1 polymorphisms on warfarin metabolism: a review of the literature. *Endocr Pract.* 2013;19:1–27.
20. **Yiu KH, Jim MH, Siu CW, et al.** Amiodarone-induced thyrotoxicosis is a predictor of adverse cardiovascular outcome. *J Clin Endocrinol Metab.* 2009;94:109–114.
21. **O'Sullivan AJ, Lewis M, Diamond T.** Amiodarone-induced thyrotoxicosis: left ventricular dysfunction is associated with increased mortality. *Eur J Endocrinol.* 2006;154:533–536.
22. **Wang TJ, Evans JC, Benjamin EJ, et al.** Natural history of asymptomatic left ventricular systolic dysfunction in the community. *Circulation.* 2003;108:977–982.
23. **Tomisti L, Materazzi G, Bartalena L, et al.** Total thyroidectomy in patients with amiodarone-induced thyrotoxicosis and severe left ventricular systolic dysfunction. *J Clin Endocrinol Metab.* 2012;97: 3515–3521.
24. **Houghton SG, Farley DR, Brennan MD, van Heerden JA, Thompson GB, Grant CS.** Surgical management of amiodarone-associated thyrotoxicosis: Mayo Clinic experience. *World J Surg.* 2004;28:1083–1087.
25. **Gough J, Gough IR.** Total thyroidectomy for amiodarone-associated thyrotoxicosis in patients with severe cardiac disease. *World J Surg.* 2006;30:1957–1961.
26. **Pierret C, Tourtier JP, Pons Y, Merat S, Duverger V, Perrier E.** Total thyroidectomy for amiodarone-associated thyrotoxicosis: should surgery always be delayed for pre-operative medical preparation? *J Laryngol Otol.* 2012;126:701–705.
27. **Bogazzi F, Miccoli P, Berti P, et al.** Preparation with iopanoic acid rapidly controls thyrotoxicosis in patients with amiodarone-induced thyrotoxicosis before thyroidectomy. *Surgery.* 2002;132:1114–1117; discussion 1118.
28. **Albino CC, Paz-Filho G, Graf H.** Recombinant human TSH as an adjuvant to radioiodine for the treatment of type 1 amiodarone-induced thyrotoxicosis (AIT). *Clin Endocrinol (Oxf).* 2009;70:810–811.
29. **Bogazzi F, Tomisti L, Ceccarelli C, Martino E.** Recombinant human TSH as an adjuvant to radioiodine for the treatment of type 1 amiodarone-induced thyrotoxicosis: a cautionary note. *Clin Endocrinol (Oxf).* 2010;72:133–134.

CHAPTER 13

Thyrotoxic Periodic Paralysis

Chih-Jen Cheng and Shih-Hua Lin

ABSTRACT

Thyrotoxic periodic paralysis (TPP) characterized by a triad of muscle paralysis, acute hypokalemia, and hyperthyroidism is a potentially life-threatening but reversible medical emergency. Due to subtle thyrotoxic symptoms in most TPP patients, the assessment of electrolyte and acid-base status in blood and urine, electrocardiography, and the potassium chloride (KCl) dosage required to recover from paralysis are valuable in diagnosing TPP. Regarding acute therapy, the dose of KCl should be minimized to avoid rebound hyperkalemia. The judicious use of nonselective beta blockers may help terminate the attack, especially for those who developed paradoxical hypokalemia associated with hyperadrenergic activity.

INTRODUCTION

Hypokalemic periodic paralysis (HypoPP) is characterized by muscle weakness or paralysis associated with acute hypokalemia due to a sudden shift of potassium (K^+) into cells without a total K^+ deficit (1). Among the etiologies of HypoPP, familial periodic paralysis (FPP) due to voltage-gated sodium (Nav 1.4) and calcium (Cav1.1) channel mutations is most common in individuals of Asian descent, and nonfamilial thyrotoxic periodic paralysis (TPP) is most common in individuals of non-Asian descent (2). In the United States, the incidence of TPP in a non-Asian ethnic population is approximately one tenth (0.1%–0.2%) of that found in Asian countries (3). With immigration and globalization, TPP has been increasingly encountered worldwide (4,5). It is crucial to recognize and treat TPP promptly in order to avoid life-threatening complications such as cardiac arrhythmias and respiratory failure. Nevertheless, TPP is still fraught with emergent challenges concerning correct diagnosis and more appropriate management (6).

PATHOGENESIS

The pathogenesis of TPP remains incompletely understood. The severity of muscle paralysis seems to be correlated with the degree of hypokalemia rather than that of elevated thyroid hormone (1,2), suggesting the role of acute hypokalemia in the mechanisms of muscle paralysis. In skeletal muscle, Na-K-ATPase and potassium channels provide the main access for inward (uptake) and outward (release) potassium fluxes, respectively (7). Accordingly, the stimulation of Na-K-ATPase or inhibition of K^+ channels can be critical to the pathogenesis of acute hypokalemia in TPP. An increased Na^+-K^+ ATPase pump activity stimulated by thyroid hormone and/or by hyperadrenergic activity and hyperinsulinemia has been long thought to be a major mechanism of TPP (8). The role of insulin in TPP was revealed by the findings that hyperinsulinemia was observed during acute attacks of TPP and that TPP patients had exaggerated insulin responses to oral glucose challenge in comparison with hyperthyroidism patients without TPP (9,10). The hyperinsulinemic response may account for the association of TPP with high-carbohydrate ingestion. However, only 0%–30% of TPP patients receiving an oral glucose load to examine the role of endogenous hyperinsulinemia in precipitating attacks developed glucose-induced acute hypokalemia with paralysis (11). TPP patients with provocable attacks had similar insulin responses to those without induced paralysis. Based on the infrequency of glucose load-induced paralysis, other insulin-independent factors must also be involved in the pathogenesis of TPP. Recent elegant studies have shown that reduced outward K^+ efflux in the skeletal muscle-specific inward rectifying K^+ (Kir) channel also plays a critical role in increasing the susceptibility of hypokalemia-induced paradoxical depolarization, in turn leading to Na^+ channel inactivation and the resultant muscle excitability and paralysis (12–14).

CLINICAL FEATURES

TPP is known to occur predominately in males despite a higher incidence of thyrotoxicosis in women (1). TPP attacks are most common in hot weather during summer and autumn. Increased consumption of sweet drinks, increased outdoor activities and exercise, and increased K^+ loss in sweat are possible factors explaining the seasonal pattern. Most attacks occur in the early morning or late evening. The first episode of TPP usually occurs between the ages of 20 and 40 years in contrast to the younger onset (under 20 years) of FPP (1,15). The clinical features of TPP are virtually indistinguishable from those of FPP. Prodromal symptoms include muscle aches, cramps, and muscle stiffness. Weakness usually begins in the proximal muscles of the lower extremities and can progress to flaccid quadriplegia. The paralysis is usually symmetrical but bulbar, respiratory, and ocular muscles are usually spared. Serum K^+ concentration decreases but not always below the normal range during the attack. Although spontaneous resolution of attacks will occur within a few hours to 2 days, patients with unrecognized TPP or without K^+ supplementation may die of the life-threatening cardiac arrhythmias and respiratory failure under a hypokalemic state. One has to separate TPP from thyrotoxic myopathy characterized by persistent muscle weakness and soreness of proximal muscles and normokalemia (1).

SYMPTOMS AND SIGNS OF HYPERTHYROIDISM

Thyrotoxicosis is a prerequisite for the diagnosis of TPP. However, it is often stated in the literature that typical clinical symptoms of thyrotoxicosis such as weight loss, heat intolerance, palpitations, increased appetite, excitability, and diaphoresis may be subtle, and periodic paralysis may precede these symptoms in TPP (3,16,17). Because thyroid hormone measurement is not often available in the emergency department, prompt diagnosis of thyrotoxicosis primarily relies on family and personal histories, as well as on clinical assessment of hyperthyroid signs/symptoms. It was recently reported that only one third of TPP patients had a known personal or family history of hyperthyroidism (11). Using the Wayne's index (a reliable quantitative score of hyperthyroid severity), only 17% of TPP patients had toxic thyrotoxicosis (score >19) at the time of presentation, supporting the notion that most TPP patients have mild to equivocal hyperthyroid symptoms (11). For those who did not have known personal/family history or overt clinical thyrotoxicosis, the rapid and correct diagnosis of TPP relies on some distinct clinical and laboratory findings characteristic of TPP.

PRECIPITANTS

Precipitating factors, including high-carbohydrate loads, strenuous exercise, trauma, acute upper respiratory tract infection (URI), high-salt diet, emotional stress, exposure to cold, alcohol ingestion, menstruation, and use of drugs such as corticosteroids, epinephrine, acetazolamide, and nonsteroidal anti-inflammatory drugs, have been reported to induce attacks of TPP (1–3,11,19,20). However, an extensive review of precipitating factors in a recent TPP prospective study has found that only the minority of TPP attacks (34%) had identifiable precipitants (11). High-carbohydrate loads and strenuous exercise, the 2 most-recognized precipitating factors in TPP and FPP, were implicated in only 12% and 7% of TPP patients, respectively. The low frequency of high-carbohydrate load-provoked TPP may be related to the westernization of the Asian diet with declining rice intake and increasing protein consumption. Nevertheless, other potential provocative factors still need to be scrutinized in TPP patients whose attacks lack currently identifiable precipitants.

DIAGNOSIS

TPP is a hyperthyroidism-related acute hypokalemia with muscle weakness or paralysis resulting from a sudden shift of K^+ into cells without a total K^+ deficit. Unawareness or delayed treatment of TPP often leads to serious consequences, such as rhabdomyolysis, respiratory failure, or cardiac arrhythmia. As mentioned previously, typical clinical symptoms of hyperthyroidism are often subtle, and thyroid function tests are usually not available in the emergency room. It should be also noted that the findings of thyrotoxicosis and hypokalemia do not guarantee the diagnosis of TPP. For instance, patients with hyperthyroidism can develop hypokalemic paralysis caused by diuretic-induced or coexisting renal tubular disorders with renal K^+ wasting. The first assessment of renal K^+ excretion and acid-base status at presentation, as well as the amount of KCl supplement to correct hypokalemia, are always required for the diagnosis of TPP (21). Low renal K^+ excretion in response to acute hypokalemia and relatively normal acid-base status are characteristic findings in TPP in contrast to non-HypoPP disorders, which usually have metabolic acidosis or alkalosis associated with large total K^+ deficits (Table 13-1). Because one cannot await a 24-hour urine collection to assess urine K^+ excretion in emergent conditions, a spot urine sample should be used to estimate urinary K^+ excretion rate (22).

Other distinct findings of TPP can also help establish TPP. These include adult males without a family history of periodic paralysis, systolic hypertension, tachycardia, and high QRS voltage or first-degree atrioventricular (AV) block on electrocardiography (ECG), as well as low serum creatinine concentration, hypophosphatemia with hypophosphaturia, and hypercalciuria (Table 13-1) (21,23–25). A low to normal serum creatinine concentration was primarily related to the increased renal function due to hyperdynamic changes rather than low lean muscle mass due to hypercatabolism in hyperthyroidism. Enhanced renal reabsorption of phosphate with chronic normal to increased blood phosphate concentration is well known in hyperthyroidism. However, acute hypophosphatemia with low urine phosphate excretion, similar to the mechanisms of acute hypokalemia, was frequently observed in acute attacks of TPP. An increased urine calcium excretion rate due to the direct or indirect effect of thyroid hormone on bone and kidney was also common in TPP. The findings of hypercalciuria and hypophosphaturia are unique in an acute attack of TPP and may be used as an early index to suggest TPP.

TPP can occur with any causes of hyperthyroidism. Once TPP is established, the underlying etiology for hyperthyroidism must be identified and effectively treated to avoid missing a potentially curable cause of TPP. In addition to history and physical examination, the assessment of serum thyroid-stimulating hormone (TSH), autoantibodies to thyroid, and thyroglobulin concentration, as well as radioiodine uptake, can easily identify the underlying causes.

Table 13-1. Distinct Clues for the Diagnosis of TPP

A. Gender: adult males >> females
B. History: nonfamilial paralysis but familial hyperthyroidism
C. Clinical thyrotoxic symptoms and signs (Wayne's index score >19)
D. ECG findings
  - Sinus tachycardia or sinus arrhythmia
  - First-degree atrioventricular (AV) block
  - Left ventricular hypertrophy (LVH) pattern
E. Electrolyte, acid-base, and biochemistry in blood and urine
  - Hypokalemia with low urine K^+ excretion rate
  - Relatively normal blood acid-base balance
  - Hypophosphatemia with low urine phosphate excretion
  - Normal or increased serum calcium with hypercalciuria
  - Hypocreatinemia (increased glomerular filtration rate)
F. Therapeutic course
  - Lower K^+ dose to achieve recovery
  - Rebound hyperkalemia if high K^+ dose is given

MANAGEMENT

Acute Emergent Therapy

K⁺ supplementation. Due to acute hypokalemia, close cardiac monitoring is absolutely warranted. K^+ replacement has been advocated for the treatment of paralysis and prevention of a fatal cardiac arrhythmia in patients with TPP. Unlike non-HypoPP disorders due to a large K^+ deficit (26), patients with TPP do not have K^+ deficit. The aim of K^+ supplementation is to raise serum K^+ concentration rather than to fill a large K^+ deficit (26). It has been shown that intravenous (IV) KCl therapy (10 mEq/hr [10 mmol/hr]) is associated with a more rapid recovery of muscle strength (2 times shorter) than controls (27). The mechanism is still unclear, but the slight correction of hypokalemia may stop the hypokalemia-induced paradoxical depolarization of skeletal muscles and reactivate the voltage-gated Na^+ channel (21). However, exogenous KCl administration carries a risk of rebound hyperkalemia because K^+ is released from cells rapidly when the paralysis subsides (Figure 13-1) (1,26). Rebound hyperkalemia (>5.0 mEq/L [5 mmol/L]) on recovery has been reported in approximately 40%–70% of patients with TPP receiving KCl therapy and is correlated with the dose of KCl administered (27,28). Severe rebound hyperkalemia with ventricular arrhythmia needs to be emergently treated with rapid calcium and insulin infusion, followed by the administration of loop diuretics and exogenous mineralocorticoid. However, the risk of rebound hyperkalemia is markedly reduced if the total KCl dose given is less than 50 mEq (50 mmol) (27). Based on the previous reports and our experience, we suggest that the KCl dose should be given at the rate of no more than 10 mEq/hr (10 mmol/hr).

Of note, "paradoxical hypokalemia" defined as a further fall in plasma K^+ concentration (>0.1 mEq/L [0.1 mmol/L]) is not uncommon (approximately 25%) during KCl therapy (28). Patients developing paradoxical hypokalemia during treatment are associated with more severe hyperthyroidism and hyperadrenergic activity. They usually need a higher KCl dosage to restore muscle strength and consequently develop more severe rebound hyperkalemia after recovery. Those who do not develop paradoxical hypokalemia usually need a smaller KCl dose to achieve recovery and have a much lower risk of rebound hyperkalemia.

Some cautionary notes are in order when KCl is administered to treat patients with TPP (26,27). First, parenteral KCl might be administered in saline instead of glucose solution, which may cause redistribution of K^+ from extracellular into intracellular space via enhanced insulin secretion. Second, if bowel sounds are absent or diminished, the oral route for K^+ administration should be avoided. When oral KCl is given, the intestinal K^+ absorption could be late when bowel

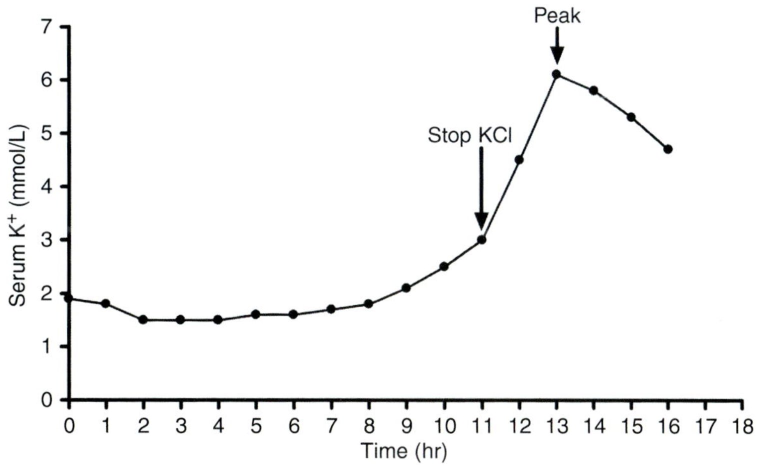

Figure 13-1. Illustration for the paradoxical hypokalemia during treatment and rebound hyperkalemia on recovery. KCl is intravenously administered at a rate of 10 mEq/hr (10 mmol/hr).

motility is compromised by hypokalemia (so-called *hypokalemia-induced pseudointestinal obstruction*). Furthermore, these patients are prone to develop hyperkalemia secondary to enhanced KCl reabsorption hidden in the gastrointestinal tract after hypokalemia is corrected on recovery (26). Third, clinicians may be inclined to administer more K^+ to patients who develop paradoxical hypokalemia (29). Although this management increases the risk of rebound hyperkalemia and life-threatening ventricular arrhythmias upon recovery, a higher dose of K^+ is still urgently warranted in patients who develop life-threatening ventricular arrhythmias and impending respiratory failure. A more rapid KCl 3–6 mEq (3–6 mmol) can be administered intravenously in 1 minute or more to transiently raise K^+ concentration by 1–2 mEq/L (1–2 mmol/L) (cardiac output, 5 L/min; plasma volume, 3 L) (30). The maximum dose of KCl should be kept at 20–40 mEq/hr (20–40 mmol/hr) (30,31).

Nonselective beta blockers. High-dose nonselective beta blockers via the suppression of β_2 adrenergic activity and inhibition of insulin secretion have reportedly been used as an alternate therapy based on the implication of hyperadrenergic activity and hyperinsulinemia in the pathogenesis of TPP (32). Nonselective beta blockers (eg, propranolol: oral 3–4 mg/kg or IV 1–2 mg) but not the selective β_1 receptor blocker (eg, metoprolol) have been shown to shorten the duration of attack and promote recovery in patients with TPP (33,34) and TPP-like disorders (eg, amphetamine-induced TPP-like features and hypokalemic paralysis following a convulsion due to alcohol abstinence) (35,36). Patients with paradoxical hypokalemia may be more suited for the use of nonselective beta blockers to block K^+ uptake via Na-K-ATPase. However, large-scale controlled trials are required to legitimate the use of nonselective beta blockers in TPP. The combined therapy with low-dose KCl and nonselective beta blockers in fostering the recovery and abating rebound hyperkalemia merits further investigation.

The therapeutic algorithm for TPP is shown in Figure 13-2.

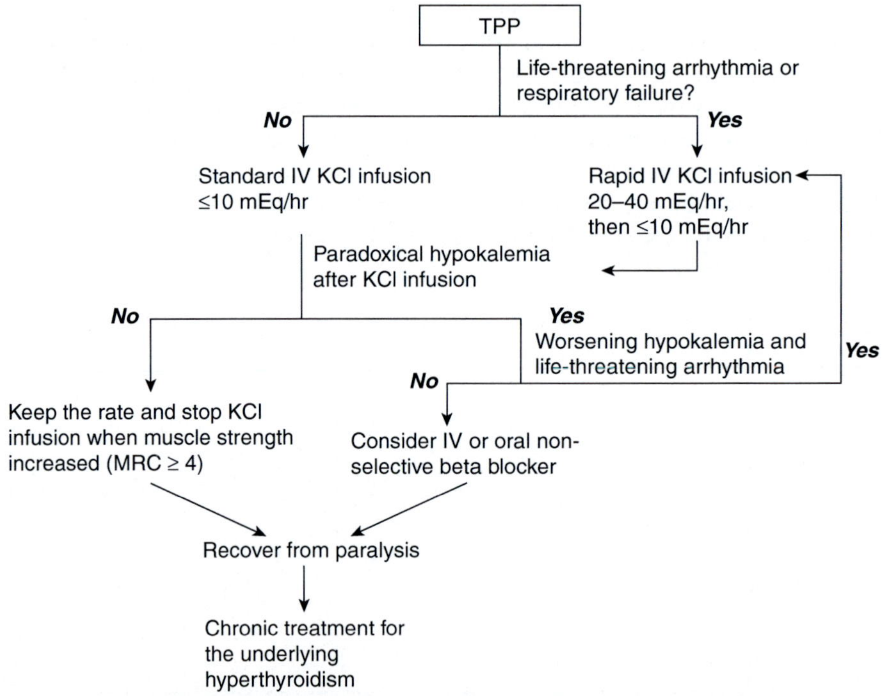

Figure 13-2. The therapeutic algorithm for TPP: IV KCl infusion is generally given at a rate of 10 mEq/hr for TPP patients. This rate can be elevated to 20–40 mEq/hr if life-threatening arrhythmia or respiratory failure occurs. Patients who develop paradoxical hypokalemia after KCl infusion often need more and faster K supplementation, especially when hypokalemia worsens and life-threatening events occur. Judicious use of IV or oral nonselective beta blockers may help facilitate the recovery of paralysis. The definite therapy of TPP relies on the effective control of the underlying etiology of hyperthyroidism. Medical Research Council (MRC) scale for assessment of muscle power (MRC ≥ 4, can move against gravity and some resistance exerted by examiner).

Chronic Therapy

Patients should be advised to avoid any identifiable precipitating factors such as a high-carbohydrate diet, exercise, and stress. The control of underlying causes of hyperthyroidism is the definitive therapy to completely abolish TPP attacks. These therapies include antithyroid drugs, surgical thyroidectomy, and radioiodine therapy. Radioiodine is the preferred mode of therapy for toxic multinodular goiter or toxic adenoma as well as for relapses after antithyroid medications. Nonselective beta blockers are also efficacious in preventing recurrent attacks of TPP via blocking the effect of the thyroid hormone (37). Acetazolamide, which is commonly used in patients with FPP, can precipitate recurrent attacks of TPP and should not be used in TPP (38). Based on the pathogenic role of reduced K^+ channel efflux in TPP, drugs that specifically increase Kir outward current in skeletal muscle, albeit unavailable now, could be potentially effective in the prevention and treatment of TPP, especially in those patients carrying Kir2.1 polymorphism or Kir2.6 mutations (21,39).

CONCLUSIONS

Thyrotoxic periodic paralysis (TPP) is fraught with pathogenetic, diagnostic, and therapeutic challenges. Besides the increased Na^+-K^+ ATPase pump activity, reduced outward K^+ efflux in skeletal muscle-specific Kir channel also plays a critical role in the pathogenesis. Although most patients with TPP do not manifest typical symptoms and signs related to hyperthyroidism, blood and urine electrolyte and acid-base, ECG, and the KCl dose required to correct hypokalemia all help establish the diagnosis of TPP. In acute therapy, the dose of KCl should be minimal to avoid rebound hyperkalemia, except in cases of ventricular arrhythmia and impending respiratory insufficiency. Alternatively, high-dose nonselective beta blockers may be used to help terminate muscle paralysis, especially for those who developed paradoxical hypokalemia associated with evidence of hyperadrenergic activity. Chronic therapy relies on avoiding precipitating factors, the preemptive use of nonselective beta blockers, and definitive control of hyperthyroidism.

ACKNOWLEDGMENTS

The authors have nothing to disclose.

REFERENCES

1. **Lin SH.** Thyrotoxic periodic paralysis. *Mayo Clin Proc.* 2005;80:99–105.
2. **Maciel RM, Lindsey SC, Dias da Silva MR.** Novel etiopathophysiological aspects of thyrotoxic periodic paralysis. *Nat Rev Endocrinol.* 2011;7:657–667.
3. **Ober KP.** Thyrotoxic periodic paralysis in the United States: report of 7 cases and review of the literature. *Medicine.* 1992;71:109–120.
4. **Tran HA, Kay SE, Kende M, Doery JC, Colman PG, Read A.** Thyrotoxic, hypokalaemic periodic paralysis in Australasian men. *Intern Med J.* 2003;33:91–94.
5. **Kilpatrick RE, Seiler-Smith S, Levine SN.** Thyrotoxic hypokalemic periodic paralysis: reports of four cases in black American males. *Thyroid.* 1994;4: 441–445.
6. **Kung AW.** Clinical review: thyrotoxic periodic paralysis: a diagnostic challenge. *J Clin Endocrinol Metab.* 2006;91:2490–2495.
7. **Clausen T.** Hormonal and pharmacological modification of plasma potassium homeostasis. *Fundam Clin Pharmacol.* 2010;24:595–605.
8. **Chan A, Shinde R, Chow CC, Cockram CS, Swaminathan R.** In vivo and in vitro sodium pump activity in subjects with thyrotoxic periodic paralysis. *Br Med J.* 1991;303:1096–1099.
9. **Lee KO, Taylor EA, Oh VM, Cheah JS, Aw SE.** Hyperinsulinaemia in thyrotoxic hypokalaemic periodic paralysis. *Lancet.* 1991;337:1063–1064.
10. **Chan A, Shinde R, Chow CC, Cockram CS, Swaminathan R.** Hyperinsulinaemia and Na^+-K^+-ATPase activity in thyrotoxic periodic paralysis. *Clin Endocrinol.* 1994;41:213–216.
11. **Chang CC, Cheng CJ, Sung CC, et al.** A 10-year analysis of thyrotoxic periodic paralysis in 135 patients: focus on symptomatology and precipitants. *Eur J Endocrinol.* 2013;169:529–536.
12. **Ryan DP, da Silva MR, Soong TW, et al.** Mutations in potassium channel Kir2.6 cause susceptibility to thyrotoxic hypokalemic periodic paralysis. *Cell.* 2010;140:88–98.
13. **Cheng CJ, Lin SH, Lo YF, et al.** Identification and functional characterization of Kir2.6 mutations associated with non-familial hypokalemic periodic paralysis. *J Biol Chem.* 2011;286:27425–27435.
14. **Cheung CL, Lau KS, Ho AY, et al.** Genome-wide association study identifies a susceptibility locus for thyrotoxic periodic paralysis at 17q24.3. *Nat Genet.* 2012;44:1026–1029.
15. **Matthews E, Labrum R, Sweeney MG, et al.** Voltage sensor charge loss accounts for most cases of hypokalemic periodic paralysis. *Neurology.* 2009;72: 1544–1547.
16. **Kelley DE, Gharib H, Kennedy FP, Duda RJ Jr, McManis PG.** Thyrotoxic periodic paralysis: report of 10 cases and review of electromyographic findings. *Arch Intern Med.* 1989;149:2597–2600.

17. **Goh SH.** Thyrotoxic periodic paralysis: reports of seven patients presenting with weakness in an Asian emergency department. *Emerg Med J.* 2002;19:78–79.
18. **Crooks J, Murray IPC, Wayne EJ.** Statistical methods applied to the clinical diagnosis of thyrotoxicosis. *QJM.* 1959;28:211–234.
19. **McFadzean AJ, Yeung R.** Periodic paralysis complicating thyrotoxicosis in Chinese. *Br Med J.* 1967;1:451–455.
20. **Hsieh MJ, Lyu RK, Chang WN, et al.** Hypokalemic thyrotoxic periodic paralysis: clinical characteristics and predictors of recurrent paralytic attacks. *Eur J Neurol.* 2008;15:559–564.
21. **Lin SH, Huang CL.** Mechanism of thyrotoxic periodic paralysis. *J Am Soc Nephrol.* 2012;23:985–988.
22. **Lin SH, Lin YF, Chen DT, Chu P, Hsu CW, Halperin ML.** Laboratory tests to determine the causes for hypokalemia and paralysis. *Arch. Intern. Med.* 2004;164:1561–1566.
23. **Hsu YJ, Lin YF, Chau T, Liou JT, Kuo SW, Lin SH.** Electrocardiographic manifestations in patients with thyrotoxic periodic paralysis. *Am J Med Sci.* 2003;326:128–132.
24. **Lin YF, Wu CC, Pei D, Chu SJ, Lin SH.** Diagnosing thyrotoxic periodic paralysis in the ED. *Am J Emerg Med.* 2003;21:339–342.
25. **Lin SH, Chu P, Cheng CC, Chu SJ, Hung YJ, Lin YF.** Early diagnosis of thyrotoxic periodic paralysis: urine calcium to phosphate ratio. *Crit Care Med.* 2006;34:2984–2989.
26. **Lin SH, Davis MR, Halperin ML.** Hypokalemia and paralysis. *QJM.* 2003;96: 161–169.
27. **Lu KC, Hsu YJ, Chiu JS, Hsu YD, Lin SH.** Effects of potassium supplementation on the recovery of thyrotoxic periodic paralysis. *Am J Emerg Med.* 2004;22:544–547.
28. **Manoukian MA, Foote JA, Crapo LM.** Clinical and metabolic features of thyrotoxic periodic paralysis in 24 episodes. *Arch Intern Med.* 1999;159: 601–606.
29. **Shiang JC, Cheng CJ, Tsai MK, et al.** Therapeutic analysis in Chinese patients with thyrotoxic periodic paralysis over six years. *Eur J Endocrinol.* 2009;161:911–916.
30. **Halperin ML, Kamel KS.** Potassium. *Lancet.* 1998;352:135–140.
31. **Alfonzo AV, Isles C, Geddes C, Deighan C.** Potassium disorder—clinical spectrum and emergency management. *Resuscitation.* 2006;70:10–25.
32. **Tassone H, Moulin A, Henderson SO.** The pitfalls of potassium replacement in thyrotoxic periodic paralysis: a case report and review of the literature. *J Emerg Med.* 2004;26:157–161.
33. **Shayne P, Hart A.** Thyrotoxic periodic paralysis terminated with intravenous propranolol. *Ann Emerg Med.* 1994;24:736–740.
34. **Birkhahn RH, Gaeta TJ, Melniker L.** Thyrotoxic periodic paralysis and intravenous propranolol in the emergency setting. *J Emerg Med.* 2000;18: 199–202.
35. **Lin SH, Lin YF.** Propranolol rapidly terminates the hypokalemia, hypophosphatemia and paralysis in thyrotoxic periodic paralysis. *Am J Kidney Dis.* 2001;37:620–623.
36. **Alazami M, Lin SH, Cheng CJ, Davids MR, Halperin ML.** Unusual causes of hypokalemia and paralysis. *QJM.* 2006;99:181–192.
37. **Chen WH, Yin HL, Lin HS, Chen SS, Liu JS.** Delayed hypokalemic paralysis following a convulsion due to alcohol abstinence. *J Clin Neurosci.* 2006;13: 453–456.
38. **Yeung RT, Tse TF.** Thyrotoxic periodic paralysis: effect of propranolol. *Am J Med.* 1974;57:584–590.
39. **Cheng CJ, Kuo E, Huang CL.** Extracellular potassium homeostasis: insights from hypokalemic periodic paralysis. *Semin Nephrol.* 2013;33:237–247.

CHAPTER 14

Sight-Threatening Graves' Ophthalmopathy

Rebecca S Bahn and James A Garrity

ABSTRACT

Graves' ophthalmopathy (GO) is an autoimmune disease with heterogeneous expression ranging from mild ocular discomfort to severe disease. In 3%–5% of patients with GO, sight-threatening corneal breakdown or dysthyroid optic neuropathy (DON) may develop. The rare patient experiences anterior displacement or subluxation of the globe. Prompt recognition of the signs and symptoms of these sight-threatening conditions allows the clinician to arrange appropriate urgent or emergent referral to a specialist ophthalmologist.

INTRODUCTION

Graves' ophthalmopathy (GO), also known as Graves' orbitopathy or thyroid eye disease, is an autoimmune disorder with heterogeneous expression ranging from mild ocular discomfort to sight-threatening disease (1). Almost half of all patients with hyperthyroidism due to Graves' disease can be identified as having some degree of ocular involvement. Patients may report a sensation of ocular "grittiness," diplopia, or eye redness and periorbital edema that can fluctuate in degree during the course of a single day or from day to day (2). The disease progresses in approximately 20% of patients who may experience eye pain, frequent diplopia, severe periorbital erythema and swelling, or excessive proptosis. In 3%–5% of patients, sight-threatening corneal breakdown or compressive optic neuropathy, a condition termed dysthyroid optic neuropathy (DON), may develop (3). Although the management of patients with mild GO is generally supportive, disease that is moderate to severe may require immunosuppressive therapy or surgical intervention (4). Sight-threatening disease requires urgent or emergent evaluation. Early intervention is especially important for corneal ulcers because these can lead to globe perforation with loss of vision and potential loss of the eye itself. Although treatment of DON is less urgent, case series suggest that about 20% of untreated eyes may be left with visual acuity of 20/100 or less, with most having vision ranging from finger counting to no light perception (5). In our experience, orbital decompression improved or stabilized visual acuity by at least 3 lines of Snellen visual acuity in only 110 of 205 eyes having visual acuity of 20/40 or less, and improved or resolved field defects in 246 of 291 eyes (6).

Patients with GO, except those with the mildest of manifestations, are optimally evaluated and cared for jointly by an endocrinologist and an ophthalmologist with special expertise in the treatment of patients with GO. However, most endocrinologists do not care for a large number of patients with this disorder, and few practice in the setting of a thyroid eye clinic where ophthalmological expertise is readily available. This chapter focuses on the key features of impending or established sight-threatening GO that clinicians should recognize in order that appropriate urgent or emergent referral to a specialist ophthalmologist can be made.

DYSTHYROID OPTIC NEUROPATHY

DON is multifactorial in etiology and occurs secondary to the orbital tissue remodeling that characterizes the disease. The neuropathy results from direct compression of the optic nerve or less likely impingement of its vascular supply by enlarged extraocular muscles at the orbital apex (7). A contributing factor in some patients is a tight orbital septum preventing the auto-decompression of orbital pressures by forward protrusion of the globe. Rarely, DON develops in the setting of extreme proptosis caused by a stretching of the optic nerve between the orbital apex and the globe. Men, older patients of either gender, smokers, and patients with diabetes mellitus are at particular risk for the development of DON (8).

Clinical characteristics were studied in 47 patients considered to have features suspicious for DON who were evaluated at 7 European centers during a 1-year period (9). Although most patients had moderate to severe inflammatory signs and symptoms with excessive proptosis at presentation, 25% had only modest inflammation, and a third had proptosis of <21 mm on exophthalmometry. Visual acuity was reduced in 75% (6/9 Snellen or worse), and formal color vision assessment showed abnormalities in essentially all patients. Double vision was present in most patients and was frequently inconstant (present with side gaze) or constant in primary gaze. Keratopathy was evident in 20 patients, and corneal ulceration was found in 3 patients. DON was unilateral in about half of the patients.

Because changes in visual acuity and color vision may be insidious, many patients with DON may not complain of any visual changes. Subtle color vision issues in association with a unilateral optic neuropathy can be identified with a red-desaturation test where a red-colored object is shown to each eye independently. The eye with optic neuropathy will appear washed-out and less intense. The report of new onset blurred or dimmed vision that is not corrected by blinking (which regenerates the tear film) or by closing one eye (which distinguishes the visual changes from incipient diplopia) should alert the physician to the possibility of DON (10). Similarly, the presence of optic nerve involvement should be suspected in patients who show "frozen eyes" or significant restriction of eye movement, particularly to upward gaze, or who suffer from constant diplopia (9).

The finding of a relative afferent pupillary defect (RAPD; asymmetrical pupillary response to a light stimulus, often tested using a "swinging flashlight") is very suggestive of DON. However, the RAPD may be absent if DON is bilateral and symmetrical. Although the presence of disc edema can be one of the cardinal features of DON, about 50%–75% of patients with this diagnosis show normal optic disc morphology or only minimal retinal venous congestion (Figure 14-1). The signs with the greatest specificity for DON are impairment of color perception and optic disc swelling (9). Ballottement of the globe revealing a tense, rather than a soft, consistency is not a sensitive test but may occasionally be useful.

Once DON is suspected, the patient should be referred urgently to a specialist ophthalmologist who can obtain and interpret additional testing. Because no single test confirms or refutes the diagnosis, the decision either to immediately treat or closely observe a patient is based on a constellation of findings. Further assessment generally includes formal visual acuity assessment, determination of pupillary responses, and color vision

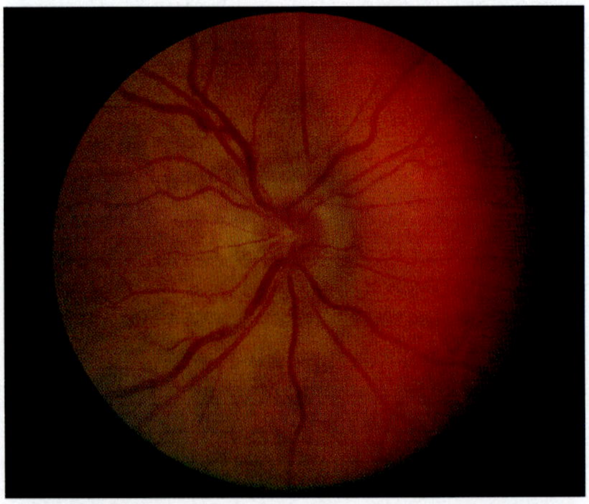

Figure 14-1. Optic disc edema (right eye) in a patient with DON showing elevation of the optic disc with indistinct margins. Retinal veins are congested.

testing, although this latter test will not be helpful in the 10% of males who are congenitally color-blind. Automated perimetry is performed to identify visual field defects, which are generally central, paracentral, and/or inferior when DON is present (2). However, these tests may be difficult to interpret in the setting of visual impairment caused by confounding ocular pathology, such as glaucoma, cataracts, or macular degeneration. Imaging with computed tomography (CT) scanning or magnetic resonance imaging (MRI) is commonly used to support the diagnosis of DON in patients who have shown impairment in any of these parameters (Figure 14-2). The combination of apical crowding (effacement of perineural fat at the apex) and evidence of fat herniation through the superior orbital fissure seen on axial images has a specificity of 91% and a sensitivity of 94% for DON (11).

Therapy for DON involves intravenous (IV) pulse therapy with methylprednisolone, orbital decompression surgery, or both modalities. Orbital radiotherapy is not recommended in this setting except as an adjunct to these 2 proven therapies (4). Perhaps because of the rarity of the condition and the lack of well-defined diagnostic criteria, only one randomized controlled trial (15 patients) comparing the 2 modalities has been performed (12). In this study, 5 of 6 patients who initially underwent orbital decompression surgery subsequently deteriorated or failed to improve visual acuity and subsequently required treatment with IV methylprednisolone (1.0 g daily for 3 consecutive days, repeated once after 1 week) followed by a 4-month course of oral prednisone (2 weeks of 40 mg daily, 4 weeks of 30 mg, 4 weeks of 20 mg, tapering by 2.5 mg per week until finished). Conversely, 4 of 9 IV methylprednisolone-treated patients subsequently required orbital decompression. Although neither approach was uniformly successful as an initial therapy, DON ultimately resolved in all cases because patients failing one approach responded to the other. Case studies report some visual function improvement in 76%–90% of patients within a few days of orbital decompression surgery (12).

Pulse therapy with IV methylprednisolone has been reported to be effective in 94%, while 73% of patients improve within 1–2

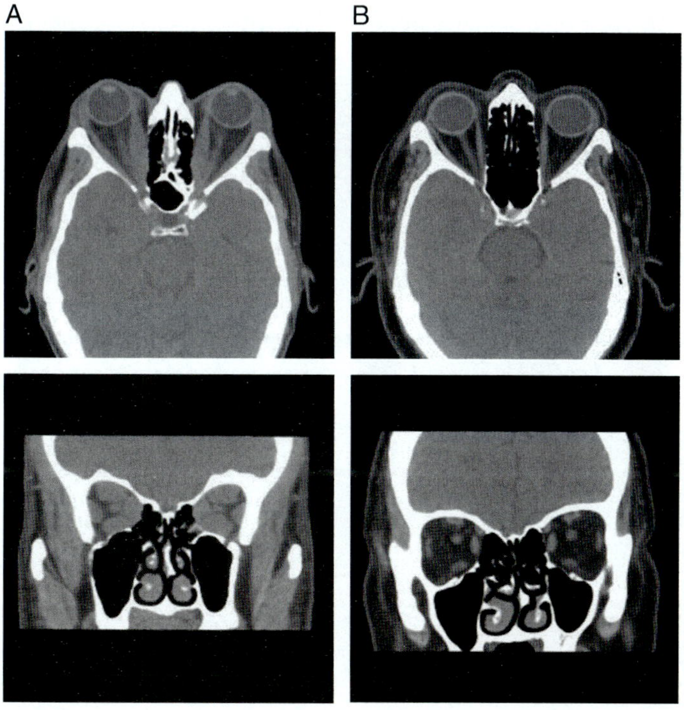

Figure 14-2. Axial (A, top) and coronal (A, bottom) CT scans of a patient (also shown in Figure 14-1) with DON showing compression of the optic nerve at the apex of the orbit by enlarged extraocular muscles with apical crowding (effacement of perineural fat at the apex). Axial (B, top) and coronal (B, bottom) CT scans of a normal orbit are shown for comparison.

weeks with oral glucocorticoid therapy alone (prednisone 80–120 mg daily) (13). The consensus statement from the European Group on Graves' Orbitopathy (EUGOGO) advises starting with IV methylprednisolone therapy in most patients and observing the response over 2–3 weeks' time (4). If no improvement is seen or deterioration ensues, prompt orbital decompression surgery is indicated. Surgery may be indicated as first-line therapy if visual acuity is <20/200, the corneal exposure from proptosis is significant, congestive features are prominent, or steroid side effects are to be avoided (6).

CORNEAL BREAKDOWN

Severe eye pain in a patient with GO, especially if new in onset, sharp in quality, and associated with blurred vision, is a worrisome feature suggestive of corneal breakdown. Although much less common than DON, suspicion of corneal breakdown requires emergent, rather than urgent, referral to an ophthalmologist (4). Corneal ulceration can develop when corneal protection is limited (Figure 14-3). This can result from extreme proptosis, excessive eyelid retraction, ineffective blinking with poor tear production, or incomplete eyelid closure. In some patients with GO, the cornea remains exposed when the eyelids are approximated because the reflex upward motion of the globe is prevented by a tight inferior rectus muscle (absent Bell's phenomenon). Such patients, especially those unable to completely close their eyes (lagophthalmos) owing to excessive lid retraction, are particularly at risk for corneal breakdown (2).

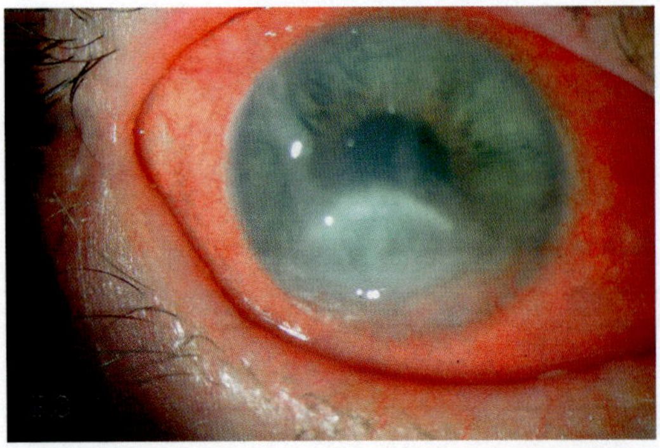

Figure 14-3. Slit-lamp photograph showing a corneal ulcer in a patient with lid retraction and lagophthalmos.

Initial treatment for corneal breakdown includes the frequent use of topical lubricants and intensive topical antibiotics where appropriate. Eyelids may be taped closed or a moisture chamber may be used for protection of the healing cornea. When corneal breakdown is more severe, temporary globe coverage may be achieved by injecting botulinum toxin into the levator (although there is typically a 3–4 day delay in therapeutic effect) or surgically by tarsorrhaphy. IV pulse therapy with methylprednisolone or orbital decompression surgery may be considered in refractory cases. In the setting of severe corneal ulcer, corneal transplant or amniotic membrane grafts may be required (4).

SUBLUXATION OF THE GLOBE

Axial globe subluxation is defined as anterior displacement of the globe equator beyond the orbital rim, lid retraction behind the equator, and tethering of the optic nerve. A retrospective study of 4,000 patients with GO found the incidence of globe subluxation to be 0.01% (14). Examination of the CT scans of these 4 patients uniformly revealed increased orbital fat without significant extraocular muscle enlargement. The authors concluded that the increased orbital fat content results in increased compliance of the soft tissues and the normal caliber of the muscles allows them to be more extensible, permitting acute contraction of the eyelids posterior to the equator of the globe. With subluxation, vision is acutely threatened by exposure keratopathy and optic neuropathy, which is generally treated with IV methylprednisolone. Tarsorrhaphy may be performed at presentation as a temporary measure prior to orbital decompression surgery. Patients with significant proptosis and lid retraction, particularly those with excessive orbital fat enlargement, should be made aware of this condition and instructed regarding manual repositioning of the globe with axial pressure should it occur.

CONCLUSIONS

Optimum care of the patient with GO is achieved through team work between endocrinologist and ophthalmologist. Because

Table 14-1. Features of Sight-Threatening Graves' Ophthalmopathy

Sight-Threatening Condition	Risk Factors	Suggestive Signs/Symptoms	Referral to Ophthalmologist
Dysthyroid optic neuropathy	Diabetes mellitus Smoking Older patients Severe inflammation (but may occur in patients with little inflammation)	Complaint of blurry vision not corrected by blinking Dulling of color vision Constant diplopia Optic disc edema Relative afferent pupillary defect	Urgent
Corneal ulcer	Extreme proptosis Lagophthalmos/excessive lid retraction Absent Bell's phenomenon	Severe eye pain, especially if new in onset; sharp in quality and associated with blurry vision	Emergent
Subluxation of the globe	Extreme proptosis with lid retraction Excessive orbital fat enlargement with relatively normal extraocular muscle volume	Patient may describe an episode compatible with subluxation	Urgent

sight-threatening GO may require prompt intervention by an ophthalmologist, at each visit the endocrinologist should assess key clinical and historical features in the context of the patient's risk factors (Table 14-1). In particular, a patient who describes severe eye pain, especially if new in onset, sharp in nature, and associated with visual blurring, should be emergently referred to an ophthalmologist for possible corneal breakdown. Reported deterioration in vision that does not clear with blinking, especially if disc edema is detected, suggests impending or established DON and requires urgent referral to an ophthalmologist. A history compatible with subluxation of the globe warrants urgent ophthalmological referral to prevent recurrent episodes.

ACKNOWLEDGMENTS

The authors have nothing to disclose.

REFERENCES

1. **Bahn RS.** Graves' ophthalmopathy. *N Engl J Med.* 2010;362:726–738.
2. **Dickinson AJ, Perros P.** Controversies in the clinical evaluation of active thyroid associated orbitopathy: use of a detailed protocol with comparative photographs for objective assessment. *Clin Endocrinol (Oxf).* 2001;55:283–303.
3. **Ben Simon GJ, Syed HM, Douglas R, Schwartz R, Goldberg RA, McCann JD.** Clinical manifestations and treatment outcome of optic neuropathy in thyroid-related orbitopathy. *Ophthalmic Surg Lasers Imaging.* 2006;37:284–290.
4. **Bartalena L, Baldeschi L, Dickinson A, et al.** Consensus statement of the European Group on Graves' orbitopathy (EUGOGO) on management of GO. *Eur J Endocrinol.* 2008;158:273–285.
5. **Trobe JD, Glaser JS, Laflamme P.** Dysthyroid optic neuropathy: clinical profile and rationale for management. *Arch Ophthalmol.* 1978;96:1199–1209.
6. **Soares-Welch CV, Fatourechi V, Bartley GB, et al.** Optic neuropathy of Graves' disease: results of transantral orbital decompression and long-term follow-up in 215 patients. *Am J Ophthalmol.* 2003;136:433–441.
7. **Dosso A, Safran AB, Sunaric G, Burger A.** Anterior ischemic optic neuropathy in Graves' disease. *J Neuroophthalmol.* 1994;14:170–174.
8. **Kalmann R, Mourits MP.** Diabetes mellitus: a risk factor in patients with Graves' orbitopathy. *Br J Ophthalmol.* 1999;83:463–465.
9. **McKeag D, Lane C, Lazarus JH, et al.** Clinical features of dysthyroid optic neuropathy: a European Group on Graves' Orbitopathy (EUGOGO) survey. *Br J Ophthalmol.* 2007;91:455–458.
10. **Bahn RS, Bartley GB, Gorman CA.** Emergency treatment of Graves' ophthalmopathy. *Baillieres Clin Endocrinol Metab.* 1992;6:95–105.
11. **Birchall D, Goodall KL, Noble JL, Jackson A.** Graves' ophthalmopathy: intracranial fat prolapse on CT images as an indicator of optic nerve compression. *Radiology.* 1996;200:123–127.
12. **Wakelkamp IM, Baldeschi L, Saeed P, Mourits MP, Prummel MF, Wiersinga WM.** Surgical or

medical decompression as a first-line treatment of optic neuropathy in Graves' ophthalmopathy? A randomized controlled trial. *Clin Endocrinol (Oxf).* 2005;63: 323–328.

13. **Wiersinga WM, Prummel MF.** An evidence-based approach to the treatment of Graves' ophthalmopathy. *Endocrinol Metab Clin North Am.* 2000;29:297–319.
14. **Rubin PA, Watkins LM, Rumelt S, Sutula FC, Dallow RL.** Orbital computed tomographic characteristics of globe subluxation in thyroid orbitopathy. *Ophthalmology.* 1998;105:2061–2064.

CHAPTER 15

Acute Medical Aspects Related to Advanced Thyroid Cancer

Michael E Menefee and Robert C Smallridge

ABSTRACT

The last 2 decades have seen a substantial escalation in the number of cases of thyroid cancer. Given the relatively long survival associated with thyroid cancer, even in its most advanced stages, it is becoming increasingly important for clinicians to be aware of the acute risks that may affect patients with advanced thyroid cancer. Several of these acute medical problems related to advanced thyroid cancer will be briefly outlined.

INTRODUCTION

The last 2 decades have seen a substantial escalation in the number of cases of thyroid cancer; in 2014, approximately 63,000 cases are anticipated in the United States alone (1). More recently, we have also seen a concomitant increase in the number of approved therapeutics for advanced thyroid cancer, as well as a surge in thyroid cancer-directed clinical trials with novel therapeutics. Given the relatively long survival associated with thyroid cancer, even in its most advanced stages, it is becoming increasingly important for clinicians to be aware of the acute risks that may affect patients with advanced thyroid cancer, whether related directly to their underlying disease or to the therapeutics used to treat it.

ACUTE AIRWAY OBSTRUCTION

Although most individuals who develop thyroid malignancy can anticipate an excellent chance for cure, patients with anaplastic thyroid cancer (ATC) have an ominous prognosis, even when detected early. The 2012 American Thyroid Association guidelines for management of patients with ATC discussed many detailed recommendations for this condition, including airway management (2). Patients with ATC are at risk for airway obstruction due to local progression of the primary tumor; accordingly, a tracheostomy may be required to avoid asphyxia. Airway obstruction may occur as a direct consequence of a large obstructing mass, tracheal compression, direct infiltration of the tumor through the tracheal wall, or from massive hemorrhage into the trachea (2,3).

The benefits of preserving the airway have to be weighed against the overall prognosis of the patient. Palliative interventions with good intent, such as tracheostomy, may ultimately result in not only the prolongation of life, but also prolongation of the anguish the patient may be experiencing. Therefore, the advantages and disadvantages of tracheostomy tube placement need to be weighed carefully. Accordingly, in most circumstances, a surgical airway can be avoided in the management of patients with advanced, unresectable disease. Exceptions to this general principle include the presence of stridor or other acute airway distress, particularly if it is the presenting sign or symptom of ATC (3).

EFFECTS OF SYSTEMIC THERAPEUTICS

Radioiodine

Patients with well-differentiated thyroid malignancies (papillary, follicular, Hürthle cell) have an excellent prognosis. Even the presence of distant metastases does not have the same negative impact on overall survival that we typically associate with disseminated metastatic disease. Most patients who are not cured by surgical resection alone are cured with the use of I^{131} radioiodine (RAI), which can serve to ablate any remnant thyroid tissue, or be used in an adjuvant fashion for micrometastatic disease or detectable, disseminated metastases. Although RAI is used commonly in this patient population, and is generally well tolerated, it can be associated with a number of chronic, as well as acute, toxicities (4).

Sialadenitis results from the preferential uptake of RAI in the salivary glands. The resulting xerostomia, which is often accompanied by dysgeusia and/or ageusia, can be either an acute or chronic problem for patients. Preventative measures to reduce the incidence and severity of sialadenitis include using lower doses of RAI, maintaining adequate hydration, and using sialogogues. Once sialadenitis has developed, it tends to be permanent, although the changes in taste and smell are generally transient, resolving within 1 to 2 months in most circumstances (5). There are limited prospective data to guide treatment recommendations; however, the following interventions have anecdotally been found to be useful for some patients:

1. Salivary substitutes
2. Candies (hard candies, chewing gum, lozenges, etc.)
3. Humidification of air
4. Dietary modification (moist, non-acidic foods)
5. Avoidance of medications that promote xerostomia (eg, clonidine, diphenhydramine)
6. Avoidance of caffeine
7. Avoidance of ethanol
8. Muscarinic agonists (eg, pilocarpine)
9. Meticulous dental hygiene with frequent dental examinations

Another acute but less frequent toxicity of RAI affecting the oral cavity is stomatitis. This is less frequent than sialadenitis, typically occurring within the first week after receiving RAI. Management is largely symptomatic, utilizing compound rinses used in chemotherapy- or radiation-induced mucositis (eg, viscous lidocaine, diphenhydramine, sucralfate).

Epiphora, or nasolacrimal duct obstruction (unilateral or bilateral) with excessive tearing, has been described after RAI. This has typically been observed in individuals receiving either a large solitary dose of I^{131} or after a large cumulative exposure. Epiphora is usually managed with dilation of the tear duct or stent placement; however, if complete obstruction has occurred, surgical diversion of the tear duct may be required for resolution.

Pulmonary pneumonitis and fibrosis are well-established, albeit rare, complications of RAI therapy for metastatic thyroid cancer. These complications are associated both with the extent of pulmonary metastases and the amount of RAI exposure. The use of dosimetry to limit the amount of radioiodine uptake in radioiodine-avid lung metastases may reduce the risk of these complications of treatment. As in more conventional forms of radiation-induced lung damage, glucocorticoids have been used empirically, with some success; however, there is a lack of prospective data in the literature to confirm the benefit of their use.

Because thyroid cancer tends to affect younger adults, counseling regarding the potential impact of therapy on fertility and pregnancy needs to be discussed with all patients of reproductive potential. In general, it is recommended that pregnancy be delayed for at least 1 year after receiving a therapeutic dose of RAI. However, there are no available data to indicate that RAI is an abortifacient at clinically relevant doses, nor are there data to suggest perinatal morbidity or mortality to the fetus. RAI does not appear to result in premature menopause nor does it cause any significant changes in the menstrual cycle, although there have been case reports of transient amenorrhea (6).

Bone marrow suppression is an adverse event more commonly associated with cytotoxic chemotherapeutics. However, when patients are examined closely, declines in blood counts occur in most patients receiving RAI who had any of the following:

1. Extensive bone metastases
2. Prior bone irradiation
3. >200 cGy of whole body radiation exposure

Most of the declines in blood counts, when present, are asymptomatic and no specific intervention is required other than observation, although the presence of 1 or more of these risk factors may factor into the dosimetry considerations.

Cytotoxic Chemotherapy-Related Adverse Events

Three classes of cytotoxic compounds routinely are used in thyroid cancer: the anthracyclines, the taxanes (paclitaxel and docetaxel), and the platinum compounds (cisplatin and carboplatin). Many of the toxicities of cytotoxic agents are overlapping and cumulative. For example, all of these agents can be expected to produce myelosuppression to varying degrees. Most will cause some degree of nausea and vomiting or other gastrointestinal disturbance if appropriate prophylaxis is not implemented. However, each class of drug has particular acute toxicities that present challenges in the successful delivery of therapy.

Doxorubicin, an anthracycline that received regulatory approval in 1974, was the first and only FDA-approved drug for advanced thyroid malignancies for over 36 years (7). Its labeling allows its use in all forms of thyroid cancer; however, in practice its use is largely limited to a couple of settings: as a radiosensitizer for ATC; and as a palliative measure for patients with refractory disease, often in combination with a platinum compound or a taxane. The benefit of doxorubicin is quite marginal in most individuals with aggressive thyroid cancer, and, at the same time, it exposes patients to significant toxicity, including myelosuppression, myriad gastrointestinal disturbances, and the potential for cardiac toxicity with depressed left ventricular function. Furthermore, it causes alopecia, which may have a negative psychosocial effect on patients. The limited efficacy, coupled with the significant toxicity, has largely limited the use of doxorubicin and other cytotoxic chemotherapeutics for patients with advanced, aggressive thyroid cancers.

The taxanes are similarly used for both radiosensitization and for patients with metastatic disease (8). Prolonged use of taxanes, particularly when given at full dose on an every 21 days schedule, will often result in the development of peripheral neuropathy. Peripheral neuropathy is a common occurrence with cytotoxic agents that affect the microtubule (eg, taxanes, vinca alkaloids, epothilones), though it is well described with other classes of chemotherapy as well (eg, platinum compounds, proteasome inhibitors). The most common manifestation is sensory peripheral neuropathy, often involving the fingers/hands and toes/feet, though other areas of the body may be affected. Patients often report numbness and/or tingling, but also may report pain. It is also important to keep in mind that motor neuropathic symptoms and signs may develop and, even much more rarely, autonomic neuropathy. For patients with low-grade neuropathy, therapy with the offending agent can often be continued successfully without interruption or dose modification. Conversely, when progressively worsening symptoms persist, an interruption may be required. A rechallenge with the offending agent may be considered if symptoms improve promptly, with likely consideration for a dose modification. The therapeutic intent may also influence the tolerance of such adverse events.

As noted previously, the platinum compounds are commonly used in patients with advanced thyroid cancer and, moreover, they are also potentially neurotoxic. However, the spectrum of serious adverse events also includes nephrotoxicity and ototoxicity. Cisplatin is the most commonly used platinum drug in advanced thyroid cancer. It appears from the available data in this setting, as well as in other tumor types, to have slightly superior anticancer activity. Nonetheless, it also appears to be slightly more toxic than carboplatin. Although carboplatin tends to be more myelosuppressive, cisplatin predisposes to nephrotoxicity and ototoxicity (hearing impairment and tinnitus). Cisplatin-induced nephrotoxicity can span asymptomatic elevations in creatinine to permanent renal failure requiring hemodialysis. Although many of the acute adverse events associated with platinum compounds are transient and potentially reversible, great thought needs to be given to implementing them in a patient population with ATC.

Targeted Chemotherapy-Related Adverse Events

In 2011, the first FDA approval for a thyroid cancer drug since doxorubicin occurred. Vandetanib, a tyrosine kinase inhibitor (TKI) targeting the vascular endothelial growth factor receptor (VEGFR), the epidermal growth factor receptor (EGFR), and the RET tyrosine kinase, was approved for the treatment of symptomatic or progressive medullary thyroid cancer (MTC) in patients with *unresectable*, locally advanced, or metastatic disease (9). This was followed in rapid succession by the approval of cabozantinib, also designated for patients with advanced MTC. Like vandetanib, cabozantinib is a multi-targeted TKI. It shares VEGFR and RET inhibition with vandetanib; however, in contrast, it also targets the hepatocyte growth factor receptor (MET), whereas vandetanib targets EGFR.

Even more recently, in 2013, we saw yet another TKI receive approval; this time for patients with differentiated thyroid cancer (10). Sorafenib was among the first generation of TKIs in the clinic, receiving initial FDA approval for renal cell carcinoma in 2005 before going on to receive approval for hepatocellular carcinoma in 2008. Sorafenib ushered in a wave of novel, multi-targeted TKIs, which largely had VEGFR inhibition in common, with most agents also having secondary or "off target" effects that may have contributed to the efficacy, as well as toxicity, of the drug.

Although there are only 3 FDA-approved TKIs for thyroid cancer, a much larger number of agents have been evaluated in the clinic, expanding our understanding of how this class of agents works in thyroid cancer, but also contributing substantially to our knowledge of treatment-related adverse events. In particular, familiarity with the toxicities associated with these novel therapeutics is critical to providing patients with adequate informed consent prior to initiation of such therapies. Although it is essential that medical oncologists be familiar with this information, it is also important for endocrinologists, primary care physicians, and emergency medical personnel to be familiar with these drugs and their accompanying toxicities. Given the often indolent natural history of thyroid cancers and the prolonged clinical benefit observed with TKI, it is very possible that multiple practitioners spanning multiple specialties may be involved in the management of the acute and chronic adverse events associated with such therapy.

When approaching TKI-related adverse events, it is often most optimal to evaluate according to the effect of a drug on a particular target, rather than looking at each drug individually (Table 15-1). However, in clinical practice, most of the drugs in use have overlapping targets and mechanisms of action, and, consequently, overlapping side effects. Therefore, it is important to be familiar with all of the targets being engaged by the drug to fully understand the spectrum of toxicity the patient can expect to experience (Table 15-2).

CONCLUSIONS

Thyroid cancer is the most common cancer affecting the endocrine system (1). Given the relatively long survival associated with thyroid

Table 15-1. Selected Therapeutics for Advanced Thyroid Cancers

	Agent	Molecular Target(s)
Differentiated thyroid cancer	Axitinib	VEGFR, PDGFRβ, KIT
	Pazopanib	VEGFR, PDGFRβ, KIT
	Motesanib	VEGFR, KIT, SCF
	Sorafenib	VEGFR, BRAF, PDGFRβ, KIT, FLT3
	Sunitinib	VEGFR, KIT, PDGFRβ, FLT3
Medullary thyroid cancer	Vandetanib	VEGFR, RET, EGFR
	Cabozantinib	VEGFR, RET, MET

Table 15-2. TKI-Related Toxicities

Target	Toxicities
VEGFR	Fatigue Hypertension Arterial/venous thromboembolic events Hemorrhage Bowel perforation Left ventricular dysfunction Diarrhea Poor wound healing Cardiac repolarization abnormalities
EGFR	Fatigue Diarrhea Acneiform rash Asymptomatic left ventricular dysfunction
RET	???
PDGFR	Hypopigmentation? Cardiac repolarization abnormalities
RAF	Palmar-plantar erythrodysesthesia (hand-foot syndrome)
KIT	Hypopigmentation? Cardiac repolarization abnormalities

cancer, even in its most advanced stages, it is increasingly important for clinicians to be aware of the acute medical risks that may affect patients with advanced thyroid cancer, whether related directly to their underlying disease (eg, airway management) or to the therapeutics used to treat it.

ACKNOWLEDGMENTS

The authors have nothing to disclose.

REFERENCES

1. **Siegal R, Ma J, Zou Z, et al.** Cancer statistics, 2014. *CA Cancer J Clin.* 2014;64:9–29.
2. **Smallridge RC, Ain KB, Asa SL, et al.** American Thyroid Association guidelines for management of patients with anaplastic thyroid cancer. *Thyroid.* 2012;22:1104–1139.
3. **Shaha AR, Ferlito A, Owen RP, et al.** Airway issues in anaplastic thyroid carcinoma. *Eur Arch Otorhinolaryngol.* 2013;270:2579–2583.
4. **Lee S.** Complications of radioactive iodine treatment of thyroid carcinoma. *J Natl Compr Canc Netw.* 2010;8:1277–1287.
5. **Dingle IF, Mishoe AE, Nguyen SA, Overton LJ, Gillespie MB.** Salivary morbidity and quality of life following radioactive iodine for well-differentiated thyroid cancer. *Otolaryngol Head Neck Surg.* 2013;148:746–752.
6. **Van Nostrand D.** The benefits and risks of I-131 therapy in patients with well-differentiated thyroid cancer. *Thyroid.* 2009;19:1381–1391.
7. **Gottlieb J, Hill CS.** Chemotherapy of thyroid cancer with adriamycin: experience with 30 patients. *N Engl J Med.* 1974;290:193–197.
8. **Ain K, Egorin MJ, DeSimone PA.** Treatment of anaplastic thyroid carcinoma with paclitaxel: phase 2 trial using ninety-six-hour infusion. *Thyroid.* 2000;10:587–594.
9. **Wells S, Robinson BG, Gagel RF, et al.** Vandetanib in patients with locally advanced or metastatic medullary thyroid cancer: a randomized, double-blind phase III trial. *J Clin Oncol.* 2012;30(2):134–141.
10. **Brose M, Nutting CM, Sherman SI, et al.** Rationale and design of DECISION: a double-blind, randomized, placebo-controlled phase III trial evaluating the efficacy and safety of sorafenib in patients with locally advanced or metastatic radioactive iodine (RAI)-refractory, differentiated thyroid cancer. *BMC Cancer.* 2011;11:349.

SECTION VI

Adrenal Disorders

SECTION INTRODUCTION

Emergent Management of Adrenal Disorders

Paul M Stewart

The ongoing advances in endocrinology have also encompassed the adrenal gland and its associated disorders. Over 60 years ago, Hench, Kendall, and Reichstein won the Nobel Prize for the isolation and purification of cortisone and in a quite beautiful paradigm for translational medicine went on to demonstrate its anti-inflammatory properties in patients with rheumatoid arthritis. The rest is history—"physiological" glucocorticoid replacement therapy now saves thousands of lives of patients with primary and secondary adrenal insufficiency. Synthetic corticosteroids save more lives in patients with underlying inflammation—be it asthma, Crohn's disease, polymyalgia rheumatica, urticaria, or vasculitides. But these advances have brought accompanying problems. Despite much effort it has been impossible (at least in clinical studies) to dissect out the transrepressive, anti-inflammatory effects of glucocorticoids from the transactivating "cushingoid" effects. Glucocorticoid-induced side effects with so-called "tertiary adrenal suppression" now contribute to morbidity and premature mortality in the 3% or so of western populations taking exogenous steroids; its diagnosis and management remain challenging.

Turning to replacement therapy in adrenal insufficiency, many of us have questioned over the years how "physiological" this really is. It certainly fails to mimic normal circadian secretion patterns and undoubtedly earlier regimens did result in over-replacement with all the added risks of long-term, albeit mild, Cushing's syndrome. This together with the ongoing and unacceptable management of patients with adrenal crises, even in Centres of Excellence, is likely to explain the increased mortality (standardized mortality ratio [SMR] ~2.1) in patients with primary and secondary adrenal insufficiency. It remains to be seen whether exciting new developments in hydrocortisone therapies that deliver closer "physiological" replacement (eg, Plenadren, which is available in several countries but awaiting US approval) impact upon failure of care. Primary and secondary adrenal failure management is discussed in various chapters and is summarized in Table VI-1.

We have made headway in the management of endogenous Cushing's with the approval of the very first pituitary-targeted medical therapy for Cushing's disease—pasireotide. Other medical therapies, notably the glucocorticoid receptor (GR) antagonist mifepristone, have also been licensed and other metyrapone-like compounds are on the way, but sadly these will not yet replace surgical expertise in terms of efficacy and chance of "cure."

Phenotype-genotype advances have significantly impacted this field, no more so than in the field of adrenal-based hypertension. The realization that primary aldosteronism is no longer a "rare" disease, but one that explains 10% of all cases of hypertension, is a message that is still not instilled across primary care and cardiovascular clinicians. Clinical guidelines have given us sensible criteria on who we screen, and

Table VI-1. Recommended Therapeutic Approach to Adrenal Insufficiency

Acute adrenal insufficiency	
Glucocorticoid replacement	Start on physiological saline infusions, initial rate 1 L/hr under continuous cardiac monitoring conditions
	Administer 100 mg hydrocortisone as an IV injection followed by 100–200 mg hydrocortisone in glucose 5% per continuous IV infusion (alternatively, administer hydrocortisone IM at a dose of 25–50 mg 4 times daily)
Mineralocorticoid replacement	Only in primary adrenal insufficiency
	Not required as long as hydrocortisone dose >50 mg per 24 hr
Adrenal androgen replacement	Not required
Chronic adrenal insufficiency	
Glucocorticoid replacement	Primary adrenal insufficiency: start on 20–25 mg hydrocortisone per 24 hr
	Secondary adrenal insufficiency: 15–20 mg hydrocortisone per 24 hr; if borderline-fail in short-ACTH (cosyntropin or Synacthen) stimulation test consider 10 mg or stress dose cover only
	Administer in 2–3 divided doses; administer first dose immediately after waking up
	Consider modified-release hydrocortisone formulation where approved
	Monitoring • Check body weight; calculate body mass index (BMI) • Check for signs of under-replacement (weight loss, fatigue, nausea, myalgia, lack of energy) • Check for signs of over-replacement (weight gain, central obesity, stretch marks, osteopenia/osteoporosis, prediabetes/diabetes, hypertension) • Take a detailed account of stress-related glucocorticoid dose self-adjustments since last visit and potential adverse events, including emergency treatment and/or hospitalization
Mineralocorticoid replacement	Only required in primary adrenal insufficiency
	Not required as long as hydrocortisone dose >50 mg per 24 hr
	Start on 100 µg fludrocortisone (doses vary between 50 and 250 µg per 24 hr) administered as a single dose in the morning immediately after waking up
	Monitoring • Blood pressure sitting and erect (postural drop ≥20 mm Hg indicative of under-replacement; high blood pressure may indicate over-replacement) • Check for peripheral edema (indicative of over-replacement) • Check serum sodium and potassium • Check plasma renin activity (at least every 2–3 yr upon clinical suspicion of over- and under-replacement and after significant changes in the hydrocortisone dose (40 mg hydrocortisone = 100 µg fludrocortisone)
Adrenal androgen replacement	Consider in patients with impaired well-being and mood despite apparently optimized glucocorticoid and mineralocorticoid replacement and in women with symptoms and signs of androgen deficiency (dry, itchy skin; reduced libido)
	25–50 mg DHEA as a single morning dose; in women also consider using transdermal testosterone (300 µg/d; ie, 2 patches per week)
	Monitoring • In women, serum testosterone and SHBG (to calculate free androgen index) • In men and women on DHEA replacement, serum DHEAS, and androstenedione levels • Blood should be sampled at steady state (ie, 12–24 hr after the last preceding DHEA dose)

(Continued)

Table VI-1. Recommended Therapeutic Approach to Adrenal Insufficiency (Continued)

Additional monitoring requirements	Regular follow-up in specialist center every 6–12 months
	In primary adrenal insufficiency of autoimmune origin (isolated Addison or APS)
	• Serum TSH every 12 months
	In female patients: Check regularity of menstrual cycle; consider measurement of ovarian autoantibodies if family planning not finalized
	Check emergency bracelet/steroid card; update as required
	Check knowledge of "sick day rules" and reinforce emergency guidelines involving partner/family members
	Consider prescription of a hydrocortisone emergency self-injection kit, particularly if delayed access to acute medical care is likely (rural areas, travel)
	Check if other medication includes drugs known to induce (eg, rifampicin; mitotane; anticonvulsants such as phenytoin, carbamazepine, oxcarbazepine, phenobarbital, and topiramate) or inhibit (eg, antiretroviral gents) hepatic cortisol inactivation by CYP3A4, which may require glucocorticoid dose adjustment

Abbreviations: ACTH = adrenocorticotropic hormone; APS = autoimmune polyglandular syndromes; CYP3A4 = cytochrome P450 3A4; DHEA(S) = dihydroepiandrosterone (sulfate); IM = intramuscular; IV = intravenous; SHBG = sex hormone-binding globulin; TSH = thyroid-stimulating hormone.

Adapted with permission from Arlt W. The approach to the adult with newly diagnosed adrenal insufficiency. J Clin Endocrinol Metab. *2009;94:1059–1067.*

this is important because it may target monotherapy with mineralocorticoid receptor blockade rather than empirical and often triple therapy. Additional cardiovascular protection may be conferred through such therapy. Elegant genetic studies have helped explain the basis for aldosterone-secreting adrenal adenomas (*KCNJ5* mutations), but it is in the field of catecholamine-secreting pheochromocytomas/paragangliomas where the genetic basis for disease has had its greatest impact both diagnostically and clinically. Mutation analysis of several candidate genes (eg, *RET, SDHB, SDHD, NF-1, VHL*) is positive in over 30% of cases, even in patients labeled as having "sporadic disease," and now dictates therapy and earlier intervention through family screening. Diagnostic advances, notably in the measurement of highly sensitive plasma metanephrines, have assisted these pathways. Other genetic studies continue to shed light on defects in adrenal steroidogenesis, adrenal androgen excess, and adrenal hypoplasia; it is hoped that such technological advances will impact upon the devastating disease adrenal cancer where, unlike breast and prostate cancer, we remain relatively ignorant of underlying causative gene mutations.

Technology brings unexpected clinical burdens. The earlier postmortem findings that in excess of 5% of elderly patients harbor incidental adrenal adenomas has now emerged as major endocrine referral with the widespread introduction of abdominal computed tomography (CT) and magnetic resonance imaging (MRI) scanning for unrelated issues. Two questions are posed when evaluating such patients—malignancy or functionality? Again, clinical guidelines are in place based on imaging findings (size, Hounsfield units) and endocrine testing to help the differential diagnosis. Fortunately, most patients harbor completely innocent adenomas, but the clinical and patient demand is significant. Urinary steroidobolomics—in effect evaluating a patient's individual adrenal steroid metabolome—may offer a future diagnostic advance in this arena.

From the dizzy heights of innovation 60 years ago, Hench, Kendall, and Reichstein would be delighted to see the advances in our understanding of the pathogenesis of adrenal disorders and the improvements in diagnosis and therapy, but 60 years on, nothing has really matched the immense impact of glucocorticoid replacement therapy and therapeutic corticosteroids in human disease. We all have work still to do.

ACKNOWLEDGMENTS

The author has nothing to disclose.

CHAPTER 16

Emergency Treatment of Florid Cushing's Syndrome

Krystallenia I Alexandraki and Ashley B Grossman

ABSTRACT

Cushing's syndrome (CS) may occasionally present as an acute emergency and would then require urgent and appropriate management. In general, clinical suspicion is followed by a step-by-step diagnostic work-up starting from the confirmation of endogenous hypercortisolemia, followed by the localization of the source of cortisol hypersecretion, with both biochemical investigations and imaging studies. In suspected cases of CS caused by exogenous glucocorticoid exposure, a detailed drug history is mandatory and any relevant drug-drug interactions should be addressed. However, in an emergency situation treatment focuses on the management of severe metabolic disturbances, followed by rapid resolution of the excess glucocorticoid exposure, and subsequent confirmation of the cause and its treatment. Meticulous evaluation has to be instituted during follow-up.

INTRODUCTION

Cushing's syndrome (CS) is defined by long-standing exposure to supraphysiological concentrations of circulating glucocorticoids (1). Untreated CS results in high morbidity and mortality rates, mainly because of its metabolic abnormalities and the risk of overwhelming infection. In certain cases, CS presents as an emergency, and its prompt diagnosis should be followed by urgent therapy to normalize the excess glucocorticoid state, which may take precedence over establishing the cause.

ETIOLOGY

The most common cause of CS is the exogenous iatrogenic administration of glucocorticoids for medical reasons; a detailed drug history is extremely important to establish whether any medications are involved, which should include questioning regarding topical, inhaled, or injected preparations as well as other possible remedies obtained outside of a medical setting. Typically, the doses used in these cases of exogenous glucocorticoids result in more chronic problems and are rarely a medical emergency. However, drug interactions can cause iatrogenic CS, and in particular alterations in the metabolism of synthetic glucocorticoids by antiretroviral drugs can be very problematic and present as an emergency (2–4).

In terms of endogenous CS, recent reports suggest an incidence of 2.3 per million per year, including 1.2–1.7 per million per year for adrenocorticotropic hormone (ACTH)-secreting pituitary adenomas (defined as Cushing's disease [CD]), 0.6 per million per year for adrenal adenomas, and 0.2 per million per year for adrenal carcinomas (5). ACTH-dependent CS is more frequently present in 80%–85% of patients with CS, compared to ACTH-independent CS, which is present in only 20%. In adults, ACTH-dependent CS includes CD (80%) and the ectopic CS (ECS), including both ectopic ACTH (20%) and very rarely ectopic corticotropin-releasing hormone (CRH) (<1%) syndromes (1). CD is mainly caused by microadenomas, defined as adenomas with a size less than 1 cm in diameter, and less often by macroadenomas (5%–10%), with or without extrasellar extension or invasion; pituitary corticotroph carcinomas are defined by extra-pituitary metastases (6). CD is more common in women and tends to present between the ages of 25 and 40 years, while ECS is more common in men, and usually presents 1 decade older than CD, after the age of 40 years (7). The tumors associated with ECS are those arising from the lung, including small cell lung carcinoma (3.3%–50%) and bronchial carcinoids (5%–40%), islet cell tumors/pancreatic carcinoids (7.5%–25%), thymic carcinoids (5%–42%), pheochromocytomas (5%), and medullary thyroid carcinoma (2%–8%). In 12%–37.5% of cases a tumor cannot be identified (7). ECS is usually associated with tumors sited in the thorax and the neck, and in only one third of cases in the abdomen. A further classification regards the identification of the primary site of the source of ECS, resulting in *overt* ECS when the tumoral source is present, *covert* ECS when the tumor is identified at a later evaluation or follow-up, and *occult* ECS when the tumoral source cannot be identified even over time.

ACTH-independent CS is usually due to a unilateral tumor, in 60% by a cortisol-secreting adrenal adenoma (AA) and 40% by a cortisol-secreting adrenal carcinoma (AAC). Adrenal adenomas occur most often around 35 years of age and are significantly more common in women, while adrenal carcinoma is slightly more common in women and has a bimodal age distribution, with peaks in childhood and adolescence and then later in life.

In an emergency situation the cause is likely to be severe hypercortisolemia secondary to a macroadenoma causing CD, the ectopic ACTH syndrome, or an adrenal carcinoma.

PATHOPHYSIOLOGY

The pituitary adrenal axis is regulated by CRH and vasopressin secretion from the hypothalamus, which in turn stimulate the secretion of ACTH from the pituitary gland, and this in turn acts on both zona fasciculata and reticularis of the adrenal gland inducing cortisol and androgen secretion. This cycle is completed by the feedback that cortisol exerts at both hypothalamic and pituitary levels. Moreover, normal individuals exhibit a circadian rhythm in ACTH and cortisol secretion (ie, cortisol levels present a peak at 07.00h–09.00h falling during the day to a nadir at around midnight, and start rising again at 02.00h). Both these features of cortisol physiology (loss of normal suppression to the exogenous administration of glucocorticoids and loss of circadian rhythm) are distorted and, along with the increased levels of cortisol, are included as pathophysiological features of CS and are used in the diagnostic work-up of CS.

Additionally, regarding drug-drug interactions, the concomitant use of synthetic glucocorticoids, such as triamcinolone, budesonide, fluticasone, dexamethasone, and prednisolone, and antiretroviral agents used in the medical therapy of human immunodeficiency virus (HIV), such as ritonavir and atazanavir, results in increased serum concentrations of glucocorticoids. This is due to the inhibition of hepatic enzyme CYP3A4 and P-glycoprotein (PGP) export pump by the protease inhibitors, because both mediators participate in the metabolism of glucocorticoids (2–4).

CLINICAL SIGNS AND FEATURES

The most important step for the diagnosis of CS is the clinical suspicion along with a detailed past medical and drug history (8). This is usually straightforward when CS is florid. The only exception is the paraneoplastic wasting syndrome, which can mask the hypercortisolism in cases of ECS that usually have a rapid onset with severe features, most often secondary to small cell lung cancers (SCLCs). In this case a patient may be admitted as a matter of emergency.

A vast range of signs, symptoms, and other comorbidities, along with a wide range in severity, can be seen in CS (1,8). The presentation is obvious when central obesity, a buffalo hump, purplish skin striae, hyperpigmentation, limb wasting and muscle weakness, a plethoric red face with hirsutism, frontal balding, spontaneous bruising along with metabolic abnormalities (hypertension, prediabetes, or diabetes), and osteoporotic fractures are present. Psychiatric features, sometimes a severe psychosis, may be the presenting feature. In addition, although specific clinical features may suggest one rather than another etiology, the *degree* of hypercortisolemia seems to be the major determinant of the clinical features rather than its duration. Severe hirsutism and virilization strongly suggest an adrenal carcinoma and are relatively uncommon with adrenal adenomas. A gradual onset of signs may be seen with neuroendocrine tumors (NETs) as opposed to SCLCs, which usually have a more rapid onset with symptoms of profound weakness, hyperpigmentation, little or no weight gain, and an absence of overt cushingoid features. The rapidity of onset and the severity of the syndrome have been both implicated as the cause of the more frequent presence of skin pigmentation and ankle edema in SCLCs compared with other causes of ECS. On the other hand, in ECS psychiatric disorders are more prominent with NETs than with SCLCs.

DIAGNOSTIC CONSIDERATIONS

As noted previously, the most important step for the diagnosis of CS is the clinical suspicion along with a detailed past medical and drug history (8). This is usually straightforward when CS is florid.

When endogenous CS is suspected, hypercortisolemia must be established before any attempt at differential diagnosis. Hypercortisolemia can be established by the combination of the following tests: (i) a 24-hr urinary free cortisol (UFC; at least 2 measurements) that confirms the increased synthesis of cortisol exceeding the binding capacity of cortisol-binding globulin (CBG); (ii) the low-dose dexamethasone suppression test (LDDST, 0.5 mg every 6 hr for 2 days) or overnight dexamethasone test (ODST, 1 mg the previous night at midnight), which confirms resistance of the hypothalamo-pituitary-adrenal axis to glucocorticoid feedback; and (iii) midnight serum cortisol (MSeC) or late-night salivary cortisol (LNSaC) assessment confirming the loss of circadian rhythmicity (1,8–10). Recent studies suggest that the 3 screening diagnostic tests are complementary, and their diagnostic performance may increase by their combination, while in specific cases some tests may be superior to others (11). Once the diagnosis of CS is unequivocal, ACTH levels and CRH testing, together with appropriate imaging, are the most useful noninvasive investigations to determine the etiology. However, it should be emphasized that the presence of clear clinical features of CS, plus a massively elevated random serum cortisol (more than 36 mcg/dL [1,000 nmol/L]) at any time, or a 24-hr urinary cortisol more than 4 times the upper limit of normal, is usually sufficient to establish the diagnosis, and no further tests to diagnose CS may be necessary.

When endogenous hypercortisolemia has been confirmed the diagnostic cascade moves to the differential diagnosis to establish the cause of CS by measuring plasma ACTH. A plasma ACTH greater than 30 pg/mL will immediately establish ACTH-dependence, while levels consistently less than 5 pg/mL will indicate primary adrenal pathology. When ACTH is readily detectable, then the patient either has CD or ECS. A positive ACTH and/or cortisol response to the CRH test will suggest CD. Direct sampling of pituitary venous blood by bilateral inferior petrosal sinus sampling (BIPSS) with CRH stimulation may be needed to clarify the diagnosis. We recommend its use in all situations of ACTH-dependent CS except when there is an obvious pituitary macroadenoma or ectopic source. Axial imaging with thin-cut multislice-computed tomography (CT) of the chest and abdomen and pelvic MRI have the highest detection rate for the identification of an ectopic source. The appearance of the adrenals on CT scanning may also support a diagnosis, such as the possibility of a pheochromocytoma as the ECS source; the adrenals may be enlarged in patients with CD but this is almost invariable in ECS. Somatostatin receptor (SSTRs) scintigraphy may prove helpful because ECS may be caused by a small NET expressing SSTRs, adding supportive functional data to conventional imaging techniques. Positron emission tomography (PET) with 18-fluorodeoxyglucose (FDG-PET) is of limited utility except in very occasional cases because these tumors usually show low metabolic activity. Whole-body PET with ^{11}C-5-hydroxytryptophan has been proposed as a universal imaging technique for NETs, in particular for identifying an otherwise occult NET. Its experience is limited, however, because it is not generally available. The same applies to ^{131}I- and ^{123}I-meta-iodobenzylguanidine scans, which have been also used in only small series. Despite all this diagnostic work-up, the definitive proof of an ACTH-dependent tumor requires complete resolution of the clinical and biochemical features after tumor resection or partial resolution after tumor debulking, and/or demonstration of ACTH immunohistochemical staining in the tumor tissue or in metastatic deposits.

If ACTH is very low or undetectable, the next step is imaging of the adrenals. High-resolution CT scanning of the adrenal glands provides the best resolution of adrenal anatomy; this is accurate for masses over 1 cm allowing evaluation of the contralateral gland. A mass over 5 cm in diameter is considered to be malignant until proven otherwise.

In suspected cases of exogenous CS caused by excess glucocorticoid exposure, a detailed drug history (including over-the-counter agents) is mandatory.

MANAGEMENT OF CUSHING'S SYNDROME

The goals of treatment of CS are the normalization of glucocorticoid levels with a reversal of clinical symptoms with the long-term objective to avoid the consequences of excess glucocorticoid exposure. For endogenous CS, surgical removal of the tumor of ACTH-dependent or ACTH-independent origin is the first-line therapeutic approach in the long-term. However, medical treatment aimed at reducing glucocorticoid levels/effects may be required before surgery to reverse the metabolic consequences and poor healing, in patients who cannot be submitted to surgical procedures because of comorbidities, in patients who are unwilling to receive other types of treatments, or finally as an alternative when surgical treatment fails. Bilateral adrenalectomy may also be used in this latter scenario. For exogenous CS, a detailed drug history is mandatory and any relevant drug-drug interactions should be identified and addressed.

Acute Intervention in Florid Cushing's Syndrome

In severe cases of endogenous CS, as noted previously, the diagnosis may be established by florid clinical features in the presence of severe hypercortisolemia. It should be emphasized that clinical features must be present given that ACTH and cortisol are stress hormones and may be elevated during any severe metabolic or systemic stressor such as sepsis, myocardial infarction, and in patients in intensive care. The only exception is the patient with an SCLC when the systemic features of CS may be minimal, but in this scenario the lung lesion should be obvious. For severe cases of exogenous CS, any relevant drug-drug interactions should be addressed urgently.

Having established the diagnosis, establishing the cause is less important than treatment of the acute problem(s). The metabolic derangements should be attended to urgently, and then measures taken to lower the cortisol levels. Diabetes needs to be controlled, often requiring insulin, while the medication may be discontinued after control of the CS. Hypertension will require urgent control in a conventional manner, and no specific agents are recommended, but the combination of fluid retention and hypertension may be associated with cardiac failure; this must be evaluated, especially in the older patient. Hypokalemia is present in almost all patients with ECS and some 10% of patients with other etiologies; we would start therapy with spironolactone and, at a dose of 50 or 100 mg daily, with triamterene or amiloride as alternatives (together with initial potassium replacement as indicated). In recent years it has been realized that CS is associated with a significant prothrombotic tendency, mainly due to an increase in circulating von Willebrand factor, such that subcutaneous heparin should be used at prophylactic doses. Where the mental changes are severe and causing problems in management, haloperidol may be necessary to calm the patient, although there is also some experience with olanzapine. If there are significant osteoporotic fractures then adequate pain relief is necessary and other supportive measures as indicated. It is important to note that many of these aberrations are acute effects of the excess glucocorticoid state and may rapidly reverse with subsequent lowering of glucocorticoid levels, so constant careful monitoring (including for development of acute adrenal failure) is mandatory.

One of the most feared complications of fulminating CS is sepsis, because this may be life-threatening and lack some of the usual indicators and signs of its presence. Hence, any bacterial, fungal, and viral infection must be vigorously treated as soon as possible when recognized, as with other immune-suppressed patients. Prophylaxis with trimethoprim-sulfamethoxazole is highly effective for pneumocystis pneumonia (PCP) in patients receiving a glucocorticoid dose equivalent to ≥20 mg of prednisone daily for 1 month or longer, if they have an additional cause for immunocompromise. The same is valid for patients with rheumatological diseases in combination with a second immunosuppressive drug. However, patients with polymyositis/dermatomyositis who have interstitial pulmonary fibrosis may be at increased risk for PCP with glucocorticoids alone (12). Nevertheless, for patients with endogenous CS it is more imperative simply to treat the hypercortisolemia per se. In patients with severe infection, the serum cortisol should be lowered to a level compatible with that seen in other patients with life-threatening infection, which we take as 22–36 mcg/dL (600–1,000 nmol/L). In addition, perforation of a viscus may occur, with minimal evidence of peritonitis, especially in the elderly with underlying diverticular disease; vigorous resuscitation should be undertaken, and surgery performed as indicated.

When drug interactions are involved in the etiology of CS, it is worth considering alternative therapeutic options (eg, substituting with beclomethasone as an inhaled glucocorticoid because it is not metabolized by CYP3A4). However, if there is no substitute, such as with the intra-articular administration of triamcinolone, meticulous follow-up of the patient along with appropriate cover with glucocorticoids to avoid an adrenal crisis is essential. Furthermore, changing ritonavir-containing antiretroviral therapy to a noninteracting compound, such as an integrase inhibitor, may also be considered (2–4).

Adrenal-Specific Therapy

Lowering of the elevated serum cortisol levels should be attempted as soon as the urgent measures noted previously have been initiated. This is usually best accomplished by using drugs directed at adrenal steroidogenesis. Metyrapone is the optimal initial choice because it is rapid in onset and highly effective, but doses up to 1 g four times a day may be required. The effect is usually seen within hours, and we would generally start with 500–750 mg three times daily; paradoxically, lower doses may be required for the ECS or adrenal tumors because in this situation there is no feedback that might overcome the blockade. Metyrapone is an 11β-hydroxylase inhibitor, which leads to the accumulation of androgenic and some mineralocorticoid precursors, but in the acute situation these should not be problematic. Ketoconazole, an imidazole blocking cytochrome P450 enzymes, can be used additionally or in place of metyrapone, although its onset of action is slower, occurring over several days or possibly longer. Up to 400 mg three times a day may be required. Ketoconazole may cause mild liver enzyme elevation, and very rarely acute liver failure, so this needs to be monitored; mild elevations of liver enzymes need not require cessation of therapy. Where neither drug alone or in combination is effective or tolerated, then one can try the glucocorticoid antagonist mifepristone 400–800 mg daily, which may rapidly reduce the symptoms and signs of CS (off-label use). However, the *serum cortisol cannot be used as a marker of efficacy,* and the patient can become addisonian unless care is taken; severe hypokalemia often follows, but this should respond to spironolactone. If all else fails, intravenous etomidate, an imidazole potently blocking 11β-hydroxylase and side chain cleavage enzyme, but also aldosterone synthase, at sub-anesthetic doses, may be life-saving: it acts within hours and is almost always highly effective. This drug may be used as first-line treatment in severely ill patients, and we would start with 2.5–3 mg/hr as an infusion with dose titration according to serum cortisol if cortisol levels are not falling within 12–24 hr. If complete rather than partial blockade is desired ("block and replace"), a hydrocortisone infusion may be added. It should be noted that in adrenal CS, or ECS, patients are more sensitive to the blocking effect of etomidate resulting in adrenal insufficiency in lower doses compared to patients with CD. However, it needs to be very carefully monitored, and unless the clinicians and their service are highly experienced in its use, we would recommend that it only be used in an intensive care unit (ICU) or high-dependency unit (HDU) setting. Care should be taken because of sedation that may be apparent in higher doses, and adjustments should be made with regard to renal failure and stressed situations such as sepsis (13).

For any cause of ACTH-dependent CS, bilateral adrenalectomy induces rapid resolution of the clinical features after first-line treatment failure or when drugs are not effective or tolerated, or when the rapid control of hypercortisolemia is crucial; however, patients will need lifelong treatment with glucocorticoids and mineralocorticoids along with careful education to prevent adrenal insufficiency. On the other hand, this may be first-line treatment of an uncontrolled hypercortisolemia in an emergency care setting when everything else fails, and the clinical situation of the patient is deteriorating. Nevertheless, even with a good laparoscopic technique, surgery in the presence of severe hypercortisolemia is far from ideal, and every attempt should be made to lower the cortisol levels preoperatively with medical therapy.

CONCLUSIONS

In an acute situation in a patient with clinically obvious endogenous CS, this can be confirmed in most instances with a single grossly elevated serum cortisol level taken at any time of the day. In suspected cases of CS caused by exogenous glucocorticoid exposure, a detailed drug history is mandatory and any relevant drug-drug interactions should be addressed urgently. The most urgent priority in florid CS is to treat the metabolic complications such as diabetes and hypertension, stabilize any psychotic state, and vigorously treat any suspected sepsis or perforated viscus. Emergency lowering of the elevated serum cortisol in endogenous CS is most rapidly achieved with oral metyrapone, but if parenteral therapy is required then intravenous etomidate is rapidly effective in almost all cases, but all measures require careful supervision and monitoring.

ACKNOWLEDGMENTS

ABG has received lecture and advisory board fees from Novartis, Ipsen, HRA Pharma, and Viropharma. This work was not supported by any outside funding.

REFERENCES

1. **Newell-Price J, Bertagna X, Grossman AB, Nieman LK.** Cushing's syndrome. *Lancet.* 2006;367:1605–1617.
2. **Eeftinck Schattenkerk JK, Lager PS.** Cushing's syndrome during HIV treatment: pharmacological interaction during use of ritonavir. *Ned Tijdschr Geneeskd.* 2013;157:A5509. [Article in Dutch]
3. **From HIV i-Base.** Case reports: Cushing's syndrome with atazanavir/ritonavir. http://www.thebody.com/content/63748/case-reports-cushings-syndrome-with-atazanavirrito.html.
4. **Hall JJ, Hughes CA, Foisy MM, Houston S, Shafran S.** Iatrogenic Cushing syndrome after intra-articular triamcinolone in a patient receiving ritonavir-boosted darunavir. *Int J STD AIDS.* 2013;24:748–752.
5. **Steffensen C, Bak AM, Rubeck KZ, Jørgensen JO.** Epidemiology of Cushing's syndrome. *Neuroendocrinology.* 2010;92(suppl 1):1–5.
6. **Kaltsas GA, Nomikos P, Kontogeorgos G, Buchfelder M, Grossman AB.** Clinical review: diagnosis and management of pituitary carcinomas. *J Clin Endocrinol Metab.* 2005;90:3089–3099.
7. **Alexandraki KI, Grossman AB.** The ectopic ACTH syndrome. *Rev Endocr Metab Disord.* 2010;11:117–126.
8. **Alexandraki KI, Grossman AB.** Cushing's syndrome. In: Bandeira F, Gharib H, Golbert A, Griz L, Faria M, eds. *Endocrinology and Diabetes: A Problem Oriented Approach.* New York: Springer Science+Business Media; 2014: 99–111.
9. **Nieman LK, Biller BM, Findling JW, et al.** The diagnosis of Cushing's syndrome: an Endocrine Society Clinical Practice Guideline. *J Clin Endocrinol Metab.* 2008;93:1526–1540.
10. **Alexandraki KI, Grossman AB.** Novel insights in the diagnosis of Cushing's syndrome. *Neuroendocrinology.* 2010;92(suppl 1):35–43.
11. **Arnaldi G, Angeli A, Atkinson AB, et al.** Diagnosis and complications of Cushing's syndrome: a consensus statement. *J Clin Endocrinol Metab.* 2003;88:5593–5602.
12. **Thomas CF, Limper AH.** Treatment and prevention of pneumocystis pneumonia in non-HIV-infected patients. *UpToDate.* Marr KA, Thorner AR, eds. http://www.uptodate.com/contents/treatment-and-prevention-of-pneumocystis-pneumonia-in-non-hivinfectedpatients.
13. **Preda VA, Sen J, Karavitaki N, Grossman AB.** Etomidate in the management of hypercortisolaemia in Cushing's syndrome: a review. *Eur J Endocrinol.* 2012;167:137–143.

CHAPTER 17

Endocrine Hypertensive Emergencies

Graeme Eisenhofer, Andrzej Januszewicz,
Christina Pamporaki, and Jacques WM Lenders

ABSTRACT

Endocrine causes of hypertensive emergencies are easily overlooked when patients present with uncontrolled hypertension in association with end-organ damage. Emergencies arising from hypertensive crises due to pheochromocytoma can be particularly dangerous. To ensure appropriate therapeutic countermeasures and a favorable outcome, the presence of a catecholamine-producing tumor should be distinguished from more common etiologies as well as other uncommon endocrine causes, such as primary hyperaldosteronism, Cushing's syndrome, and thyrotoxicosis. However, diagnosis at the time of the emergency can be made difficult by activation of the sympathoadrenal system resulting from the physiological stress of the clinical condition. Tests of catecholamine excess are, therefore, rendered problematic to interpret, with reliable diagnosis often only possible once and if the patient recovers. Because of this and time delays in obtaining test results, recognition of a possible endocrine cause in the emergency setting requires careful attention to patient history, presentation, and precipitating causes that may provide clues to underlying etiologies for guiding therapeutic interventions.

INTRODUCTION

Hypertensive emergencies are defined by situations of uncontrolled hypertension resulting in acute or looming end-organ damage (1). Such end-organ involvement includes serious cardiac, vascular, cerebral, and renal complications (Table 17-1). In severest forms a hypertensive emergency can present as or progress to multi-organ failure, cardiovascular collapse, and death. Presence of acute life-threatening end-organ damage distinguishes hypertensive emergency, requiring rapid therapeutic intervention, from hypertensive urgency, which does not involve end-organ damage and may be managed by slower acting agents without the necessity for transfer of the patient to an intensive care unit (2,3).

In general for the patient with a hypertensive emergency, fast-acting antihypertensive drugs are required to bring blood pressure down and prevent progression of target organ damage. The nature of end-organ involvement dictates the choice of antihypertensive agent and targeted blood pressure falls. Endocrine causes of hypertensive emergencies require specific drug considerations in view of the underlying pathology. For the patient with pheochromocytoma, certain agents, such as beta-adrenergic receptor blockers, are contraindicated. Thus, management of the patient presenting with a hypertensive emergency is not only directed at safely lowering blood pressure, but also must be tailored according to affected end-organs and underlying etiology (4).

Table 17-1. Spectrum of Cardiovascular End-Organ Damage in Patients with Hypertensive Emergencies

- Acute left ventricular failure
- Acute coronary syndrome
- Aortic dissection
- Encephalopathy
- Intracerebral hemorrhage
- Subarachnoidal hemorrhage
- Acute ischemic stroke
- (Sub)acute renal failure
- Eclampsia
- Advanced retinopathy[a]

[a] *Defined as grade III or IV.*

HYPERTENSIVE EMERGENCIES

Hypertensive emergencies presenting as acute coronary syndromes or left ventricular failure are the most common presentation (5). Even in patients without coronary artery disease, myocardial ischemia may result from acute large increases in blood pressure that evoke increases in cardiac oxygen consumption and left ventricular wall stress. Patients presenting with severe hypertension and stroke represent another common emergency situation in which severe elevations of blood pressure may represent the acute precipitating cause overlaying other contributing pathogenic causes. Such emergency conditions are relatively easily identified by standard history, as well as physical and laboratory evaluations (Table 17-2).

Hypertensive encephalopathy can occur even with mild hypertension (4), and this may be evoked when the mean arterial blood pressure level exceeds the upper blood pressure limit of cerebral blood flow autoregulation. In normotensive individuals this upper limit of mean arterial blood pressure is around 150 mm Hg (6). Above that blood pressure level autoregulation can become overwhelmed, leading to increases in cerebral blood flow proportional to those in blood pressure. This induces cerebral vasodilation, cerebral edema, and subsequent clinical characteristics of acute lethargy, confusion, headache, visual disturbances, and seizures. In patients with established hypertension the window for cerebral blood flow autoregulation is shifted upward so that a much higher blood pressure may be required to evoke breakthrough of the blood-brain barrier. If untreated, cerebral edema can progress to cerebral hemorrhage, coma, and death.

Among less common hypertensive emergencies, aortic dissection carries the highest risk for rapid fatality (Figure 17-1). Rapid onset of severe, sharp, or tearing pain in the chest or back is the most common presenting symptom. Patients may have aortic regurgitation, widened pulse pressure, and discrepancies in right- and left-arm blood pressure readings. In case of a large dissection or rupture, patients can even present with syncope, hypotension, or shock. With low cardiac output patients may present with acute myocardial infarction, stroke, paraplegia, renal failure, or limb and visceral ischemia.

In addition to a history of hypertension, evidence of atherosclerotic disease, a vascular inflammatory disorder, cocaine use, pregnancy, or previously diagnosed vascular abnormalities (eg, aortic aneurysm, bicuspid aortic valve, aortic coarctation) are all risk factors to consider when evaluating the possibility of aortic dissection. Other risk factors include connective tissue diseases, such as Marfan or Ehlers-Danlos syndrome. Aortic dissection may also occur as a result of trauma following surgery or an accident. Definitive diagnosis requires transesophageal echocardiography, magnetic resonance angiography, or a computed tomography angiogram.

Table 17-2. Tests for Patients with Hypertensive Emergencies

Initial tests for all patients in the emergency situation
- Serum creatinine, plasma sodium and potassium, glucose
- Urinanalysis: protein, cells, and cell casts
- Blood count/smear for microangiopathic hemolysis
- Electrocardiogram
- Chest X-ray
- Fundoscopy to document advanced stage retinopathy

Optional when indicated in the emergency situation
- Troponin in case of ischemic heart disease
- Echocardiography in case of suspicion of heart failure
- CT or MRI of the brain in case of neurological signs/symptoms
- Transesophageal echocardiography, magnetic resonance angiography, or computed tomography angiogram of thorax and abdomen when aortic dissection suspected
- CT of abdomen when pheochromocytoma suspected

Tests for endocrine pathologies (for the stabilized patient)
- Plasma metanephrines or 24-hr urinary excretion of metanephrines
- Plasma aldosterone and plasma renin concentration or activity
- 24-hr urinary excretion of cortisol or midnight salivary cortisol

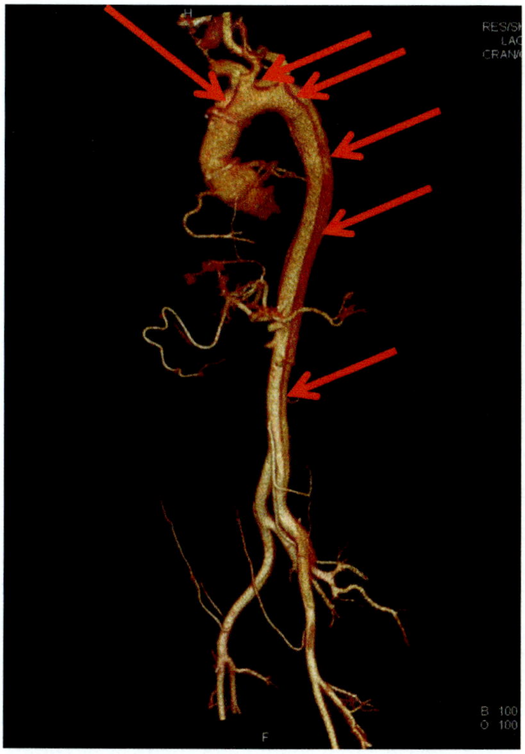

Figure 17-1. Aortic dissection (red arrows) in a 37-year-old male patient with severe hypertension. Computed tomographic volume rendering projection shows aortic dissection type A Stanford after surgical repairment of ascending aorta.

PATHOGENESIS

Beyond the originating cause of increased blood pressure, the pathogenesis of end-organ damage in many cases of hypertensive emergency is suggested to involve disruption of vascular endothelial integrity, increased endothelial permeability with edema, and associated inflammatory responses (1). This may be accompanied by arteriolar fibrinoid necrosis and thrombotic microangiopathic hemolysis. Disseminated intravascular coagulation may also follow from loss of endothelial fibrinolytic activity combined with activation of coagulation. It has been postulated that endothelial damage from high blood pressure also triggers release of the prothrombotic von Willebrand factor, which activates intravascular coagulation.

The previously discussed pathological processes are considered to follow abrupt vasoconstrictor responses as the initiating step, which may follow impact of endogenous vasoconstrictors, such as norepinephrine or angiotensin II. Activated sympathoadrenal-medullary, hypothalamo-pituitary-adrenocortical, and renin-angiotensin-aldosterone systems underlie endocrine hypertensive emergencies. However, the same systems may also be involved in other situations, such as psychogenic stress leading to severe hypertension and takotsubo cardiomyopathy. Drugs such as cocaine, which alter the disposition of endogenous vasoconstrictors, represent other situations whereby neuronal or endocrine systems may act as mediators of initiating vasoconstrictor responses.

Autocrine/paracrine release of nitric oxide and other vasodilators by the vascular endothelium helps to buffer vasoconstrictor responses. However, these compensatory responses can be overwhelmed when hypertension is severe or sustained. The result can be ischemia with failure of affected end-organs; this may involve proinflammatory responses with secretion of cytokines and further endothelial damage and vasoconstrictor responses. Breakdown in endothelial integrity may primarily manifest as edema, such as that affecting pulmonary and cerebral organs. Increased platelet aggregation may further promote vasoconstriction and inflammation and lead to thrombosis and ischemic injury to end-organs.

HYPERTENSIVE EMERGENCIES ASSOCIATED WITH PHEOCHROMOCYTOMA

Pheochromocytoma stands out from primary hyperaldosteronism, Cushing's syndrome, and thyrotoxicosis as the most prominent endocrine cause of hypertensive emergencies (Figure 17-2). The literature is replete with case reports involving highly diverse situations in which a pheochromocytoma hypertensive crisis involves serious end-organ involvement, in many instances culminating in death (7,8). Hypertension due to pheochromocytoma results in more severe end-organ damage than that resulting from similarly increased blood pressure in patients with essential hypertension (9).

As reviewed in detail elsewhere (10), hypertensive emergencies due to pheochromocytoma are wide ranging. Severe hypertension may be accompanied by myocardial ischemia or infarction (11,12) and

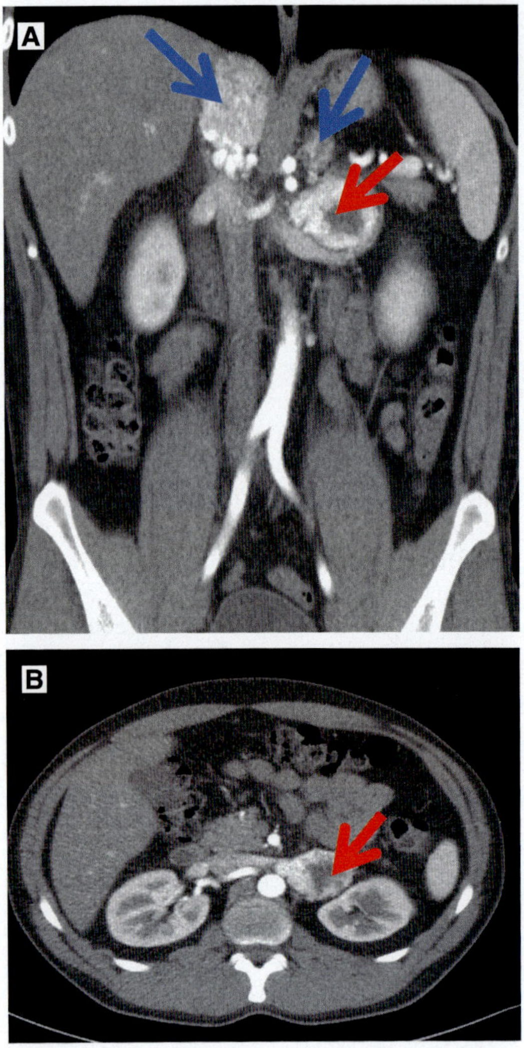

Figure 17-2. Paragangliomas (indicated by arrows) associated with paraganglioma syndome 1 (due to a mutation of the succinate dehydrogenase subunit D gene) in a 39-year-old male patient with severe hypertension. Computed tomographic multiplanar reconstruction of upper abdomen scans show multiple contrast enhanced periaortic masses (A). An axial scan at the level of the kidneys and the lower of the three paragangliomas is shown in B.

bradyarrhythmias or tachyarrhythmias (13,14), as well as hypertrophic cardiomyopathy and heart failure (15,16). Strokes and other cerebrovascular accidents have also been reported repeatedly (17–20), including their combination with hypertrophic cardiomyopathy (21,22). In the previously discussed situations, an underlying pheochromocytoma is often difficult to recognize, but should always be considered when acute heart failure is not accompanied by evidence of valvular or coronary artery disease.

Increasingly now described in conjunction with pheochromocytoma are cases of takotsubo cardiomyopathy (Figure 17-3). This form of cardiomyopathy may present with signs and symptoms of an acute coronary syndrome but without significant obstructive coronary artery disease. It has been postulated that pheochromocytoma-related takotsubo cardiomyopathy is mediated by excessive local myocardial levels of catecholamines, resulting in hyperkinesis of the basal part of the ventricle with apical ballooning. The shape of the left ventricle resembles a Japanese octopus fishing pot, a so-called takotsubo. In patients diagnosed with symptoms of acute coronary syndrome without coronary artery stenosis or spasm, pheochromocytoma-induced takotsubo cardiomyopathy should be considered, particularly when accompanied by pronounced blood pressure variability or shock (8,23,24).

Pheochromocytomas occurring in association with acute aortic dissection pose a particularly difficult dilemma, with the need for rapid aortic repair balanced against adequate adrenergic blockade in preparing the patient for surgery (25,26). If immediately operated

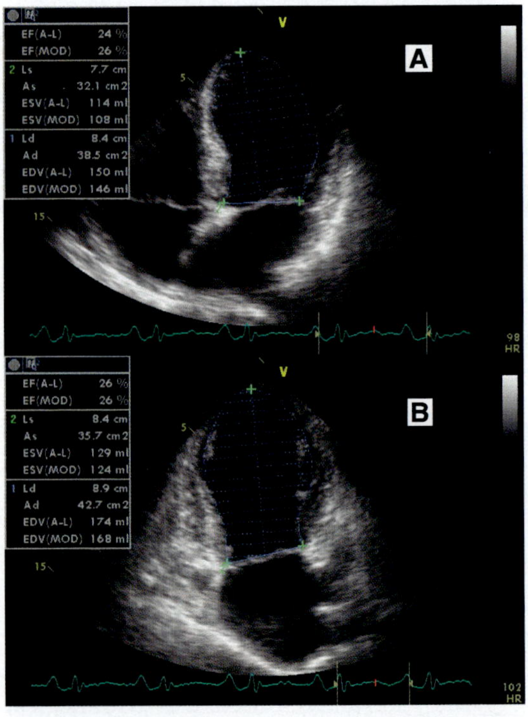

Figure 17-3. Echocardiagraphic evidence by apical four chamber (A) and two chamber (B). Views of systolic ballooning of the apical and midportions of the left ventricle and significant systolic dysfunction in 53-year-old patient with takotsubo cardiomyopathy.

on without blockade, there is a high risk of life-threatening complications secondary to tumoral catecholamine release. Thus, when evaluating imaging studies carried out to diagnose aortic dissection it is important not to dismiss any adrenal or abdominal mass that could represent the underlying endocrine cause of the condition.

Pulmonary edema, either cardiac or noncardiac and presenting as severe respiratory distress, is a particularly common emergency condition associated with pheochromocytoma that may present either with other life-threatening conditions or alone as the primary feature of the tumor (27,28). Presumably as a reflection of the vasoconstriction-associated reduced vascular perfusion, pheochromocytomas can also present as acute renal failure or reversible functional renal artery stenosis (29–31). Ischemia combined with actions of catecholamines to reduce intestinal peristalsis and motility is also believed responsible for emergency presentations of intestinal pseudo-obstruction, megacolon, and ischemic colitis in other cases of pheochromocytoma (32–34). In some cases peripheral ischemia may be severe enough to result in gangrene and tissue necrosis (35,36).

Presentation as unexplained shock is one of the most dangerous situations for a patient with an unsuspected pheochromocytoma (37–39). Pheochromocytoma in such situations should be suspected when accompanied by significant abdominal pain, pulmonary edema, intense mydriasis unresponsive to light stimulation, profound weakness, diaphoresis, cyanosis, hyperglycemia, and leukocytosis. Abrupt cessation of catecholamine secretion by the tumor in a patient with a constricted circulatory volume and desensitized adrenoceptors, following prolonged exposure to catecholamines, is thought to represent the main mechanism responsible for shock in this setting. Decreased cardiac output due to catecholamine-induced cardiomyopathy or myocardial infarction may also be contributing factors.

Shock in patients with pheochromocytoma may be accompanied or followed by multiple organ dysfunction syndrome, where early detection of the tumor can be crucial to improve a patient's chances of survival (40–42). Pheochromocytoma multisystem crisis is defined as multiple organ failure, lactic acidosis, temperature often greater than 40°C, encephalopathy, and hypertension and/or hypotension (43). The presentation can easily be mistaken for septicemia, delaying appropriate treatment. Fever and acute inflammatory symptoms may be due to interleukin-6 production by the tumor (44). Therefore, pheochromocytoma should be included in the differential diagnosis of patients with shock.

The hypertensive emergency in a pregnant patient with pheochromocytoma, a situation frequently mistaken for preeclampsia, carries a particularly high risk of both maternal and fetal mortality if the tumor remains undiagnosed (45,46). However, if pheochromocytoma is recognized and appropriate countermeasures are made the prognosis is considerably improved with now close to an 85%–90% chance of survival for both mother and neonate. Potentially fatal hypertensive crises in unrecognized pregnancies may be precipitated by anesthesia, vaginal delivery, mechanical effects of the gravid uterus, uterine contractions, and vigorous fetal movements.

OTHER ENDOCRINE CAUSES OF HYPERTENSIVE EMERGENCIES

Hypertensive emergencies due to Cushing's syndrome can be as dangerous as those occurring with pheochromocytoma, but are more rarely described. Patients with hypertension due to hypercortisolism can present with left ventricular failure, pulmonary edema, and other end-organ complications (47,48). Cushing's syndrome during pregnancy with uncontrolled hypertension, masquerading as preeclampsia, has also been described (49,50). Associated clinical conditions of hypercortisolism, also requiring immediate therapeutic attention, can exacerbate dangers and further increase the high risk of mortality. Such conditions that may contribute to morbidity include electrolyte and metabolic imbalances as well as opportunistic infections or even sepsis related to immunosuppression.

Primary hyperaldosteronism (Figure 17-4) carries a high risk for end-organ damage not only due to the resulting hypertension, but also resulting from direct deleterious effects of high levels of circulating aldosterone as well as from downstream actions on electrolyte balance (51). Thus, patients with hypertension due to hyperaldosteronism have more severe

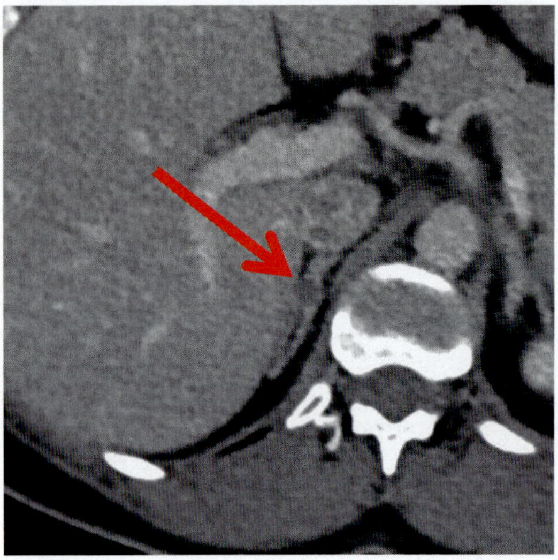

Figure 17-4. Computed tomographic scan of a 43-year-old male patient with primary hyperaldosteronism showing a small hypodense mass in the right adrenal gland.

end-organ damage than those with essential hypertension and similar increases in blood pressure. The mechanism is thought to involve mineralocorticoid receptor activation, which induces oxidative stress, dysfunction, inflammation, and fibrosis of the vascular wall (52).

Despite significant end-organ damage in patients with hyperaldosteronism, reports of hypertensive emergencies in the condition are relatively rare (53). This may reflect the typically sustained nature of the associated blood pressure increases and the chronically progressive rather than acute nature of end-organ damage resulting from primary hyperaldosteronism, particularly common in patients with resistant hypertension (54).

Acute emergencies that do occur in patients with hyperaldosteronism may relate to associated hypokalemia leading to arrhythmias, ventricular fibrillation, and, rhabdomyolysis, the latter usually presenting as muscular weakness, limb pain, and, in severe cases, as muscular paralysis. Pulmonary edema has also been reported in isolated cases of severe hypertension in patients with primary hyperaldosteronism (55).

Thyrotoxicosis, presenting in its extreme form as a thyrotoxic crisis (or thyroid storm), can be accompanied by hypertension, though this is not a consistent or a usually primary feature. The more usual key manifestations include fever, often with profuse sweating, tachycardia, arrhythmias, and respiratory distress (56). The latter may reflect pulmonary hypertension and right ventricular failure, other manifestations increasingly reported in patients with severe thyrotoxicosis (57–59). The etiology is most commonly Graves' disease, with transition to thyrotoxic crisis usually requiring a secondary contributing cause, such as infection, trauma, or surgery. The condition can involve multi-organ failure with mortality rates reaching 10%–20%.

DIAGNOSTIC CONSIDERATIONS

In addition to standard laboratory studies (eg, urinalysis, serum electrolytes, creatinine, urea or blood urea nitrogen, blood count) useful to pinpoint end-organ involvement, blood or urine specimens may also be collected for measurements of specific hormones should an endocrine cause of the hypertensive emergency be suspected (Table 17-2). Recommended tests for diagnosis of pheochromocytoma include plasma or urinary fractionated metanephrines (60). For primary aldosteronism, measurements of plasma aldosterone and renin, to yield a ratio of aldosterone to renin, is the recommended first-line test (61). First-line diagnostic tests for Cushing's syndrome include urinary or salivary measurements of cortisol (62).

For patients presenting with hypertensive emergencies the requirement to immediately institute therapeutic countermeasures supersedes requirements for any useful information that might be provided by endocrine diagnostic testing. Availability of results for these tests invariably involves considerable delay. Some tests, such as those involving 24-hour urine collections for measurements of metanephrines or cortisol, are moreover impractical in the emergency setting for timely delivery of diagnostic test results. Furthermore, because the compounds measured are either stress hormones or metabolites of stress hormones, the very nature of the acute emergency situation renders a high likelihood of false-positive results.

Problems with stress-associated influences on diagnostic test results are particularly problematic for measurements of catecholamines and their *O*-methylated metabolites, the metanephrines (Figure 17-5). Although the metanephrines are produced within chromaffin cells and chromaffin cell tumor derivatives by a process that is independent of exocytotic release, the metabolites can also be produced by

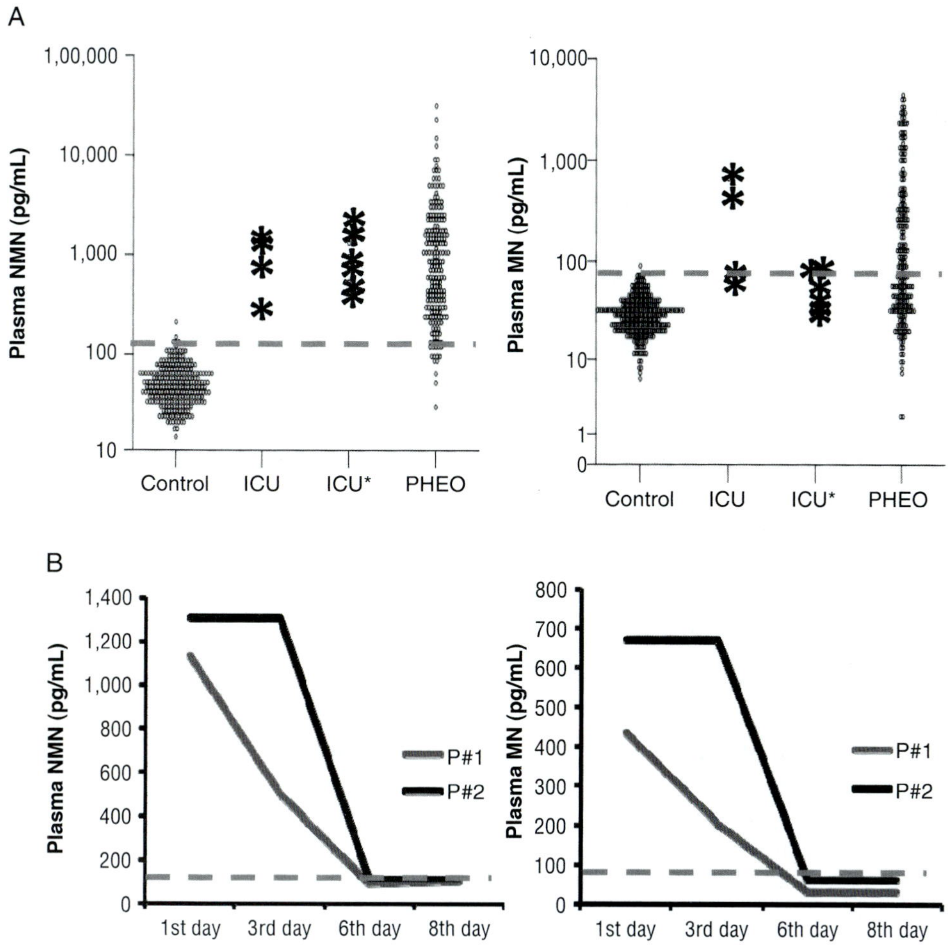

Figure 17-5. (A) Dot-plot logarithmic distributions of plasma concentrations of free normetanephrine (NMN) and metanephrine (MN) in a reference population (Control; $n = 262$) and a population of patients with pheochromocytoma (PHEO; $n = 198$) compared to patients without pheochromocytoma sampled in an intensive care unit (ICU) with (ICU*; $n = 7$) and without (ICU; $n = 4$) norepinephrine infusions. Dashed horizontal lines show the upper cut-offs (97.5 percentiles) for the reference population. Note that both groups of ICU patients have concentrations of NMN well above the upper cut-offs of reference intervals that are indistinguishable from concentrations in patients with pheochromocytoma. In addition, 2 of the 4 ICU patients not receiving IV norepinephrine also had plasma concentrations of MN well above the upper cut-offs. (B) Repeated measurements of plasma free NMN and MN in 2 of the 4 ICU patients not receiving IV norepinephrine over the 8 days of hospitalization. Note normalization of plasma concentrations of NMN and MN with clinical stabilization.

extraneuronal metabolism of norepinephrine released by sympathetic nerves and to a minor extent from epinephrine released from the adrenal medulla (63). From this understanding it can be appreciated that there is absolutely no benefit in measurements performed during hypertensive crises. In fact, blood sampling for measurements of plasma metanephrines is most ideally performed under conditions of minimal stress; patients should be lying supine for 30 minutes before blood sampling to minimize sympathoadrenal activation and reduce the likelihood of false-positive results (64).

Precautions to minimize false-positive results are largely impractical in the acute emergency setting. As a result, plasma concentrations of normetanephrine, metanephrine, and parent amines in blood samples collected during hypertensive emergencies in patients without pheochromocytoma can run well into the range of concentrations commonly observed in patients with the tumor (Figure 17-5). Plasma levels reaching 10-fold or more above upper cut-offs of reference intervals in such patients without pheochromocytoma can make interpretation of positive test results nearly impossible. Confirming any endocrine cause of a hypertensive emergency by biochemical testing invariably also requires follow-up testing, also impractical in the acute emergency setting.

Endocrine diagnostic testing may, of course, yield negative results that can be used to rule out the tumors. Nevertheless, such results are likely to remain unavailable during the critical time of the acute emergency when initial decisions about best management practices must be made.

Taking into account the previously outlined considerations, the acute hypertensive emergency represents one situation where imaging studies to locate a tumor may be carried out directly, without adhering to recommendations that imaging should only be carried out once biochemical evidence is clear. Such imaging studies, nevertheless, are only reasonable to consider when there is sufficient evidence to suspect an endocrine cause or when carried out as part of other investigations into associated pathology (eg, investigation of an aortic dissection). For suspicion of an underlying endocrine cause, awareness of clinical clues is essential.

Table 17-3. Clinical Clues for Considering Pheochromocytoma When a Patient Presents with a Hypertensive Emergency

- Previous history of pheochromocytoma
- Presence of paroxysmal signs and symptoms known to be associated with pheochromocytoma
- Use of a medication known to elicit a pheochromocytoma crisis
- Pheochromocytoma in first- or second-degree relatives
- Presence of an adrenal incidentaloma
- Family history of hereditary syndromes known to be associated with pheochromocytoma: von Hipple-Lindau syndrome, multiple endocrine neoplasia type 2, neurofibromatosis type 1, familial paraganglioma syndromes
- Diagnosed mutation in a known pheochromocytoma- or paraganglioma-susceptibility gene

CLUES TO ENDOCRINE CAUSES OF HYPERTENSIVE EMERGENCIES

Apart from sustained or episodic hypertension, patients with pheochromocytoma often present with symptoms of catecholamine excess. Although knowledge of the classic symptoms of pheochromocytoma—such as diaphoresis, palpitations, and headaches—may be useful general pointers, such symptoms also commonly occur in patients with hypertensive emergencies. Consideration of familial disease, preceding history, and precipitating factors are more important than symptoms alone for raising the level of suspicion for an underlying pheochromocytoma (Table 17-3).

Among the previously mentioned considerations, any knowledge gained from the patient or family members for the presence of a mutation in a pheochromocytoma or paraganglioma tumor-susceptibility gene should immediately arouse strong suspicion that the hypertensive emergency results from a catecholamine-producing tumor. Such suspicion need not just require knowledge of a diagnosed mutation in the patient, but can also include a previous history of pheochromocytoma or associated clinical syndrome (eg, multiple endocrine neoplasia type 2, neurofibromatosis type 1, von Hippel-Lindau syndrome) in family members. If the patient has a history of pheochromocytoma, this should also raise immediate suspicion that the emergency reflects residual or recurrent disease. A previous history of paroxysmal hypertension or other clinical conditions such as panic attacks can also raise the level of suspicion for a catecholamine-producing tumor.

Among precipitating factors, considerations of medications and drugs known to provoke tumoral catecholamine release can provide particularly useful clues to the possibility of an underlying pheochromocytoma (65). D2-dopamine-receptor antagonists, such as metoclopramide, and beta-adrenergic receptor blockers are the better known classes of drugs established to provoke hypertensive emergencies in patients with pheochromocytoma. Features of hypertensive emergencies due to pheochromocytoma precipitated by beta-adrenergic receptor blockers commonly include severe hypertension and/or pulmonary edema, in some cases progressing to shock. When such adverse reactions occur in a patient taking beta-adrenergic receptors blockers, pheochromocytoma should be suspected immediately.

Other drugs documented to result in hypertensive emergencies in patients with pheochromocytoma include tricyclic antidepressants, monoamine oxidase inhibitors, and sympathomimetics (65). Corticosteroids, including dexamethasone, prednisone, and hydrocortisone, are also agents now increasingly recognized to cause hypertensive crises in patients with an unsuspected pheochromocytoma, in some cases culminating in multi-organ failure and death (66). Thus, pheochromocytoma should be strongly suspected in any patient presenting with a hypertensive emergency after administration of steroids.

Other emergencies where pheochromocytoma should be strongly suspected are those occurring during surgical anesthesia or physical procedures, insults, or changes in physiology that involve compression of an unsuspected catecholamine-producing tumor. Included among the latter are pregnancy, childbirth, and micturition-induced hypertensive emergencies in cases of patients with bladder paraganglioma.

Clues to other endocrine causes of hypertensive emergencies, such as Cushing's syndrome, primary hyperaldosteronism, and thyrotoxicosis are in most cases best provided from physical and routine laboratory evaluations. For Cushing's syndrome, features such as the classic moon face, buffalo hump, abdominal striae, ecchymoses, osteoporosis, depression, and hirsutism in women should arouse suspicion. Extremely low potassium should arouse suspicion of primary hyperaldosteronism, but apart from this there are only a few clear physical or laboratory findings that might immediately signal aldosterone excess in such patients. Plasma potassium is, however, decreased only in 1 out of every 3 patients with primary hyperaldosteronism. Another factor complicating the use of potassium is the fact that when the patient presents with a hypertensive emergency, potassium is usually low due to the activation of the renin-aldosterone-angiotensin system. An enlarged thyroid gland, extreme tachycardia, history of weight loss, diarrhea, and exophthalmos can signal thyrotoxicosis, but often there should also be a history of Graves, disease or another recognized contributing condition.

TREATMENT OF HYPERTENSIVE EMERGENCIES

In most cases of hypertensive emergencies, the first goal is a partial reduction and not necessarily normalization of blood pressure (67). Guidelines recommend that treatment of hypertensive emergencies should take into consideration the nature of associated organ damage, with a range in treatment from no or extremely cautious lowering of blood pressure in acute stroke to prompt and aggressive blood pressure reduction in acute pulmonary edema or aortic dissection. Except for acute stroke, these recommendations are not based on randomized controlled trials comparing aggressive with conservative blood pressure lowering but only on long-standing clinical experience.

Rapid lowering of blood pressure is particularly contraindicated in patients with cerebrovascular end-organ involvement, in whom excessive reduction of blood pressure can lead to extension of stroke (68). In contrast, in the patient with aortic dissection rapid lowering of systolic blood pressure to at least 120 mm Hg within 20 minutes has been advocated.

There are a number of parenteral agents that may be used for first-line acute lowering of blood pressure, with choice tailored according to the presentation, type of emergency, and etiology (Table 17-4). In acute coronary syndrome, the use of intravenous (IV) nitroglycerine as vasodilator can be combined with a beta-adrenergic receptor blocker such as esmolol or metoprolol to reduce heart rate and myocardial oxygen consumption. Among these agents, esmolol is most useful due to its rapid onset and short duration of action allowing titration of dosage. The combined alpha- and beta-adrenergic blocking agent, labetalol, is an alternative.

For control of volume overload in patients with a hypertensive emergency and left ventricular heart failure, IV nitroglycerine or sodium nitroprusside should be combined with a loop diuretic. In cases of aortic dissection, labetalol or the combination of esmolol and nitroprusside can be used to minimize stress on the aortic wall and prevent spread of the dissection.

Use of antihypertensives in acute stroke can be complicated by impaired autoregulation of cerebral blood flow in ischemic areas such that blood pressure reduction may further reduce flow to affected brain areas and expand the size of the infarct. Because of this it has been suggested to consider antihypertensive therapy in patients with ischemic stroke only when blood pressures exceed 220/120 mm Hg (68). Even then blood pressure should be reduced only gradually. Labetalol is most commonly used for this indication. Lower

Table 17-4. Available Drugs for Acute Treatment of Hypertensive Emergencies

Drug	Indication	Dose	Adverse Effects
Sodium nitroprusside	Most hypertensive emergencies except in ischemic heart disease and eclampsia. Not when renal or liver failure is present	Start: 0.3–10 ug/kg/min; increase by 0.5 ug/kg/min every 5 minutes	Cyanide toxicity, methemoglobin-emia; increased intracranial pressure
Nitroglycerine	Ischemic heart disease	Start: 5–100 ug/min; increase by 5 ug/min every 5 minutes	Flushing; headache; tolerance
Nicardipine	Most hypertensive emergencies; not for ischemic heart disease and heart failure	Start: 5 mg/hr, increase by 2.5 mg every 15–30 minutes until 15 mg/hr	Reflex tachycardia; increased intracranial pressure
Clevidipine	Most hypertensive emergencies; not for ischemic heart disease and heart failure	Start: 1–2 mg/hr then titrate to maximum of 16 mg/hr	Reflex tachycardia; increased intracranial pressure; soy allergy
Labetalol	Most hypertensive emergencies except pheochromocytoma, acute heart failure, 2nd-or 3rd-degree AV block, broncho-constrictive disease	Start: 1–2 mg/min; increase every 10 minutes by 1 mg/min until maximum dose of 20 mg/hr	
Esmolol	Most hypertensive emergencies except for pheochromocytoma, acute heart failure, 2nd-or 3rd-degree AV block, and bronchoconstrictive disease	Start: 80 mg bolus in 30 seconds, then 150 ug/kg/min	
Phentolamine	Hypertensive emergencies due to catecholamine excess, eg, pheochromocytoma	2.5–5 mg bolus and repeat after 5–10 minutes; Continuous: 0.5–1.0 mg/hr	Flushing; headache; tachycardia
Fenoldopam	Most hypertensive emergencies, in particular acute renal failure	0.1–0.6 ug/kg/min	Flushing; headache; tachycardia
Urapidil	Hypertensive emergencies due to catecholamine excess, eg, pheochromocytoma	12.5–50 mg as bolus; Continuous: 1–10 ug/kg/min	Headache

blood pressure thresholds (systolic >180 mm Hg) for initiating antihypertensive therapy are, however, called for in patients with cerebral hemorrhage. Nicardipine or labetalol and sodium nitroprusside can be used for patients with acute hemorrhagic stroke. In case of hypertensive encephalopathy, either labetalol or nicardipine can be used.

TREATMENT OF PHEOCHROMOCYTOMA-RELATED HYPERTENSIVE EMERGENCIES

Hypertensive emergencies in patients with pheochromocytoma are best treated with IV infusions of rapidly acting alpha-adrenergic receptor antagonists such as phentolamine or urapidil, but sodium nitroprusside and nicardipine are reasonable alternatives. More recently employed antihypertensive agents include clevidipine, an ultra-short acting IV dihydropyridine calcium channel blocker recently approved by the Food and Drug Administration for use in treatment of hypertensive emergencies (69). The agent has some unique pharmacodynamic and pharmacokinetic properties that in clinical trials have shown promise in comparison to other agents, including nicardipine, nitroglycerin, and sodium nitroprusside. Use of the drug during intraoperative management of patients with pheochromocytoma has been described (70,71). Phentolamine may be given as an IV bolus of 2.5 mg to 5 mg at 1 mg/min, with the dose repeated every 5–10 minutes, or as a continuous infusion (100 mg of phentolamine in 500 mL of 5% dextrose in water) of 0.5–1.0 mg/hr with doses adjusted to the blood pressure response. Urapidil, a selective alpha$_1$-adrenoceptor blocker, can also be administered in IV bolus doses or by infusion (Table 17-4).

Beta-adrenergic blockers may be used to treat arrhythmias or tachycardia, the latter often arising as a reflex to vasodilators, but only after adequate blockade of alpha-adrenoceptor-mediated vasoconstriction. The danger of using beta-adrenergic receptor blockers without first blocking alpha-adrenergic receptors has been documented in numerous case studies of hypertensive emergencies in patients with unsuspected pheochromocytoma receiving beta-adrenergic receptor blockers (for review see [65]). The mechanism is believed to involve inhibition of beta$_2$-adrenoceptor-mediated vasodilation, leaving alpha-adrenoceptor-mediated vasoconstrictor responses to catecholamines unopposed. Importantly, such adverse reactions have been documented in numerous reports for the mixed adrenoceptor blocker, labetalol (72–78). This is likely due to the fact that the nonselective beta-adrenergic receptor blocking actions of labetalol predominate over the alpha-adrenergic receptor blocking actions at a 7:1 ratio (when used intravenously). Therefore, labetalol should not be used in any patient with a hypertensive emergency when there is real suspicion of pheochromocytoma.

For patients presenting with shock and multi-organ failure, therapeutic options are limited in circumstances when an underlying pheochromocytoma is suspected. In some patients with catecholamine-induced shock, vasoconstriction may be so severe that reliable blood pressure measurements are compromised, obscuring severe central hypertension. In this situation, assessment of volume status and cardiac function is critical. Volume expansion becomes important once hypovolemic shock is clearly identified.

For the patient with multisystem crisis or shock, it is imperative to correct metabolic acidosis and improve peripheral perfusion with judicious use of colloids and/or crystalloids. Renal function should also be assessed and protected as necessary. Identification and correction of hypocalcemia may also be particularly important in patients with pheochromocytoma-associated cardiogenic shock (79). In such situations, replacement of ionized calcium may preserve cardiac function and reduce mortality.

Pulmonary edema is common in cases of pheochromocytoma-associated hypertensive emergencies and may require intubation and lung-protective ventilatory strategies to maintain oxygenation. Hypertensive encephalopathy, hyperthermia, hyperglycemia, and hepatic failure may further complicate prognosis and therapeutic options in patients with multisystem organ failure and add to the high mortality of this condition.

If pheochromocytoma is suspected in a patient with a hypertensive emergency, any requirement for biochemical confirmation of catecholamine excess is largely made impractical by the seriousness of the patient's condition and likely delay in obtaining laboratory results. Immediate attempts are better made to localize the lesion, with abdominal CT the most practical imaging option in patients on cardiac and ventilatory support. Carefully considered and planned surgery may present the only chance for a successful outcome in patients with multisystem crisis (38,42,80,81). However, emergency resection of pheochromocytoma without adequate preoperative preparation is associated with high surgical morbidity and mortality and thus remains controversial (82). If the patient can be stabilized, it is preferable that surgery be carried out after preparation with recommended alpha-adrenergic receptor blockers or other agents to block the hemodynamic effects of catecholamines produced by the tumors.

Treatment of a hypertensive emergency in a pregnant patient with a pheochromocytoma remains one of the most difficult therapeutic challenges for a clinician because the life of both mother and fetus is at stake. Once the pheochromocytoma is discovered, acute treatment of the hypertensive crisis, with some caveats, is not different from a nonpregnant woman with pheochromocytoma. Nicardipine might be the drug to start with but some prefer phentolamine. In pregnancy the use of IV magnesium sulfate has been advocated, with a mechanism of action thought to involve vasodilation as well reductions in the release and effects of catecholamines (83). Combined administration of nicardipine and magnesium sulfate might act synergistically and cause unwanted excessive blood pressure reductions. Some drugs, such as sodium nitroprusside, are not desirable due to the risk of fetal cyanide intoxication. A multidisciplinary approach by obstetrician, surgeon, endocrinologist, and anesthesiologist is essential to achieve optimal outcome.

TREATMENT OF OTHER ENDOCRINE HYPERTENSIVE EMERGENCIES

In severe enough cases of hypertensive emergency in Cushing's syndrome, IV etomidate or administration of other fast-acting steroidogenesis inhibitors may be initiated to provide immediate relief, but as in pheochromocytoma, surgical intervention provides the only cure (47,84). Bilateral adrenalectomy may be employed as an emergency surgical procedure even in the more common cases of ACTH-dependent Cushing's syndrome (85). In such cases steroid replacement therapy must be initiated immediately during surgery to avoid associated dangers of adrenal insufficiency, particularly cardiovascular collapse.

CONCLUSIONS

Most of the numerous blood pressure lowering drugs can be used to treat patients with hypertensive emergencies, with treatment practices varying considerably due to a paucity of evidence-based randomized trials to support use of one agent over another (86). Nevertheless, lower level evidence and inferential reasoning strongly suggest that choice of therapeutic agents and mode of therapy should be tailored according to clinical presentation and affected end-organs, with additional considerations of etiology. The latter can be particularly important in endocrine causes of hypertensive emergencies in which additional therapeutic strategies may be considered (steroidogenesis inhibitors in Cushing's syndrome) or in which other therapies are contraindicated (eg, beta-adrenergic blockers in pheochromocytoma). Standard blood or urine tests to diagnose endocrine causes of hypertensive emergencies are rendered largely irrelevant due to issues of time and stress-associated false-positive results. Rather, recognition of endocrine causes of hypertensive crises primarily requires appreciation of clinical features and precipitating stimuli.

ACKNOWLEDGMENTS

The authors have nothing to disclose.

REFERENCES

1. **Vaughan CJ, Delanty N.** Hypertensive emergencies. *Lancet.* 2000;356:411–417.
2. **Moser M, Izzo JL Jr, Bisognano J.** Hypertensive emergencies. *J Clin Hypertens* (Greenwich). 2006;8: 275–281.
3. **Rosei EA, Salvetti M, Farsang C.** European Society of Hypertension Scientific Newsletter: treatment of hypertensive urgencies and emergencies. *J Hypertens.* 2006;24:2482–2485.
4. **Kaplan NM.** Management of hypertensive emergencies. *Lancet.* 1994;344:1335–1338.
5. **Zampaglione B, Pascale C, Marchisio M, Cavallo-Perin P.** Hypertensive urgencies and emergencies. Prevalence and clinical presentation. *Hypertension.* 1996;27:144–147.
6. **Strandgaard S, Jones JV, MacKenzie ET, Harper AM.** Upper limit of cerebral blood flow autoregulation in experimental renovascular hypertension in the baboon. *Circ Res.* 1975;37:164–167.
7. **Brouwers FM, Eisenhofer G, Lenders JW, Pacak K.** Emergencies caused by pheochromocytoma, neuroblastoma, or ganglioneuroma. *Endocrinol Metab Clin North Am.* 2006;35:699–724.
8. **Prejbisz A, Lenders JW, Eisenhofer G, Januszewicz A.** Cardiovascular manifestations of phaeochromocytoma. *J Hypertens.* 2011;29:2049–2060.
9. **Stolk RF, Bakx C, Mulder J, Timmers HJ, Lenders JW.** Is the excess cardiovascular morbidity in pheochromocytoma related to blood pressure or to catecholamines? *J Clin Endocrinol Metab.* 2013;98:1100–1106.
10. **Whitelaw BC, Prague JK, Mustafa OG, et al.** Phaeochromocytoma crisis [published online ahead of print October 17, 2013]. *Clin Endocrinol* (Oxf). 2014;80:13–22.
11. **Garg A, Banitt PF.** Pheochromocytoma and myocardial infarction. *South Med J.* 2004;97:981–984.
12. **Brown H, Goldberg PA, Selter JG, et al.** Hemorrhagic pheochromocytoma associated with systemic corticosteroid therapy and presenting as myocardial infarction with severe hypertension. *J Clin Endocrinol Metab.* 2005;90:563–569.
13. **Petit T, de Lagausie P, Maintenant J, Magnier S, Nivoche Y, Aigrain Y.** Thoracic pheochromocytoma revealed by ventricular tachycardia. Clinical case and review of the literature. *Eur J Pediatr Surg.* 2000;10:142–144.
14. **Tzemos N, McNeill GP, Jung RT, MacDonald TM.** Post exertional broad complex tachycardia in a normotensive patient: a rare presentation of phaeochromocytoma. *Scott Med J.* 2001;46:14–15.
15. **Wood R, Commerford PJ, Rose AG, Tooke A.** Reversible catecholamine-induced cardiomyopathy. *Am Heart J.* 1991;121:610–613.
16. **Giavarini A, Chedid A, Bobrie G, Plouin PF, Hagege A, Amar L.** Acute catecholamine cardiomyopathy in patients with phaeochromocytoma or functional paraganglioma. *Heart.* 2013;99:1438–1444.
17. **Moritani H, Sakamoto M, Yoshida Y, Nasu H, Nemoto R, Nakamura I.** Pheochromocytoma of the urinary bladder revealed with cerebral hemorrhage. *Intern Med.* 2001;40:638–642.
18. **Van YH, Wang HS, Lai CH, Lin JN, Lo FS.** Pheochromocytoma presenting as stroke in two Taiwanese children. *J Pediatr Endocrinol Metab.* 2002;15: 1563–1567.
19. **Chuang HL, Hsu WH, Hsueh C, Lin JN, Scott RM.** Spontaneous intracranial hemorrhage caused by pheochromocytoma in a child. *Pediatr Neurosurg.* 2002;36:48–51.
20. **Petramala L, Cavallaro G, Polistena A, et al.** Multiple catecholamine-secreting paragangliomas:

diagnosis after hemorrhagic stroke in a young woman. *Endocr Pract.* 2008;14:340–346.
21. **Cohen JK, Cisco RM, Scholten A, Mitmaker E, Duh QY.** Pheochromocytoma crisis resulting in acute heart failure and cardioembolic stroke in a 37-year-old man. *Surgery.* 2013; pii:S0039-6060(12)00713-1. doi: 10.1016/j.surg.2012.11.013. [Epub ahead of print]
22. **Vindenes T, Crump N, Casenas R, Wood K.** Pheochromocytoma causing cardiomyopathy, ischemic stroke and acute arterial thrombosis: a case report and review of the literature. *Conn Med.* 2013;77:95–98.
23. **Gianni M, Dentali F, Grandi AM, Sumner G, Hiralal R, Lonn E.** Apical ballooning syndrome or takotsubo cardiomyopathy: a systematic review. *Eur Heart J.* 2006;27:1523–1529.
24. **De Backer TL, De Buyzere ML, Taeymans Y, Kunnen P, Rubens R, Clement DL.** Cardiac involvement in pheochromocytoma. *J Hum Hypertens.* 2000;14:469–471.
25. **Triplett JC, Atuk NO.** Dissecting aortic aneurysm associated with pheochromocytoma. *South Med J.* 1975;68:748, 753.
26. **Bowen FW, Civan J, Orlin A, Gleason T.** Management of type A aortic dissection and a large pheochromocytoma: a surgical dilemma. *Ann Thorac Surg.* 2006;81:2296–2298.
27. **de Leeuw PW, Waltman FL, Birkenhager WH.** Noncardiogenic pulmonary edema as the sole manifestation of pheochromocytoma. *Hypertension.* 1986;8: 810–812.
28. **Desai AS, Chutkow WA, Edelman E, Economy KE, Dec GW Jr.** Clinical problem-solving. A crisis in late pregnancy. *N Engl J Med.* 2009;361:2271–2277.
29. **Shemin D, Cohn PS, Zipin SB.** Pheochromocytoma presenting as rhabdomyolysis and acute myoglobinuric renal failure. *Arch Intern Med.* 1990;150:2384–2385.
30. **Kuzmanovska D, Sahpazova E, Kocova M, Damjanovski G, Popov Z.** Phaeochromocytoma associated with reversible renal artery stenosis. *Nephrol Dial Transplant.* 2001;16:2092–2094.
31. **Gillett MJ, Arenson RV, Yew MK, Thompson IJ, Irish AB.** Diagnostic challenges associated with a complex case of cystic phaeochromocytoma presenting with malignant hypertension, microangiopathic haemolysis and acute renal failure. *Nephrol Dial Transplant.* 2005;20:1014.
32. **Turner CE.** Gastrointestinal pseudo-obstruction due to pheochromocytoma. *Am J Gastroenterol.* 1983;78: 214–217.
33. **Sweeney AT, Malabanan AO, Blake MA, de las Morenas A, Cachecho R, Melby JC.** Megacolon as the presenting feature in pheochromocytoma. *J Clin Endocrinol Metab.* 2000;85:3968–3972.
34. **Wu HW, Liou WP, Chou CC, Chen YH, Loh CH, Wang HP.** Pheochromocytoma presented as intestinal pseudo-obstruction and hyperamylasemia. *Am J Emerg Med.* 2008;26:971.e1–971.e4.
35. **Tack CJ, Lenders JW.** Pheochromocytoma as a cause of blue toes. *Arch Intern Med.* 1993;153:2061.
36. **Lutchman D, Buchholz S, Keightley C.** Phaeochromocytoma-associated critical peripheral ischaemia. *Intern Med J.* 2010;40:150–153.
37. **Bergland BE.** 1989. Pheochromocytoma presenting as shock. *Am J Emerg Med.* 1989;7:44–48.
38. **Mohamed HA, Aldakar MO, Habib N.** Cardiogenic shock due to acute hemorrhagic necrosis of a pheochromocytoma: a case report and review of the literature. *Can J Cardiol.* 2003;19:573–576.
39. **Hanna JS, Spencer PJ, Savopoulou C, Kwasnik E, Askari R.** Spontaneous adrenal pheochromocytoma rupture complicated by intraperitoneal hemorrhage and shock. *World J Emerg Surg.* 2011;6:27.
40. **Kolhe N, Stoves J, Richardson D, Davison AM, Gilbey S.** Hypertension due to phaeochromocytoma—an unusual cause of multiorgan failure. *Nephrol Dial Transplant.* 2001;16:2100–2104.
41. **Herbland A, Bui N, Rullier A, Vargas F, Gruson D, Hilbert G.** Multiple organ failure as initial presentation of pheochromytoma. *Am J Emerg Med.* 2005;23:565–566.
42. **Moran ME, Rosenberg DJ, Zornow DH.** Pheochromocytoma multisystem crisis. *Urology.* 2006;67:846. e819–846.e820.
43. **Newell KA, Prinz RA, Pickleman J, et al.** Pheochromocytoma multisystem crisis. A surgical emergency. *Arch Surg.* 1988;123:956–959.
44. **Kang JM, Lee WJ, Kim WB, et al.** Systemic inflammatory syndrome and hepatic inflammatory cell infiltration caused by an interleukin-6 producing pheochromocytoma. *Endocr J.* 2005;52:193–198.
45. **Mannelli M, Bemporad D.** Diagnosis and management of pheochromocytoma during pregnancy. *J Endocrinol Invest.* 2002;25:567–571.
46. **Lenders JW.** Pheochromocytoma and pregnancy: a deceptive connection. *Eur J Endocrinol.* 2012;166:-143–150.
47. **Kamenicky P, Droumaguet C, Salenave S, et al.** Mitotane, metyrapone, and ketoconazole combination therapy as an alternative to rescue adrenalectomy for severe ACTH-dependent Cushing's syndrome. *J Clin Endocrinol Metab.* 2011;96:2796–2804.
48. **von Stempel C, Perks C, Corcoran J, Grayez J.** Cardio-respiratory failure secondary to ectopic Cushing's syndrome as the index presentation of small-cell lung cancer. *BMJ Case Rep.* 2013; doi:10.1136/bcr-2013-009974.
49. **Choi WJ, Jung TS, Paik WY.** Cushing's syndrome in pregnancy with a severe maternal complication: a case report. *J Obstet Gynaecol Res.* 2011;37: 163–167.
50. **Lim WH, Torpy DJ, Jeffries WS.** The medical management of Cushing's syndrome during pregnancy. *Eur J Obstet Gynecol Reprod Biol.* 2013;168:1–6.
51. **Born-Frontsberg E, Reincke M, Rump LC, et al.** Cardiovascular and cerebrovascular comorbidities of hypokalemic and normokalemic primary aldosteronism: results of the German Conn's Registry. *J Clin Endocrinol Metab.* 2009;94:1125–1130.
52. **Marney AM, Brown NJ.** Aldosterone and end-organ damage. *Clin Sci (Lond).* 2007;113:267–278.
53. **Labinson PT, White WB, Tendler BE, Mansoor GA.** Primary hyperaldosteronism associated with hypertensive emergencies. *Am J Hypertens.* 2006;19:623–627.
54. **Calhoun DA.** Aldosteronism and hypertension. *Clin J Am Soc Nephrol.* 2006;1:1039–1045.
55. **Prejbisz A, Klisiewicz A, Januszewicz A, et al.** 22-Year-old patient with malignant hypertension

associated with primary aldosteronism. *J Hum Hypertens.* 2013;27:138–140.

56. **Carroll R, Matfin G.** Endocrine and metabolic emergencies: thyroid storm. *Ther Adv Endocrinol Metab.* 2010;1:139–145.
57. **Soroush-Yari A, Burstein S, Hoo GW, Santiago SM.** Pulmonary hypertension in men with thyrotoxicosis. *Respiration.* 2005;72:90–94.
58. **Paran Y, Nimrod A, Goldin Y, Justo D.** Pulmonary hypertension and predominant right heart failure in thyrotoxicosis. *Resuscitation.* 2006;69:339–341.
59. **Suk JH, Cho KI, Lee SH, et al.** Prevalence of echocardiographic criteria for the diagnosis of pulmonary hypertension in patients with Graves' disease: before and after antithyroid treatment. *J Endocrinol Invest.* 2011;34:e229-e234.
60. **Pacak K, Eisenhofer G, Ahlman H, et al.** Pheochromocytoma: recommendations for clinical practice from the First International Symposium. *Nat Clin Pract Endocrinol Metab.* 2007;3:92–102.
61. **Funder JW, Carey RM, Fardella C, et al.** Case detection, diagnosis, and treatment of patients with primary aldosteronism: an Endocrine Society Clinical Practice Guideline. *J Clin Endocrinol Metab.* 2008;93:3266–3281.
62. **Nieman LK, Biller BM, Findling JW, et al.** The diagnosis of Cushing's syndrome: an Endocrine Society Clinical Practice Guideline. *J Clin Endocrinol Metab.* 2008;93:1526–1540.
63. **Eisenhofer G, Huynh TT, Hiroi M, Pacak K.** Understanding catecholamine metabolism as a guide to the biochemical diagnosis of pheochromocytoma. *Rev Endocr Metab Disord.* 2001;2:297–311.
64. **Grossman A, Pacak K, Sawka A, et al.** Biochemical diagnosis and localization of pheochromocytoma: can we reach a consensus? *Ann N Y Acad Sci.* 2006;1073:332–347.
65. **Eisenhofer G, Rivers G, Rosas AL, Quezado Z, Manger WM, Pacak K.** Adverse drug reactions in patients with phaeochromocytoma: incidence, prevention and management. *Drug Saf.* 2007;30:1031–1062.
66. **Rosas AL, Kasperlik-Zaluska AA, Papierska L, Bass BL, Pacak K, Eisenhofer G.** Pheochromocytoma crisis induced by glucocorticoids: a report of four cases and review of the literature. *Eur J Endocrinol.* 2008;158:423–429.
67. **Elliott WJ.** Management of hypertension emergencies. *Curr Hypertens Rep.* 2003;5:486–492.
68. **Bath P, Chalmers J, Powers W, et al.** International Society of Hypertension (ISH): statement on the management of blood pressure in acute stroke. *J Hypertens.* 2003;21:665–672.
69. **Sarafidis PA, Georgianos PI, Malindretos P, Liakopoulos V.** Pharmacological management of hypertensive emergencies and urgencies: focus on newer agents. *Expert Opin Investig Drugs.* 2012;21:1089–1106.
70. **Kline JP.** Use of clevidipine for intraoperative hypertension caused by an undiagnosed pheochromocytoma: a case report. *AANA J.* 2010;78: 288–290.
71. **Bettesworth JG, Martin DP, Tobias JD.** Intraoperative use of clevidipine in a patient with von Hippel-Lindau disease with associated pheochromocytoma. *J Cardiothorac Vasc Anesth.* 2013;27:749–751.
72. **Briggs RS, Birtwell AJ, Pohl JE.** Hypertensive response to labetalol in phaeochromocytoma. *Lancet.* 1978;1:1045–1046.
73. **FitzGerald GA.** Hypertensive response to labetalol in phaeochromocytoma. *Lancet.* 1978;1:1259.
74. **Feek CM, Earnshaw PM.** Hypertensive response to labetalol in phaeochromocytoma. *Br Med J.* 1980;281:387.
75. **Sheaves R, Chew SL, Grossman AB.** The dangers of unopposed beta-adrenergic blockade in phaeochromocytoma. *Postgrad Med J.* 1995;71:58–59.
76. **Chung PC, Li AH, Lin CC, Yang MW.** Elevated vascular resistance after labetalol during resection of a pheochromocytoma (brief report). *Can J Anaesth.* 2002;49:148–150.
77. **Petrie J, Lockie C, Paolineli A, et al.** Undiagnosed phaeochromocytoma masquerading as eclampsia. *BMJ Case Rep.* 2012;pii: bcr1020114922. doi: 10.1136/bcr.10.2011.4922.
78. **Kuok CH, Yen CR, Huang CS, Ko YP, Tsai PS.** Cardiovascular collapse after labetalol for hypertensive crisis in an undiagnosed pheochromocytoma during cesarean section. *Acta Anaesthesiol Taiwan.* 2011;49:69–71.
79. **Olson SW, Deal LE, Piesman M.** Epinephrine-secreting pheochromocytoma presenting with cardiogenic shock and profound hypocalcemia. *Ann Intern Med.* 2004;140:849–851.
80. **Uchida N, Ishiguro K, Suda T, Nishimura M.** Pheochromocytoma multisystem crisis successfully treated by emergency surgery: report of a case. *Surg Today.* 2010;40:990–996.
81. **Salinas CL, Gomez Beltran OD, Sanchez-Hidalgo JM, Bru RC, Padillo FJ, Rufian S.** Emergency adrenalectomy due to acute heart failure secondary to complicated pheochromocytoma: a case report. *World J Surg Oncol.* 2011;9:49.
82. **Scholten A, Cisco RM, Vriens MR, et al.** Pheochromocytoma crisis is not a surgical emergency. *J Clin Endocrinol Metab.* 2013;98:581–591.
83. **James MF, Cronje L.** Pheochromocytoma crisis: the use of magnesium sulfate. *Anesth Analg.* 2004; 99:680–686, table of contents.
84. **Lutgers HL, Vergragt J, Dong PV, et al.** Severe hypercortisolism: a medical emergency requiring urgent intervention. *Crit Care Med.* 2010;38:1598–1601.
85. **Biller BM, Grossman AB, Stewart PM, et al.** Treatment of adrenocorticotropin-dependent Cushing's syndrome: a consensus statement. *J Clin Endocrinol Metab.* 2008;93:2454–2462.
86. **Perez MI, Musini VM.** Pharmacological interventions for hypertensive emergencies: a Cochrane systematic review. *J Hum Hypertens.* 2008;22:596–607.

SECTION VII

Calcium, Phosphate, and Metabolic Bone Diseases

SECTION INTRODUCTION

Emergent Management of Calcium, Phosphate, and Metabolic Bone Diseases

John P Bilezikian

The field of bone and mineral metabolism has become established, over the past 3 decades, as a key endocrinological discipline. With the great Fuller Albright leading the way even earlier, clinical disorders of calcium metabolism are now being defined in biochemical, structural, and molecular terms. The most prevalent of these diseases is osteoporosis, a disorder of skeletal microstructure and bone mineral density leading to an increased risk of fracture. The diagnosis of osteoporosis can be made either by the occurrence of the fragility fracture itself or by a bone density measurement. The advent of dual energy X-ray absorptiometry (DXA) in the late 1980s ushered in a new era in this field because now the diagnosis of osteoporosis could be made before the fracture event by measuring bone density. Osteoporosis is defined according to the World Health Organization (WHO) guidelines as a bone density that is 2.5 standard deviations lower than young, gender-matched values (eg, T-score <−2.5). The other seminal moment in this field was a therapeutic one, namely the development of safe and effective drugs that prevent the occurrence of fragility fractures. One can point to the approval of the bisphosphonate, alendronate, for the prevention and treatment of osteoporosis in 1995 as a watershed event in our field. Since then there have been other bisphosphonates that have become available in formulations that permit weekly or monthly (oral) or quarterly or yearly (intravenous) administration. The therapeutic landscape of osteoporosis continues to be exciting with the approval of other molecular classes such as teriparatide, (a fully active N-terminal fragment [1-34] of human recombinant parathyroid hormone) and denosumab (human anti-Rank Ligand antibody). In development are 2 additional classes based upon the molecular targets of cathepsin K (odanacatib) and sclerostin (romosozumab and blosozumab).

Although osteoporosis dominates the field of bone and mineral metabolism, because of its worldwide prevalence in the hundreds of millions, and because of the devastating effects of its most important consequence, the hip fracture, other abnormalities of bone and mineral metabolism are also of importance. For example, disorders of the parathyroid glands, as seen in primary and secondary hyperparathyroid states and in hypoparathyroidism, have led to new insights into how parathyroid hormone controls mineral metabolism. Primary hyperparathyroidism is a relatively common disorder characterized usually by hypercalcemia and elevated levels of parathyroid hormone. Even if the parathyroid hormone does not happen to be elevated, its presence is abnormal in the setting of hypercalcemia. Primary hyperparathyroidism is seen most often among postmenopausal women, but it occurs in men and in both sexes at any age. We have gained new insights through the study of primary hyperparathyroidism with regard to parathyroid hormone's target effects at bone and the kidney as well as off-target effects that conceivably could be seen as vascular or neurocognitive dysfunction. The secondary hyperparathyroid states are seen when the parathyroid glands respond appropriately to a lowering of the serum calcium. Most commonly, secondary hyperparathyroidism is associated with kidney or gastrointestinal disorders. Management of secondary hyperparathyroidism associated with gastrointestinal disease (eg, malabsorption) is handled by treating the gastrointestinal tract disorder. With regard to chronic kidney disease, guidelines are established as to how to deal with that form of secondary hyperparathyroidism.

Hypoparathyroidism occurs when the parathyroid glands are no longer functional because they have all been removed or they have been irreversibly damaged. This is due most commonly to their removal in the course of parathyroid, thyroid, or other neck surgery. The serum calcium is below normal while the parathyroid hormone level is below the limits of assay detection. The hypocalcemia can present as a medical emergency with life-threatening neuromuscular irritability such as laryngeal spasm and seizures. Recent advances in the therapeutic use of parathyroid hormone in hypoparathyroidism may signal a new era in which this disorder, the only one in which the deficient hormone is not available as an approved agent, can be managed by replacement therapy.

Paget's disease of bone is a focal or multifocal disorder of excessive osteoclast-mediated bone resorption. It can be treated effectively with amino-substituted bisphosphonates (eg, zoledronic acid). In some cases, patients achieve a remission that appears to be permanent. Although Paget's disease has diminished in incidence and is generally now rather easily treatable, it is important to note that it can also present as an emergent problem. If the Pagetic bone is in a vulnerable site, such as the femur, or the cervical vertebrae, it may be urgent to treat, thus preventing devastating orthopedic and/or neurological sequellae.

Nutritional issues are becoming more noteworthy in the field of bone and mineral metabolism. Vitamin D sufficiency is a key physiological requirement for normal bone and mineral metabolism. Sufficient vitamin D helps to optimize calcium and phosphate absorption. When the vitamin D level is insufficient, for whatever reason, the serum calcium will tend to be in the lower range of normal, and the parathyroid hormone level will rise. The serum phosphate will also be low. The definition of vitamin D insufficiency is a matter of debate, but most experts agree that levels <20 ng/mL (50 nmol/L) are deficient. The controversy centers on whether the standard for normalcy should be set at 20 ng/mL (>50 nmol/L) or >30 ng/mL (>75 nmol/L). Whatever the outcome of this uncertainty turns out to be, no one disagrees that vitamin D insufficiency is detrimental to bone and must be corrected.

In the context of nutrition, it is also important to mention phosphate. Circulating phosphate is in steady state with the circulating calcium level with one often affecting the other. The serum phosphate can be very low in the context of vitamin D deficiency, malabsorption syndromes, or renal tubular abnormalities. When the serum phosphate is exceedingly low (<1.5 mg/dL [<0.48 mmol/L]), musculoskeletal weakness, platelet and white cell dysfunction, and reduced oxygen delivery to tissues can be present.

These various disorders will be discussed in this section, with attention given to those presentations requiring urgent attention.

ACKNOWLEDGMENTS

The author has nothing to disclose.

CHAPTER 18

Hypocalcemia

Richard Quinton, Muhammad Asam, and Glenn Matfin

ABSTRACT

Hypocalcemia is a common electrolyte disturbance, especially in the inpatient setting. There are a wide variety of causes of hypocalcemia, and correct management depends on the underlying diagnosis. However, symptomatic acute hypocalcemia is associated with significant morbidity and mortality and should be managed as a medical emergency. Chronic care of the hypocalcemic patient is also briefly described, because this is an important opportunity to reduce further admissions related to both hypocalcemic and hypercalcemic presentations.

INTRODUCTION

Hypocalcemia is a common electrolyte disturbance complicating approximately 26% of hospital admissions and up to 88% of patients admitted to an intensive care unit (ICU) (1). There are a large number of recognized causes (see Table 18-1), and though much of the acute management is generic, the overall quality of management is greatly enhanced by an appropriate diagnosis (2,3). Chronic hypocalcemia may be asymptomatic even at very low levels of serum calcium, but severe or acute hypocalcemia is associated with predictable signs. Hypocalcemia with neurological, muscular, or cardiac dysfunction is associated with significant morbidity and mortality and should be managed as a medical emergency.

PATHOPHYSIOLOGY

Calcium, phosphate, and magnesium are the major divalent cations in the body (4). They are ingested in the diet, absorbed from the intestine, filtered in the glomerulus of the kidney, reabsorbed in the renal tubules, and eliminated in the urine. Only a small amount of these 3 ions is present in extracellular fluid (ECF). Calcium is regulated within a narrow range by vitamin D and parathyroid hormone (PTH) through their action on bowel, skeleton, and kidneys.

Vitamin D

Vitamin D is structurally akin to steroid and retinoid hormones and actually functions itself as a prohormone (5–7). It contributes to maintenance of plasma levels of calcium and phosphate, by increasing their absorption from the intestine, and is also necessary for normal bone formation. Vitamin D_3 (cholecalciferol) is predominantly synthesized by ultraviolet irradiation (UVB: around 300 nm wavelength) of 7-dehydrocholesterol in the skin, though in winter dietary sources may predominate. Some foods are statutorily fortified with vitamin D, but this varies hugely from country to country.

Once it enters the circulation from the skin or intestine, it is concentrated in the liver and hydroxylated to form 25-hydroxyvitamin D_3 (25-[OH]D_3 [calcidiol]. It is then transported to the kidney, where it is transformed into active 1,25-dihydroxyvitamin D_3 (1,25-[OH]2D_3, or calcitriol). However,

Table 18-1. Etiology of Hypocalcemia

Reduced Entry of Calcium into Circulation	Increased Movement of Calcium out of Circulation
Parathyroid dysfunction	**Movement into bone stores**
Hypoparathyroidism	"Hungry bone" syndrome
Autoimmune	Osteoblastic metastases (eg, prostate, breast)
Autoimmune polyglandular syndrome	**Chelation of ionized calcium**
Postoperative	Acute pancreatitis
Infiltrative (eg, hemochromatosis, amyloidosis)	Hyperphosphatemia
Hypomagnesemia	Renal impairment
Hypermagnesemia	Tumor lysis syndrome
Congenital disorders of the parathyroid glands	Rhabdomyolysis
DiGeorge syndrome	Citrate or EDTA in context of transfusions and phlebotomy
Defects in calcium-sensing receptor	**Miscellaneous**
Pseudohypoparathyroidism secondary to G-protein defects	Sepsis
	Drugs (including chemotherapeutic agents and foscarnet)
Drugs (including cinacalcet)	
Vitamin D deficiency	
Dietary or malabsorption	
Lack of sunlight exposure	
Renal impairment	
Reduced bone resorption	
Drugs (including bisphosphonates and denosumab)	

some 1-alpha hydroxylation also takes place in macrophages and, in a paracrine manner, in peripheral tissues (8). The major action of calcitriol is to increase the absorption of calcium from the intestine, but it also sensitizes bone to the resorptive actions of PTH, limits parathyroid gland growth, and suppresses the synthesis and secretion of PTH. Calcitriol formation is regulated in feedback fashion by plasma levels of calcium, phosphate, fibroblast growth factor 23 (FGF23, a potent phosphaturic agent, or phosphatonin), and calcitriol itself. Hyperphosphatemia is sensed by osteocytes, which respond by secreting FGF23. High levels of FGF23, as found in chronic kidney disease (or rarely tumor-induced osteomalacia), block 1 alpha hydroxylation of vitamin D, thereby contributing to hypocalcemia in these patients (9).

Parathyroid Hormone

Parathyroid hormone (PTH), a major regulator of plasma calcium and phosphate, is secreted by the 4 parathyroid glands located on the posterior surface of the thyroid gland. The dominant regulator of PTH is the ECF calcium concentration. A unique receptor on the parathyroid cell membrane (calcium-sensing receptor; CaSR) responds rapidly to changes in ECF calcium levels (10). The main function of PTH is to maintain the calcium concentrations in the ECF. It performs this function by promoting the release of calcium from bone, increasing the activation of vitamin D as a means of enhancing intestinal absorption of calcium, and by stimulating calcium conservation by the kidney while increasing phosphate excretion. Most renal calcium conservation is through reabsorption at proximal tubule level (65%). By promoting phosphate excretion, PTH keeps the calcium-phosphate product low, so as to prevent calcium phosphate salt formation in the ECF. When the plasma calcium level is high, PTH secretion is inhibited and vice versa; the PTH response to a change in plasma calcium is prompt, occurring within seconds. There is also a direct, calcium-independent effect of calcitriol to inhibit PTH secretion (9).

ETIOLOGY OF HYPOCALCEMIA

Calcium homeostasis is maintained through interactions involving the parathyroid glands, kidneys, bones, and vitamin D metabolism (4). Hypocalcemia occurs with either decreased entry of calcium into the blood supply, or through sequestration and effective removal of calcium (see Table 18-1).

The most frequent cause of chronic hypocalcemia in the general population and among hospitalized patients is vitamin D deficiency. However, the most commonly encountered cause of acute symptomatic hypocalcemia is postoperative hypoparathyroidism in the context of recent head and neck surgery (11). In practice, many cases are multifactorial, comprising 2 or more different risk factors (eg, vitamin D deficiency +/− drug-induced hypomagnesemia +/− parathyroid surgery effect) (6). Reversible hypoparathyroidism is also seen in severe hypomagnesemia (mild hypomagnesemia tends to promote PTH secretion), which can thereby predispose to hypocalcemia.

Rare causes of hypocalcemia include genetic/epigenetic, autoimmune, and infiltrative conditions (12). The latter include amyloidosis and iron/copper overload from hemochromatosis and Wilson's disease, respectively. Genetic disorders cause hypocalcemia through defects in calcium- or PTH-signaling. Inactivating CaSR mutations cause autosomal dominant hypocalcemia with hypercalciuria, which is usually asymptomatic (10). Pseudohypoparathyroidism typically arises from epigenetic G-protein defects causing postreceptor inhibition of PTH action. Patients have hypocalcemia and hyperphosphatemia as per true hypoparathyroidism, but a high PTH level. They may also exhibit syndromic features of Albright's osteodystophy syndrome, such as moon facies and short fourth and fifth metacarpals. Autoimmune hypoparathyroidism can be an isolated autoimmune process or part of polyglandular autoimmune syndrome type 1 (AIRE1 gene), which is a familial disorder associated with adrenal insufficiency, fulminant liver disease, and mucocutaneous candidiasis.

Hypocalcemia arising from "hungry bone syndrome" (due to excessive movement of ECF calcium into bone) can occur with osteoblastic bone disease including metastatic cancer (eg, breast or prostate cancer), following correction of long-standing hypercalcemia due to hyperparathyroidism (though this seems to have become a very rare occurence in modern times), and even less commonly with treatment of hyperthyroidism and osteomalacia due to rapid remineralization (13). Routine post-thyroidectomy prophylactic vitamin D and calcium supplementation may be helpful in reducing the occurrence of transient symptomatic hypocalcemia (14), and seems to be more cost-effective than calcitriol in this context and also improves quality of life (15). However, at least some postoperative hypocalcemic crises ascribed to hungry bone syndrome may simply reflect undiagnosed severe vitamin D deficiency.

Hyperphosphatemia, most commonly seen in renal impairment, but also a feature of tumor lysis syndrome and rhabdomyolysis, causes hypocalcemia through sequestration and complexing of ionized calcium. Acute pancreatitis is associated with the formation of calcium complexes within the abdominal cavity. Calcium chelation can occur with ethylenediaminetetraacetic acid (EDTA), or citrate, but is rare in patients being transfused with normal renal and hepatic function. Sepsis-related hypocalcemia is multifactorial, but significant factors include renal impairment, magnesium abnormalities, release of inflammatory cytokines, and frequent transfusions. It is particularly associated with gram-negative septicemia. Mortality rates are increased compared with matched septic patients without hypocalcemia (16).

Finally, a number of medications are associated with hypocalcemia (reviewed elsewhere, eg, [17]). These include inhibitors of bone turnover, such as high-dose bisphosphonates and denosumab; the CaSR-agonist cinacalcet; drugs causing renal tubular magnesium loss, either reversibly (diuretics) or potentially irreversibly (cisplatin, carboplatin, aminoglycosides); proton pump inhibitors (PPI), which seem to cause a dose-dependent gastrointestinal magnesium leak; and calcium chelation by foscarnet and fluoride. Finally, phenytoin, rifampicin, theophylline, and phenobarbital cause vitamin D deficiency through induction of cytochrome P450 enzyme activity, which accelerates calcidiol metabolism.

DIAGNOSTIC CONSIDERATIONS

ECF calcium is normally maintained within a narrow reference range (2.1–2.6 mmol/L;

8.5–10.5 mg/dL). Hypocalcemia is defined as a serum calcium level of less than 2.1 mmol/L (<8.5 mg/dL) or an ionized calcium level of less than 1.0 mmol/L (<4 mg/dL). Forty percent of total serum calcium is protein bound with the majority bound to albumin, while 50% is ionized and active. Alkalosis tends to decrease ionized calcium levels due to increased binding to albumin. Albumin levels should, therefore, be considered when assessing possible hypocalcemia, although most laboratories now provide a corrected, or adjusted, calcium (ACa) level. However, in states of acute albumin fluctuation, such as sepsis, measurement of ionized calcium is a more reliable assessment of calcium status. Apparent hypocalcemia after gadolinium-based magnetic resonance imaging (MRI) contrasts is due to assay interference and, as contrast is rapidly excreted in urine, the effect is transient with normal renal function (18).

Although not delaying the emergent treatment outlined below, the finding of acute hypocalcemia should always prompt biochemical testing to elicit a cause, comprising renal function, PTH, phosphate, alkaline phosphatase (ALP), magnesium, bicarbonate, and vitamin D levels (Table 18-2). Measurement of PTH level is crucial in identifying the underlying cause, as inappropriately low levels suggest hypoparathyroidism, whereas high levels confirm physiological PTH response to hypocalcemia arising from other etiology. Exceptions to this rule include severe magnesium deficiency or excess, both of which can impair PTH release.

Measurement of calcidiol (25OHD) level is crucial, because deficiency thereof is one of the most common causes of hypocalcemia. Why some patients with hypovitaminosis D develop hypocalcemia and others do not is unclear, but likely reflects the interplay of dietary calcium intake, concomitant medication(s), and individual factors including robustness of PTH response. Measurement of serum calcitriol is surprisingly unhelpful in this context, possibly because paracrine effects predominate. In vitamin D deficiency, both hypocalcemia and hypophosphatemia may be present, whereas patients with hypoparathyroidism, tumor lysis syndrome, and renal failure tend to have hypocalcemia with hyperphosphatemia.

Both hypo- and hypermagnesemia can be associated with hypocalcemia due to inhibition of PTH release from the parathyroid. High urinary magnesium excretion levels point toward renal magnesium wasting. Acid-base assessment is also important because alkalosis can cause reduction in ionized calcium due to increased protein binding. Amylase/lipase should be measured in suspected pancreatitis.

Finally, detailed physical examination and diagnostic imaging are crucial to the assessment of patients with osteoblastic metastases. High bone turnover may be associated with elevated levels of ALP and other serum or urine bone turnover markers.

Table 18-2. Investigation of Hypocalcemia

Routine investigations
• Corrected calcium, phosphate
• Parathyroid hormone
• Alkaline phosphatase
• Magnesium
• Vitamin D level
• BUN (urea)/creatinine
• Liver function tests
• Bicarbonate level
• ECG—looking for prolonged QTc or arrhythmia
Other investigations
• Amylase/lipase—if pancreatitis suspected
• Fecal elastase/bowel investigation—if malabsorption suspected
• Urinary magnesium—if urinary magnesium loss suspected.
• X-rays—to look for osteomalacia due to vitamin D deficiency
• Bone scan and other imaging—for malignancy-related hypocalcemia
• Genetic tests—if genetic causes of hypocalcemia suspected
• Special investigations like c-AMP measurement in urine in pseudohypoparathyroidism

Clinical Assessment

Clinical manifestations of hypocalcemia. It is crucial to identify these, because if present, they identify symptomatic patients who may require urgent corrective measures. The severity of signs and symptoms depends both on the absolute degree of hypocalcemia and the rapidity of its onset, with the majority of features relating to neuromuscular dysfunction. Perioral tingling and acral paresthesia are the earliest symptoms and almost always present in symptomatic cases, while other frequently reported features include muscle stiffness, myalgia, and confusion (Table 18-3).

Chvostek's sign describes ipsilateral twitching of the facial muscle groups including the perioral, nasal, and ocular regions, when the facial nerve is tapped 2 cm anterior to the earlobe beneath the zygomatic bone. However, perioral twitching is also seen in up to 25% of normal individuals and, conversely, this sign is negative in approximately 30% of those with hypocalcemia (19). However, Trousseau's sign is more sensitive (94%) and specific for hypocalcemia and describes flexion of the wrist and metacarpophalangeal joints, hyperextension of the fingers, and flexion of the thumb producing a characteristic deformity known as *main d'accoucheur*. It is elicited by occluding the brachial artery 20 mm Hg above systolic pressure for 3 minutes and is positive in only 1% of normocalcemic patients (20).

Table 18-3. Assessment of the Hypocalcemic Patient

Features of acute hypocalcemia
• Arrhythmias—check pulse and ECG
• Tetany
• Chvostek's sign—less specific (present in 25% normocalcemic subjects)
• Trousseau's sign—more specific (present in 1% normocalcemic subjects)
• Shortness of breath/stridor
• Seizure (partial or generalized)
• Acute confusion
• Cardiac failure
Features of chronic hypocalcemia
• Features of parkinsonism/other movement disorders
• Dementia
• Nail dystrophy
• Hair loss
• Dry skin
• Papilledema
• Cataract
Features of underlying cause
• Evidence of neck surgery—suggestive of primary hypoparathyroidism
• Abdominal tenderness (pancreatitis); previous surgery (malabsorption); hepatic failure (hemochromatosis)
• Proximal muscle weakness—suggestive of osteomalacia
• Syndromic features (eg, moon facies, short fourth/fifth metacarpals)—suggestive of genetic cause
• Evidence of malignancy such as breast or prostate
• Features of infiltrative diseases, such as skin discoloration (hemochromatosis) or Kayser-Fleischer rings (Wilson's disease)
• Features of Addison's disease, mucocutaneous candidiasis—autoimmune polyglandular syndrome type 1

Neurological manifestations of acute hypocalcemia include irritability, confusion, and seizures. In known epilepsy, hypocalcemia lowers the threshold for seizure activity. Features of chronic hypocalcemia include depression, dementia, extrapyramidal features, hair and nail changes, cataracts, and papilledema. Patients who present with acute-on-chronic hypocalcemia can exhibit both sets of features.

Cardiac features of hypocalcemia include electrocardiographic (ECG) changes and cardiac failure (21). The ECG hallmark of hypocalcemia is prolongation of the corrected QT interval, the duration of which is proportional to the degree of hypocalcemia. The more prolonged the QTc interval, the more likely an arrhythmia. The most common arrhythmia associated with prolonged QTc is *torsades de pointes* which, if untreated, can progress to ventricular fibrillation and cardiac arrest. Other recognized abnormalities include reduced voltage or negative T waves, although T waves are normal in more than half of those with hypocalcemia, and changes that mimic acute anterior myocardial infarction. Low calcium levels may cause resistance to digoxin. Hypocalcemia can lead to cardiac failure, particularly if associated with severe hypovitaminosis D.

Medical history. Medical history is central to the initial assessment of hypocalcemia and helps to mark key priorities in the diagnostic work-up.

Onset in childhood is obviously consistent with congenital etiology, although environmental factors must also be considered, such as severe hypovitaminosis D in the breastfed child of a dark-skinned mother living at high latitudes. A family history raises the possibility of autosomal dominant hypocalcemia/hypercalciuria, or of autoimmune polyglandular syndrome type 1. Abdominal pain or jaundice suggests the possibility of pancreatitis, whereas a history of massive/multiple transfusions, particularly in trauma patients, points toward transfusion-related hypocalcemia. Risk factors should also be identified (or a defined history established) for malabsorption of calcium, vitamin D, and/or magnesium (eg, Crohn's, celiac disease, chronic pancreatitis, and malabsorptive bariatric surgery). A history of renal disease, liver disease, and/or anticonvulsant therapy might indicate a defect of vitamin D hydroxylation/metabolism. Recent neck surgery, particularly thyroidectomy or parathyroidectomy, suggests acute hypoparathyroidism due to removal/devascularization of parathyroid glands, though other risk factors might also coexist.

Hyperventilation and history of anxiety disorder are compatible with a (reversible) fall in ionized calcium due to induced respiratory alkalosis, and recent contrast MRI with gadolinium-induced pseudohypocalcemia due to assay interference. Drug history is also important as noted previously. Hypoalbuminemia associated with malnutrition and/or chronic illness may lead to apparently low total and ACa levels—hence the need for measurement of ionized calcium. Finally, a history of malignancies with propensity for osteoblastic metastases, such as breast and prostate cancer, should not be missed.

In summary, a full medical history and traditional "head to toe" examination may not only elicit signs of hypocalcemia but also help differentiate acute from chronic and syndromic from nonsyndromic hypocalcemia and will usually indicate other underlying diagnoses.

Acute Interventions

Intravenous calcium. Symptomatic patients (eg, tetany, seizures, laryngospasm, and cardiac arrhythmias or dysfunction) or those with an ACa below 2 mmol/L (<8 mg/dL) should prompt urgent intervention with intravenous (IV) calcium replacement (see Table 18-1). This treatment should be given in the hospital and calcium levels carefully monitored (usually 4–6 hourly). Ten to twenty mL (1–2 standard ampoules) 10% calcium gluconate should be infused slowly in 50–100 mL 0.9% saline (or 5% dextrose) over 10–20 minutes (with cardiac monitoring) (Figure 18-1).

Calcium gluconate is the preferred formulation for acute calcium replacement and should be repeated until the patient is symptom-free. Ten milliliters of 10% calcium gluconate contains 93 mg of elemental calcium, and a similar quantity and concentration of calcium chloride contains 273 mg of elemental calcium. Ten milliliters of 10% calcium chloride can also be used but is more irritating to the veins than calcium gluconate, and

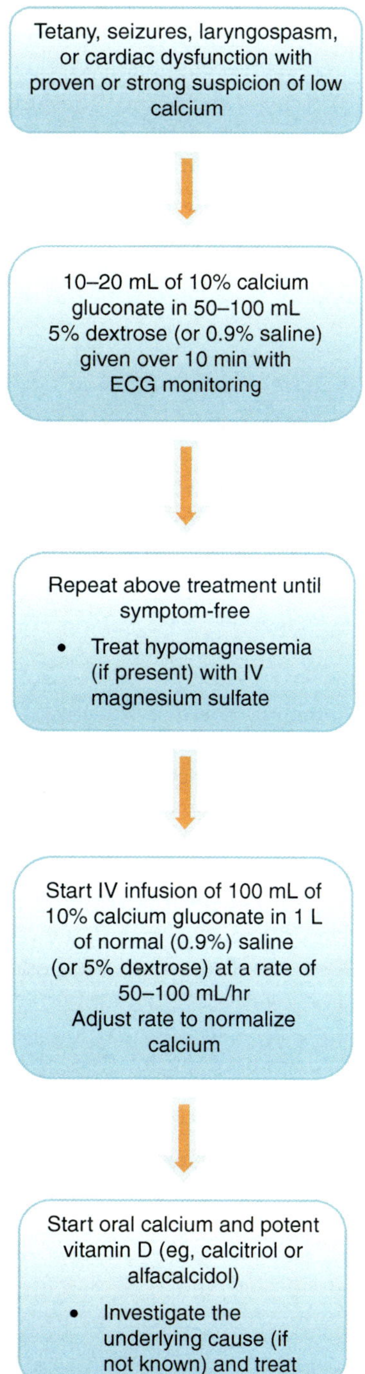

Figure 18-1. Management of acute hypocalcemia.

extravasation can lead to tissue necrosis. This will increase the serum calcium levels for 2–3 hours and should be followed by a slow infusion of 100 mL (10 standard ampoules) of 10% calcium gluconate in 1 L 0.9% saline (or 5% dextrose). The infusion should be commenced at 50–100 mL/hr and titrated to normalize serum calcium.

A solution of 10% calcium gluconate contains 10 g of calcium gluconate in 100 mL, and 10 g of calcium gluconate contains about 900 mg of elemental calcium. Therefore, adding 100 mL of 10% calcium to 1 L of fluid gives a preparation close to 1 mg/mL of elemental calcium. Calcium infusion is usually given at 0.5–1.5 mg/kg per hour of elemental calcium. Infusion of calcium compounds is occasionally associated with the induction of cardiac arrhythmias and infarction (hence, the need for cardiac monitoring) and may cause chelation with resultant end-organ deposition if hyperphosphatemia is present and not addressed. Care should be taken if the patient has a known history of coronary artery disease or arrhythmias, but in most situations correction of severe hypocalcemia would take priority. Oral calcium should be started as soon as possible so that the calcium level can be maintained once IV calcium is stopped.

Hypomagnesemia should always be corrected because it causes inhibition of PTH secretion as well as resistance to its action; correction of hypocalcemia may be difficult with uncorrected hypomagnesemia. Administer IV Mg^{2+}, 24 mmol/24 hr, made up as 6 g of magnesium sulfate (30 mL of 20%, 800 mmol/L, $MgSO_4$) in 500 mL normal (0.9%) saline or 5% dextrose. Monitor serum Mg^{2+} and aim to achieve a normal serum magnesium level (22). The underlying cause of hypomagnesemia should be diagnosed and treated. Specifically, PPIs should always be stopped unless absolutely necessary and diuretics replaced with alternative agents wherever feasible. Even if cessation is not possible, any dose reduction will be useful.

There are 3 situations where extra caution must be observed with parenteral drug administration (22). First, patients taking digoxin (whose action is blunted by hypocalcemia) might develop clinical digoxin toxicity as calcium levels improve. Second, aggressive calcium replacement in patients with hyperphosphatemia can lead to precipitation of calcium phosphate salts and metastatic calcification, most typically in tumor lysis syndrome. Finally, correction of acidemia in renal failure patients with hypocalcemia can result in tetany due to increased protein binding of calcium, so hypocalcemia should always be corrected before correction of acidemia.

Oral therapies. Oral calcium replacement therapy should be initiated as soon as possible, within the limits of patient tolerability, so as to facilitate independence from parenteral replacement. Vitamin D deficiency should also be corrected as soon as possible, because this will facilitate subsequent stabilization of patients on oral replacement. Although there are no protocols specific to the context of acute hypocalcemia, pharmacokinetic studies in patients with severe vitamin D deficiency indicate that a single oral dose of 200,000–300,000 IU normalizes serum calcidiol levels within 48–72 hours, without risk of "overshoot-hypercalcemia," whereas the same dose given intramuscularly can take weeks to achieve this (23). Meanwhile, calcitriol (1,25-[OH]2D3), which has a more rapid onset of action than unhydroxylated D3, should be started immediately at an initial dose of 0.5–1 mcg per day.

Maintenance therapy. This may not be required for vitamin D-replete patients who merely experienced transient postoperative hypoparathyroidism. Indeed, it may even be possible to gradually wean off therapy patients who have been taking oral replacement for many years after neck surgery. For patients with intact parathyroid function, but prior hypovitaminosis D, avoidance of other precipitating factors, or drugs and maintenance therapy with oral vitamin D so as to achieve optimum serum levels of 25OHD will suffice. The prolonged effective half-life and large volume of distribution of vitamin D, necessarily arising from its marked lipophilicity (24), means that repeat assessment of 25OHD levels should be deferred for around 3 months after commencing therapy (7). Due to the impossibility of monitoring any meaningful serum levels, its comparative expense, and risk of overtreatment (ie, hypercalcemia), calcitriol/alfacalcidol should not be used for replacement therapy. However, these short-acting (~6 hr) agents are really useful for patients with permanent hypoparathyroidism who require a more nuanced approach.

Having achieved consistent target-range 25OHD levels through supplementation and/or lifestyle adjustments, the dose of short-acting agents, calcitriol/alfacalcidol +/− oral calcium, should be adjusted so as to maintain appropriate serum calcium levels. Because deficiency of PTH action at the renal tubule predisposes to unopposed calciuria, repletion of calcium in these patients to levels within the upper half of the normal range reported by most laboratories will lead to excessive urinary calcium excretion, hence favoring nephrolithiasis or nephrocalcinosis. Thus, a serum ACa level at, or just below, the lower end of the normal range and that relieves the patient's symptoms should, therefore, be the therapeutic goal. Urinary calcium excretion and calcium/creatinine ratio should be measured once a satisfactory serum level has been achieved, ideally on a 24-hour collection of urine or, failing that, a "spot" urine sample. If excessive excretion is detected, a lower serum calcium target should be set. If use of a lower target is associated with hypocalcemic symptoms, a low dose of thiazide diuretic could potentially be beneficial due to the reduced tubular calcium excretion. Even in stable patients, serum and urinary calcium levels should be monitored every 6 months to check for hypercalcemia and hypercalciuria (12).

Management of hypoparathyroidism in pregnancy requires more frequent calcium monitoring and dose-adjustment (11). Calcium levels should be kept at the lower end of the normal range. Replacement doses may need to be reduced during the third trimester, perhaps due to enhanced hydroxylation of vitamin D to its active form by placental 1 alpha hydroxylase activity.

Emerging Therapies

Hypoparathyroidism is currently the only life-threatening hormone deficiency for which bioidentical replacement therapy is not routinely available, but this may be about to change (11). Teriparatide, a synthetic injectable human PTH(1-34), is currently licensed only for the treatment of osteoporosis. However, several randomized controlled trials have shown that when compared with conventional therapies (ie, calcium and vitamin D), administration of teriparatide achieves similar restoration of normal calcium levels and prevents bone demineralization in patients with hypoparathyroidism (25). In addition, urinary calcium levels remain normal in the teriparatide group in contrast to the frequent hypercalciuria observed (with consequent increased risk of renal disease) in conventionally treated patients. Furthermore, case reports suggest there may be a role for teriparatide in patients who fail to become asymptomatic on conventional therapies (26). Patients with negligible or nonexistent endogenous PTH hormone secretion, such as postparathyroidectomy patients, may benefit from use of this agent, although current high costs preclude routine use. Typically, patients are treated with 20 mg of teriparatide subcutaneously, twice a day, or up to 2 mg/kg per day.

There is also growing evidence for the efficacy of PTH(1-84) in the treatment of primary hypoparathyroidism. Results from the recent REPLACE study, which was a large randomized placebo-controlled double-blind trial, are encouraging in this regard (27). In this 6-month trial PTH(1-84) added to standard treatment was compared with standard treatment with calcitriol and calcium supplements. Adding PTH(1-84) at a dose between 25 and 100 mcg once daily to a standard regimen resulted in more than a 50% reduction in doses of vitamin and calcium with reduction in phosphate levels but no significant change in urinary calcium. Urinary calcium did not rise despite improvement in plasma calcium. Only 2% of patients in the placebo arm achieved dose reduction of vitamin and calcium. PTH(1-84) treatment of hypoparathyroidism is associated with increases in histomorphometric and biochemical indices of skeletal dynamics. Structural changes are consistent with an increased remodeling rate in both trabecular and cortical compartments. These changes suggest that PTH(1-84) may improve abnormal skeletal properties in hypoparathyroidism by restoring bone metabolism toward normal euparathyroid levels (28). However, it is not yet approved for use in hypoparathyroidism due to its cost implications and need for more safety data.

Finally, drugs that antagonize the calcium-sensing receptor (termed *calcilytics*), thereby increasing PTH secretion, are in early phase development and may also have a role in the management of hypoparathyroidism (29).

CONCLUSIONS

Hypocalcemia is a common electrolyte disturbance, especially in the inpatient setting. Acute hypocalcemia is associated with significant morbidity and mortality and should be managed as a medical emergency. Management of chronic hypocalcemia can seem complex due to the varying underlying diagnoses and different calcium and vitamin D formulations available, but there is an underlying logic that is based on physiological first principles. Patients on long-term, potent hydroxylated vitamin D-analog products (calcitriol/alfacalcidol) should be closely monitored for complications of therapy (ie, hypercalcemia, hypercalciuria, nephrocalcinosis). These products should not be used to replace vitamin D deficiency itself, for which cholecalciferol, or ergocalciferol is logical, safer, and cheaper (7,24).

ACKNOWLEDGMENTS

The authors have nothing to disclose.

REFERENCES

1. **Zivin J, Gooley T, Zager R, Ryan M.** Hypocalcemia: a pervasive metabolic abnormality in the critically ill. *Am J Kidney Dis.* 2001;37:689–698.
2. **Murphy E, Williams G.** Hypocalcaemia. *Medicine.* 2009;37:465–468.
3. **Schafer AL, Schoback D.** Hypocalcemia: definition, etiology, pathogenesis, diagnosis, and management. In: Rosen CJ, ed. *Primer on the Metabolic Bone Diseases and Disorders of Mineral Metabolism.* 8th ed. Washington DC: American Society for Bone and Mineral Research; 2013:572–578.
4. **Favus MJ, Goltzman D.** Regulation of calcium and magnesium. In: Rosen CJ, ed. *Primer on the Metabolic Bone Diseases and Disorders of Mineral Metabolism.* 8th ed. Washington DC: American Society for Bone and Mineral Research; 2013: 173–179.
5. **Holick MF.** Vitamin D deficiency. *N Engl J Med.* 2007; 357:266–281.
6. **Pearce SHS, Cheetham TD.** Diagnosis and management of vitamin D deficiency. *BMJ.* 2010;340: 142–147.
7. **National Osteoporosis Society.** Vitamin D and bone health: a practical clinical guideline for patient management. http://www.nos.org.uk/document.doc?id=1352.
8. **Monkawa T, Yoshida T, Hayashi M, Saruta T.** Identification of 25-hydroxyvitamin D3 1alpha-hydroxylase gene expression in macrophages. *Kidney Int.* 2000; 58:559–568.
9. **Jüppner H.** Phosphate and FGF-23. *Kidney Int.* 2011;79:S24–S27.
10. **Egbuna OI, Brown EM.** Hypercalcaemic and hypocalcaemic conditions due to calcium-sensing receptor mutations. *Best Pract Res Clin Rheumatol.* 2008;22:129–148.
11. **Bilezikian JP, Khan A, Potts JT Jr, et al.** Hypoparathyroidism in the adult: epidemiology, diagnosis, pathophysiology, target-organ involvement, treatment, and challenges for future research. *J Bone Miner Res.* 2011;26:2317–2337.
12. **Shoback D.** Hypoparathyroidism. *N Engl J Med.* 2008; 359:391–403.
13. **Brasier AR, Nussbaum SR.** Hungry bone syndrome: clinical and biochemical predictors of its occurrence after parathyroid surgery. *Am J Med.* 1988;84:654–660.
14. **Alhefdhi A, Mazeh H, Chen H.** Role of postoperative vitamin D and/or calcium routine supplementation in preventing hypocalcemia after thyroidectomy: a systematic review and meta-analysis. *Oncologist.* 2013;18:533–542.
15. **Wang TS, Roman SA, Sosa JA.** Postoperative calcium supplementation in patients undergoing thyroidectomy. *Curr Opin Oncol.* 2012;24:22–28.
16. **Desai TK, Carlson RW, Geheb MA.** Prevalence and clinical implications of hypocalcemia in acutely ill patients in a medical intensive care setting. *Am J Med.* 1988;84:209–214.
17. **Liamis G, Milionis H, Elisaf M.** A review of drug induced hypocalcemia. *J Bone Miner Metab.* 2009;27:635–642.
18. **Doorenbos CJ, Ozyilmaz A, van Wijnen M.** Severe pseudohypocalcemia after gadolinium-enhanced magnetic resonance angiography. *N Engl J Med.* 2003;349:817–818.
19. **Hoffman E.** The Chvostek sign: a clinical study. *Am J Surg.* 1958;96:33–37.
20. **Jesus JE, Landry A.** Chvostek's and Trousseau's signs. *N Engl J Med.* 2012;367:e15.
21. **Hurley K, Baggs D.** Hypocalcemic cardiac failure in the emergency department. *J Emerg Med.* 2005; 28(2):155–159.
22. **Society for Endocrinology 2013.** Acute hypocalcemia. http://www.endocrinology.org/policy/docs/13-02_EmergencyGuidance-AcuteHypocalcaemia_(inAdults).pdf.
23. **Romagnoli E, Mascia ML, Cipriani C, et al.** Short and long-term variations in serum calciotropic hormones after a single very large dose of ergocalciferol (vitamin D2) or cholecalciferol (vitamin D3) in the elderly. *J Clin Endocrinol Metab.* 2008;93: 3015–3020.
24. **Holick MF, Brinkley NC, Bischoff-Ferrari HA, et al.** Evaluation, treatment, and prevention of vitamin D deficiency: an Endocrine Society Clinical Practice Guideline. *J Clin Endocrinol Metab.* 2011; 96:1911–1930.

25. **Winer KK, Ko CW, Reynolds JC, et al.** Long-term treatment of hypoparathyroidism: a randomized controlled study comparing parathyroid hormone-(1-34) versus calcitriol and calcium. *J Clin Endocrinol Metab.* 2003;88:4214–4220.
26. **Hall L, Gallacher SJ.** Primary hypoparathyroidism resistant to conventional therapy. *Scot Med J.* 2006;51:54.
27. **Mannstadt B, Clarke BL, Vokes T, et al.** Efficacy and safety of recombinant human parathyroid hormone (1–84) in hypoparathyroidism (REPLACE): a double-blind, placebo-controlled, randomised, phase 3 study. *Lancet Diabetes Endocrinol.* 2013;1:275–283.
28. **Rubin MR, Dempster DW.** PTH(1-84) administration reverses abnormal bone-remodeling dynamics and structure in hypoparathyroidism. *J Bone Miner Res.* 2011;26:2727–2736.
29. **Saidek Z, Brazier M, Kamel S, Mentaverri R.** Agonists and allosteric modulators of the calcium-sensing receptor and their therapeutic applications. *Mol Pharmacol.* 2009;76;1131–1144.

CHAPTER 19

Hypercalcemia

William D Fraser and Glenn Matfin

ABSTRACT

Hypercalcemia is commonly seen in the context of parathyroid dysfunction and malignancy and, when severe, can be life-threatening. The differential diagnosis of hypercalcemia can be broadly categorized based on parathyroid hormone measurement. The investigation and acute management of severe hypercalcemia are discussed along with a brief review of therapeutic advances in the field.

INTRODUCTION

Hypercalcemia (serum calcium >10.5 mg/dL [2.6 mmol/L], measured on at least 2 occasions), affects about 0.5% of hospitalized patients and is usually well tolerated if adjusted calcium concentrations are <12 mg/dL (3.0 mmol/L). Adjusted calcium (ACa) above this threshold is associated with nephrogenic diabetes insipidus, and increasingly severe volume contraction, as well as neurological, cardiac, and gastrointestinal dysfunction, and requires urgent treatment to prevent life-threatening consequences.

PATHOPHYSIOLOGY

Calcium, phosphate, and magnesium are the major divalent cations in the body (1). Calcium is ingested in the diet, absorbed from the intestine, filtered in the glomerulus of the kidney, reabsorbed in the renal tubules, and eliminated in the urine. Approximately 99% of total body calcium (1 kg) is found in bone. Most of the remainder is located in the intracellular compartment with only a small amount present in extracellular fluid (ECF). Calcium homeostasis is directly or indirectly regulated by vitamin D metabolites and parathyroid hormone (PTH) (2–4).

PTH is secreted by the chief cell of the parathyroid glands. A unique calcium receptor on the cell membrane (extracellular calcium-sensing receptor [CaSR]) responds rapidly to changes in serum ionized calcium (5). When the ionized calcium is high, appropriate inhibition of PTH synthesis and release occurs, while a decrease in ionized calcium prompts a rapid adaptive increase in PTH release. The main function of PTH is to maintain the calcium concentration of the ECF by promoting the release of calcium from bone by osteoclast resorption, increasing the activation of 25-hydroxyvitamin D to 1,25-dihydroxyvitamin D, which increases calcium absorption from the intestine plus sensitizes bone to the resorptive actions of PTH, and stimulating calcium conservation by the kidney while increasing phosphate excretion (Figure 19-1).

At least 1 of the following mechanisms is involved in the pathophysiology of hypercalcemia: (1) increased intestinal calcium absorption; (2) increased bone resorption; and (3) increased renal calcium reabsorption or decreased calcium excretion. Hypercalcemia predominantly results from increased mobilization of calcium from bone with consequent increased delivery of calcium to the nephron with reduced excretion via the kidneys. When the urinary calcium concentration exceeds 10 mmol/L (plasma concentration ~3.0 mmol/L), nephrogenic diabetes insipidus results with impaired

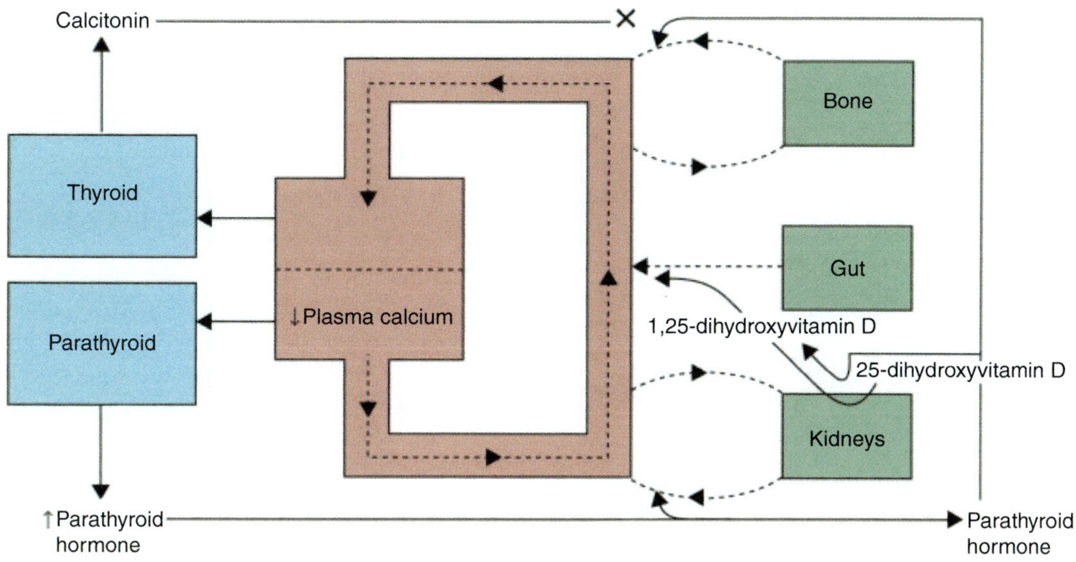

Figure 19-1. Parathyroid hormone response to a fall in ionized calcium. A decrease in ionized calcium is detected by the calcium-sensing receptor on the chief cells of the parathyroid gland to stimulate PTH release and synthesis. PTH acts on the osteoblasts and osteoclasts promoting calcium release via bone resorption and on the kidneys that promote calcium reabsorption and 1,25-dihydroxyvitamin D production, which stimulates calcium absorption via the intestine, thereby increasing circulating ionized calcium. Adapted from Fraser WD. Hyperparathyroidism. Lancet. 2009;11;374:145–158. Copyright from Lancet.

urine concentrating ability, due to both effects on vasopressin binding, with aquaporin downregulation and altered renal interstitial sodium concentration. Volume depletion can also result from associated vomiting. The resultant intravascular volume contraction and subsequent reduction in glomerular filtration rate (GFR) severely limit the ability of the kidneys to excrete calcium. If continued calcium mobilization from bone occurs, hypercalcemia can rapidly increase. This chain of events highlights the extreme importance of volume resuscitation in the management of hypercalcemia.

ETIOLOGY

The causes of hypercalcemia can be conveniently divided into those associated with an elevated or inappropriately normal PTH level, and those where PTH output is appropriately suppressed (Table 19-1). Notable exceptions to this paradigm include hypercalcemia due to familial hypocalciuric hypercalcemia (FHH), where PTH output is appropriate to the level of ambient calcium sensed by the abnormal CaSR or treatment with thiazide diuretics or lithium (5). In an ambulatory population, primary hyperparathyroidism (PHPT) accounts for the vast majority of detected hypercalcemia (>90%) (6,7). Inappropriate autonomous PTH secretion is found in the context of parathyroid adenomas, which may be solitary or multiple (3). Parathyroid adenomas are most commonly sporadic, but may be part of an endocrine neoplastic syndrome such as multiple endocrine neoplasia (MEN)-1, especially if numerous or found in the young. Parathyroid hyperplasia without an obvious physiological stimulus can also occur, and usually involves all 4 glands. Rarely, inappropriate PTH secretion may result from a parathyroid carcinoma. Secondary hyperparathyroidism (SHPT) is an appropriate physiological adaptation to many situations in which hypocalcemia is seen, including vitamin D deficiency, advanced chronic kidney disease (CKD), and gastrointestinal malabsorption of calcium (3,4). However, parathyroid autonomy often develops if the stimulus persists, and when hypercalcemia results the condition is redefined as tertiary hyperparathyroidism (THPT). Vitamin D deficiency is typically severe and long-standing before THPT develops. Lithium therapy produces biochemistry that mimics FHH as the intracellular calcium concentration threshold at which PTH continues to be produced and secreted is raised, while hypocalciuria is also seen.

Table 19-1. Etiology of Hypercalcemia

Elevated or Inappropriately Normal PTH	Suppressed PTH
PHPT Solitary adenoma Multiple adenoma Parathyroid hyperplasia Parathyroid carcinoma	**Malignancy** Humoral mediators (eg, PTHrP) Vitamin D-mediated Multiple myeloma Lytic bone metastases
THPT Advanced CKD Severe vitamin D deficiency Malabsorption of calcium (eg, celiac disease)	**Drug-induced** Calcium supplementation Milk-alkali syndrome Vitamin D intoxication Vitamin A intoxication Thiazide diuretics Lithium therapy
Miscellaneous FHH	**Endocrinopathies** Thyrotoxicosis Addison's disease Pheochromocytoma VIPoma **Immobilization** Granulomatous disorders, including sarcoidosis

Abbreviations: CKD = chronic kidney disease; FHH = familial hypocalciuric hypercalcemia; PHPT = primary hyperparathyroidism; PTH = parathyroid hormone; PTHrP = parathyroid hormone-related protein; THPT = tertiary hyperparathyroidism.

Hypercalcemia of malignancy (HCM) is the most common cause of inpatient hypercalcemic crises (>50%) and complicates 10%–30% of malignancies. Hypercalcemia secondary to malignancy usually presents in the context of advanced clinically obvious disease. It results either from humoral-mediated bone resorption, increased calcitriol production due to increased 1α-hydroxylase activity in some lymphomas, or direct destruction of bone either in myeloma or lytic metastatic disease. The majority of humoral hypercalcemia of malignancy (>80%) is induced by parathyroid hormone-related protein (PTHrP), a peptide with significant amino terminal homology to PTH (8). PTHrP induces bone resorption by binding to PTH receptor type 1 and can also induce phosphaturia/hypophosphatemia. Increased expression of 1α-hydroxylase by lymphoproliferative tissues, including lymphoma, occasionally results in clinically significant hypercalcemia as a result of significantly increased synthesis of 1,25-dihydroxyvitamin D (9). Many solid tumors are associated with hypercalcemia and include squamous cell carcinomas of the lung, head and neck, and esophagus, renal cell carcinoma, and breast carcinoma. Humoral-mediated bone resorption stimulated by PTHrP accounts for the majority of hypercalcemia in these malignancies (10) even when lytic metastatic bone disease is present. Hematological malignancies such as multiple myeloma can be associated with hypercalcemia via locally produced osteolytic peptides, which can include PTHrP.

A number of administered drugs can cause hypercalcemia. Thiazide diuretics reduce renal calcium excretion, increase renal calcium reabsorption, and, as a result, mild hypercalcemia is frequently seen; they also can unmask PHPT. The effect of lithium is discussed previously. Calcium supplementation rarely causes hypercalcemia if normal physiological mechanisms of calcium regulation are intact. In milk-alkali syndrome, a high intake of milk or calcium carbonate (used to treat dyspepsia or more commonly now osteoporosis) may lead to hypercalcemia mediated by the high calcium intake plus metabolic alkalosis, which augments calcium reabsorption in the distal tubule. This is usually happening in the presence of renal impairment and reducing GFR, which decreases calcium excretion while increasing serum adjusted calcium. Hypercalcemia in the context of vitamin D intoxication is recognized but rare (2), but treatment with vitamin D metabolites (alfacalcidol, calcitriol), especially in CKD and osteoporosis, is increasingly recognized as a cause of hypercalcemia. Prolonged immobilization may be associated with hypercalcemia due to marked increase in bone resorption. Patients with underlying high bone turnover states are at particular risk. Granuloma-associated macrophages occasionally express 1α-hydroxylase with consequent increased active 1,25-dihydroxyvitamin D concentrations (calcitriol), and hypercalcemia will complicate over 10% of cases of sarcoidosis. A number of endocrinopathies are associated with hypercalcemia. Hypercalcemia in thyrotoxicosis is postulated to be secondary to increased bone resorption (11,12). Volume depletion in Addison's disease is claimed to promote hypercalcemia, while PTHrP secretion by pheochromocytomas occasionally results in clinically significant hypercalcemia. The very rare vasoactive intestinal peptide (VIP)-secreting tumor, VIPoma, is associated with hypercalcemia possibly through VIP-mediated stimulation of the PTH receptor.

DIAGNOSTIC CONSIDERATIONS

Severe hypercalcemia is defined as a serum calcium >14 mg/dL (3.5 mmol/L) (13). Forty percent of total serum calcium is protein bound with the majority bound to albumin, while 50% is ionized and active. Albumin concentrations should, therefore, be considered when assessing hypercalcemia; most laboratories provide calcium adjusted for the prevailing albumin (ACa). However, in states of acute albumin fluctuations such as sepsis, infections such as meningitis, and in many emergency situations, measurement of ionized calcium (hypercalcemia >5.6 mg/dL [1.4 mmol/L]) is a more reliable assessment of calcium status.

Severe hypercalcemia, suspected clinically or detected biochemically, should prompt immediate treatment. The first step in the evaluation of hypercalcemia, which must be performed prior to commencing any treatment, is to obtain samples for PTH measurement and establish whether the hypercalcaemia is PTH-dependent (14). Other tests include measurement of serum creatinine, 25-hydroxyvitamin D, thyroid function, serum electrophoresis and urinary Bence-Jones protein, and bone markers such as alkaline phosphatase, performed as soon as possible to direct specific treatment. PTHrP can be measured but adds little to the management if malignancy-associated hypercalcemia is already obvious. Assessment of 1,25-dihydroxyvitamin D is required if the patient is receiving vitamin D metabolites, or has a confirmed or suspected diagnosis of granulomatous disease or lymphoproliferative disorders.

PTH can be unstable in serum and, therefore, blood samples should be taken into the appropriate preservative and delivered to the laboratory promptly. The "intact" molecule (PTH (1-84)) is now assayed routinely and was thought to have eliminated the problems of measured bio-inactive C-terminal fragments (especially in patients with impaired renal function). It has become clear that the "intact" assays measure some PTH fragments (particularly PTH (7-84)), which are biologically inactive but accumulate with impaired renal function. The percentage of PTH (7-84) fragments increase proportionally with decreasing renal function. New "whole" PTH assays have been developed that do not cross react with the PTH (7-84) fragments, but these have not been shown to offer any major clinical usefulness when investigating calcium abnormalities compared to the "intact" assays. It should be remembered that PHPT is a common condition and is, therefore, occasionally (12%–15% of patients with HCM) the cause of hypercalcemia in patients with concurrent cancer (10,13).

Other investigations should be directed by the clinical situation and include electrocardiogram (ECG) and imaging tests as required.

CLINICAL SIGNS AND FEATURES

The symptoms and signs of hypercalcemia predominantly relate to the rapidity of onset or chronicity of the abnormality and the effects on volume contraction that accompany increased adjusted calcium, as well as the neuromuscular dysfunction that occurs. Aside from underlying specific features (ie, bone pain in metastatic neoplastic disease), the symptoms can be the same irrespective of the etiology, and relate more to the level of hypercalcemia. Overt symptoms are unlikely to occur if the ACa is <12 mg/dL (3.0 mmol/L), although a thorough search for symptoms in patients with milder degrees of hypercalcemia will often elicit abdominal or neuropsychiatric features not necessarily initially volunteered by the patient. While the differential diagnosis of hypercalcemia is broad, a finding of ACa increased to the extent that overt symptoms are present nearly always indicates either PHPT or malignancy. Acute onset of hypercalcemia and rapidly increasing calcium strongly favors a diagnosis of neoplastic disease, although sudden volume contraction secondary to diarrhea, vomiting, surgery, or immobilization can dangerously exacerbate preexisting hypercalcemia.

As a consequence of hypercalcemia-induced nephrogenic diabetes insipidus, the initial symptoms relate to polyuria and the resultant adaptive increased thirst. Neurological dysfunction, secondary to the central neuronal depressant effect of increased calcium, is prominent and may manifest as confusion, drowsiness, agitation, stupor, or coma. Myopathy is occasionally seen. Polyuria, with an adaptive increase in thirst, is the result of calcium-induced nephrogenic diabetes insipidus. Hypertension as a consequence of calcium-mediated vasoconstriction can occur in chronic disease but is less likely in the acute volume contracted state. Bradyarrhythmias or heart block are frequently seen in severe hypercalcemia, however, and relate to detrimental effects on the cardiac action potential as a consequence of increased extracellular calcium. Gastrointestinal symptoms resulting in part from reduced smooth muscle hypotonicity include constipation, nausea, anorexia, vomiting, and abdominal pain, which are often severe. Renal stones and pancreatitis can occur. The term hypercalcemic crisis is frequently used to describe the severely compromised patient with profound volume depletion; altered sensorium, which may be manifest as coma; cardiac decompensation; and abdominal pain that may mimic an acute abdomen.

The diagnosis of hypercalcemic crisis can sometimes be difficult to make clinically when associated with malignancy. This is because the patient may already be debilitated, anorexic, nauseated, constipated, weak, and confused from the underlying malignancy, concurrent medications, and complications of chemo- or radiotherapy, as well as comorbid disorders. Clinical vigilance in this setting is crucial to prevent unnecessary morbidity and mortality.

ACUTE INTERVENTION

Once severe hypercalcemia is recognized, the patient should be managed in an appropriate emergency setting, such as an acute medical unit (AMU), high-dependency area (HDU), or intensive care unit (ICU). As with all acute medical patients, prompt assessment and management of the ABCDEs should occur (ie, airway, breathing, circulation, disability [ie, conscious level], and exposure [ie, examination and evaluation]).

The acute management of hypercalcemia will depend on a number of factors, including severity of symptoms, comorbidities that may affect treatment options, and the patient's prognosis. In malignancy-related severe hypercalcemia it may be appropriate to adopt a palliative approach that will emphasize comfort cares and symptom control.

General Supportive Care

The cornerstone of acute management of hypercalcemia is fluid resuscitation with correction of the volume state. As described previously, hypercalcemia potently induces a diuresis, and the subsequent volume contraction and reduction in GFR compound renal calcium clearance. Appropriate fluid administration should depend on an assessment of volume depletion, but in most situations of hypercalcemic crisis, 500–1,000 mL of 0.9% saline (NaCl) should be given over the first hour, and 2–6 L over the first 24 hours. This regimen should be continued for several days with careful monitoring of cardiac status and total body hydration. Although historical approaches advocated the use of loop diuretics (eg, furosemide) to induce further renal calcium losses in the acute management, more recent treatment strategies have warned of the risk of aggravating volume contraction if these medications are used (15). However, loop diuretics do have a role in those patients where vigorous fluid resuscitation may provoke cardiogenic fluid overload. In these situations, once euvolemia has been attained, aggressive fluid administration (ie, 3 L 0.9% saline over 24 hr) should be balanced with intravenous (IV) furosemide treatment (20–40 mg every 2–4 hr) to maintain a neutral fluid balance. In most circumstances this can be achieved by inducing a forced diuresis of 2.5 L over 24 hours and allowing for 500 mL of insensible fluid loss. Potassium and magnesium levels should be cautiously monitored whenever furosemide is used, and replaced appropriately if required. Central line insertion with central venous pressure (CVP) measurements should be considered in patients where external features of fluid state are difficult to assess, or in those who poorly tolerate initial attempts at aggressive fluid administration.

Any possible agents causing hypercalcemia should be discontinued as soon as possible. Immobilization promotes osteoclastic bone resorption; hence, early ambulation should be encouraged if possible. Dietary calcium restriction is only rarely warranted in patients with vitamin D/vitamin D metabolite-dependent hypercalcemia.

For treatment of severe hypercalcemia, where possible the cause should be identified and multiple therapies started as soon as possible. In the shorter term, rapid-acting (hours) approaches, including rehydration, possibly forced diuresis, and short-term calcitonin, should be considered, and in the longer term, the most effective antiresorptive agents (ie, bisphosphonates) should be considered. If the diagnosis is PHPT then surgical removal of parathyroid adenoma(s) should be planned (Figure 19-2).

Calcium-Specific Therapy

Irrespective of the etiology, severe hypercalcemia predominantly results from increased mobilization of calcium from bone. Bisphosphonate therapy directly addresses this feature by inhibiting osteoclast activity (16). Several IV bisphosphonate formulations are licensed; in order of potency, they are the nitrogen-containing zoledronate, pamidronate, and ibandronate, and the non-nitrogen-based clodronate. Zoledronate and pamidronate are the most potent and are licensed in the United States. Analyses of randomized controlled trials (RCTs) suggest a superior effect of zoledronate over pamidronate in the management of HCM (17). Intravenous bisphosphonates (Table 19-2) should be administered as soon as possible following rehydration (12 hr) for severe hypercalcemia because there is latency until peak effect of 2–5 days. The dose of pamidronate depends on the level of hypercalcemia (ie, 30 mg over 2 hours with calcium <12 mg/dL [<3 mmol/L] or significant renal impairment [see following sentence]; 60 mg over 4 hr with calcium 12–14 mg/dL [3.0–3.4 mmol/L]; and 90 mg over 6 hr with calcium >14 mg/dL [3.4 mmol/L]). Caution should be exercised in renal impairment, and both pamidronate and zoledronate

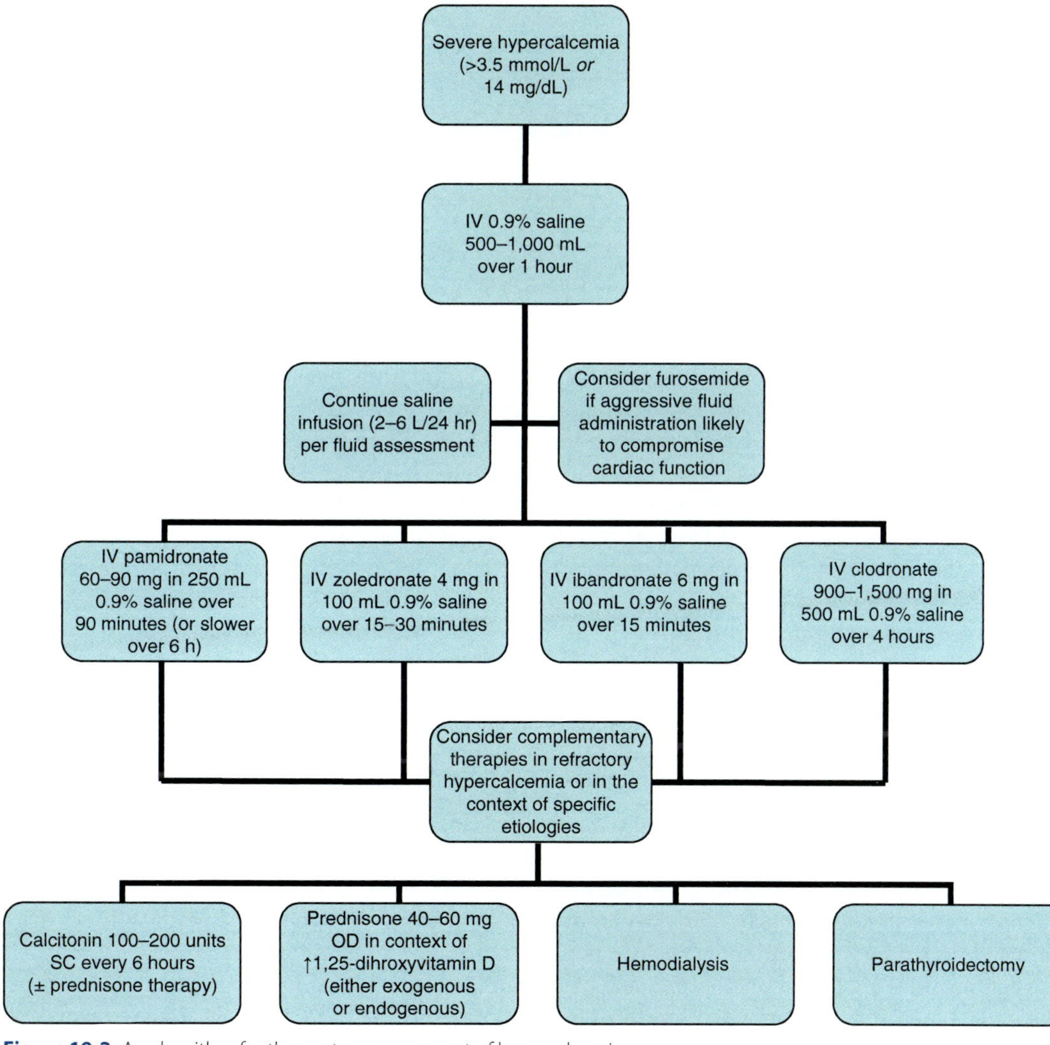

Figure 19-2. An algorithm for the acute management of hypercalcemia.

Table 19-2. Medical Therapy in Severe Hypercalcemia

Drug	Dose	Infusion Rate	Notes
Bisphosphonates			
Pamidronate	30–90 mg	1 mg/min in 250 mL 0.9% saline (or slower over 6 hr)	Flu-like symptoms; calcium-lowering effect may last 2–6 weeks
Zoledronate	4 mg	15–30 min in 100 mL 0.9% saline	Flu-like symptoms (30% of patients); hypocalcemia (check vitamin D status); calcium-lowering effect may last 2–8 weeks
Ibandronate (18)	6 mg	15 min in 100 mL 0.9% saline	Flu-like symptoms, nausea, vomiting; calcium-lowering effect may last 2–4 weeks (19)
Clodronate (20)	900–1,500 mg	4 hr in 500 mL 0.9% saline	Nausea, diarrhea, skin reactions, bronchospasm; calcium-lowering effect may last 2 weeks (21)
Additional options			
Calcitonin (19)	100–200 units 4× daily (test dose of 10–50 units essential)	IM/SC	Hypersensitivity reaction (test dose required); flushing, nausea, vomiting
	10 units/kg	6 hr in 500 mL 0.9% saline IV	Hyperglycemia, neutrophilia, adrenal suppression, psychosis
Prednisone	40–60 mg once daily	Oral	
Hydrocortisone	100–300 mg/day	IV	

All bisphosphonates are more effective when given following 12–24-hour saline rehydration as described in the text.

are relatively contraindicated if the GFR is less than 30 mL/min/1.73 m^2. However, the clinician should assess the perceived benefit of treatment in severe hypercalcemia, and must also consider that renal impairment may be a consequence of the hypercalcemia and dehydration. In such cases, renal impairment may be seen to improve as the hypercalcemia abates. Some 60%–90% of patients will have a significant decrease in ACa following a bisphosphonate infusion, and ongoing treatment should be considered if the hypercalcemia is likely to recur at a later date (usually in HCM). Due to the long duration of effect of these agents, second doses are usually not required for some time (at least 7–14 days) and should be based on the prescribing information for the agent used.

Bisphosphonates are not generally necessary in patients with PHPT because these patients often respond to rehydration alone. Bisphosphonates should be particularly avoided if parathyroid surgery is imminent because their use can result in profound postoperative hypocalcemia. Lowering calcium with cinacalcet is a better option in these circumstances.

Calcitonin acts by inhibiting osteoclast action and, thereby, calcium mobilization from bone (22). It can be given as a subcutaneous (SC) or intramuscular (IM) injection (100–200 units every 6 hr) or as an IV infusion in emergencies (10 units/kg over 6 hr). A test dose (10–50 units) should precede a treatment because hypersensitivity reactions have been reported. Flushing, nausea, and vomiting can occur as milder side effects. Tachyphylaxis is often seen with calcitonin administration (within 5 days) and can be reduced by the coadministration of glucocorticoid therapy. Calcitonin administration can result in more rapid decreases in adjusted calcium, and so it can be used early in treatment to get a more rapid decrease in calcium while waiting for the bisphosphonate therapy to take effect and in patients with refractory hypercalcemia, given that the absolute effect on ACa is small (13).

Glucocorticoid therapy may also be useful in cases of hypercalcemia resulting from increased exogenous (ie, vitamin D toxicity) or endogenous 1,25-dihydroxyvitamin D (ie, granulomatous or lymphoproliferative disorders) due to increased metabolism of vitamin D in the context of glucocorticoid therapy (2). Prednisone can be prescribed at a dose of 40–60 mg once daily, or if IV therapy is required, hydrocortisone at a dose of 100–300 mg/day. Glucocorticoids may also be useful in HCM involving cytokine release (eg, some myelomas).

Medications that interfere with osteoclast action and, therefore, bone resorption include gallium nitrate and mithramycin. These preparations are associated with significant side effects and are very rarely used. Gallium nitrate appears to be at least as effective as pamidronate in achieving decreases in ACa, but is limited by the long duration of infusion (23). Customarily, 200 mg per square meter of body surface is administered over 24 hours for 5 consecutive days. Significant nephrotoxicity seen with rapid infusions is ameliorated by the longer duration of infusion (24). Mithramycin (plicamycin) is a tumoricidal antibiotic that has significant renal and hepatic toxicity. It is currently only available for research purposes but has significant hypocalcemic properties. Phosphate infusion efficiently reduces the serum calcium level within minutes of administration, but the resultant tissue deposition of calcium phosphate makes it inappropriate for use in most hypercalcemia. The only indications are for life-threatening cardiac arrhythmias or severe encephalopathy when dialysis is not immediately available.

Hemodialysis against a low calcium bath diasylate is effective and should be considered in any patient already on dialysis therapy. In refractory hypercalcemia it should be considered as an additional therapy even in those without underlying renal dysfunction. Urgent parathyroidectomy can be considered in all patients with hypertensive crises as a result of hyperparathyroidism but is more safely performed in the stabilized elective patient. However, initial curative success rates differ only marginally between elective and urgent cases, and long-term outcomes appear similar (25).

TREATMENT OF PRECIPITATING ILLNESS

After the acute treatment of severe hypercalcemia (ACa can be decreased by 3–9 mg/dL [0.7–2.2 mmol/L] within 24–48 hr in most patients), the underlying cause should be established. Further therapy will be determined by the diagnosis.

All patients with underlying parathyroid disease (eg, parathyroid adenoma or carcinoma), who present with hypercalcemic crisis, should be considered for elective parathyroidectomy at the earliest safest opportunity unless there is good reason not to (ie, comorbidities, poor prognosis, nonlocalizable disease, or strong patient preference). Definitive treatment of a primary solid tumor with expression of PTHrP may prevent further hypercalcemic events. PTHrP secretion by a tumor significantly decreases bisphosphonate efficacy restoring normocalcemia and will result in earlier rebound hypercalcemia (Figure 19-3). Occasionally patients with nonhumoral hypercalcemia as a result of lytic bone metastases may find improvement with radiation therapy directed at the lesion. Treatment of granulomatous disorders with standard therapy, including glucocorticoids and immunosuppressants, may reduce circulating 1,25-dihydroxyvitamin D concentrations resulting in decreased ACa.

In the rare occasions where severe hypercalcemia is felt to be secondary to drug therapy, the offending drug must be stopped and ACa monitored for 3–6 months. This may be particularly difficult in those on lithium therapy. However, newer psychotropic agents effective in bipolar disease can effect this change more safely than in the past. Drug cessation must also occur in the more common scenario where a drug is felt to have contributed to the hypercalcemic state (ie, thiazide therapy in a patient with HCM), unless significant benefit to risk ratios can be demonstrated.

EMERGING TREATMENTS

Cinacalcet, a calcimimetic that activates the CaSR and thereby reduces parathyroid hormone secretion, is currently being used in the treatment of PHPT, SHPT, and THPT (3). It is licensed in the United States for THPT in the context of advanced CKD, parathyroid carcinoma, and additionally PHPT deemed unsuitable for surgery. It decreases ACa significantly in most patients with PHPT, and in approximately two thirds of those with parathyroid carcinoma (26,27). The use of

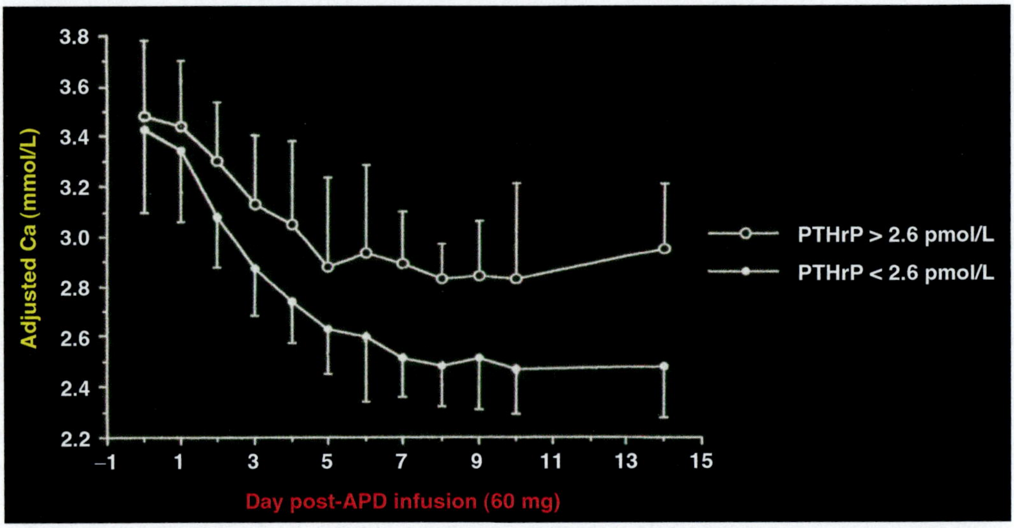

Figure 19-3. The effect of parathyroid hormone-related peptide (PTHrP) on the response to bisphosphonate. Circulating PTHrP greater than 2.6 pmol/L (Nichols Institute Assay) significantly decreases the percentage of patients normalizing adjusted calcium and shortens the length of time of response to a 60-mg pamidronate (APD) infusion.

cinacalcet in the management of hypercalcemic crisis has not yet to our knowledge been the subject of a RCT, but many case studies and reports demonstrate safety and effectiveness of its application in the context of refractory hyperparathyroid disease. It is commenced at a dose of 30 mg once-daily orally and titrated to a maximum dose of 90 mg every 6 hours (180 mg per day in renal dialysis patients).

Osteoclast recruitment with resultant bone resorption is in part mediated by the receptor activator of nuclear factor-kappa B ligand (RANKL) system (28). Activation of the RANK receptor located on immature osteoclasts by osteoblast-derived RANKL promotes maturation and differentiation of the osteoclast. Denosumab (Prolia), a monoclonal antibody that binds to RANKL preventing binding to the RANK receptor, has been shown to decrease bone resorption in metastatic bone disease and in osteoporosis with a good safety profile (29). A recent report has demonstrated the efficacy of denosumab in patients with HCM who have become "resistant" to bisphosphonates (30). Monoclonal antibodies directed against PTHrP have been produced and have been shown to be useful for controlling bone metastases in patients with small cell lung cancer (31). Whether this will translate into a useful additional treatment for the management of severe hypercalcemia secondary to humoral mechanisms remains to be seen.

CONCLUSIONS

Severe hypercalcemia is an endocrine emergency that requires prompt action to prevent severe neurological, cardiac, and renal consequences. The diagnosis should be considered in any patient with known parathyroid disease or neoplasm who presents with acute deterioration, especially in the context of neurological dysfunction. The cornerstone of management is to perform appropriate investigations to make an accurate diagnosis, followed by volume resuscitation, then the administration of calcium-specific therapies such as bisphosphonates. Additional therapies, including calcimimetics in certain situations and drugs that affect the RANKL system, are likely to become more widely used in the future, although further studies are required to define their role.

ACKNOWLEDGMENTS

The authors have nothing to disclose.

REFERENCES

1. **Favus MJ, Goltzman D.** Regulation of calcium and magnesium. In: Rosen CJ, ed. *Primer on the Metabolic Bone Diseases and Disorders of Mineral Metabolism.* 8th ed. Washington DC: American Society for Bone and Mineral Research;2013:173–179.
2. **Holick MF.** Vitamin D deficiency. *N Engl J Med.* 2007;357:266–281.

3. **Fraser WD.** Hyperparathyroidism. *Lancet.* 2009;11; 374:145–158.
4. **Holick MF, Brinkley NC, Bischoff-Ferrari HA, et al.** Evaluation, treatment, and prevention of vitamin D deficiency: an Endocrine Society Clinical Practice Guideline. *J Clin Endocrinol Metab.* 2011;96: 1911–1930.
5. **Egbuna OI, Brown EM.** Hypercalcaemic and hypocalcaemic conditions due to calcium-sensing receptor mutations. *Best Pract Res Clin Rheumatol.* 2008;22:129–148.
6. **Joshie D, Center, JR, Eisman JA.** Investigation of incidental hypercalcaemia. *BMJ.* 2009;339:b4613.
7. **Marcocci C, Cetani F.** Clinical practice. Primary hyperparathyroidism. *N Engl J Med.* 2011;365: 2389–2397.
8. **Broadus AE, Mangin M, Ikeda K, et al.** Humoral hypercalcemia of cancer: identification of a novel parathyroid hormone-like peptide. *N Engl J Med.* 1988;319:556–563.
9. **Hewison M, Burke F, Evans KN, et al.** Extra-renal 25-hydroxyvitamin D3-1-hydroxylase in human health and disease. *J Steroid Biochem.* 2007;103: 316–321.
10. **Fraser WD, Robinson J, Lawton R, et al.** Clinical and laboratory studies of new immunoradiometric assay of parathyroid hormone related protein. *Clin Chem.* 1993;39:414–419.
11. **Igbal AA, Burgess EH, Gallina DL, et al.** Hypercalcemia in hyperthyroidism: patterns of serum calcium, parathyroid hormone, and 1,25-dihydroxyvitamin D3 levels during management of thyrotoxicosis. *Endocr Pract.* 2003;9:517–521.
12. **Fraser WD, Logue FC, MacRitchie K, et al.** Intact parathyroid hormone concentration and cyclic AMP metabolism in thyroid disease. *Acta Endocrinology.* 1991;124:652–657.
13. **Stewart A.** Hypercalcaemia associated with cancer. *N Engl J Med.* 2005;352:373–379.
14. **Fraser WD, Logue FC, Gallacher SJ, et al.** Direct and indirect assessment of the parathyroid hormone response to pamidronate therapy in Paget's disease of bone and hypercalcaemia of malignancy. *Bone & Mineral.* 1991;12:113–121.
15. **LeGrand SB, Leskuski D, Zama I.** Narrative review: furosemide for hypercalcemia: an unproven yet common practice. *Ann Intern Med.* 2008;149;259–263.
16. **Reszka AA.** Bisphosphonate mechanisms of action. In: Alder RA, ed. *Contemporary Endocrinology: Osteoporosis.* 2nd ed. New York: Humana Press; 2010;443–468.
17. **Major P, Lortholary A, Hon J, et al.** Zoledronic acid is superior to pamidronate in the treatment of hypercalcemia of malignancy: a pooled analysis of two randomized, controlled clinical trials. *J Clin Oncol.* 2001;19:558–567.
18. **von Moos R, Caspar CB, Thurlimann B, et al.** Renal safety profiles of ibandronate 6 mg infused over 15 and 60 min: a randomized, open-label study. *Ann Oncol.* 2008;19:1266–1270.
19. **Ralston SH, Thiebaud D, Herrmann Z, et al.** Dose-response study of ibandronate in the treatment of cancer-associated hypercalcaemia. *Brit J Cancer.* 1997;75:295–300.
20. **Atula ST, Tahtela RK, Nevalainen JI, Pylkkanen LH.** Clodronate as a single-dose intravenous infusion effectively provides short-term correction of malignant hypercalcemia. *Acta Oncologica.* 2006;42;735–740.
21. **Purohit OP, Radstone CR, Anthony C, Kanis JA, Coleman RE.** A randomised double-blind comparison of intravenous pamidronate and clodronate in the hypercalcaemia of malignancy. *Brit J Cancer.* 1995;72:1289–1293.
22. **Chesnut CH, Azria M, Silverman S, Engelhardt M, Olson M, Mindeholm M.** Salmon calcitonin: a review of current and future therapeutic indications. *Osteoporos Int.* 2008;19:479–491.
23. **Cvitkovic F, Armand J-P, Tubiana-Hulin M, Rossi J-F, Warrell R.** Randomized, double-blind, phase II trial of gallium nitrate compared with pamidronate for acute control of cancer-related hypercalcemia. *Cancer J.* 2006;12:47–53.
24. **Chitambar CR.** Medical applications and toxicities of gallium compounds. *Int J Environ Res Public Health.* 2010;7:2337–2361.
25. **Cannon J, Lew J, Solorzano J.** Parathyroidectomy for hypercalcemic crisis: 40 years' experience and long-term outcomes. *Surgery.* 2010;148:807–813.
26. **Marcocci C, Chanson P, Shoback D, et al.** Cinacalcet reduces serum calcium concentrations in patients with intractable primary hyperparathyroidism. *J Clin Endocr Metab.* 2009;94:2766–2772.
27. **Silverberg SJ, Rubin MR, Faiman C, et al.** Cinacalcet hydrochloride reduces the serum calcium concentration in inoperable parathyroid carcinoma. *J Clin Endocr Metab.* 2007;92:3803–3808.
28. **Tanaka S, Nakamura K, Takahasi N, Suda T.** Role of RANKL in physiological and pathological bone resorption and therapeutics targeting the RANKL–RANK signaling system. *Immunol Rev.* 2005;208: 30–49.
29. **Body JJ, Lipton A, Gralow J, et al.** Effects of denosumab in patients with bone metastases with and without previous bisphosphonate exposure. *J Bone Miner Res.* 2010;25:440–446.
30. **Hu MI, Glezerman I, Leboulleux S, et al.** Denosumab for patients with persistent or relapsed hypercalcemia of malignancy despite recent bisphosphonate treatment. *J Natl Cancer Inst.* 2013;105(18): 1417–1420.
31. **Yamada T, Muguruma H, Yano S, et al.** Intensification therapy with anti-parathyroid hormone-related protein antibody plus zoledronic acid for bone metastases of small cell lung cancer cells in severe combined immunodeficient mice. *Mol Cancer Ther.* 2009;8:119–126.

CHAPTER 20

Acute Medical Aspects Related to Phosphate Disorders

Barton S Levine and Arnold J Felsenfeld

ABSTRACT

Acute hypophosphatemia with phosphate depletion is common in the hospital setting and results in significant morbidity and mortality. Acute hypophosphatemia may be mild (2–2.5 mg/dL [0.65–0.81 mmol/L]), moderate (1–1.9 mg/dL [0.32–0.61 mmol/L]), or severe (<1 mg/dL [0.32 mmol/L]) and commonly occurs in clinical settings such as refeeding, alcoholism, diabetic ketoacidosis, malnourishment/starvation, postoperatively (particularly after partial hepatectomy), and in the intensive care unit. Phosphate replacement can be given orally, intravenously, in dialysate, or in TPN solutions. The rate and amount of replacement are empiric, and several algorithms are available. Treatment should be tailored to symptoms, severity, anticipated duration of illness, and presence of comorbid conditions such as renal failure, volume overload, hypo- or hypercalcemia, hypo- or hyperkalemia, and acid-base status. Mild/moderate acute hypophosphatemia can usually be corrected with increased dietary phosphate or oral supplementation, but intravenous replacement is generally needed when significant comorbid conditions or severe hypophosphatemia with phosphate depletion exists. Acute hyperphosphatemia associated with tumor lysis syndrome and phosphate bowel preparations can also be a medical emergency requiring prompt treatment.

INTRODUCTION

Unlike serum calcium, which is tightly regulated throughout the day and during a lifetime, serum phosphorus values are greater in infancy and childhood than in adulthood, show considerable diurnal variation, and decrease postprandially. The range of normal values for serum phosphorus for adults is wide, 2.5–4.5 mg/dL (0.8–1.4 mmol/L). Hypophosphatemia is generally divided into acute and chronic. Acute hypophosphatemia with phosphate depletion is common in the hospital setting and when severe can result in significant morbidity (1,2). Chronic hypophosphatemia usually results in abnormal growth presenting as rickets in children and osteomalacia in adults and is generally associated with genetic or acquired renal phosphate-wasting disorders. Acute hypophosphatemia with severe phosphate depletion often is a metabolic emergency and will be the focus of this chapter. Although chronic hypophosphatemia requires treatment, it generally is not a metabolic emergency and will not be discussed in this review. Details of its pathophysiology and treatment can be found elsewhere (3–5). Although hyperphosphatemia is commonly seen in chronic kidney disease, hypoparathyroidism/pseudohypoparathyroidism, and tumoral calcinosis, hyperphosphatemia is not a metabolic emergency in these disorders and will not be discussed. However, acute hyperphosphatemia, which develops after endogenous phosphate release in tumor lysis syndrome or after exogenous use of phosphate bowel preparations, is often a metabolic emergency and its management will be reviewed.

PATHOPHYSIOLOGY OF PHOSPHATE

Maintenance of phosphate balance is critical for survival. Phosphate plays a vital role in physiological processes such as nucleic acid synthesis, cell membrane structure, intracellular signaling, protein synthesis, energy stores via adenosine triphosphate (ATP), oxygen delivery via 2,3-diphosphoglycerate (2,3-DPG), acid excretion, and bone structure. Approximately 85% of body phosphate is located in bone with the remainder in the intracellular pool except for less than 1% in the extracellular pool. Phosphate balance is maintained by ingestion/intestinal absorption and renal excretion. Important hormonal regulators of phosphate include parathyroid hormone (PTH) and fibroblast growth factor 23 (FGF23), both of which increase renal excretion, and 1,25-vitamin D (1,25D), which increases intestinal absorption. Finally, because approximately 60%–80% of ingested dietary phosphate presented to the small intestine is absorbed, excessive oral loads of phosphate can result in a large burden of absorbed phosphate that can overcome regulatory processes, especially if renal function is impaired.

Unlike serum calcium, which is regulated by PTH, serum phosphorus is not tightly regulated by any hormone. However, serum phosphorus is affected by serum calcium modulation of PTH. Phosphate loading decreases serum calcium by reducing calcium efflux from bone resulting in an increased demand for PTH, which besides correcting serum calcium increases renal phosphate excretion lowering serum phosphorus, which in turn increases the calcemic action of PTH. Hyperphosphatemia may also directly stimulate PTH secretion (6). In contrast, phosphate depletion increases calcium efflux from bone, decreasing PTH values, and decreases PTH secretion in the parathyroid gland via a post-transcriptional effect (6). Moreover, changes in the phosphate status directly affect production of 1,25D. Hypophosphatemia stimulates 1,25D production increasing intestinal phosphate absorption, while hyperphosphatemia suppresses 1,25D production decreasing intestinal phosphate absorption. Phosphate loading has been associated with increases in FGF23, but the response is not immediate and less robust than expected (7). Moreover, a reciprocal pathway is present between FGF23 and 1,25D with FGF23 suppressing 1,25D production and 1,25D stimulating FGF23 secretion (8). Also, a gut-renal phosphate axis has been shown in experimental studies in which phosphate instilled into the duodenum rapidly increases renal phosphate excretion by a mechanism not due to FGF23 or other known phosphatonins (9).

HYPOPHOSPHATEMIA AS A METABOLIC EMERGENCY

Etiology of Acute Hypophosphatemia

In adults, hypophosphatemia occurs in up to 5% of hospitalized patients, and its incidence may be as high as 30%–50% in clinical settings such as alcoholism, sepsis, or intensive care unit (ICU) admissions (1). Other medical conditions in which acute hypophosphatemia is commonly seen include refeeding after starvation/malnutrition or large weight losses, in anorexia nervosa, and with kwashiorkor/marasmus (Figure 20-1) (2). Postsurgical conditions associated with hypophosphatemia include hepatic surgery, possibly because the liver may metabolize phosphotonins such as matrix extracellular phosphoglycoprotein (known as MEPE), and after parathyroidectomy for severe primary or secondary hyperparathyroidism due to hungry bone syndrome. Finally, hypophosphatemia is commonly seen in the ICU during continuous renal replacement therapy (CRRT).

Phosphate depletion results from decreased intake/absorption, renal/extracorporeal losses, and shifts of phosphate into bone (hungry bone syndrome), while transcellular shifts of phosphate are a major cause of hypophosphatemia (Figure 20-1). Although severe hypophosphatemia is often associated with phosphate depletion, the serum phosphorus value especially on presentation may not be representative of total body phosphorus. An example of the failure of serum phosphorus to indicate phosphate depletion is the poorly controlled diabetic patient who presents to the emergency department with a normal or even elevated serum phosphorus value

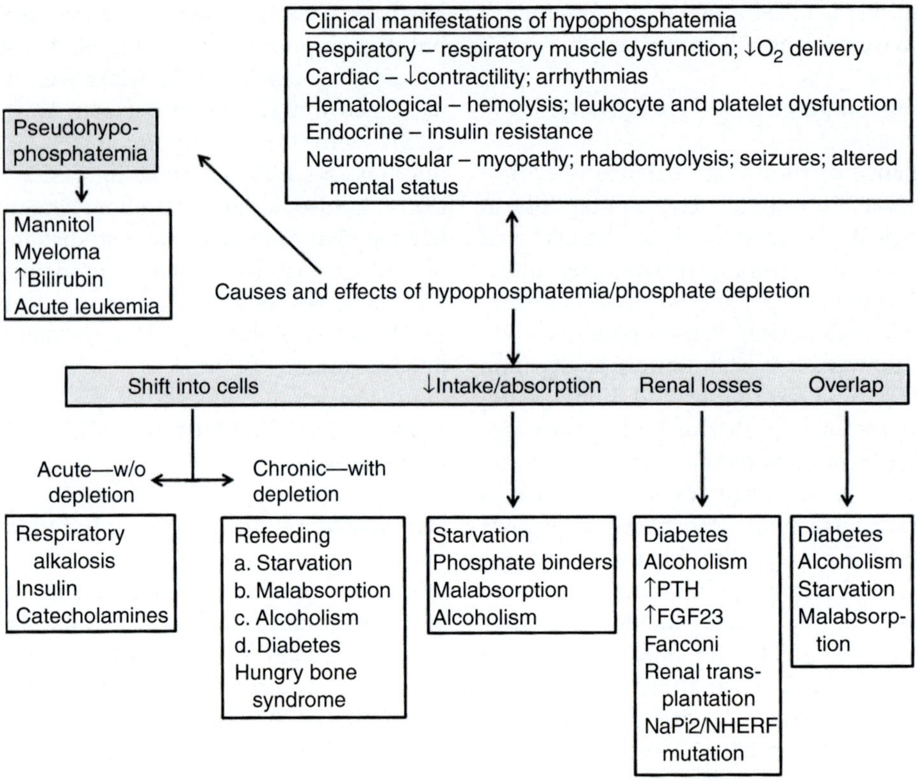

Figure 20-1. Causes and effects of hypophosphatemia/phosphate depletion. Hypophosphatemia may be acute or chronic and results from decreased intake and/or absorption, gastrointestinal and renal/extracorporeal losses, internal redistribution, or a combination of these factors. Pseudohypophosphatemia may occur in acute leukemias from increased uptake of phosphate by leukemic cells in vitro or may result from interference with the phosphate assay by mannitol, bilirubin, or dysproteinemia. Abbreviations: FGF23 = fibroblast growth factor 23; NaPi2/NHERF = sodium-phosphate 2 cotransporter/sodium-hydrogen exchanger regulatory factor; PTH = parathyroid hormone.

despite continuous renal phosphate losses and decreased phosphate intake (2).

Hypophosphatemia only develops after treatment with insulin results in a marked shift of phosphate into the intracellular compartment. Another cause of hypophosphatemia is that associated with the infusion of fructose, which results in sequestration of phosphate in extracellular sites or intracellular pathways that do not produce ATP or 2,3-DPG. Finally, awareness of factors that can cause pseudohypophosphatemia is important because phosphate treatment is not necessary and can be harmful. Mannitol, myeloma protein, and hyperbilirubinemia can interfere with the colorimetric assay for serum phosphorus. In acute leukemia, phosphate uptake by abundant white cells in the test tube can cause a hypophosphatemic reading (Figure 20-1).

Transcellular shifts of phosphate are an interesting phenomenon because they can occur with or without phosphate depletion. When free intracellular phosphate is moved into glycolytic or protein synthesis pathways, free intracellular phosphate concentrations decrease, and extracellular phosphate shifts into cells (10). Examples include the decrease in serum phosphorus from insulin and glucose infusion and from respiratory alkalosis (Figure 20-1). Treatment of hypophosphatemia is not necessary in these situations because ATP and 2,3-DPG concentrations are maintained. Of interest, a precipitous decrease in serum phosphorus after initiating glucose-containing solutions may indicate phosphate depletion (11).

Clinical Manifestations

Acute hypophosphatemia with phosphate depletion is associated with many clinical manifestations (Figure 20-1) and increases morbidity. In the ICU setting, hypophosphatemia has been associated with longer durations of mechanical ventilation and hospitalization, decreased left ventricular stroke index and blood pressure, an increased incidence of ventricular tachycardia, and postoperative complications (1,2,12). The primary mechanism responsible for acute symptoms with hypophosphatemia is depletion of ATP and 2,3-DPG, which results, respectively, in reduced energy stores and impaired oxygen delivery (2,10). Correction of severe hypophosphatemia improves myocardial and respiratory performance (2,10).

Treatment of Hypophosphatemia

In certain situations, hypophosphatemia may be anticipated and prevented by judicious phosphate supplementation. During refeeding in malnutrition, the intake of fluids, electrolytes, and energy should be introduced gradually (2). Careful monitoring of serum phosphorus is important. During hyperalimentation, symptomatic hypophosphatemia can be prevented by administering 11–14 mmol of potassium phosphate per 1,000 calories in the parenteral feeding. In patients undergoing CRRT, hypophosphatemia can be prevented by adding phosphate to the dialysate or administering phosphate when serum phosphorus falls below normal (2).

Phosphate repletion for acute hypophosphatemia associated with phosphate depletion can be given orally or intravenously, with the former route safer (Table 20-1). IV repletion corrects hypophosphatemia more rapidly, but adverse effects may include hypocalcemia, arrhythmias, ectopic calcification, and acute kidney injury (AKI). The severity of hypophosphatemia is important in determining the urgency and mode of treatment. In most instances, mild (serum phosphorus 2–2.5 mg/dL, 0.65–0.81 mmol/L) or moderate (serum phosphorus 1–1.9 mg/dL, 0.32–0.61 mmol/L) hypophosphatemia can be treated by increasing dietary phosphate or giving oral phosphate supplementation (Table 20-1). In severe acute hypophosphatemia (<1 mg/dL, <0.32 mmol/L) with phosphate depletion, treatment with IV phosphate is generally necessary, especially in patients in the ICU. IV therapy also is indicated in hypophosphatemic patients unable to tolerate or ingest oral phosphate.

The amount of phosphate needed to restore serum phosphorus and/or replete

Table 20-1. Oral and Intravenous Phosphate Preparations and Replacement Guidelines

Preparation	Phosphate Content (g)		Sodium (mEq)	Potassium (mEq)
	Oral Preparations			
Skim milk (1 L)	1.0		28	38
Phospho-soda (1 mL)	0.150		4.8	0
K-phos original #1 (1 tablet)	0.114		0	3.70
K-phos original #2 (1 tablet)	0.250		5.80	2.80
K-phos neutral (1 tablet)	0.250		13.0	1.10
	Commonly Used Intravenous Preparations			
Sodium phosphate (1 mL)	0.011		4.0	0
Potassium phosphate (1 mL)	0.011		0	4.4
	Intravenous Replacement Guidelines			
Serum Phosphorus (mg/dL)	Intensive Care Unit Setting		Ward Setting	
	Amount[a] (mmol/kg bwt)	Duration (hr)	Amount[a] (mmol/kg bwt)	Duration (hr)
<1	0.6	6	0.64	24–72
1–1.7	0.4	6	0.32	24–72
1.8–2.2	0.2	6	0.16	24–72

Complications may include diarrhea (oral), thrombophlebitis (K-phos infusion), hypocalcemia, acute kidney injury, nephrocalcinosis, hyperkalemia, hypernatremia/volume overload, hyperphosphatemia, and metabolic acidosis. Conversion factor for phosphorus in mg/dL to mmol/L, × 0.3229. No conversion necessary for sodium and potassium in mEq/L mmol/L.

[a] In patients who are >130% of their ideal body weight, an adjusted body weight should be used.

total-body phosphate is empirical because the volume of distribution is highly variable (13). When giving oral supplementation for mild to moderate hypophosphatemia, 32–65 mmol/day of phosphate for 7–10 days is usually adequate to replenish stores. However, doses as high as 97 mmol/day may be needed initially for severe deficiency. Cow milk, preferably skim milk to avoid diarrhea, is a good source of phosphate containing 1 mg/mL. Oral sodium and potassium-based phosphate preparations are also available (Table 20-1).

In the first studies with IV phosphate replacement in severely hypophosphatemic patients (<1 mg/dL), 9 mmol (~0.14 mmol/kg) of IV phosphate was administered every 12 hours. Three additional doses were needed to achieve normal serum phosphorus at 48 hours (2). In a subsequent study, a 0.32 mmol/kg per 12 hours dose was given, which was increased to 0.48 mmol/kg per 12 hours if serum phosphorus did not increase by 0.2 mg/dL (0.065 mmol/L) at 6 hours (2). Seven of 10 patients attained a serum phosphorus ≥2 mg/dL (≥0.65 mmol/L) by 24 hours and all 10 by 48 hours. Because the hypophosphatemic patient in the ICU with myocardial or respiratory compromise may need more rapid correction, higher doses of IV phosphate have been used. In severe hypophosphatemia, doses as high as 10–20 mmol/hr given for 1–3 hours have been used without reported adverse effects (2). Perhaps in a better-suited approach, doses of 42–67 mmol have been given over 6–9 hours (Table 20-1) (2). In moderate hypophosphatemia, lower doses of IV phosphate have been used. In most studies, either potassium or sodium phosphate was used based on a pre-infusion serum potassium value of 4 mEq/L (4 mmol/L). Finally, in the presence of decreased renal function, the dose of phosphate replacement should be reduced, serum phosphorus should be carefully monitored during repletion, and the use of potassium phosphate replacement should be minimized. Key considerations for treatment of hypophosphatemia are shown in Table 20-2.

HYPERPHOSPHATEMIA AS A METABOLIC EMERGENCY

In several settings acute hyperphosphatemia is a metabolic emergency (Table 20-2). These include the endogenous release of phosphate in tumor lysis syndrome (TLS) and after exogenous administration of phosphate bowel

Table 20-2. Key Considerations for Treatment of Hypophosphatemia and Hyperphosphatemia

- Severity: Mild (2–2.5 mg/dL, 0.65–0.81 mmol/L) or moderate (1–1.9 mg/dL, 0.32–0.61 mmol/L) hypophosphatemia can usually be treated with increased dietary phosphate or oral phosphate supplements. Severe acute hypophosphatemia (<1mg/dL, <0.32 mmol/L) with phosphate depletion, particularly in the ICU setting, is often a metabolic emergency requiring IV phosphate replacement.
- Comorbid conditions: When the contribution of hypophosphatemia to symptoms is unclear, the severity of illness should be a determining factor in deciding whether oral or IV treatment is preferred.
- Hypocalcemia, hypercalcemia: Phosphate therapy can exacerbate hypocalcemia. In hypercalcemic patients, phosphate therapy can lead to calcium-phosphate precipitation, nephrocalcinosis, and AKI.
- Renal failure: In renal failure, the dose of phosphate replacement should be reduced by at least 50%.
- Use of potassium or sodium phosphate treatment: With hypokalemia, potassium containing phosphate supplements are preferred, but with hyperkalemia, sodium containing supplements should be used. With volume overload avoid sodium containing phosphate supplements if possible. In CKD, sodium phosphate replacement is generally preferred.
- Pseudohypophosphatemia: Pseudohypophosphatemia is important to recognize because treatment is not needed and can result in hyperphosphatemia (see Figure 20-1 for causes).
- Hyperphosphatemia in TLS: When severe, hyperphosphatemia in TLS is a metabolic emergency because of the risk of acute kidney injury. The decision to treat with CRRT depends on the magnitude of hyperphosphatemia, rate of increase in serum phosphorus, deterioration in renal function, and adequacy of urine output.
- Hyperphosphatemia from phosphate bowel preparations: Severe hyperphosphatemia from phosphate enemas and OSPs is associated with acute kidney injury and catastrophic effects such as hypotension and severe metabolic acidosis. The risk is greatest in elderly patients and anyone with decreased kidney function. Awareness of potential toxicity is the best prevention.

Abbreviations: AKI = acute kidney injury; CKD = chronic kidney disease; CRRT = continuous renal replacement therapy; IV = intravenous; OSP = oral sodium phosphate purgative; TLS = tumor lysis syndrome.

preparations, especially phosphate-containing enemas. These disorders are briefly discussed in the following two sections.

Tumor Lysis Syndrome

Several recent comprehensive reviews of TLS are available (14,15). TLS occurs when bulky, rapidly growing tumors with high sensitivity to cytotoxic chemotherapy are treated. Heading the list of these tumors are hematological malignancies such as acute lymphoblastic/cytic and myeloid leukemias and Burkitt lymphoma. However, treatment of other rapidly growing, chemosensitive tumors can also result in TLS. Besides tumor bulk and chemosensitivity, a preexisting decrease in renal function (serum creatinine >1.4 mg/dL, >123 μmol/L) increases the risk of TLS (15). Rapid destruction of cells releases uric acid and phosphate, both of which are nephrotoxic to renal tubules. Until recently the decision whether to treat the hyperuricemia or hyperphosphatemia could be problematic because a posttreatment observation period was needed to decide whether hyperuricemia or hyperphosphatemia predominates. Hydration with IV crystalloid, at least 3 L per day as long as urine output is adequate, is recommended treatment for TLS. For marked hyperuricemia, IV sodium bicarbonate was recommended to alkalinize the urine, which greatly increases solubility of uric acid. However, if hyperphosphatemia predominated, solubility of calcium-phosphate is greater in acid urine, and IV sodium chloride is recommended. With the current availability of rasburicase, a recombinant form of urate oxidase, which lowers serum uric acid dramatically by converting insoluble uric acid into the more soluble allantoin, hyperuricemia is now treatable. Because of the high cost of rasburicase, our approach is not to administer it prophylactically, but rather to observe uric acid values after completion of chemotherapy and to give a single dose of rasburicase if marked hyperuricemia develops. Because rasburicase also generates hydrogen peroxide, patients should be tested for glucose-6-phosphatase deficiency before treatment. Besides causing AKI, hyperphosphatemia can also result in profound hypocalcemia, which can cause tetany, cardiac arrhythmias, hypotension, and seizures. The decision to treat the hyperphosphatemia depends on the magnitude of hyperphosphatemia, the rate of rise of serum phosphorus, adequacy of urine output, and the deterioration of renal function. Because phosphate clearance is time dependent, phosphate removal is best accomplished with CRRT rather than intermittent hemodialysis.

Nephropathy from Phosphate Bowel Preparations

Acute phosphate nephropathy has been observed after both oral sodium phosphate (OSP) purgatives for colonoscopy and phosphate enemas. The former often results in subacute kidney injury without obvious clinical symptomatology in which the patient presents several months later with decreased kidney function (16). In one study, 28% of patients receiving OSP (11.6 grams of phosphate) for colonoscopy had serum phosphorus values >8 mg/dL (2.58 mmol/L) after taking the OSP (16). Kidney biopsies obtained when serum creatinine was discovered to be increased several months later showed calcium phosphate deposition in the tubular epithelial cells. Preexisting risk factors for nephrotoxicity include decreased kidney function, volume depletion, age, female gender, hypertension, diabetes, and use of ACE-inhibitors/angiotensin receptor blockers, diuretics, and nonsteroidals.

Acute phosphate nephropathy associated with phosphate enemas often presents as a metabolic emergency. In a recent retrospective study of 11 patients hospitalized after a sodium phosphate (Fleet) enema, 7 patients presented in the first 24 hours (17). Mean age of the patients was 80 years and 10 patients received the Fleet enema for constipation. Presenting findings included hypotension, volume depletion, severe hyperphosphatemia, profound hypocalcemia, metabolic acidosis, hypernatremia, and both hypo- and hyperkalemia. The mean serum phosphorus and calcium on presentation were 18.8 mg/dL (6.06 mmol/L) and 5.9 mg/dL (1.47 mmol/L), respectively. Five patients died, and three patients required prolonged hospitalizations. Eight patients received the standard Fleet enema dose of 250 mL, which contains 10.7 grams elemental phosphorus, and 3 patients received doses between 500 and 798 mL. Awareness that phosphate enemas in the elderly population can result in a metabolic emergency is the most important preventive. Preexisting chronic kidney disease, common in the elderly, magnifies the risk for developing phosphate nephropathy. Key considerations for the development and treatment of hyperphosphatemia are presented in Table 20-2.

In summary, treatment of hypophosphatemia has largely been based on empirical administration of different doses of oral and IV phosphate. In the setting of severe hypophosphatemia especially in the ICU, IV phosphate administration is generally necessary. Hyperphosphatemia and the severe metabolic toxicities associated with phosphate bowel preparations can be prevented by awareness of the patient population at risk. Hyperphosphatemia associated with TLS requires prompt treatment to prevent renal toxicity.

ACKNOWLEDGMENTS

The authors have nothing to disclose.

REFERENCES

1. **Brunelli SM, Goldfarb S.** Hypophosphatemia: clinical consequences and management. *J Am Soc Nephrol.* 2007;18:1999–2003.
2. **Felsenfeld AJ, Levine BS.** Approach to treatment of hypophosphatemia. *Am J Kidney Dis.* 2012;60:655–661.
3. **Levine BS, Kleeman CR, Felsenfeld AJ.** The journey from vitamin D-resistant rickets to the regulation of renal phosphate transport. *Clin J Am Soc Nephrol.* 2009;4:1866–1877.
4. **Imel EA, Econs MJ.** Approach to the hypophosphatemic patient. *J Clin Endocrinol Metab.* 2011;97: 696–706.
5. **Prie D, Friedlander G.** Genetic disorders of renal phosphate transport. *N Engl J Med.* 2010;362:2399–2409.
6. **Silver J, Naveh-Many T.** Phosphate and the parathyroid. *Kidney Int.* 2009;75:898–905.
7. **Nishida Y, Taketani Y, Yamanaka-Okumura H, et al.** Acute effect of oral phosphate loading on serum fibroblast growth factor 23 levels in healthy men. *Kidney Int.* 2006;70:2141–2147.
8. **Quarles LD.** Endocrine functions of bone in mineral metabolism regulation. *J Clin Invest.* 2008;118: 3820–3828.
9. **Berndt T, Thomas LF, Craig TA, et al.** Evidence for a signaling axis by which intestinal phosphate rapidly modulates renal phosphate reabsorption. *Proc Natl Acad Sci (USA).* 2007;104:11085–11090.
10. **Rubin MF, Narins RG.** Hypophosphatemia: pathophysiological and practical aspects of its therapy. *Semin Nephrol.* 1990;10:536–545.
11. **Ritz E.** Acute hypophosphatemia. *Kidney Int.* 1982; 22:84–94.
12. **Bacchetta J, Salusky IB.** Evaluation of hypophosphatemia: lessons from patients with genetic disorders. *Am J Kidney Dis.* 2012;59:152–159.
13. **Lentz RD, Brown DM, Kjellstrand CM.** Treatment of severe hypophosphatemia. *Ann Intern Med.* 1978; 89:941–944.
14. **Coiffier B, Altman A, Pui C-H, Younes A, Cairo MS.** Guidelines for the management of pediatric and adult tumor lysis syndrome: an evidence-based review. *J Clin Oncol.* 2008;26:2767–2778.
15. **Wilson FP, Berns JS.** Onco-nephrology: tumor lysis syndrome. *Clin J Am Soc Nephrol.* 2012;7:1730–1739.
16. **Markowitz GS, Perazella MA.** Acute phosphate nephropathy. *Kidney Int.* 2009;76:1027–1034.
17. **Ori Y, Rozen-Zvi B, Chagnac A, et al.** Fatalities and severe metabolic disorders associated with the use of sodium phosphate enemas. *Arch Intern Med.* 2012; 172:263–265.

CHAPTER 21

Acute Medical Aspects Related to Osteoporosis and Its Therapy

Dima L Diab and Nelson B Watts

ABSTRACT

There are several safety concerns with the use of nonpharmacological and pharmacological agents for the treatment of osteoporosis. Excessive calcium and vitamin D intake have been linked to an increased risk of renal calculi. Safety issues with bisphosphonate therapy include gastrointestinal side effects, acute phase reaction, hypocalcemia, musculoskeletal pain, renal safety, osteonecrosis of the jaw, and atypical fractures. Safety concerns with denosumab include hypocalcemia, infections, skin reactions, malignancy, osteonecrosis of the jaw, and atypical femur fractures. The main acute adverse events with teriparatide use are hypercalcemia and hypercalciuria. In the event of an acute fragility fracture, patients should undergo proper evaluation, and pain control should be achieved with the resumption of physical activity as soon as possible.

INTRODUCTION

Osteoporosis is a generalized skeletal disorder characterized by compromised bone strength, which predisposes to an increased risk of fractures (1). Osteoporosis has no clinical manifestations until there is a fracture. The annual incidence of osteoporotic fractures in the United States is greater than 2 million, which is expected to rise to more than 3 million by the year 2020 (2). The gold standard for establishing the diagnosis of osteoporosis is the measurement of bone mineral density (BMD) by dual-energy X-ray absorptiometry (DXA) of the spine, hip, and/or forearm, where a T-score of −2.5 or lower is consistent with this condition. A clinical diagnosis of osteoporosis can be made in individuals who sustain a fragility fracture regardless of the T-score. There are numerous effective pharmacological treatment options for osteoporosis, with different safety profiles (3). This chapter provides a thorough updated review of the safety of osteoporosis therapy, with a focus on the acute medical aspects related to such therapy. This chapter also discusses the work-up and management of the acute fragility fracture.

SAFETY CONCERNS WITH OSTEOPOROSIS THERAPY

Calcium

Adequate intake of calcium is an important component in the prevention and treatment of osteoporosis. The recommended calcium intake for postmenopausal women is 1,200 mg daily, with the preferred source being dietary (4,5). Supplementation is recommended if this cannot be obtained through diet alone. Excessive calcium supplementation may cause hypercalcemia, hypercalciuria, and kidney stones. In general, the concern that high dietary calcium increases the risk of nephrolithiasis is unfounded, because the incidence of stone formation appears to be reduced in both men and women (6). However, calcium supplements have been associated with an increased risk of kidney stones in randomized clinical trials. The Women's Health Initiative (WHI) trial reported an increased risk of kidney stones in postmenopausal women who were supplemented with calcium and vitamin D when compared with placebo (2.5% vs 2.1%, HR 1.17, 95% CI 1.02–1.34), although the total calcium intake in the intervention group exceeded 2,000 mg/day (7).

The effect of calcium supplementation on risk of cardiovascular disease is controversial. In the WHI trial described previously, there was no effect of calcium and vitamin D supplementation on cardiovascular disease (8). However, the findings of 2 meta-analyses evaluating calcium or calcium with or without vitamin D supplementation raised some concern about an increased risk of myocardial infarction in patients randomly assigned to calcium versus placebo (9,10). Some prospective studies also showed an increased cardiovascular risk with calcium supplements, but no relationship between dietary calcium intake and cardiovascular disease (11,12). On the other hand, data from a 5-year randomized, controlled trial and 4.5 years of post-trial follow-up revealed that daily calcium supplementation of 1,200 mg does not increase the risk of atherosclerotic vascular disease in elderly women (13).

In summary, the total intake of calcium (diet plus supplements) should not exceed 1,500 mg/day because of the possibility of such adverse effects.

Vitamin D

Vitamin D deficiency is common and supplementation is essential for the maintenance of bone and muscle strength. Vitamin D status is assessed by measurement of its major circulating metabolite, 25-hydroxyvitamin D or 25-(OH) D, with the minimum desirable 30 ng/mL (75 nmol/L) (14,15). Many patients require supplements of vitamin D, 2,000 IU daily or more, to achieve this level. The Endocrine Society Task Force, in July 2011, published guidelines for the evaluation, treatment, and prevention of vitamin D deficiency (14). Based on these guidelines, patients with confirmed vitamin D deficiency should be treated with 50,000 IU of vitamin D2 weekly for 8 weeks, followed by maintenance therapy of 50,000 IU every other week or 1,500–2,000 IU daily to achieve and maintain a blood level of 25-(OH) D above 30 ng/mL (75 nmol/L). It is important to use the available expert recommendations in conjunction with clinical judgment to determine the proper vitamin D requirement for any given patient. For example, obese patients, patients with malabsorption, and patients on medications affecting vitamin D metabolism may require higher doses of vitamin D to maintain a normal 25-(OH) D level. A repeat 25-(OH) D level should be obtained approximately 3 months after initiating therapy in patients being treated for vitamin D deficiency to assure obtaining the goal serum 25-(OH) D level. Based on the result, the dose of vitamin D may require further adjustment and additional measurements of 25-(OH) D.

Excessive vitamin D, especially combined with calcium supplementation, may cause hypercalcemia, hypercalciuria, and kidney stones. High-dose vitamin D (300,000 to 500,000 units) administered once yearly is not recommended due to an increase in the risk of falls and fracture (16,17). Furthermore, chronically high levels of 25-(OH) D (exceeding 50 ng/mL [125 nmol/L]) have been found in some association studies to be linked to a modest increase in the risk of some cancers (such as pancreatic) and all-cause mortality (18–20).

Bisphosphonates

Bisphosphonates reduce osteoclastic bone resorption by entering the osteoclast, causing loss of resorptive function and accelerating osteoclast apoptosis. Alendronate was the first bisphosphonate approved by the Food and Drug Administration (FDA) in 1995 for the treatment of osteoporosis, followed by risedronate in 1998, zoledronic acid in 2001, and ibandronate in 2005. Approval of bisphosphonates in the United States was based on studies of 3 to 4 years' duration, although some of these studies have been extended, with zoledronic acid, risedronate, and alendronate suggesting efficacy for up to 6 years, 7 years, and 10 years, respectively (21–24).

Gastrointestinal side effects have been the primary concern for patients taking oral bisphosphonates, which may irritate the esophagus and cause reflux, esophagitis, or esophageal ulcers. The incidence of these side effects is low if proper instructions for administration are followed. Bisphosphonates should not be given orally to patients who cannot remain upright, who have active upper gastrointestinal symptoms, or have delayed esophageal emptying such as in patients with strictures, achalasia, or severe dysmotility.

Intravenous (IV) bisphosphonates are often associated with an acute-phase reaction within 24 to 72 hours of the infusion, characterized by fever, myalgias, and arthralgias (25–27). Treatment with antipyretic agents generally improves the symptoms, and these rarely recur with subsequent infusions.

Hypocalcemia may occur with bisphosphonate use but is usually mild and not clinically important except in patients with hypoparathyroidism, calcium deficiency, or vitamin D deficiency (28). Disturbances of mineral metabolism should be corrected before initiating bisphosphonate therapy.

In terms of renal safety, bisphosphonates appear to be safe and effective in individuals with mild or moderate renal impairment and no dosage adjustment is recommended for these patients. It also appears that the risk of kidney damage in patients receiving IV bisphosphonates is very small and can be reduced further by adequate hydration and the use of longer infusion times. However, there is a dearth of data on use of bisphosphonates in patients with severe renal impairment and in end-stage renal disease (ESRD) (29). Despite the lack of evidence regarding the use of bisphosphonates in patients with chronic kidney disease (CKD) stage 5 (eGFR <15mL/min), one approach based on the known pharmacokinetics of bisphosphonates in subjects with normal renal function (30) suggests treating patients suffering fragility fractures with half the usual dose of bisphosphonates for up to 3 years, only after the diagnosis of osteoporosis is confirmed by a bone biopsy, because patients with ESRD may have fractures due to other forms of metabolic bone disease, such as osteomalacia or adynamic bone disease, for which bisphosphonate use is contraindicated (29,31).

Cases of severe musculoskeletal pain (bone, joint, and/or muscle pain) in adults on bisphosphonates have been reported to the FDA (32). In this series of 117 cases, pain was not isolated to a particular anatomical site and could occur at any time after starting bisphosphonate therapy. Some patients experienced immediate improvement in their symptoms after discontinuation of the offending drug, although for most patients the improvement was gradual or partial. The frequency and mechanism for this adverse effect are not known. Likewise, there is no evidence supporting a causal relationship between this side effect and bisphosphonate use.

In terms of long-term safety, concerns about 2 uncommon but possibly time-related adverse events have emerged: osteonecrosis of the jaw (ONJ) and atypical femur fractures (AFF) (33,34).

ONJ is defined as exposed necrotic bone in the maxillofacial region, not healing after 8 weeks in patients with no history of craniofacial radiation. ONJ appears as areas of exposed yellow-white hard bone with smooth or ragged borders and can be associated with pain, swelling, paresthesias, suppuration, soft tissue ulceration, intra- or extraoral sinus tracks, and loosening of teeth. This can occur spontaneously but is generally associated with invasive dental procedures such as tooth extraction. ONJ has been described in patients receiving chronic bisphosphonate therapy (23) but appears to be much more common in cancer patients receiving bisphosphonates in 10–12 times higher doses than those used to treat osteoporosis (35). In patients already receiving oral bisphosphonates, there is concern for patients scheduled for invasive dental procedures that involve the jaw, such as extractions or implants. Guidelines for oral surgeons have also been published by the American Association of Oral and Maxillofacial Surgeons (36), who suggest performing dentoalveolar surgery as usual in patients who have been treated with oral bisphosphonates for less than 3 years, and to discontinue the oral bisphosphonate for 3 months prior to performing the dental surgery if a patient has been treated for more than 3 years, aiming to restart it when the bone has healed. However, there is no evidence to support that this would lower ONJ risk, especially since bisphosphonates stay in bone for years. In fact, the most recent guidelines from the American Dental Association state that the benefit provided by antiresorptive therapy outweighs the low risk of developing osteonecrosis of the jaw, and that discontinuing bisphosphonate therapy may not lower the risk but may have a negative effect on low bone mass treatment outcomes (37). Useful information for patients is also available on the ADA Web site (http://www.ada.org) (37,38).

AFF are thought to be stress fractures that are frequently bilateral. These are typically associated with minimal or no trauma and often present with prodromal pain in the region of the fracture (39,40). These fractures had been described in patients who have not received any treatment for osteoporosis. A case-control study found that longer use of bisphosphonates (5–9 years) was associated with a greater risk of atypical fractures (OR 117, 95% CI 34–402) compared with shorter use (<2 years) (OR 35, 95% CI 10–124) (41). A 2013 systematic review and meta-analysis of 11 published studies examining the association of bisphosphonates with AFF showed that bisphosphonate exposure was associated with an increased risk of AFF with an adjusted RR of 1.70 (95% CI 1.22–2.37) (42). The FDA currently recommends that bisphosphonate-users with new-onset groin or thigh pain be further evaluated (43). Conventional radiography is usually the initial imaging procedure of choice, followed by magnetic resonance imaging (MRI) or bone scintigraphy if clinical suspicion is high and conventional radiography is unrevealing. In patients confirmed to have an atypical fracture, antiresorptive medications should be discontinued and these fractures should be reported. A high index of suspicion for a contralateral fracture should be maintained in patients with such fractures.

No causal relationship has been established between prolonged bisphosphonate exposure and either of these outcomes. Even though the risks of ONJ and AFF may increase after 5 years of bisphosphonate therapy, the likelihood remains low. The FDA suggests reevaluation of the need for continuing bisphosphonate therapy beyond 3 to 5 years in individual patients (44).

Denosumab

Denosumab is a fully human monoclonal antibody to the receptor activator of nuclear factor-kappa B ligand (RANKL), an osteoclast differentiating factor. It inhibits osteoclast formation resulting in decreased bone resorption (45). Denosumab was approved by the FDA in 2010 for the treatment of postmenopausal women with osteoporosis. It is administered as a subcutaneous injection every 6 months. Six years of denosumab exposure in postmenopausal women with osteoporosis in the Fracture Reduction Evaluation of Denosumab in Osteoporosis Every 6 Months (FREEDOM) Extension trial was associated with a favorable risk/benefit profile (46). Denosumab was also generally safe and well-tolerated after 8 years of exposure in an open-label phase 2 clinical trial (47).

The FDA label includes a caution about the possibility of hypocalcemia after denosumab administration, and there have been postmarketing reports of severe, symptomatic hypocalcemia after denosumab injection (48–51). Although all antiresorptive agents may induce a small and transient hypocalcemic effect after administration, clinically significant hypocalcemia is not typically observed in patients with adequate calcium and vitamin D intake. Thus, it is important to ensure that patients maintain an adequate amount of calcium and vitamin D supplementation, especially with conditions that predispose to hypocalcemia, such as CKD or malabsorption syndromes. Denosumab should not be given to patients with preexisting hypocalcemia until it is corrected. In the FREEDOM trial discussed previously, there was no difference in reported hypocalcemia between the treated and the placebo groups either in the registration (first 3 years: 3 cases in the placebo group and none with denosumab) or the extension trial (2 more years).

The major safety concerns with denosumab have been the potential risks for infections and malignancy because of the ubiquitous presence of RANKL throughout many tissues, including cells of the immune system. In the FREEDOM trial discussed previously, there was no increase in the overall risk of infection, or cancer; however, serious adverse events of cutaneous infections, namely cellulitis and erysipelas, occurred in 1 (<0.1%) placebo subject and 12 (0.3%) denosumab subjects (P = 0.002). Dermatological adverse events such as dermatitis, eczema, and rashes also occurred at a significantly higher rate in the treated versus placebo groups (10.8% vs 8.2%, $P < 0.0001$) (52). A detailed post hoc analysis of this trial examining the incidence and types of infections revealed that serious adverse events of infections (namely skin, gastrointestinal, ear, urinary, and cardiac valvular infections) were numerically higher in the denosumab group, although the number of events was small and the differences between groups were not statistically significant (53).

The 3-year FREEDOM trial reported no cases of ONJ in either the denosumab or placebo group. There have been 8 adjudicated cases of ONJ in the FREEDOM extension trial in both the cross-over group and long-term group (54). Good oral hygiene and regular dental visits should be recommended for everyone.

In addition, 2 cases of atypical subtrochanteric femur fractures have been reported in the denosumab osteoporosis clinical trials (55). Further studies of long-term treatment with denosumab are needed to evaluate the possible occurrence of atypical fractures with the use of this agent.

Teriparatide

In contrast to the other available therapies for osteoporosis, all of which reduce bone resorption, teriparatide (recombinant form of parathyroid hormone) is an anabolic agent that stimulates bone remodeling, preferentially increasing bone formation over resorption. Teriparatide was approved by the FDA in 2002 for the treatment of postmenopausal women with osteoporosis. It is administered as a subcutaneous injection daily.

Hypercalcemia and hypercalciuria are the 2 most common short-term side effects of parathyroid hormone treatment. Following once-daily subcutaneous administration, teriparatide produces a modest but transient increase in serum calcium, consistent with the known effects of endogenous PTH on mineral metabolism. The excursion in serum calcium is brief, due to the short length of time that teriparatide concentrations are elevated (56). Significant hypercalcemia rarely occurs, and persistent hypercalcemia after discontinuation of therapy should lead to an evaluation for other causes. There are small increases from baseline in urinary calcium excretion, which are clinically not significant for the majority of patients, although it may be prudent to consider urinary calcium monitoring for patients with a history of nephrolithiasis (57).

The most theoretically worrisome long-term adverse event with teriparatide use is the development of osteosarcoma. There have been only 3 cases of osteosarcoma reported in over 1 million subjects who have received teriparatide since 2002, which is lower than epidemiological expectations (58,59). Furthermore, in a recent postmarketing study where 549 of 1,448 patients diagnosed with osteosarcoma in the United States between 2003 and 2009 were interviewed, none reported a history of teriparatide use (60). Nevertheless, the drug carries a "black box warning" and is contraindicated in patients with existing risk factors for osteosarcoma, including Paget's disease of bone, prior skeletal radiation, and children with open epiphyses. The FDA recommends that teriparatide therapy be limited to 2 years in a lifetime.

WORK-UP AND MANAGEMENT OF THE ACUTE FRAGILITY FRACTURE

Osteoporotic fractures (fragility fractures, low-trauma fractures) are those occurring from a fall from a standing height or less, without major trauma. Vertebral compression fractures are the most common type of osteoporotic fracture. About two thirds of vertebral fractures are asymptomatic and are diagnosed as an incidental finding on imaging. In some patients, the presence of vertebral fractures may become apparent because of height loss or kyphosis. In patients who have a symptomatic vertebral fracture, there is often no history of preceding trauma. Typically patients present with acute back pain after bending, coughing, or lifting. The pain from a vertebral compression fracture may be sharp or dull and often radiates bilaterally into the anterior abdomen in the distribution of contiguous nerve routes. Sitting and movement aggravate the discomfort. Acute episodes of pain usually resolve after 4 to 6 weeks, but mild pain may persist for up to 3 months (61). In some patients, the pain may persist beyond 3 months, sometimes due to paraspinal spasm. However, severe back pain that persists longer should raise the question of more fractures or another diagnosis (eg, osteomalacia, infections, or malignancy). Posterior wedging is uncommon and may indicate an underlying destructive lesion. A solitary vertebral fracture in vertebrae higher than T4 is also unusual and should prompt further evaluation. The patient should be assessed for neurological findings, which may indicate fracture fragments in the spinal canal that demand surgical intervention. A bone density scan should be performed on a nonurgent basis if not already done.

Initial laboratory testing for osteoporosis should include the following:

- Complete (full) blood count
- Complete metabolic panel, including creatinine, calcium, phosphorus, alkaline phosphatase, and liver function tests
- 25-OH D to evaluate for vitamin D deficiency
- Testosterone in men to test for hypogonadism
- 24-hour urine calcium, sodium, and creatinine to check for calcium malabsorption or hypercalciuria

This work-up identifies about 90% of occult disorders at a reasonable cost (62). Patients who have abnormalities on the initial laboratory testing or who have suspicious findings on history and physical examination may also require additional laboratory tests (63).

Initial management of osteoporotic vertebral compression fractures should include pain control—with resumption of activity as quickly as possible—and physical therapy. Acute pain requires nonopioid or opioid analgesics and may require some limitation of activity. Options include acetaminophen (paracetamol), nonsteroidal anti-inflammatory medications, or opioids combined with acetaminophen (paracetamol). A short course of calcitonin, 200 units (1 spray) once daily alternating nostrils, can be a useful adjunct to traditional analgesics in the acute setting for patients who do not have adequate pain relief with oral analgesics.

Treatment should be aimed at the underlying disease, and, with osteoporosis, medications such as bisphosphonates, denosumab, or teriparatide should be initiated. Muscle relaxants, back braces, vertebroplasty, and/or kyphoplasty are not recommended for the routine management of acute pain due to osteoporotic compression fractures (64–66). The American Academy of Orthopedic Surgeons recommends against vertebroplasty and provides only a limited recommendation for kyphoplasty as an option for neurologically intact patients due to the quality of the evidence available (67). These modalities have also not been adequately evaluated for the treatment of chronic pain. Exercise has beneficial effects on BMD and an exercise program can be initiated when pain has diminished.

Hip fractures are the most devastating osteoporotic fractures and are associated with increased morbidity and mortality. Initial care of the patient with a hip fracture consists primarily of providing adequate analgesia and consulting an orthopedic surgeon. Because the occurrence of fall and fracture often signals underlying ill health, a comprehensive multidisciplinary approach is required from presentation to subsequent follow-up, including the transition from hospital to community.

CONCLUSIONS

There are several treatment options for osteoporosis with different side effect profiles and safety concerns. The evaluation of an osteoporotic compression fracture includes assessment for neurological findings and laboratory evaluation to assess for causes of secondary osteoporosis. Oral analgesics are first-line therapy for the relief of acute pain due to vertebral compression fractures. Calcitonin may be a useful adjunct. Muscle relaxants, back braces, vertebroplasty, and/or kyphoplasty are not recommended for the routine management of acute pain due to osteoporotic compression fractures. Osteoporosis therapy should be initiated to decrease the risk of new fractures.

ACKNOWLEDGMENTS

NBW has received honoraria from Amgen and Merck and consulting fees from the following: AbbVie, Amarin, Amgen, Bristol-Meyers Squibb, Corcept, Endo, Imagepace, Janssen, Lilly, Merck, Novartis, Noven, Pfizer/Wyeth, Radius, and Sanofi-Aventis. He has also received research report from Merck and NPS Pharmaceuticals. DLD has nothing to disclose.

REFERENCES

1. Osteoporosis prevention, diagnosis, and therapy. *NIH Consens Statement.* 2000;17:1–45.
2. http://www.surgeongeneral.gov/library/reports/bonehealth/full_report.pdf.
3. **Diab DL, Watts NB.** Postmenopausal osteoporosis. *Curr Opin Endocrinol Diabetes Obes.* 2013;20(6):501–509.
4. **Tang BM, Eslick GD, Nowson C, et al.** Use of calcium or calcium in combination with vitamin D supplementation to prevent fractures and bone loss in people aged 50 years and older: a meta-analysis. *Lancet.* 2007; 370:657–666.
5. **Verbrugge FH, Gielen E, Milisen K, Boonen S.** Who should receive calcium and vitamin D supplementation? *Age Ageing.* 2012;41:576–580.
6. **Curhan GC, Willett WC, Speizer FE, et al.** Comparison of dietary calcium with supplemental calcium and other nutrients as factors affecting the risk for kidney stones in women. *Ann Intern Med.* 1997;126: 497–504.
7. **Jackson RD, LaCroix AZ, Gass M, et al.** Calcium plus vitamin D supplementation and the risk of fractures. *N Engl J Med.* 2006;354:669–683.
8. **Hsia J, Heiss G, Ren H, et al.** Calcium/vitamin D supplementation and cardiovascular events. *Circulation.* 2007;115:846–854.
9. **Bolland MJ, Avenell A, Baron JA, et al.** Effect of calcium supplements on risk of myocardial infarction and cardiovascular events: meta-analysis. *BMJ.* 2010;341:c3691.
10. **Bolland MJ, Grey A, Avenell A.** et al. Calcium supplements with or without vitamin D and risk of cardiovascular events: reanalysis of the Women's Health Initiative limited access dataset and meta-analysis. *BMJ.* 2011;342:d2040.
11. **Xiao Q, Murphy RA, Houston DK, et al.** Dietary and supplemental calcium intake and cardiovascular disease mortality: the National Institutes of Health-AARP diet and health study. *JAMA Intern Med.* 2013;173:639–646.
12. **Van Hemelrijck M, Michaelsson K, Linseisen J, Rohrmann S.** Calcium intake and serum concentration in relation to risk of cardiovascular death in NHANES III. *PLoS One.* 2013;8:e61037.
13. **Lewis JR, Calver J, Zhu K, et al.** Calcium supplementation and the risks of atherosclerotic vascular disease in older women: results of a 5-year RCT and a 4.5-year follow-up. *J Bone Miner Res.* 2011;26:35–41.
14. **Holick MF, Binkley NC, Bischoff-Ferrari HA, et al.** Evaluation, treatment, and prevention of vitamin D deficiency: an Endocrine Society Clinical Practice Guideline. *J Clin Endocrinol Metab.* 2011; 96:1911–1930.
15. **Holick MF, Binkley NC, Bischoff-Ferrari HA, et al.** Guidelines for preventing and treating vitamin D deficiency and insufficiency revisited. *J Clin Endocrinol Metab.* 2012;97:1153–1158.
16. **Sanders KM, Stuart AL, Williamson EJ, et al.** Annual high-dose oral vitamin D and falls and fractures in older women: a randomized controlled trial. *JAMA.* 2010;303:1815–1822.
17. **Smith H, Anderson F, Raphael H, et al.** Effect of annual intramuscular vitamin D on fracture risk in elderly men and women—a population-based, randomized, double-blind, placebo-controlled trial. *Rheumatology (Oxford).* 2007;46:1852–1857.
18. **Helzlsouer KJ.** Overview of the Cohort Consortium Vitamin D Pooling Project of Rarer Cancers. *Am J Epidemiol.* 2010;172:4–9.
19. **Stolzenberg-Solomon RZ, Jacobs EJ, Arslan AA, et al.** Circulating 25-hydroxyvitamin D and risk of pancreatic cancer: Cohort Consortium Vitamin D Pooling Project of Rarer Cancers. *Am J Epidemiol.* 2010;172:81–93.
20. **Melamed ML, Michos ED, Post W, Astor B.** 25-hydroxyvitamin D levels and the risk of mortality in the general population. *Arch Intern Med.* 2008;168:1629–1637.
21. **Black DM, Reid IR, Boonen S, et al.** The effect of 3 versus 6 years of zoledronic acid treatment of osteoporosis: a randomized extension to the HORIZON-Pivotal Fracture Trial (PFT). *J Bone Miner Res.* 2012;27:243–254.
22. **Mellstrom DD, Sorensen OH, Goemaere S, et al.** Seven years of treatment with risedronate in women with postmenopausal osteoporosis. *Calcif Tissue Int.* 2004;75:462–468.
23. **Black DM, Schwartz AV, Ensrud KE, et al.** Effects of continuing or stopping alendronate after 5 years of treatment: the Fracture Intervention Trial Long-term Extension (FLEX): a randomized trial. *JAMA.* 2006;296:2927–2938.
24. **Schwartz AV, Bauer DC, Cummings SR, et al.** Efficacy of continued alendronate for fractures in women with and without prevalent vertebral fracture: the FLEX trial. *J Bone Miner Res.* 2010;25:976–982.
25. **Adami S, Bhalla AK, Dorizzi R, et al.** The acute phase response after bisphosphonate administration. *Calcif Tissue Int.* 1987;41:326–331.
26. **Gallacher SJ, Ralston SH, Patel U, Boyle IT.** Side-effects of pamidronate. *Lancet.* 1989;2:42–43.
27. **Zojer N, Keck AV, Pecherstorfer M.** Comparative tolerability of drug therapies for hypercalcaemia of malignancy. *Drug Safety.* 1999;21(5):389–406.
28. **Maalouf NM, Heller HJ, Odvina CV, Kim PJ, Sakhaee K.** Bisphosphonate-induced hypocalcemia: report of 3 cases and review of literature. *Endocrine Practice.* 2006;12:48–53.
29. **Miller PD.** Diagnosis and treatment of osteoporosis in chronic renal disease. *Semin Nephrol.* 2009;29:144–155.
30. **Miller PD.** Is there a role for bisphosphonates in chronic kidney disease? *Semin Dial.* 2007;20:186–190.
31. **Miller PD.** The role of bone biopsy in patients with chronic renal failure. *Clin J Am Soc Nephrol.* 2008; 3(suppl 3):S140–S150.
32. **Wysowski DK, Chang JT.** Alendronate and risedronate: reports of severe bone, joint, and muscle pain. *Arch Intern Med.* 2005;165:346–347.
33. **Diab DL, Watts NB.** Bisphosphonates in the treatment of osteoporosis. *Endocrinol Metab Clin North Am.* 2012;41:487–506.
34. **Watts NB, Diab DL.** Long-term use of bisphosphonates in osteoporosis. *J Clin Endocrinol Metab.* 2010; 95:1555–1565.

35. **Khosla S, Burr D, Cauley J, et al.** Bisphosphonate-associated osteonecrosis of the jaw: report of a task force of the American Society for Bone and Mineral Research. *J Bone Miner Res.* 2007;22:1479–1491.
36. American Association of Oral and Maxillofacial Surgeons position paper on bisphosphonate-related osteonecrosis of the jaws. *J Oral Maxillofac Surg.* 2007;65:369–376.
37. **Hellstein JW, Adler RA, Edwards B, et al.** Managing the care of patients receiving antiresorptive therapy for prevention and treatment of osteoporosis: executive summary of recommendations from the American Dental Association Council on Scientific Affairs. *J Am Dent Assoc.* 2011;142:1243–1251.
38. Osteoporosis medications and your dental health. *J Am Dent Assoc.* 2011;142:1320.
39. **Dell RM, Adams AL, Greene DF, et al.** Incidence of atypical nontraumatic diaphyseal fractures of the femur. *J Bone Miner Res.* 2012;27:2544–2550.
40. **Shane E, Ebeling PR, Abrahamsen B, et al.** Atypical subtrochanteric and diaphyseal femoral fractures: second report of a task force of the American Society for Bone and Mineral Research. *J Bone Miner Res.* 2014;29(1):1–23.
41. **Meier RP, Perneger TV, Stern R, et al.** Increasing occurrence of atypical femoral fractures associated with bisphosphonate use. *Arch Intern Med.* 2012; 172:930–936.
42. **Gedmintas L, Solomon DH, Kim SC.** Bisphosphonates and risk of subtrochanteric, femoral shaft, and atypical femur fracture: a systematic review and meta-analysis. *J Bone Miner Res.* 2013;28:1729–1737.
43. http://www.fda.gov/drugs/drugsafety/ucm229009.htm.
44. **Whitaker M, Guo J, Kehoe T, Benson G.** Bisphosphonates for osteoporosis—where do we go from here? *N Engl J Med.* 2012;366:2048–2051.
45. **Josse R, Khan A, Ngui D, Shapiro M.** Denosumab, a new pharmacotherapy option for postmenopausal osteoporosis. *Curr Med Res Opin.* 2013;29:205–216.
46. **Bone HG, Chapurlat R, Brandi ML, et al.** The effect of three or six years of denosumab exposure in women with postmenopausal osteoporosis: results from the FREEDOM extension. *J Clin Endocrinol Metab.* 2013;98:4483–4492.
47. **McClung MR, Lewiecki EM, Geller ML, et al.** Effect of denosumab on bone mineral density and biochemical markers of bone turnover: 8-year results of a phase 2 clinical trial. *Osteoporos Int.* 2013;24:227–235.
48. **Martin-Baez IM, Blanco-Garcia R, Alonso-Suarez M, et al.** Severe hypocalcaemia post-denosumab. *Nefrologia.* 2013;33:614–615.
49. **McLachlan JM, Marx GM, Bridgman M.** Severe symptomatic hypocalcaemia following a single dose of denosumab. *Med J Aust.* 2013;199:242–243.
50. **Okada N, Kawazoe K, Teraoka K, et al.** Identification of the risk factors associated with hypocalcemia induced by denosumab. *Biol Pharm Bull.* 2013;36(10):1622–1626.
51. **Ungprasert P, Cheungpasitporn W, Srivali N, et al.** Life-threatening hypocalcemia associated with denosumab in a patient with moderate renal insufficiency. *Am J Emerg Med.* 2013;31:756.e1–2.
52. **Cummings SR, San Martin J, McClung MR, et al.** Denosumab for prevention of fractures in postmenopausal women with osteoporosis. *N Engl J Med.* 2009;361:756–765.
53. **Watts NB, Roux C, Modlin JF, et al.** Infections in postmenopausal women with osteoporosis treated with denosumab or placebo: coincidence or causal association? *Osteoporos Int.* 2012;23:327–337.
54. **Diab DL, Watts NB.** Denosumab in osteoporosis. *Expert Opin Drug Saf.* 2014;13(2):247–253.
55. http://www.mhra.gov.uk/Safetyinformation/DrugSafetyUpdate/CON239411. Accessed August 1, 2013.
56. **Satterwhite J, Heathman M, Miller PD, et al.** Pharmacokinetics of teriparatide (rhPTH[1-34]) and calcium pharmacodynamics in postmenopausal women with osteoporosis. *Calcif Tissue Int.* 2010;87:485–492.
57. **Miller PD, Bilezikian JP, Diaz-Curiel M, et al.** Occurrence of hypercalciuria in patients with osteoporosis treated with teriparatide. *J Clin Endocrinol Metab.* 2007;92:3535–3541.
58. **Subbiah V, Madsen VS, Raymond AK, et al.** Of mice and men: divergent risks of teriparatide-induced osteosarcoma. *Osteoporos Int.* 2010;21:1041–1045.
59. **Cipriani C, Irani D, Bilezikian JP.** Safety of osteoanabolic therapy: a decade of experience. *J Bone Miner Res.* 2012;27:2419–2428.
60. **Andrews EB, Gilsenan AW, Midkiff K, et al.** The US postmarketing surveillance study of adult osteosarcoma and teriparatide: study design and findings from the first 7 years. *J Bone Miner Res.* 2012;27:2429–2437.
61. **Venmans A, Klazen CA, Lohle PN, et al.** Natural history of pain in patients with conservatively treated osteoporotic vertebral compression fractures: results from VERTOS II. *AJNR Am J Neuroradiol.* 2012;33:519–521.
62. **Tannenbaum C, Clark J, Schwartzman K, et al.** Yield of laboratory testing to identify secondary contributors to osteoporosis in otherwise healthy women. *J Clin Endocrinol Metab.* 2002;87:4431–4437.
63. **Diab D, Watts N.** Secondary osteoporosis: differential diagnosis and work-up. *Clin Obstet Gynec.* 2013; 56(4):686–693.
64. **Abudou M, Chen X, Kong X, Wu T.** Surgical versus non-surgical treatment for thoracolumbar burst fractures without neurological deficit. *Cochrane Database Syst Rev.* 2013;6:CD005079.
65. **Hoshino M, Tsujio T, Terai H, et al.** Impact of initial conservative treatment interventions on the outcomes of patients with osteoporotic vertebral fractures. *Spine (Phila Pa 1976).* 2013;38:E641–E648.
66. **Lee HM, Park SY, Lee SH, et al.** Comparative analysis of clinical outcomes in patients with osteoporotic vertebral compression fractures (OVCFs): conservative treatment versus balloon kyphoplasty. *Spine J.* 2012;12:998–1005.
67. http://www.aaos.org/research/guidelines/SCFguideline.pdf.

CHAPTER 22

Acute Medical Aspects Related to Paget's Disease of Bone

Ethel S Siris and Dorothy A Fink

ABSTRACT

Paget's disease is a localized disorder of bone remodeling that typically presents in both men and women after age 40 to 50 years and may continue to be an active, progressive process for the rest of an individual's life. The structural changes that occur with time result in a poorer quality bone that is prone to bone deformity or fracture. Paget's disease may be completely without symptoms at presentation, or it may be associated over time with a variety of complications, some of which require urgent or emergency management. The present chapter will focus on those complications that require immediate attention and treatment.

INTRODUCTION

Paget's disease is a localized disorder of bone remodeling that typically presents in both men and women after age 40 to 50 years and may continue to be an active, progressive process for the rest of an individual's life. It is initiated by excessive bone resorption caused by increased numbers of larger than normal osteoclasts. The increased bone resorption is subsequently coupled to secondary increases in new bone formation by apparently normal osteoblasts, but the new bone that is deposited at the previously resorbed sites is disorganized woven bone rather than neatly aligned lamellar bone and is thus less compact, taking up more space, and it has greater vascularity. Paget's disease may be found in a part of a single bone (monostotic disease) or in multiple bones (polyostotic disease). It is believed that once the condition declares itself to be present at specific skeletal sites it can progress within those bones but is unlikely to appear years later in previously unaffected bones. The structural changes that occur with time result in a poorer quality bone that is prone to bone deformity or fracture.

The localized increase in bone remodeling is reflected in elevations of bone turnover markers, such as the bone resorption marker serum C-telopeptide (CTX) and the bone formation marker total serum alkaline phosphatase (SAP). High turnover and increased blood flow are the basis for the increased uptake of radiotracers at pagetic sites noted on bone scans. However, neither the elevation of markers nor the increased uptake on a bone scan are specific for Paget's disease. The diagnosis should be made only when the characteristic changes seen on skeletal radiographs (and in some cases elaborated upon by magnetic resonance imaging [MRI] or computed tomography [CT] scanning) are found. These radiographic and imaging studies not only allow for a diagnosis, but help to characterize the causes of some of the complications of Paget's disease that may occur.

For example, during the osteolytic phase in the femur or tibia an advancing "blade of grass" or lytic wedge viewed on a radiograph may slowly progress along the length of the

Table 22-1. Emergencies in Paget's Disease

Orthopedic: new, severe bone pain from new or impending fracture
Oncological: new, severe bone pain from osteosarcoma, fibrosarcoma, or chondrosarcoma; benign giant cell tumor; or bone metastases from a primary cancer (eg, breast, prostate, lung)
Neurological: spinal cord compression (or vascular steal) syndrome; platybasia of the skull with basilar invagination and hydrocephalus or brain stem compression; cranial nerve compression syndromes
Metabolic: rare instances of hypercalcemia in very high turnover; polyostotic Paget's disease with immobilization
Cardiac: high-output cardiac failure in very high turnover; polyostotic Paget's disease

bone from one end, and there is the potential for fracture. After the osteoblastic phase fills in previously resorbed regions, the poor structure of the newly made bone subjects it to the potential for cortical thickening and bone enlargement, with subsequent bone deformity. Enlargement of the skull and bowing deformities of extremities are possible outcomes. Based upon the location of pagetic sites and the highly variable magnitude of the increase in bone remodeling as suggested by the levels of SAP and CTX, Paget's disease may be completely without symptoms at presentation, or it may be associated over time with a variety of complications, some of which require urgent or emergency management. A comprehensive review of Paget's disease of bone has recently been published (1). The present chapter will focus on those complications that require immediate attention and treatment (Table 22-1).

SEVERE BONE PAIN IN PERSONS WITH PAGET'S DISEASE

Severe Bone Pain That May Indicate Fracture or Impending Fracture

What patients perceive as pagetic bone pain may result from 1 or more of several causes, some of which pose acute, intermittent or chronic, nonemergency issues, and some of which are much more serious. Examples of nonemergency complaints include nonspecific aches and pains that may result from minor microfractures along the convex surfaces of bowed extremities, pain from arthritis at a major joint due to pagetic bone enlargement and/or deformity in 1 or both of the bones at that joint, headache or a band-like tightening in the skull in the setting of skull enlargement, or radiculopathy from nerve root compression by pagetic vertebrae in the lumbar spine.

However, severe new pain at a previously asymptomatic or minimally uncomfortable site of Paget's disease, with or without bone enlargement or deformity such as bowing, warrants immediate examination and imaging with radiographs to rule out fracture or impending fracture. If an X-ray is not conclusive but there is a high level of suspicion for a fracture, a CT scan should be performed, and orthopedic consultation is mandatory. The orthopedic treatment of a fracture through pagetic bone is more complex than that for normal or osteoporotic bone, and a skilled orthopedic surgeon with experience managing Paget's disease fractures—or the ability to consult with someone else who has more experience—is desirable (2). In medically untreated Paget's disease where the SAP is 2–3 or more times above the upper limit of normal, there is the potential for greater than normal bleeding at the time of a complete fracture and during an operation to internally fix the fractured bone. Thus, in some cases treatment with an infusion of 5 mg of zoledronic acid and a delay of a few days (ideally at least 3) before doing an open repair may be appropriate, if the repair can safely wait without posing other medical risks to the typically older patient. Impending fracture of a pagetic femur or tibia may sometimes require placement of orthopedic hardware to prevent a complete fracture, and the same issues regarding bleeding and bisphosphonate therapy would apply. Alternatively, medical management with an infusion of zoledronic acid and a period of non-weight bearing on an unoperated extremity, together with careful orthopedic follow-up, may be possible and safer.

A painful acute vertebral fracture at a site of Paget's disease is typically managed conservatively, with an MRI as indicated by the patient's presentation to confirm that the fracture is not causing neural entrapment. There is very little experience with kyphoplasty or vertebroplasty of a bone affected by Paget's disease (3), and it is difficult to know whether the procedure is safe and effective in this setting, especially if adjacent vertebrae also have pagetic features. If such a patient has active

Paget's disease with elevated markers of bone turnover, it may be prudent to offer an infusion of zoledronic acid to reduce vascularity. It is not proven that this will reduce pain, but it should reduce the high bone turnover and the associated increased vascularity at the site, restoring these features toward normal.

Severe Bone Pain Due to a Neoplastic Process

Bone destruction due to a neoplastic process in pagetic bone also presents with severe new pain typically at a previously quiescent site. In addition to plain radiographs, MRI scanning is critical because it will typically reveal a soft tissue mass adjacent to the affected bone. CT scanning may also be useful in some cases to evaluate the status of the bone that is being eroded.

Neoplastic changes within bone affected by Paget's disease can include any of several types of lesions. Rarely, likely in less than 1% of patients, pagetic bone is the site of an osteosarcoma, a serious malignancy with a very poor prognosis (4). Fibrosarcoma and chondrosarcoma have also been described at pagetic sites. Osteosarcoma is managed by oncologists and orthopedic oncologic surgeons with aggressive surgery and chemotherapy, sometimes adding radiation therapy even though these lesions are relatively radio-resistant. Early metastasis to the lungs is a common complication, and the condition is often fatal within a year.

A second type of neoplasm arising at a site of Paget's disease is a benign giant cell tumor, a highly vascular lesion consisting of osteoclast-like giant cells that cause aggressive bone destruction at the localized site. These tumors are relatively rare single lesions that even more uncommonly can present over time at multiple sites within more than one pagetic bone. Often initially thought to be osteosarcoma until a biopsy correctly makes the diagnosis, these benign giant cell tumors usually shrink away dramatically and fairly quickly after treatment with high doses of dexamethasone in the range of 16–24 mg per day in divided doses (5). Prolonged use of dexamethasone if the tumor recurs locally after periods of remission has led to some of the problems associated with iatrogenic Cushing's syndrome, and other approaches to management have been attempted. In our own clinical experience a course of thalidomide, 100 mg per day for up to several months, was effective in stopping the cycle of recurrence after remission of a large, locally destructive giant cell tumor in a pagetic spine, although the year-long course of treatment led to development of peripheral neuropathy. A second patient with a periodically recurring giant cell tumor, also in the spine, appears to be in a prolonged remission while receiving denosumab, currently 60 mg every 4–5 months. There is no specific protocol for use of glucocorticoids, thalidomide, or denosumab in patients with Paget's disease-associated giant cell tumors; treatment is empirical, provided by an oncologist working closely with the patient's endocrinologist.

Finally, clinical experience has demonstrated that bones affected by Paget's disease may be sites of painful bone metastases from common primary tumors such as breast or prostate cancer or other solid tumors that metastasize to bone. Whether the heightened vascularity of metabolically active, high-turnover Paget's disease makes pagetic bone more susceptible to attracting tumor cells from distant primaries is unknown. In this situation, severe, acute bone pain is the presenting complaint, and it must be addressed with imaging studies such as an MRI and possibly biopsy to determine if a neoplasm is present. A bone scan, normally useful in locating sites of malignancy in cancer patients, will not be helpful if the patient's metastatic disease is at a site of Paget's disease, because the scan is going to be positive as a consequence of the pagetic change.

A metastasis from a distant primary may also manifest itself as an "ivory vertebra," a radio-dense vertebral body that could reflect a pagetic vertebra, an osteoblastic bone metastasis from a distant primary cancer, or a hemangioma. Paget's disease is most likely if the posterior elements as well as the vertebral body light up on a bone scan. Positron-emission tomography (PET) scans of sites of active Paget's disease display substantially less activity than what is seen when there is a malignant tumor at a site, and this may be helpful in differential diagnosis (6). A full patient work-up is needed to diagnose the cause of an ivory vertebra, including the patient's history, symptoms, and other clinical and radiographic or imaging findings.

Whether the destructive bone lesion found at a severely painful site of Paget's disease is osteosarcoma, benign giant cell tumor, or bone metastasis from a remote primary, help from an oncologist is critical, and an orthopedic surgeon is required in most cases to biopsy the bone for pathological confirmation of the tumor type. Treatment will depend on that diagnosis. In the case of metastatic disease at a pagetic site, cancer doses of zoledronic acid may be used. It has not been demonstrated that bisphosphonates have any benefit in giant cell tumors at pagetic sites, though they will offer benefit in the management of the patient's underlying Paget's disease. There is limited experience with bisphosphonates as a component of the management of osteosarcoma in Paget's disease, and there is not clear evidence that there is benefit. Pamidronate is sometimes used in nonpagetic osteosarcomas, but the use of that therapy for Paget's sarcoma should be made in conjunction with the managing oncologist or oncologic orthopedic surgeon.

NEUROLOGICAL COMPLICATIONS OF PAGET'S DISEASE

Pagetic bone tends to be larger than normal bone, and with its poorer structure, hypervascularity, and potential for deformity it may give rise to a number of neurological complications (7). Some of these represent medical emergencies which, while relatively uncommon, require timely diagnosis and prompt medical and neurosurgical intervention as required.

Paget's disease of the skull may be associated with headache or hearing loss, but extensive changes in the skull and facial bones after years of progressive abnormal bone remodeling with thickening, enlargement, and deformation of these bones can also lead to a variety of less common problems that may constitute emergencies. Cranial nerve palsies from narrowing of cranial nerve foramina can acutely affect cranial nerves I, II, V, VII, and VIII. Flattening of the skull base, termed platybasia, can produce basilar invagination that uncommonly results in acute compression symptoms referable to the brain stem. Hydrocephalus can result when basilar invagination leads to obstruction of cerebrospinal fluid flow, presenting as ataxia, dementia, and urinary incontinence, and even more rarely with symptoms of parkinsonism (8).

Imaging studies of the brain are needed to characterize the process causing the symptoms, and urgent neurological and neurosurgical consultations are mandatory. In some cases, direct compression of neural tissue by thickened and deformed pagetic bone is the primary problem, in which case surgical decompression typically after acute use of high-dose glucocorticoids—at the discretion of the neurologist/neurosurgeon—will be necessary, if feasible. Hydrocephalus may be relieved through the placement of a ventricular shunt, a relatively less invasive procedure. Intravenous zoledronic acid or pamidronate should probably be empirical treatment prior to surgery. Because high-turnover pagetic bone is highly vascular, and vascular steal syndromes promote ischemia in neural structures as blood flow increases in the adjacent bone, it is reasonable to use a potent intravenous bisphosphonate such as pamidronate or zoledronic acid or possibly calcitonin if a bisphosphonate cannot be used in these circumstances. By reducing elevated bone resorption fairly quickly with a subsequent reduction in elevated formation it is possible to reduce the degree of blood flow through the pagetic bone and minimize the vascular steal phenomenon. In some cases vascular steal and not direct bony compression is causal, in which case the primary treatment would be the intravenous bisphosphonate.

For certain cranial nerve syndromes such as trigeminal neuralgia or hemi-facial spasm, carbamazepine has been described to be useful, and surgical decompression has been used successfully to alleviate facial nerve palsy (7).

Paget's disease of the vertebral bodies can be a part of the basis for spinal stenosis or nerve root compression in the lumbar spine, though this is usually a chronic nonemergent problem, managed with zoledronic acid and, if it is needed and likely to help, with surgery. Concomitant osteoarthritic changes often contribute to the problem, and the degree to which the pagetic changes causing enlarged vertebral bodies or pagetic vertebral fracture play a role in lumbar stenosis can be challenging to discern. In cases of lumbar stenosis, bisphosphonate therapy is most likely to be effective when there is high turnover and less likely to help if there is very minimal increased turnover.

Subacute or acute spinal cord compression, typically in the thoracic spine, with acute or subacute loss of motor function, is a much rarer but very serious complication that constitutes an emergency. How much of the syndrome is a result of direct pagetic bony impingement on neural structures in the thoracic area, where the spinal canal is narrow, and how much results from vascular steal can be difficult to know, even with excellent imaging. Although neurosurgical decompression has been recommended by some for acute spinal cord compression (7), experience at our institution has indicated that aggressive use of a short course of high-dose dexamethasone and immediate treatment with pamidronate or zoledronic acid—particularly when indices of turnover are high—may obviate the need for surgery.

HYPERCALCEMIA

When hypercalcemia is discovered in someone with Paget's disease, bone diagnostic testing is needed to determine if the cause is parathyroid mediated or nonparathyroid mediated; management will depend on the underlying cause. Primary hyperparathyroidism can certainly coexist with Paget's disease—and may make the pagetic process more metabolically active than it would be if parathyroid hormone (PTH) levels were normal. Clinically significant acute hypercalcemia is a very unusual complication of Paget's disease, but if a patient with polyostotic Paget's disease and very high baseline bone turnover is immobilized for some reason, such as bed rest following an illness, it may occur. With immobilization the elevated bone resorption continues and may even increase, while bone formation, previously well coupled to resorption, decreases, and hypercalcemia can develop. As with other forms of acute hypercalcemia, serum PTH should be measured, hydration initiated, and intravenous zoledronic acid, 4 or 5 mg, can be given as required.

HIGH-OUTPUT CARDIAC FAILURE

Patients with polyostotic Paget's disease and current levels of high turnover have the potential for an increased vascularity in the bone, as has been described earlier, and in some cases have been shown to have increases in cardiac output as a consequence. An echocardiographic study described lower peripheral vascular resistance and higher cardiac stroke volume in patients with Paget's disease than in controls, especially in those with more extensive bone disease and evidence of higher turnover (9). Given that Paget's disease predominantly affects older individuals who may have underlying cardiovascular disease, a high-output state may be detrimental. Thus, if a patient with Paget's disease experiences congestive heart failure, an evaluation of the possibility that high bone turnover is contributing to the condition is needed. In addition to standard medical management of the cardiac problem, zoledronic acid should be administered as needed to manage the Paget's disease process.

ACKNOWLEDGMENTS

The authors have nothing to disclose.

REFERENCES

1. **Siris ES, Roodman GD.** Paget's disease of bone. In: Rosen CJ, ed. *Primer on the Metabolic Bone Diseases and Disorders of Mineral Metabolism.* 8th ed. Washington DC: American Society for Bone and Mineral Research; 2013:659–668.
2. **Parvizi J, Klein GR, Sim FH.** Surgical management of Paget's disease of bone. *J Bone Miner Res.* 2006;21(suppl 2):75–82.
3. **Pedicelli A, Papacci F, Leone A, et al.** Vertebroplasty for symptomatic monostotic Paget disease. *J Vasc Interven Radiol.* 2011;22(3):400–403.
4. **Hansen MF, Seton M, Merchant A.** Osteosarcoma in Paget's disease of bone. *J Bone Miner Res.* 2006;21(suppl 2):P58–P63.
5. **Jacobs TP, Michelsen J, Polay JS, D'Adamo AC, Canfield RE.** Giant cell tumor in Paget's disease of bone: familial and geographic clustering. *Cancer.* 1979;44(2):742–747.
6. **Sundaram M.** Imaging of Paget's disease and fibrous dysplasia of bone. *J Bone Miner Res.* 2006;21(suppl 2):28–30.
7. **McCloskey EV, Kanis JA.** Neurological complications of Paget's disease. *Clin Rev Bone Miner Metab.* 2002;1:135–143.
8. **Botez MI, Bertrand G, Leveille J, Marchand L.** Parkinsonism—dementia complex, hydrocephalus and Paget's disease. *Can J Neuro Sci.* [Le Journal Canadien des Sciences Neurologiques]. 1977;4(2): 139–142.
9. **Morales-Piga AA, Moya JL, Bachiller FJ, Munoz-Malo MT, Benavides J, Abraira V.** Assessment of cardiac function by echocardiography in Paget's disease of bone. *Clin Exp Rheumatol.* 2000;18(1):31–37.

CHAPTER 23

Acute Medical Aspects Related to Nephrolithiasis

Hasan Fattah and David S Goldfarb

ABSTRACT

The term "renal colic" is widely used to describe the pain resulting from passage of kidney stones through the urinary tract. This "colicky" renal pain is among the most common symptoms leading to emergency care presentation and often prompts extensive differential diagnosis and work-up. In this chapter we focus on the pathophysiology of renal colic, evaluation and acute management of kidney stones, and measures taken to prevent stone recurrence. We will briefly review appropriate surgical management of ureteral stones.

INTRODUCTION

The term "renal colic" is widely used to describe the pain resulting from passage of kidney stones through the urinary tract. The severe intermittent flank pain that radiates to the lower abdomen, genitalia, and groin may be associated with other gastroenterological or urological symptoms. This "colicky" renal pain is among the most common symptoms leading to emergency care presentation and often prompts extensive differential diagnosis and work-up.

In this chapter we focus on the pathophysiology of renal colic, evaluation and acute management of kidney stones, and measures taken to prevent stone recurrence. We will briefly review appropriate surgical management of ureteral stones.

EPIDEMIOLOGY

Kidney stones are a common diagnosis in the United States, affecting approximately 1 in 11 people at least once in their lifetime (1). Although kidney stones are becoming more frequent in women, there continues to be a gender prevalence difference, with a male: female ratio of about 2:1. Some data suggest women are catching up (2). Stones affect as many as 6%–15% of American men, and up to 7% of American women. This ratio appears to be consistent with that observed in other countries (3).

Moreover, epidemiological studies suggest an increasing prevalence worldwide, best demonstrated in the United States by the National Health and Nutrition Examination Survey (NHANES) III cohort (1988–1994 and 2007–2010) (2). This increasing prevalence is of uncertain etiology but may be attributable to changing dietary practices, increasing prevalence of diabetes and obesity, migration from cooler rural settings to warmer urban settings, and even global warming. These increasing prevalence rates are also associated with an increase in the cost of kidney stone management to an estimated $2.1 billion in 2000 in the United States (4).

Renal colic affects approximately 1.2 million people each year in the United States, accounts for about 1% of all emergency department (ED) visits, and is the main diagnosis for about 1% of all hospital admissions (5). A related estimate is that urolithiasis leads to approximately 4,000 ED visits each day (6).

PATHOPHYSIOLOGY

The pain of renal colic may simply be thought to arise from the muscular contraction of the ureter in response to the irritating, descending stone. In fact, the mechanism seems to be more complicated. The ureteral smooth muscle contracts in a peristalsis-like manner, which could expel the stone. However, prolonged isotonic contraction leads eventually to increased production of lactic acid, which irritates the submucosal nerve endings located in the upper urinary tract. Pain radiates to, and can be perceived in, any organ with similar innervation, such as the gastrointestinal organs and other components of the genitourinary system (7).

Calcium Stones

The most common crystal composition of kidney stones is calcium oxalate (8). About 20% of calcium stones are predominantly calcium phosphate (9). Although calcium stones are occasionally secondary to a systemic disease, in most occasions they are idiopathic. Calcium phosphate stones should lead to consideration of primary hyperparathyroidism, when serum calcium is at the high end of the normal range or high, and renal tubular acidosis.

Uric Acid Stones

Uric acid stones occur as the result of low urine pH; hyperuricosuria is much less important as a risk factor (10). Uric acid stones have recently been associated with the metabolic syndrome, obesity, and diabetes, all of which lead to impaired ammoniagenesis and acid urine (11). The growing prevalence of diabetes and metabolic syndrome, leading to increasing prevalence of uric acid stones, likely contributes to increasing kidney stone prevalence.

Struvite Stones

Struvite stones are composed of "triple phosphate" crystals composed of calcium ammonium magnesium phosphate. They result exclusively in the presence of very high urine pH ($\geq$7.5) as the result of urease-producing organisms, particularly species of *Proteus* (12). Struvite stones are more common in women because women are more often affected by urinary tract infections.

Cystine Stones

Cystinuria is a genetic cause of stones, accounting for 1% of all stones, and up to 7% of stones in children (13).

PATHOLOGY

New ideas about the origins of calcium stones have recently resulted from a series of examinations of renal pathology obtained from renal papillary biopsies during endoscopic stone management (14). Calcium oxalate kidney stones appear to grow over deposits of "Randall's plaque" on the papillary surface exposed to urine.

The most common urinary risk factor for calcium stones remains hypercalciuria. In most cases, the etiology of hypercalciuria remains unexplained and is usually termed idiopathic hypercalciuria. One possible mechanism by which hypercalciuria occurs and causes urinary supersaturation, promoting stone formation, is reduction of proximal tubular calcium reabsorption (15). The etiology of this reduced reabsorption is unclear but has been linked to effects of insulin.

DIFFERENTIAL DIAGNOSIS

Kidney stones are the most frequent cause of flank pain in the ED. A variety of other urinary tract and extrarenal causes should also be considered when evaluating a patient with acute flank pain. In 1 study, only 25%–60% of patients with flank pain who had a noncontrast computed tomography (CT) study proved to have a stone (16). The remainder, 20%–35%, had a nonurinary cause of pain, such as appendicitis, diverticulitis, unsuspected bowel obstruction, or twisted ovarian cyst.

RISK FACTORS

Evaluation of a patient with possible kidney stones should address several important risk factors. Table 23-1 addresses many of the risk factors for stones. Kidney stones in the general population clearly result from genetic influences. About 40% of patients with renal colic in an ED have a first degree relative with stones (17). Twin studies support this genetic effect in that monozygotic twin pairs are more than twice as likely to be concordant for the condition compared with dizygotic, or nonidentical twins (18). However, the genes accounting for this significant heritability remain obscure. Polymorphisms in candidate genes coding for proteins involved in calcium metabolism such as the vitamin D receptor or the calcium sensing receptor have been demonstrated to account for only small proportions of calcium stone formers (19,20).

Environmental risk factors include low urine volume due to ambient heat, and occupational factors that cause reduced fluid intake and result in a concentrated urine. Dietary factors have been extensively studied as well (21). Increased risk arises from higher amounts of animal protein ingestion and lower quantities of ingested fruits and vegetables (22). Prospective epidemiological studies have also shown that men and women with the highest dietary calcium ingestion (mostly via dairy products, but nondairy foods contribute as well) have the lowest associated prevalence of stones (23). This effect is attributed to the ability of ingested calcium to serve as a binder of oxalate in the intestinal lumen, diminishing its absorption into the blood and subsequent excretion by the kidneys. Obesity, hypertension, metabolic syndrome, and diabetes are now recognized as important risk factors as well (24).

MEDICATIONS

A number of medications have been implicated in stone formation. Calcium supplements are consistently associated with small absolute increases in stone incidence, even when the preferred calcium citrate is used (25). Whether administration of vitamin D is associated with an increased risk of stones is uncertain, and little evidence suggests that it is. We administered 50,000 units of vitamin D_2 to hypercalciuric calcium stone formers with 25-OH-vitamin D levels less than 30 ng/mL and found that the mean urine calcium excretion did not change after 8 weeks (26). However, some patients experienced increases; we recommend repeating 24-hour urine collections after supplementing vitamin D.

EMERGENCY CARE EVALUATION

Typical presenting symptoms of urolithiasis are intermittent colicky flank pain associated with

Table 23-1. Suggested Initial Evaluation of Kidney Stone Risk Factors in Emergency Care Setting

Past medical history: • Kidney diseases like polycystic kidney disease • Anatomical abnormalities such as medullary sponge kidney, horseshoe kidney • Metabolic disorders such as gout, hyperparathyroidism, renal tubular acidosis, diabetes, obesity • Genetic disorders such as cystinuria • Short bowel syndrome, inflammatory bowel disease, ileostomy • Sarcoidosis, urinary tract infections	Increased risk of calcium and uric acid stones
Spinal cord injury requiring intermittent catheterization, bladder dysfunction, neurogenic bladder	Increased risk for struvite stones
Dietary habits: • High protein intake • Low fluid intake • High sodium intake • Any vitamin C • Low dietary calcium intake	Increased risk of calcium stones
Positive family history	Increased risk of kidney stones
Medication use	Exclude medications associated with increased risk of kidney stones
Occupational history: athletes, hot environments, teachers	Increased risk of kidney stones

an inability to find a comfortable position. This is in contrast to the lack of movement of the typical patient with peritonitis. However, we have been fooled when these stereotypical responses are reversed. The pain may radiate to the lower abdomen or groin, and later into the genitalia. Often renal colic is associated with nausea and diaphoresis, and sometimes with vomiting. As the stone descends into the distal ureter, lower genitourinary symptoms such as dysuria, urinary frequency, or urgency occur as well.

Laboratory Studies

Laboratory evaluation should include a urinalysis, complete (full) blood count, and comprehensive metabolic profile. The most important use of the urinalysis is to rule out urinary tract infection. Infection of an obstructed urinary tract is a urological emergency and requires relief of obstruction before bacteremia supervenes (27). High urine pH ($\geq$6.5) is suggestive of renal tubular acidosis and may suggest urinary tract infection as well. Values $\geq$7.5 are most consistent with urease-producing organisms such as *Proteus* species, which may be causative for destructive struvite stones. Low urine pH suggests uric acid stones but is neither sensitive nor specific. Complete blood count is useful to detect leukocytosis, which is not expected with stones without urinary tract infection, but expected with peritonitis and other abdominal pathology. A comprehensive metabolic profile is most important to assess kidney function. Significant reductions in glomerular filtration rate (GFR) may result from bilateral obstruction, obstruction of a solitary kidney, or obstruction of 1 kidney in a patient with chronic kidney disease. Hypercalcemia can suggest primary hyperparathyroidism or sarcoidosis. Low serum bicarbonate may suggest metabolic acidosis (or respiratory alkalosis due to pain and anxiety) and could be the initial presentation of renal tubular acidosis.

Radiological Studies

When newly diagnosed renal colic is suspected due to nephrolithiasis, abdominal imaging is often indicated for diagnosis. Imaging may not be necessary in every case, however. It is important to note that many patients seek emergency care knowing full well what the correct diagnosis is, based on their previous history. Our strong recommendation is to trust them! Adequate pain relief for recurrent stones is a goal worth achieving, and while "drug-seeking behavior" is often suspected, our experience is that far more stone formers are treated inadequately and with suspicion, than opiate seekers are granted their wishes.

Unenhanced, noncontrast CT is clearly today the gold standard for the initial evaluation of kidney stones. It will also provide a thorough quantitation of total stone burden, and stone characteristics that aid in planning urological interventions if warranted later. An expectation of clinicians today should be analysis of the density of stones in Hounsfield units, because that value may be useful in determining kidney stone composition (28). Lower values are most consistent with uric acid stones and higher values with calcium stones, but significant overlap reduces the accuracy of this analysis.

MANAGEMENT

Acute management of renal colic consists of pain management and medical expulsive therapy (MET). We also offer an opinion regarding intravenous (IV) fluids. We briefly review the indications for admission, for urological consultation, and the choices of urological intervention.

Pain Control

Both IV narcotics and nonsteroidal anti-inflammatory drugs (NSAIDs) lead to pain relief, with NSAIDs leading, in some studies, to better outcomes with fewer adverse effects (29). Prostaglandin E2 may play an important role in the pathogenesis of pain by increasing the intrarenal pressure from disruption of vascular autoregulation, and by increasing ureteral muscular spasm. Hence, NSAIDs may be a perfect initial acute therapy in such patients.

Most recommendations, then, are to start with NSAIDs if the patient has no history of peptic ulcer disease, or acute or chronic eGFR decline less than 50 mL/min. The usual practice is parenteral administration of ketorolac for rapid achievement of pain control. If an opioid is used, we often prescribe combinations with acetaminophen (paracetamol), which will soon be unavailable in the United States. Meperidine is associated with more nausea, and sometimes

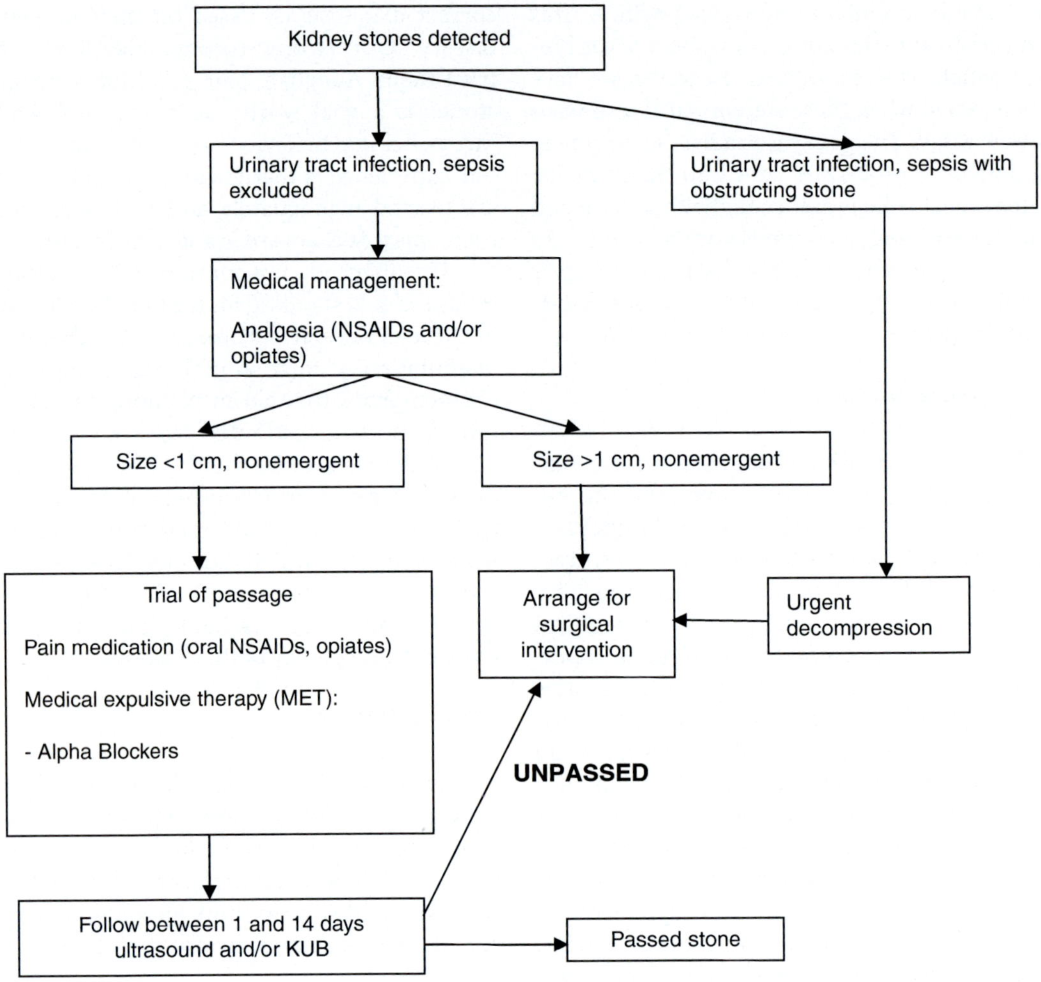

Figure 23-1. Suggested management of kidney stones causing renal colic.

vomiting, than morphine. Combining NSAIDs and opiates is also rational and may allow adverse effects of both to be avoided.

Medical Expulsive Therapy

No study has demonstrated that intravenous fluid administration has any benefit in promoting kidney stone passage. However, for various reasons it is unlikely that any significant proportion of IV fluids will find their way to the obstructed urinary tract. We suggest administration of normal saline or lactated Ringer solution only to patients with vomiting who are unable to take food or liquids by mouth.

Alpha blockers are the best studied agents for MET. The most commonly prescribed regimen currently is 0.4 mg tamsulosin each night. Occasional lowering of blood pressure occurs and normotensive patients should take it at bedtime. Larger stones and more proximal stones may be less likely to have their passage facilitated by alpha blockers. Stones less than or equal to 5 mm are more than likely to pass spontaneously, and 95% of the time will pass within 40 days, while stones greater than 7 mm will pass less than 20% of the time. MET is expected to influence these values.

Hospitalization

The most important indications for admission, and consultation with urology, are evidence of infection and renal failure. In patients with adequate pain control, effective relief of nausea and vomiting, the presence of 2 kidneys, and a normal mental status, prescription of MET and discharge is considered safe.

Urological Intervention

The decision to perform a urological procedure, and whether to perform extracorporeal shock-wave lithotripsy or laser ureteroscopy, is of course left to a urologist (30). The management of ureteral stones is comprehensively reviewed by the American Urological Association's guidelines (31). A summary of suggested management of stones is presented in Figure 23-1.

Prevention of Recurrence

Kidney stone prevention is relatively inexpensive, cost-effective, and infrequently practiced (32). Patients with stones should be notified that this is a highly recurrent disorder, and when offered therapy, many patients will indicate that episodes of renal colic, though seemingly transient and not life-threatening, are sufficiently painful, time-consuming, and humiliating to motivate them to do whatever is necessary so that "this never happens again." A recent systematic review of medical prevention of nephrolithiasis, emphasizing only RCTs, was recently published (33).

CONCLUSIONS

Kidney stones are a disorder of high and increasing prevalence. They are now linked to a wide range and diversity of disease processes making them, if not a risk factor for other significant disorders such as metabolic syndrome and diabetes, at least a warning sign of other morbidities. They account for a large number of emergency care and clinician visits. Prevention of kidney stones should not be left to the urologists, who most often see the patients, but to the internists whose responsibilities include disease prevention. This responsibility should fall to endocrinologists, as well as general internists, nephrologists, and even emergency care clinicians.

ACKNOWLEDGMENTS

DSG gratefully acknowledges support of the Rare Kidney Stone Consortium (U54KD083908), a part of NIH Rare Diseases Clinical Research Network, funded by the NIDDK and the NIH Office of Rare Diseases Research.

REFERENCES

1. **Stamatelou KK, Francis ME, Jones CA, Nyberg LM, Curhan GC.** Time trends in reported prevalence of kidney stones in the United States: 1976–1994. *Kidney Int.* 2003;63:1817–1823.
2. **Scales CD, Smith AC, Hanley JM, Saigal CS.** Prevalence of kidney stones in the United States. *Eur Urol.* 2012;62:160–165.
3. **Romero V, Akpinar H, Assimos DG.** Kidney stones: a global picture of prevalence, incidence, and associated risk factors. *Rev Urol.* 2010;12:e86–e96.
4. **Saigal CS, Joyce G, Timilsina AR.** Direct and indirect costs of nephrolithiasis in an employed population: opportunity for disease management? *Kidney Int.* 2005;68:1808–1814.
5. **Brown J.** Diagnostic and treatment patterns for renal colic in US emergency departments. *Int Urol Nephrol.* 2006;38:87–92.
6. **Foster G, Stocks C, Borofsky MS.** Emergency department visits and hospital admissions for kidney stone disease, 2009. In: *Healthcare Cost and Utilization Project (HCUP) Statistical Briefs*; 2012.
7. **Clark AJ, Norman RW.** "Mirror pain" as an unusual presentation of renal colic. *Urology.* 1998;51:116–118.
8. **Mandel NS, Mandel GS.** Urinary tract stone disease in the United States veteran population. I. Geographical frequency of occurrence. *J Urol.* 1989;142:1513–1515.
9. **Goldfarb DS.** A woman with recurrent calcium phosphate kidney stones. *Clin J Am Soc Nephrol.* 2012;7:1172–1178.
10. **Maalouf NM, Cameron MA, Moe OW, Sakhaee K.** Novel insights into the pathogenesis of uric acid nephrolithiasis. *Curr Opin Nephrol Hypertens.* 2004; 13:181–189.
11. **Maalouf NM, Cameron MA, Moe OW, Adams-Huet B, Sakhaee K.** Low urine pH: a novel feature of the metabolic syndrome. *Clin J Am Soc Nephrol.* 2007;2: 883–888.
12. **Rodman JS.** Struvite stones. *Nephron.* 1999;81(suppl 1):50–59.
13. **Mattoo A, Goldfarb DS.** Cystinuria. *Sem Nephrol.* 2008;28:181–191.
14. **Coe FL, Evan AP, Lingeman JE, Worcester EM.** Plaque and deposits in nine human stone diseases. *Urol Res.* 2010;38:239–247.
15. **Worcester EM, Coe FL.** Evidence for altered renal tubule function in idiopathic calcium stone formers. *Urol Res.* 2010;38:263–269.
16. **Talner L, Vaughan M.** Nonobstructive renal causes of flank pain: findings on noncontrast helical CT (CT KUB). *Abdom Imaging.* 2003;28:210–216.
17. **Ljunghall S, Danielson BG, Fellström B, et al.** Family history of renal stones in recurrent stone patients. *Br J Urol.* 1985;57:370–374.
18. **Goldfarb DS, Fischer ME, Keich Y, Goldberg J.** A twin study of genetic and dietary influences on nephrolithiasis: a report from the Vietnam Era Twin (VET) Registry. *Kidney Int.* 2005;67:1053–1061.
19. **Vezzoli G, Soldati L, Gambaro G.** Update on primary hypercalciuria from a genetic perspective. *J Urol.* 2008;179:1676–1682.

20. **Vezzoli G, Terranegra A, Rainone F, et al.** Calcium-sensing receptor and calcium kidney stones. *J Transl Med.* 2011;9:201.
21. **Heilberg IP, Goldfarb DS.** Optimum nutrition for kidney stone disease. *Adv Chronic Kidney Dis.* 2013;20:165–174.
22. **Taylor EN, Fung TT, Curhan GC.** DASH-style diet associates with reduced risk for kidney stones. *J Am Soc Nephrol.* 2009;20:2253–2259.
23. **Curhan GC, Willett WC, Speizer FE, Spiegelman D, Stampfer MJ.** Comparison of dietary calcium with supplemental calcium and other nutrients as factors affecting the risk for kidney stones in women. *Ann Intern Med.* 1997;126:497–504.
24. **Obligado SH, Goldfarb DS.** The association of nephrolithiasis with hypertension and obesity: a review. *Am J Hypertens.* 2008;21:257–264.
25. **Jackson RD, LaCroix AZ, Gass M, et al.** Calcium plus vitamin D supplementation and the risk of fractures. *N Engl J Med.* 2006;354:669–683.
26. **Leaf DE, Korets R, Taylor EN, et al.** Effect of vitamin D repletion on urinary calcium excretion among kidney stone formers. *Clin J Amer Soc Nephrol.* 2012;7:829–834.
27. **Borofsky MS, Walter D, Shah O, et al.** Surgical decompression is associated with decreased mortality in patients with sepsis and ureteral calculi. *J Urol.* 2013;189:946–951.
28. **Nakada SY, Hoff DG, Attai S, et al.** Determination of stone composition by noncontrast spiral computed tomography in the clinical setting. *Urology.* 2000;55:816–819.
29. **Larkin GL, Peacock WF, Pearl SM, Blair GA, D'Amico F.** Efficacy of ketorolac tromethamine versus meperidine in the ED treatment of acute renal colic. *Am J Emerg Med.* 1999;17:6–10.
30. **Aboumarzouk OM, Kata SG, Keeley FX, McClinton S, Nabi G.** Extracorporeal shock wave lithotripsy (ESWL) versus ureteroscopic management for ureteric calculi. *Cochrane Database Syst Rev.* 2012;5: CD006029.
31. **Preminger GM, Tiselius HG, Assimos DG, et al.** 2007 guideline for the management of ureteral calculi. *J Urol.* 2007;178:2418–2434.
32. **Parks JH, Coe FL.** The financial effects of kidney stone prevention. *Kidney Int.* 1996;50:1706–1712.
33. **Fink HA, Wilt TJ, Eidman KE, et al.** Medical management to prevent recurrent nephrolithiasis in adults: a systematic review for an American College of Physicians Clinical Guideline. *Ann Intern Med.* 2013;158:535–543.

SECTION VIII

Neuroendocrine Tumors

SECTION INTRODUCTION

Emergent Management of Neuroendocrine Tumors

Kjell Öberg

Neuroendocrine tumors (NETs) constitute a heterogeneous group of malignant solid tumors that arise in hormone-secreting tissues of the diffuse neuroendocrine system. Consequently, they can have various clinical presentations and courses. Some tumors present an indolent course, whereas others are more aggressive, with shorter survival. The incidence of these relatively rare tumors is estimated to be about 5.25 cases per 100,000/yr and have a prevalence of about 35 per 100,000. The overall 5-year survival for metastatic NETs is 35% (1). The major subtypes of neuroendocrine tumors are bronchial NETs (30%), small intestinal NETs (25%), rectal NETs (17%), colonic NETs (10%), pancreatic NETs (7.5%), and thymic NETs (5%).

According to the World Health Organization (WHO) 2010 classification system, NETs are divided into NET G1 with a proliferation of less than 2%, NET G2 with proliferation 3%–20%, and NET G3 with greater than 20% dividing cells. The European Neuroendocrine Tumor Society (ENETS) as well as the National Comprehensive Cancer Center (NCCN)/Union for International Cancer Control (UICC) have developed a staging system with clear features for each of the stages (2–4). In addition, all subtypes of NETs can be divided into functional tumors, which are associated with hormone-related symptoms, and nonfunctional tumors, which do not cause any clinically apparent hormone-related symptoms. The so-called functional tumors can result in various endocrine and metabolic emergencies.

Small intestinal NETs with production of serotonin, tachykinin, and bradykinin present as the carcinoid syndrome, with flushing, diarrhea, and specific carcinoid heart disease (right-sided). This syndrome can manifest as a life-threatening medical emergency during various interventional procedures, such as surgery, embolization, and biopsies. The so-called carcinoid crisis presents with tachycardia, severe flushing, and low blood pressure and is related to release of tachykinins and serotonin particularly (5). With the introduction of somatostatin analogs for treatment of patients with carcinoid tumors, this emergency is nowadays rather rare, but it is important to prepare the patient very carefully for surgery or other therapeutic and investigational interventions (5).

With regard to pancreatic NETs, the most significant clinical syndromes are the Zollinger-Ellison syndrome, insulinoma (hypoglycemia syndrome), as well as Verner-Morrison syndrome (vasoactive intestinal polypeptide [VIP] secreting tumor, termed VIPoma syndrome). The Zollinger-Ellison syndrome is related to gastrin production by the tumor resulting in high gastric acid output with repeated gastrointestinal ulcers, sometimes down to the jejunum with significant risk of bleeding. Today, these patients are treated with high doses of proton-pump inhibitors

(PPIs), sometimes in combination with somatostatin analogs to reduce this risk. For long-term management, it is important to try to find the primary tumor as well as metastases to resect as much tumor tissue as possible. Peptide receptor radionuclide therapy (PRRT) is commonly used to reduce hormone levels and clinical symptoms in these patients. The most common clinical presentation related to pancreatic NETs is hypoglycemia syndrome caused by insulinoma with production of insulin/proinsulin, resulting in hypoglycemia. This condition is sometimes missed because the symptoms are initially nonspecific, and the patient is often misdiagnosed as having psychiatric problems. The definitive diagnosis is established by demonstration of low blood glucose in the presence of high levels of insulin or proinsulin. The primary clinical objective in these patients has been to detect the primary tumor, which is usually small and located in the pancreas, and attempt resection. For malignant insulinomas, treatment with cytotoxic agents has been the standard care over the years (6). More recently, new targeted therapies such as the mTOR (mammalian target of rapamycin) inhibitor everolimus or tyrosine kinase inhibitors have also been effective. The Verner-Morrison syndrome is a severe condition with extremely high volumes of liquid stools and losses of potassium, magnesium, and bicarbonate resulting in the typical features of VIPoma syndrome. Excessive VIP secretion is the cause of this syndrome and tumors may be located either in the pancreas (most commonly) or in the lung. Surgery is important to try to reduce as much tumor bulk as possible and treatment with somatostatin analogs, alpha interferon, and everolimus can result in significant reduction of hormone levels and improvement of the clinical condition (7). The glucagonoma syndrome (related to a glucagon-producing tumor) rarely results in medical emergencies, but sometimes can cause significant hyperglycemia, anemia, and thromboembolic complications that need appropriate care (6).

Bronchial and thymic NETs can cause Cushing's syndrome due to ectopic production of adrenocorticotropic hormone (ACTH) or corticotropin-releasing hormone (CRH). This syndrome is usually difficult to treat with different steroid inhibitors, and in the end bilateral-adrenalectomy might be the solution. The ectopic Cushing's syndrome is sometimes very florid and can constitute an endocrine and metabolic emergency (8).

Ongoing challenges for clinicians caring for patients with NETs include detection of disease before metastasis, detection of tumor remnants after surgery, reliable monitoring of therapeutic efficacy, and translating research findings into clinical practice.

CONCLUSIONS

Neuroendocrine tumors can present with various types of endocrine and metabolic emergencies. A combination of different treatment modalities is necessary to control the clinical manifestations. New targeted agents (eg, mTOR and tyrosine kinase inhibitors) can facilitate the management of hormone-related emergencies. However, an unmet need exists for additional therapies that enable more personalized therapy. In addition, earlier disease detection and diagnosis may result in treatment that prevents progression to more advanced disease, which can result in the well-defined and debilitating clinical syndromes that can be associated with endocrine and metabolic emergencies.

ACKNOWLEDGMENTS

The author has nothing to disclose.

REFERENCES

1. **Yao JC, Hassan M, Phan A, et al.** One hundred years after "carcinoid": epidemiology of and prognostic factors for neuroendocrine tumors in 35,825 cases in the United States. *J Clin Oncol.* 2008;26: 3063–3072.
2. **Rindi G, Kloppel G, Couvelard A, et al.** TNM staging of midgut and hindgut (neuro) endocrine tumors: a consensus proposal including a grading system. *Virchows Arch.* 2007;451:757–762.
3. **Bosman F, Carneiro F, Hruban RH, et al.** *WHO Classification of Tumours of the Digestive System.* Lyon, France: IARC Press;2010.
4. **Strosberg JR, Cheema A, Weber JM, et al.** Relapse-free survival in patients with nonmetastatic, surgically resected pancreatic neuroendocrine tumors: an analysis of the AJCC and ENETS staging classifications. *Ann Surg.* 2012;256:321–325.
5. **Strosberg J.** Neuroendocrine tumours of the small intestine. *Best Pract Res Clin Gastroenterol.* 2012;26:755–773.
6. **Bilimoria KY, Tomlinson JS, Merkow RP, et al.** Clinicopathologic features and treatment trends of pancreatic neuroendocrine tumors: analysis of 9,821 patients. *J Gastrointest Surg.* 2007;11:1467–1469.
7. **Öberg K.** Biotherapies for GEP-NETs. *Best Pract Res Clin Gastroenterol.* 2012;26:833–841.
8. **Limper AH, Carpenter PC, Scheithauer B, et al.** The Cushing syndrome induced by bronchial carcinoid tumors. *Ann Intern Med.* 1992;117:209–214.

CHAPTER 24

Acute Endocrine and Metabolic Emergencies in Neuroendocrine Tumors

Jonathan Strosberg and Jamie Goldman

ABSTRACT

Neuroendocrine tumors (NETs) commonly secrete peptide hormones, biogenic amines, and other vasoactive substances, which can produce signs and symptoms such as flushing, diarrhea, blood pressure fluctuations, and glucose abnormalities. Some of these symptoms rise to the level of life-threatening emergencies. This chapter reviews several endocrine emergencies associated with advanced NETs, including carcinoid crisis, VIPoma syndrome, and glucagonoma syndrome. Other potentially severe endocrine abnormalities associated with NETs, such as hypoglycemia, hypertensive emergency, and Cushing's syndrome, are reviewed in other chapters.

INTRODUCTION

Neuroendocrine tumors (NETs) commonly produce peptide hormones, biogenic amines, and other vasoactive substances, including prostaglandins and tachykinins. The secretion of these substances into the circulation produces a variety of clinical signs and symptoms such as flushing, diarrhea, cardiac valvular heart disease, diabetes, hypoglycemia, rash, and bronchospasm. "Functioning" NETs produce pathologically elevated hormone levels associated with a corresponding clinical syndrome, while "nonfunctioning" tumors lack an association with a hormonal syndrome.

Over the past 3 decades, synthetic somatostatin analogs have been developed, which are used most notably in the treatment of carcinoid syndrome, as well as in syndromes associated with pancreatic NETs such as glucagonomas and vasoactive intestinal polypeptide (VIP) secreting tumors (VIPomas).

This chapter will focus on acute endocrine and metabolic emergencies in NETs, as well as emergent and palliative treatment of hormonal secretion. It is important to also take into consideration that treatment of the underlying malignancy will help ameliorate the associated hormonal syndrome.

CARCINOID SYNDROME AND CRISIS

Metastatic NETs of the distal small intestine and cecum are often associated with the carcinoid syndrome, which consists of flushing, diarrhea, bronchoconstriction, and right-sided valvular heart disease (1–3). The syndrome develops due to the secretion of serotonin and other vasoactive products, such as prostaglandins, histamine, dopamine, and tachykinins into systemic circulation (4–7). Serotonin, the primary hormonal factor responsible for carcinoid syndrome, is enzymatically inactivated in the liver into 5-hydroxyindoleacetic acid (5-HIAA), a urinary metabolite. Thus, carcinoid syndrome occurs primarily in metastatic NETs that secrete serotonin directly into the systemic, and not portal, circulation. Pulmonary, gastric, duodenal, and pancreatic NETs infrequently secrete serotonin. Carcinoid tumors of the distal colon and rectum are not associated with a hormonal syndrome (8).

The 2 most common symptoms of carcinoid syndrome are diarrhea and flushing. In an analysis of 91 patients with carcinoid syndrome, diarrhea and flushing were reported in 74% and 65% of patients, respectively, whereas carcinoid heart disease occurred in 10% and bronchospasm in 8% of cases (9). Serotonin is thought to directly stimulate peristalsis, resulting in significantly reduced colonic transit times (10). Flushing usually affects the face, neck, and upper torso and can be attributed to the multiple vasoactive substances secreted, including prostaglandins, kinins, and serotonin (11–14). Carcinoid heart disease typically occurs in patients with extreme elevations of circulating serotonin and leads to tricuspid regurgitation and pulmonic valve stenosis secondary to thickening and fibrosis of right-sided cardiac valves (15–17). The underlying mechanism of fibroblast proliferation in the cardiac valves is uncertain (18,19).

Management of carcinoid syndrome is usually accomplished via the use of somatostatin analogs octreotide or lanreotide. These analogs bind primarily to somatostatin receptor subtype 2 and inhibit the release of neuroendocrine hormones such as serotonin. They also have multiple other inhibitory effects in the digestive tract, including suppression of physiological bowel motility, secretion, and absorption. Side effects are generally mild and include nausea, bloating, and steatorrhea, along with an increased rate of biliary stone and sludge formation due to inhibitory effects on gallbladder contractility. Kvols and colleagues conducted the first clinical trial of octreotide in patients with carcinoid syndrome, finding that 88% of patients experienced amelioration of flushing and diarrhea, and 72% had major reductions in urinary 5-HIAA levels (20). Depot octreotide long-acting release (LAR) is typically administered as an intramuscular injection at doses of 20–30 mg every 4 weeks for symptom control. Use of higher doses and frequencies is common in patients who experience suboptimal control of symptoms at standard dosing levels (21). Depot lanreotide is typically given as a deep subcutaneous (SC) injection at doses of 90–120 mg every 4 weeks (22).

For patients whose diarrhea persists despite somatostatin analog therapy, loperamide or diphenoxylate/atropine may be of benefit. For severe or refractory diarrhea, tincture of opium or paregoric may be used. Somatostatin analog therapy can cause symptomatic fat malabsorption and steatorrhea, which may respond to pancreatic enzyme supplementation. Serotonin receptor antagonists, such as ondansetron, have been shown in several studies to palliate diarrhea, although the magnitude of benefit is small (23,24).

The most significant life-threatening emergency associated with carcinoid syndrome is carcinoid crisis. The term carcinoid crisis describes an episode of acute circulatory collapse caused by the massive release of serotonin and other vasoactive substances into the circulation (25,26). This event tends to occur in the perioperative setting, with triggers that include general anesthesia, epinephrine, and physical manipulation of tumors. Carcinoid crisis can lead to complete vasomotor collapse, coma, and death.

One of the first descriptions of octreotide use in humans was a case report of a patient who developed carcinoid crisis shortly after induction of anesthesia. After failure of conventional resuscitation measures, the hypotension was rapidly reversed with an intravenous (IV) infusion of octreotide (27). Ever since, standard practice has been to administer prophylactic doses of 250–500 mcg of IV or SC octreotide to carcinoid syndrome patients prior to an invasive procedure. If intraoperative hypotension develops, the patient should be given IV boluses of 500–1,000 mcg until blood pressure normalizes. Alternatively, continuous IV infusion of 50–200 mcg/hr may be given after a bolus dose. It is important to emphasize that guidelines on carcinoid crisis prophylaxis and treatment are based primarily on anecdotal experience rather than on prospective trials. One retrospective analysis has suggested that prophylactic octreotide may be ineffective at prevention of intraoperative hypotension in patients with carcinoid tumors undergoing laparotomy (28).

VIPOMA SYNDROME

VIP-secreting tumors (VIPomas) are rare, occurring in approximately 1 in 10 million people (29). VIPomas are generally solitary tumors, greater than 2 cm in diameter, and occur most commonly in the pancreas, with hepatic metastasis seen in up to 68% at diagnosis (30,31). Extrapancreatic VIPomas include ganglioneuroblastomas, ganglioneuromas, and neuroblastomas (32).

VIPoma syndrome is characterized by profuse, watery diarrhea often exceeding 3 liters/day, severe hypokalemia, and dehydration. These symptoms occur through stimulation of intestinal secretion and inhibition of electrolyte and water absorption in the bowel (33). The syndrome is also known as Verner-Morrison syndrome, pancreatic cholera, or WDHA (watery diarrhea, hypokalemia, achlorhydria) syndrome. Other clinical findings include hypercalcemia, flushing due to the vasodilatory effects of VIP, achlorhydria through inhibition of gastric acid secretion, skin erythema, abdominal distension, and myoparalysis (32,34). Hyperglycemia is less common, occurring in up to one third of patients as a result of increased hepatic glucogenolysis due to increased VIP levels (29,31).

If this syndrome is left untreated, dehydration and electrolyte disorders can lead to renal failure and shock (35). Treatment of severe diarrheal symptoms includes intensive IV fluid resuscitation and correction of electrolyte imbalances. The somatostatin analogs octreotide and lanreotide are highly effective at inhibiting serum VIP release. Use of short-acting SC octreotide is often necessary for acute control of symptoms prior to transition to long-acting somatostatin analog therapy. This allows for normalization of potassium and other electrolytes through improvement of diarrhea and VIP levels in nearly 90% of patients (22,31,32,36). The symptomatic response to octreotide use may be disproportionate to the actual reduction in plasma concentration of VIP, which suggests that direct inhibition of gastrointestinal secretion contributes to symptom palliation (37).

GLUCAGONOMA SYNDROME

Glucagonomas are rare, slow-growing tumors that arise from the alpha cells of the pancreas (38). There have been approximately 300 cases of glucagonomas published so far, with 1 in 20 million people diagnosed each year (39). Patients may present with hyperglycemia, weight loss, glossitis, anorexia, venous thrombosis, neuropsychiatric symptoms, normocytic anemia, angular stomatitis, and necrolytic migratory erythema (NME) (40). NME is an unusual rash that waxes and wanes, with painful, weeping erythematous papules or plaques involving the lower extremities, inguinal area, perineum, and perioral region (39,41). Hypoproteinemia, hypoaminoacidemia, and hypolipidemia can also be seen with glucagonomas (42).

Somatostatin analog therapy can lead to quick resolution of symptoms (39,40). Hyperglycemia can be managed with insulin or non-insulin antihyperglycemic agents (43). For patients with uncontrolled cachexia, total parenteral nutrition and other nutritional support should be considered. Zinc and essential fatty acid supplements have been shown to alleviate NME (39). Perioperative prophylactic anticoagulation should be considered in patients with glucagonomas, due to the increased risk of venous thrombosis.

CONCLUSIONS

It is important to recognize endocrine syndromes associated with NETs. Occasionally, these syndromes can manifest as life-threatening emergencies. Somatostatin analogs such as octreotide and lanreotide are often used in these hormonal syndromes due to their antisecretory effects and tolerable side-effect profile. Intravenous fluids and correction of electrolyte disorders are important in the treatment of dehydration and electrolyte and metabolic imbalances. Diarrhea can also be treated with loperamide, Lomotil, or opiate antidiarrheal drugs. Effective surgical and medical management of the underlying neuroendocrine tumor(s) is important for long-term syndrome control (44–46).

ACKNOWLEDGMENTS

JS has consulted for Novartis, Pfizer and Ipsen. JG has nothing to disclose.

REFERENCES

1. **Kvols LK.** The carcinoid syndrome: a treatable malignant disease. *Oncology (Huntingt).* 1988;2:33–41.
2. **Moertel CG, Sauer WG, Dockerty MB, Baggenstoss AH.** Life history of the carcinoid tumor of the small intestine. *Cancer.* 1961;14:901–912.
3. **Moertel CG.** Karnofsky memorial lecture. An odyssey in the land of small tumors. *J Clin Oncol.* 1987;5:1502–1522.
4. **Feldman JM.** Increased dopamine production in patients with carcinoid tumors. *Metabolism.* 1985;34:255–260.
5. **Sandler M, Karim SM, Williams ED.** Prostaglandins in amine-peptide-secreting tumours. *Lancet.* 1968;2:1053–1054.
6. **Lucas KJ, Feldman JM.** Flushing in the carcinoid syndrome and plasma kallikrein. *Cancer.* 1986;58: 2290–2293.
7. **Skrabanek P, Cannon D, Kirrane J, Powell D.** Substance P secretion by carcinoid tumours. *Ir J Med Sci.* 1978;147:47–49.
8. **Caldarola VT, Jackman RJ, Moertel CG, Dockerty MB.** Carcinoid tumors of the rectum. *Am J Surg.* 1964;107:844–849.
9. **Davis Z, Moertel CG, McIlrath DC.** The malignant carcinoid syndrome. *Surg Gynecol Obstet.* 1973;137:637–644.
10. **von der Ohe MR, Camilleri M, Kvols LK, Thomforde GM.** Motor dysfunction of the small bowel and colon in patients with the carcinoid syndrome and diarrhea. *N Engl J Med.* 1993;329:1073–1078.
11. **Cunningham JL, Janson ET, Agarwal S, Grimelius L, Stridsberg M.** Tachykinins in endocrine tumors and the carcinoid syndrome. *Eur J Endocrinol.* 2008;159:275–282.
12. **Matuchansky C, Launay JM.** Serotonin, catecholamines, and spontaneous midgut carcinoid flush: plasma studies from flushing and nonflushing sites. *Gastroenterology.* 1995;108:743–751.
13. **Vinik AI, Gonin J, England BG, Jackson T, McLeod MK, Cho K.** Plasma substance-P in neuroendocrine tumors and idiopathic flushing: the value of pentagastrin stimulation tests and the effects of somatostatin analog. *J Clin Endocrinol Metab.* 1990;70:1702–1709.
14. **Smith AG, Greaves MW.** Blood prostaglandin activity associated with noradrenaline-provoked flush in the carcinoid syndrome. *Br J Dermatol.* 1974;90:547–551.
15. **Lundin L, Norheim I, Landelius J, Oberg K, Theodorsson-Norheim E.** Carcinoid heart disease: relationship of circulating vasoactive substances to ultrasound-detectable cardiac abnormalities. *Circulation.* 1988;77:264–269.
16. **Robiolio PA, Rigolin VH, Wilson JS, et al.** Carcinoid heart disease. Correlation of high serotonin levels with valvular abnormalities detected by cardiac catheterization and echocardiography. *Circulation.* 1995;92:790–795.
17. **Pellikka PA, Tajik AJ, Khandheria BK, et al.** Carcinoid heart disease. Clinical and echocardiographic spectrum in 74 patients. *Circulation.* 1993;87:1188–1196.
18. **Waltenberger J, Lundin L, Oberg K, et al.** Involvement of transforming growth factor-beta in the formation of fibrotic lesions in carcinoid heart disease. *Am J Pathol.* 1993;142:71–78.
19. **Beauchamp RD, Coffey RJ Jr, Lyons RM, Perkett EA, Townsend CM Jr, Moses HL.** Human carcinoid cell production of paracrine growth factors that can stimulate fibroblast and endothelial cell growth. *Cancer Res.* 1991;51:5253–5260.
20. **Kvols LK, Moertel CG, O'Connell MJ, Schutt AJ, Rubin J, Hahn RG.** Treatment of the malignant carcinoid syndrome. Evaluation of a long-acting somatostatin analogue. *N Engl J Med.* 1986;315:663–666.
21. **Strosberg J, Weber J, Feldman M, Goldman J, Almhanna K, Kvols L.** Above-label doses of octreotide-LAR in patients with metastatic small intestinal carcinoid tumors. *Gastrointest Cancer Res.* 2013;6:81–85.
22. **O'Dorisio TM, Gaginella TS, Mekhjian HS, Rao B, O'Dorisio MS.** Somatostatin and analogues in the treatment of VIPoma. *Ann N Y Acad Sci.* 1988;527:528–535.
23. **Saslow SB, Scolapio JS, Camilleri M, et al.** Medium-term effects of a new 5HT3 antagonist, alosetron, in patients with carcinoid diarrhoea. *Gut.* 1998;42: 628–634.
24. **Wymenga AN, de Vries EG, Leijsma MK, Kema IP, Kleibeuker JH.** Effects of ondansetron on gastrointestinal symptoms in carcinoid syndrome. *Eur J Cancer.* 1998;34:1293–1294.
25. **Kvols LK.** Therapeutic considerations for the malignant carcinoid syndrome. *Acta Oncol.* 1989;28:433–438.
26. **Kahil ME, Brown H, Fred HL.** The carcinoid crisis. *Arch Intern Med.* 1964;114:26–28.
27. **Kvols LK, Martin JK, Marsh HM, Moertel CG.** Rapid reversal of carcinoid crisis with a somatostatin analogue. *N Engl J Med.* 1985;313:1229–1230.
28. **Massimino K, Harrskog O, Pommier S, Pommier R.** Octreotide LAR and bolus octreotide are insufficient for preventing intraoperative complications in carcinoid patients. *J Surg Oncol.* 2013;107(8):842–846.
29. **Smith SL, Branton SA, Avino AJ, et al.** Vasoactive intestinal polypeptide secreting islet cell tumors: a 15-year experience and review of the literature. *Surgery.* 1998;124:1050–1055.
30. **Shaib W, Mitchell K, Saif MW.** Amelioration of symptoms and reduction of VIP levels after hepatic artery chemoembolization in a patient with Sandostatin resistant VIPoma. *Yale J Biol Med.* 2010;83:27–33.
31. **Elshafie O, Grant C, Al-Hamdani A, Jain R, Woodhouse N.** VIPoma crisis: immediate and life saving reduction of massive stool volumes on starting treatment with octreotide. *Sultan Qaboos Univ Med J.* 2011;11:104–107.
32. **Song S, Shi R, Li B, Liu Y.** Diagnosis and treatment of pancreatic vasoactive intestinal peptide endocrine tumors. *Pancreas.* 2009;38:811–814.
33. **Verner JV, Morrison AB.** Islet cell tumor and a syndrome of refractory watery diarrhea and hypokalemia. *Am J Med.* 1958;25:374–380.
34. **Marks IN, Bank S, Louw JH.** Islet cell tumor of the pancreas with reversible watery diarrhea and achylorhydraia. *Gastroenterology.* 1967;52:695–708.

35. **Halaszlaki C, Horvath H, Kiss L, et al.** Verner-Morrison syndrome: a case study. *Orv Hetil.* 2010; 151:1111–1114.
36. **Maton PN, Gardner JD, Jensen RT.** Use of long-acting somatostatin analog SMS 201-995 in patients with pancreatic islet cell tumors. *Dig Dis Sci.* 1989;34(suppl 3):28S–39S.
37. **Oberg K, Eriksson B.** Endocrine tumours of the pancreas. *Best Pract Res Clin Gastroenterol.* 2005;19: 753–781.
38. **McGavran MH, Unger RH, Recant L, Polk HC, Kilo C, Levin ME.** A glucagon-secreting alpha-cell carcinoma of the pancreas. *N Engl J Med.* 1966;274:1408–1413.
39. **Echenique-Elizondo M, Martinez de Lizarduy I.** Glucagonoma and necrolytic migratory erythema. *Revista espanola de enfermedades digestivas: organo oficial de la Sociedad Espanola de Patologia Digestiva.* 2005;97:455–457.
40. **Wermers RA, Fatourechi V, Wynne AG, Kvols LK, Lloyd RV.** The glucagonoma syndrome. Clinical and pathologic features in 21 patients. *Medicine (Baltimore).* 1996;75:53–63.
41. **Wilkinson DS.** Necrolytic migratory erythema with carcinoma of the pancreas. *Trans St Johns Hosp Dermatol Soc.* 1973;59:244–250.
42. **Leichter SB.** Clinical and metabolic aspects of glucagonoma. *Medicine.* 1980;59:100–113.
43. **Bloom SR, Polak JM.** Glucagonoma syndrome. *Am J Med.* 1987;82(5B):25–36.
44. **Strosberg JR, Fisher GA, Benson AB, et al.** Systemic treatment in unresectable metastatic well-differentiated carcinoid tumors: consensus results from a modified delphi process. *Pancreas.* 2013;42:397–404.
45. **Kunz PL, Reidy-Lagunes D, Anthony LB, et al.** Consensus Guidelines for the Management and Treatment of Neuroendocrine Tumors. *Pancreas* 2013;42:557–577.
46. **Strosberg J.** Evolving treatment strategies for management of carcinoid tumors. *Curr Treat Options Oncol.* 2013;14:374–388.

SECTION IX

Glucose Disorders

SECTION INTRODUCTION

Emergent Management of Glucose Disorders

Richard M Bergenstal and Shaukat Sadikot

The global burden of diabetes is powerfully documented in the 2013 International Diabetes Federation (IDF) Diabetes Atlas (1); the data there are so staggering as to convey a clear message that urgent action is required. Currently, worldwide, 382 million individuals have diabetes, and by 2035 that number will rise to approximately 592 million, with a cost of 584 billion USD in 2013 (11% of health spending on adults) projected to be 627 billion USD in 2035. In the previous Atlas, it was calculated that a person dies of diabetes-related complications every 7 seconds. The current Atlas (1) shows that a person dies of diabetes-related complications every 6 seconds. Despite our increasing knowledge as well as the availability of different types of medications, things seem to be getting worse.

Eighty percent of people with diabetes live in low- and middle-income countries, yet an overwhelming proportion of the dollars that go to diabetes care are spent in a handful of the wealthier high-income countries. The IDF estimates that 175 million individuals with diabetes are undiagnosed and as many as 50 million of those may be in China alone (2). Although China, India, and the United States are the top 3 countries in terms of diabetes prevalence, its rates are increasing fastest in Africa and the Middle East.

How big a role do diabetes and chronic disease really play in the overall health care system? A recent publication, Anatomy of Health Care in the United States (3), points out that chronic illnesses account for 84% of the overall costs of health care; yet despite this the United States is falling behind other developed countries in the rate of increase in lifespan. One concerning finding in the United States is the large disparity or variation in health care outcomes state by state and even county by county. Globally, the shift from acute disease to chronic disease accounting for the bulk of health care costs and clinical suffering was acknowledged directly at the United Nations General Assembly High-level Meeting on the Prevention and Control of Non-communicable Diseases (NCDs) including cancer, cardiovascular disease (CVD), and diabetes.

Today, government and local health officials, hospitals, clinics, and funders are asking whether we are getting good outcomes for the dollars invested in diabetes care (often referred to as good value). The triple aim put forward by Berwick (4) proposes 3 essential components of an effective health care system that must be measured and optimized in order to deliver value when managing chronic diseases like diabetes. The triple aim is to improve the quality of care, to provide an excellent patient experience, and to do so at a reduced (or reasonable) cost. An individual health care system or ideally a national health care policy must come to a consensus on the definition of quality, patient experience, and cost of each disease—such as diabetes—in metrics that can be measured, tracked, compared, and rewarded in some fashion.

The most common single measure of quality diabetes care is for an individual or population to achieve a predefined hemoglobin A_{1C} (HbA_{1c} or A1c) goal or target.

Based on the DCCT/EDIC (Diabetes Control and Complications Trial/ Epidemiology of Diabetes Interventions and Complications) trial in type 1 diabetes (T1D) and the UKPDS (United Kingdom Prospective Diabetes Study) in type 2 diabetes (T2D), in the past it was common to set the target A1C goal at <7% (53 mmol/mol IFCC units) for most adults. But after a series of recent outcome trials in T2D, most quality-measure organizations and medical societies have gone away from "one size fits all" for the A1C goal and now suggest <7% (53 mmol/mol) for many individuals to reduce microvascular disease; less stringent goals such as <8% (64 mmol/mol) for those with a history of severe hypoglycemia, limited life expectancy, or advanced complications; and possibly more stringent goals such as <6.5% (48 mmol/mol) in those with early diabetes and no hypoglycemia or complications. Beyond a single A1C goal, it is now clear that quality diabetes care must be much more than a "gluco-centric measure." Most quality metrics now also include the ABCs of diabetes (ie, A1C, blood pressure, and cholesterol). Some have added not using tobacco and taking an antiplatelet agent (if one has a history of CVD) as 2 additional quality diabetes management metrics; taken together with the ABCs these are then called the D5 optimal diabetes measure. In addition, some have proposed composite index measures of quality diabetes care, such as an A1C <7% (53 mmol/mol), without severe (or significant) hypoglycemia and weight loss (or no weight gain). The US Centers for Disease Control and Prevention (CDC) recently documented that although approximately 50% of adults with diabetes were meeting generally accepted individual quality targets for the ABCs and 78% were nonsmokers, when they calculated what proportion of the population of individuals with diabetes met all 4 of these goals at the same time, the overall number was a disappointing 14.3%. In the United States and around the globe much work remains to be done on achieving and sustaining comprehensive quality diabetes metrics.

Efforts focused on improving the second component of the triple aim, the patient experience, have recently received much more attention with the new emphasis on patient-centered care or individualized/personalized care (5,6). Tools now are available to measure patient satisfaction, patient engagement, or patient-reported quality of life outcomes. Studies such as DAWN2 (the second Diabetes Attitudes Wishes and Needs study) clearly showed a need for more patient engagement. After surveying several thousand health care professionals and individuals with diabetes in 17 countries, the researchers found that 29.2% of persons with diabetes reported being asked by their health care professional for ideas when making their diabetes care plan, and 37.3% of people with diabetes felt listened to regarding how they would like to do things (7). Patient-centered team care is touted as being an essential element in reaching the triple aim, but much work remains to be done to implement such a model of diabetes care effectively.

Much of the discussion on reaching the third component of the triple aim, a reduced or reasonable cost for the care delivered, has focused on moving away from paying for procedures or visits and instead paying for quality or achieving agreed upon performance metrics. A heavy emphasis on the potential value of utilizing clinic registries (of patients with diabetes) linked to information in the electronic medical record (EMR), along with medical teams providing between-visit support and utilizing various strategies to improve medication adherence (such as shared decision making), holds all hold promise to stabilize medical costs while improving quality (adding health care value).

Reaching the triple aim in diabetes care of optimal quality and excellent patient experience at a reasonable cost will require innovative approaches to setting targets, forming teams, selecting appropriate therapies, utilizing technology, and agreeing upon a way to reimburse for the time needed to coordinate all these activities. Research and quality improvement activities are ongoing in each of these 5 T's (ie, targets, teams, therapies, technology, and time).

Targets encompass both outpatient and inpatient care because individuals with diabetes are at least twice as likely to be hospitalized as individuals in the average population (and will be the major focus in the chapters within this section). In both settings, achieving good glucose control has advantages but not at the risk of severe or frequent hypoglycemia. We must move beyond just the A1C as the only marker of glycemic control and include evaluation of actual glucose values and, in particular, glucose patterns. We are just beginning to see the potential in using risk algorithms, biomarkers, and even genotyping to personalize targets and therapies (ie, stratified medicine). Teams that include both the patient and health care professionals such as diabetes educators, dietitians, pharmacists, psychologists, and social workers appear to a have role in reaching the triple aim (8). New classes of therapies for T2D are expanding (eg, glucagon-like peptide-1 [GLP-1] agonists, dipeptidyl peptidase-4 [DPP-4], sodium-glucose cotransporter 2 [SGLT-2] inhibitors, new ultra-long acting and potentially ultra-fast acting insulins), and now the challenge is to sort out the right therapy for the right patient at the right time. Eventually, we will learn much from comparative effectiveness trials like GRADE (Glycemic Reduction Approaches in Diabetes) regarding appropriate therapy selection. In T1D management the recent 30-year anniversary of the DCCT trial is cause for celebration and reflection (9). Although there is some question today of the relative importance of glucose control in the prevention of CVD in individuals with advanced T2D, in T1D the DCCT/EDIC study clearly shows the value of early glucose control in reducing both microvascular and macrovascular disease. New technologies, such as remote access to self-monitored blood glucose (SMBG) data and utilizing real-time or retrospective continuous glucose monitoring (CGM) data, have the potential to engage patients in their own diabetes management and make it easier for patients to communicate their glucose status to the health care team and receive whatever degree of support they need. With the explosion of potential availability of glucose data it will be critical to standardize the output of these devices so patients and providers can assess one's glucose status quickly and make effective drug therapy choices or lifestyle interventions. Diabetes is the perfect disease entity to figure out the optimal health care system model that allows each team member the time needed to work with a patient and family to reduce the burden of living with diabetes.

There are solid data that social determinants of health are also critical to achieving good quality of care, particularly for chronic diseases like diabetes. The University of Wisconsin Population Health Institute (UWPHI) has collaborated with the Robert Wood Johnson Foundation to map the social determinants of health. They have shown that morbidity and mortality are influenced by the following social determinants of health: health behaviors (30%—tobacco, diet and exercise, alcohol use, and sexual activity), clinical care (20%—access to care and quality of care), social and economic factors (40%—education, employment, and income), and physical environment (10%) (10). Clinicians and other stakeholders must work closely with the public health sector to truly tackle chronic diseases like diabetes.

Given the magnitude of the diabetes epidemic, it is clear that we must not only work to improve clinical management, but we must also have a much more coordinated effort focused on diabetes prevention. Figuring out a way to make and sustain lifestyle changes, although very difficult, is ultimately essential if we are to slow the rate of diabetes development worldwide. After years of debating the best "diabetes diet," the American Diabetes Association (ADA) recently has said that just like A1C targets, there is no "one-size-fits-all" for healthy eating patterns in individuals with diabetes (11). The goal of nutrition therapy for adults with diabetes is to "promote and support healthful eating patterns, emphasizing a variety of nutrient dense foods in appropriate portions" to help achieve the ABCs of diabetes and one's body weight goals, and to help delay or prevent complications of diabetes. Some positive evidence exists for aspects of various eating patterns, including Mediterranean, vegetarian, low fat, low carbohydrate, and DASH (Dietary Approaches to Stop Hypertension). There are many recent publications on the benefits of a Mediterranean diet (particularly with added olive oil and nuts) both for prevention of CVD and even prevention of diabetes (12). The Look AHEAD trial utilized an energy-reduced low-fat eating pattern, and individuals achieved moderate success at weight loss (13). Bariatric surgery has certainly emerged as a very viable approach to improve diabetes outcomes and reduce weight in those with significant obesity, and many new classes of drugs to treat obesity are being developed and evaluated (14). How pharmacological and surgical approaches to diabetes fit into a "diabetes management" algorithm is yet to be determined.

We must combine innovative strategies in diabetes population management and personalized care with an equal focus on diabetes prevention if we are to enable individuals to live well with diabetes and slow the rate of increase in the diabetes epidemic.

ACKNOWLEDGMENTS

The authors have nothing to disclose.

REFERENCES

1. **International Diabetes Federation.** *IDF Diabetes Atlas.* 6th ed. 2013. http://www.idf.org/diabetesatlas.
2. **Yang W, LU J, Weng J, et al.** Prevalence of diabetes among men and women in China. *N Engl J Med.* 2010;362:1090–1101.
3. **Moses H 3rd, Matheson DHM, Dorsey ER, et al.** Anatomy of health care in the United States. *JAMA.* 2013;310:1947–1963.
4. **Berwick DM, Nolan TW, Whittington J.** The triple aim: care, health, and cost. *Health Aff (Millwood).* 2008;27:759–769.
5. **Inzucchi SE, Bergenstal RM, Buse JB, et al.** Management of hyperglycemia in type 2 diabetes: a patient-centered approach. Position statement of the American Diabetes Association (ADA) and the European Association for the Study of Diabetes (EASD). *Diabetes Care.* 2012;35:1364–1379.
6. **Weiner SJ, Weaver F, Yudkhowsky R, et al.** Patient-Centered Decision Making and Health Care Outcomes: an observational study. *Ann Intern Med.* 2013;158:573–579.
7. **Willaing I, Peyrot M.** Active involvement of people with diabetes and support for self-management. Abstract #0384. International Diabetes Federation, Melbourne, Australia, December 2–6, 2013.
8. **Raz I, Riddle MC, Rosenstock J, et al.** Personalized management of hyperglycemia in type 2 diabetes. *Diabetes Care.* 2013;36:1779–1788.
9. **DCCT/EDIC Trial Group.** Perspective in diabetes. The Diabetes Control and Complications Trial/Epidemiology of Diabetes Interventions and Complications Study at 30 years: advances and contributions. *Diabetes.* 2013;62:3976–3986.
10. **Bilheimer LT.** Evaluating metrics to improve population health. *Prev Chronic Dis.* 2010;7:69.
11. **Evert, AB, Boucher JL, Cypress M, et al.** Nutrition therapy recommendations for the management of adults with diabetes. *Diabetes Care.* 2014;37:S120–S143.
12. **Ramón E, Ros E, Salas-Salvado J, et al.** Primary prevention of cardiovascular disease with a Mediterranean diet. *N Engl J Med.* 2013;368:1279–1290.
13. **The Look AHEAD Research Group.** Cardiovascular effects of intensive lifestyle intervention in type 2 diabetes. *N Engl J Med.* 2013;369:145–154.
14. **Haluzík M.** Bariatric surgery and the mechanism of diabetes remission: are we getting there? *J Clin Endocrinol Metab.* 2013;98:4336–4338.

CHAPTER 25

Hypoglycemia

Elizabeth M Lamos, Lisa M Younk, and Stephen N Davis

ABSTRACT

Hypoglycemia is one of the most frequent endocrine emergencies in individuals with diabetes mellitus. However, hypoglycemia in the healthy or nondiabetic individual is rare. This review will focus on the pathophysiology, management, and etiology of hypoglycemia in persons with and without diabetes. Hypoglycemia in persons with diabetes will focus on multiple factors, including hypoglycemic unawareness, glucose monitoring, medication management, and comorbidities. Hypoglycemia in the nondiabetic individual can have multiple etiologies and poses a diagnostic challenge. It is important to respond quickly and appropriately to acute hypoglycemia in any individual. Although broad, the etiology of hypoglycemia must include a comprehensive and individualized review of medical, family, social, and pharmacological patient histories.

INTRODUCTION

Hypoglycemia represents one of the most common endocrine emergencies that clinicians are likely to encounter routinely. Relatively rare in nondiabetic individuals, hypoglycemia frequently occurs in persons with diabetes (1). In both type 1 diabetes (T1DM) and type 2 diabetes (T2DM), acute hypoglycemia is associated with increased morbidity and in some individuals even death. Hypoglycemia is a significant cost burden and is the major limiting factor for short- and long-term improved glycemic control (2,3). Hypoglycemia in persons without diabetes often presents a complex diagnostic challenge. The definition, mechanism(s), diagnostic pathways, and acute management of hypoglycemia in persons with and without diabetes in outpatient and inpatient settings will be discussed.

DEFINITION OF HYPOGLYCEMIA

The threshold value for the definition of hypoglycemia remains debated. For this review we will adopt the American Diabetes Association (ADA) and European Association for the Study of Diabetes (EASD) guidelines that hypoglycemia occurs below a plasma glucose level of <70 mg/dL (3.9 mmol/L) (3). Endocrine Society guideline recommendations for all individuals cite any glucose concentration below which symptoms are evident (4). A recent workgroup from the ADA and Endocrine Society defines iatrogenic hypoglycemia in patients with diabetes as the glucose level that exposes the individual to potential harm (5). Subclasses of hypoglycemia include severe, symptomatic, asymptomatic, probable, and pseudohypoglycemia (Table 25-1). Severe hypoglycemia is defined as hypoglycemia resulting in the requirement of assistance of another individual to administer rescue therapy (5).

Most recommend documentation of Whipple's triad (ie, low plasma glucose, symptoms or signs consistent with hypoglycemia, and resolution of those symptoms after the plasma glucose has been raised) to confirm hypoglycemia, especially in persons without

Table 25-1. Classification of Hypoglycemia in Individuals with Diabetes (5)

Severe	Requiring the assistance of another individual to administer rescue therapy
Symptomatic	Typical symptoms, plasma glucose <70 mg/dL (3.9 mmol/L)
Asymptomatic	No symptoms, plasma glucose <70 mg/dL (3.9 mmol/L)
Probable	Typical symptoms, no plasma glucose available
Pseudohypoglycemia	Typical symptoms, plasma glucose >70 mg/dL (>3.9 mmol/L)

diabetes (6). This allows clinicians to reduce unnecessary evaluation and potential harm in those situations where Whipple's triad is not observed. However, in an individual diagnosed and treated for diabetes, the probability of hypoglycemia is high, and treatment should be initiated without deferring evaluation even when a plasma glucose is unavailable for documentation.

EPIDEMIOLOGY

Hypoglycemia occurs predominantly in patients with T1DM or T2DM treated with insulin or with combination therapy involving insulin and an insulin secretagogue. In a large 1-year study that included more than 8,500 people with diabetes, 7.1% of persons with T1DM and 7.3% with insulin-treated T2DM experienced at least 1 episode of severe hypoglycemia (1). In the same study, the incidence of severe hypoglycemia in T2DM patients treated with sulfonylureas was 0.8% per year. Older individuals are at increased risk for hypoglycemia. Recent large randomized controlled trials of intensive glycemic therapy in T2DM patients, including ACCORD (7) and ADVANCE (8), reported progressive increases in risk of ~3% per year with advancing age. In addition, the T1D Exchange study in T1DM patients demonstrated a 12-month frequency of severe hypoglycemia of 19% in patients aged ≥65 years (9). In pregnant women with diabetes, severe hypoglycemia increases nearly 3-fold during the first trimester compared to prepregnancy, with rates of hypoglycemia declining with each successive trimester, from 5.3 to 2.4 to 0.5 events per patient-year in the first, second, and third trimesters, respectively (10). For critically ill patients treated with intensive insulin therapy in the intensive care unit (ICU), rates of hypoglycemia range from 2.1% to 11.5% (11).

In the United States, from 1993 to 2005, ~5 million emergency department visits were due to hypoglycemic events, 25% of which led to hospitalization (12). This is especially common in elderly patients with diabetes (more than 25% of the US population aged ≥65 years has diabetes), where hospital admissions for severe hypoglycemia were 2-fold higher than admissions for hyperglycemia among nearly 34 million Medicare beneficiaries in patients with T2DM aged 85 years and older compared with younger (65–84 years old) beneficiaries (13). Overall, hypoglycemia in patients treated with insulin is associated with a 2-fold increase in hospitalizations and emergency department visits for any reason (12). Hypoglycemia confers a large financial burden, costing over $3,200 per patient that experiences a hypoglycemic event. Absenteeism and use of short-term disability compensation are also drastically increased (14,15).

Reports suggest that 2%–13% of deaths in patients with T1DM are attributable to hypoglycemia (4,16,17). Hypoglycemia may be involved in "dead in bed" syndrome, perhaps through cardiac conduction system effects. Continuous electrocardiographic (ECG) monitoring has revealed sinus bradycardia, atrial, and ventricular ectopic beats, and P-wave abnormalities, as well as significant QT-interval prolongation during episodes of spontaneous nocturnal hypoglycemia (18,19). Under controlled insulin-induced hypoglycemia, bradycardia, ventricular ectopic beats, ST-segment depression, and T-wave flattening were observed in a portion of subjects with T2DM (20). Long-term cardiovascular damage may also be attributed to hypoglycemia, given that single and repeated hypoglycemic events induce acute inflammation, oxidative stress, leukocytosis, endothelial dysfunction, and prothrombogenic and atherogenic mechanisms (21–23). A history of repeated mild and severe hypoglycemia has also been associated with increased inflammation, endothelial dysfunction, and intima-media thickness and reduced flow-mediated arterial dilatation (24). In large intervention trials, hypoglycemia was associated with increased hazard ratios for major macro- and microvascular events, as well as cardiovascular-related and all-cause mortality (8,25). Additionally, the NICE-SUGAR trial demonstrated that critically ill patients who are intensively controlled had an increased risk of moderate-to-severe hypoglycemia and an increased risk of death (26).

GLUCOSE MEASUREMENTS

The accuracy of measured glucose samples should be considered when evaluating acute hypoglycemia. Plasma glucose samples are up to 15% higher than mixed venous whole blood glucose samples (27). Thus, knowing if a blood glucose meter is providing blood or plasma values is important for interpretation, because the lower limit of normal would be approximately 60 mg/dL (3.3 mmol/L) for a mixed venous whole blood glucose sample. Glucose meters can be imprecise, especially at low blood glucose levels (27). The correct calibration of the meter should always be ensured, especially if the blood glucose reading is low but the individual lacks corresponding symptoms.

Additionally, mixed venous blood glucose values can be considerably lower than arterial or capillary levels. Thus, under high physiological insulinemia, a venous plasma glucose value in an insulin-sensitive individual can be up to 25 mg/dL (1.5 mmol/L) lower than an arterial level, thereby resulting in a spuriously low level. Many other factors can influence the accuracy of glucose sampling. These include collection in a nonfluoride and/or oxalate containing tube (blood glucose can decrease by 10–20 mg/dL [0.5–1 mmol/L]/hr at room temperature), long duration till sample is tested, high triglyceride content, altitude, temperature, humidity, prolonged exercise exposure, and hemoglobin level (28).

PHYSIOLOGY OF GLUCOSE METABOLISM

In healthy humans, multiple mechanisms have evolved to defend against a falling plasma glucose. A coordinated interplay of insulin inhibition and release of the powerful counter-regulatory hormones, including glucagon and epinephrine, form the acute defense against hypoglycemia. Cortisol and growth hormone (GH) have a limited role in the homeostatic (counter-regulatory) response to acute hypoglycemia. However, chronic deficiencies of cortisol and/or GH can present as hypoglycemic emergencies (Figure 25-2) (29).

Postprandial glucose levels are maintained by nutrient entry from the gut. In the postabsorptive state, plasma glucose is maintained by the balance of glucose release from the liver (initially glycogenolysis and then gluconeogenesis) and uptake by peripheral tissues (predominantly peripheral muscle). Hepatic glucose production is acutely regulated by the inhibitory action of insulin and the stimulatory signals of glucagon and the autonomic nervous system (ANS). Peripheral glucose uptake is regulated by insulin levels, degree of insulin resistance, and catecholamine levels (predominantly epinephrine). Glucagon has a very limited effect, if at all, on influencing peripheral glucose uptake.

As glucose levels fall, the first counter-regulatory response is to inhibit endogenous insulin release. This occurs at plasma glucose levels below 80 mg/dL (4.5 mmol/L). At ~70 mg/dL (3.9 mmol/L), the powerful anti-insulin counter-regulatory hormones (glucagon, epinephrine, cortisol, growth hormone) are released "in concerto." Hepatic glycogenolysis and gluconeogenesis increase. The "threshold" level of norepinephrine release during a falling plasma glucose is difficult to determine. Hyperinsulinemia, even during euglycemic conditions, will stimulate ANS activity and norepinephrine release. If hypoglycemia is prolonged (>4 hr), then GH and cortisol begin to play a role in the counter-regulatory metabolic defense. Both can stimulate hepatic glucose production (gluconeogenesis) and inhibit glucose uptake. However, the contribution of both of these hormones is only about 20% that of epinephrine. The combined adrenomedullary and direct neural ANS effects on lipolysis are an additional important counter-regulatory mechanism. In fact, lipolysis provides ~25% of the defense against a falling glucose by providing glycerol and free fatty acids (FFAs) as substrate and energy, respectively, for gluconeogenesis. Furthermore, elevated FFA levels provide an alternative fuel substrate for muscle, thereby preserving circulating glucose.

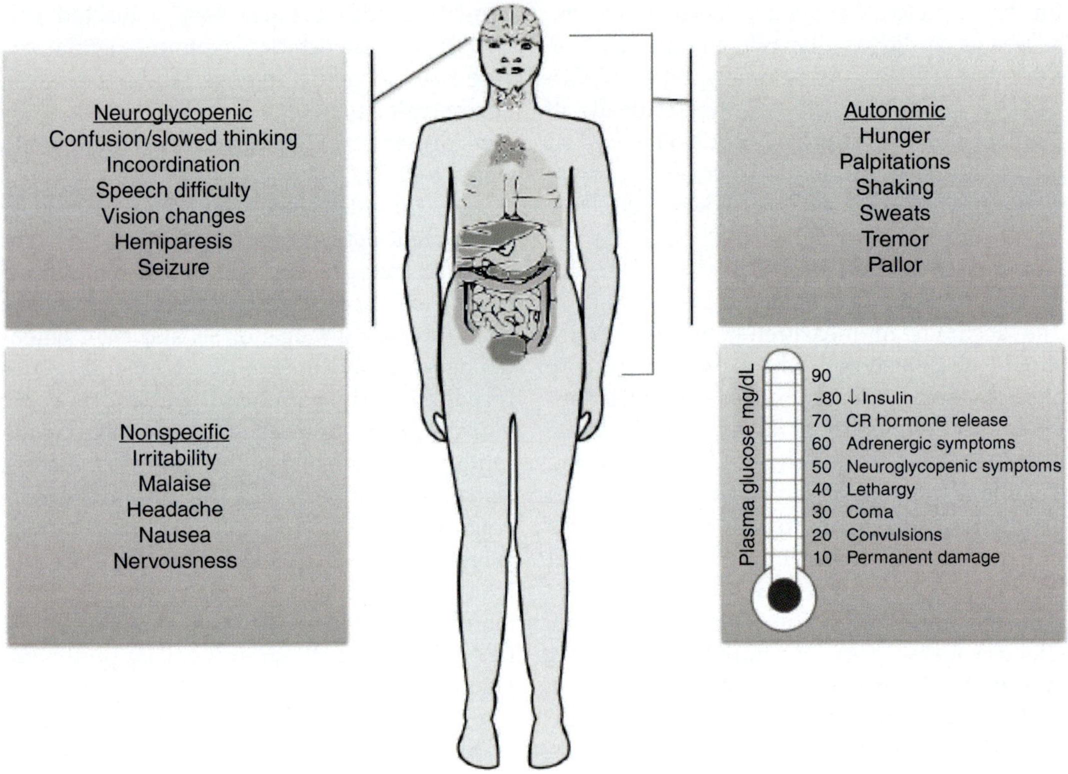

Figure 25-1. Symptoms of hypoglycemia.

Epinephrine has a complementary and multifaceted role in the defense against hypoglycemia by stimulating hepatic glucose production (initially via glycogenolysis then gluconeogenesis from liver and kidney), adipose tissue lipolysis, and skeletal muscle glycogenolysis and proteolysis, while inhibiting glucose uptake by insulin-responsive tissues.

Hypoglycemia manifests as an array of autonomic (ie, palpitations, tremor, sweating, pallor, and anxiety) and neuroglycopenic (ie, behavior changes, fatigue, seizure, loss of consciousness) signs and symptoms (Figure 25-1). The glucose threshold for the generation of autonomic signs and symptoms is plastic in nature but is typically ~60 mg/dL (3.3 mmol/L). Neuroglycopenic signs and symptoms arising from a central nervous system glucose deficit occur at lower blood glucose levels (~50 mg/dL [2.8 mmol/L]). It should be noted that hunger, per se, is a poor symptom discriminator for hypoglycemia. The origins of autonomic signs and symptoms are complex but sympathoadrenal output appears to be the primary driver. Epinephrine is responsible for ~20%–25% of the symptoms of hypoglycemia, suggesting that a large portion of signs and symptoms arise from sympathetic neural activation (30). The ability to recognize hypoglycemic symptoms within oneself is known as hypoglycemia awareness. Autonomic signs and symptoms are the indicators most recognizable to the patient, but the specific combination of symptoms experienced during a hypoglycemic episode varies inter- and intraindividually.

Hormonal counter-regulatory responses and hypoglycemic symptoms occur at similar thresholds in men and women, but in women peak counter-regulatory hormone levels are lower (31,32). The reason for these gender differences is not well-understood, but increased levels of estrogen may play an important role (33).

Pathophysiology of Glucose Metabolism in Diabetes

In T1DM and insulin-deficient T2DM individuals, a number of pathophysiological defects reduce the counter-regulatory response to hypoglycemia. These include the following:

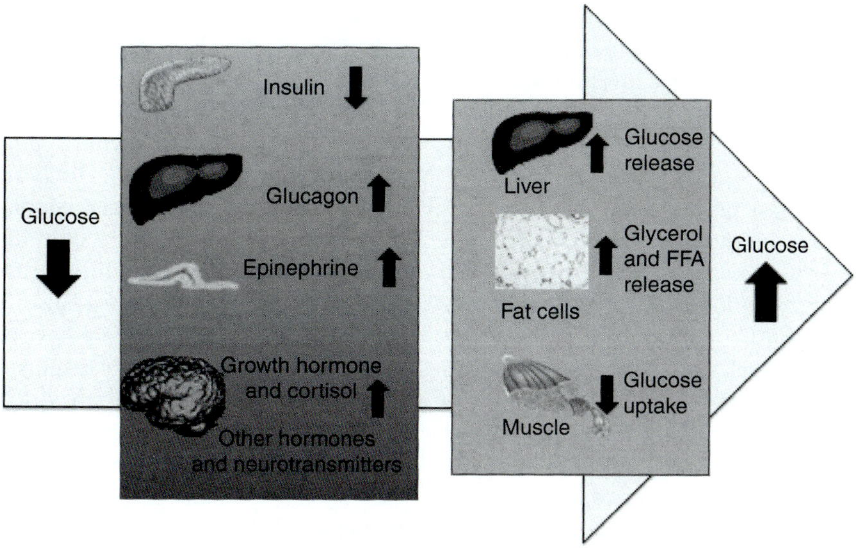

Figure 25-2. Normal counter-regulatory hormonal and metabolic responses to declining blood glucose level.

1. *First defense*: Inhibition of endogenous insulin secretion is lost. Absolute insulin deficiency precludes a physiological mechanism to reduce insulin levels, leaving the diabetic individual defenseless to previously dosed long-acting insulin or residual insulin within the subcutaneous depot, which will sustain circulating insulin levels in the face of a falling blood glucose. Residual, albeit impaired, insulin secretion in shorter-duration T2DM provides a buffer against decreasing blood glucose levels, as insulin secretion can still be physiologically inhibited.
2. *Secondary defense*: After about 5 years there is a loss of glucagon response to hypoglycemia in T1DM. It is postulated that the glucagon response may be lost either as a result of a signaling defect within the pancreatic alpha cell due to a lack of a reduction in endogenous insulin and/or ANS input. However, alpha cells in T1DM are present in normal number and size and respond appropriately to other physiological stresses (ie, exercise, amino acids). Without adequate glucagon secretion, the usual rapid response (10–15 min) of glucose production from the liver is reduced. Glycogenolysis and later gluconeogenesis (if glycerol, lactate, pyruvate, and amino acids are available) may also be impaired.
3. *Third defense*: Reduction of epinephrine response occurs. The ability to promote glucose recovery from hypoglycemia is dependent upon epinephrine-mediated beta-adrenergic mechanisms in the glucagon deficient state (34). This is especially prominent after antecedent hypoglycemia or associated with classic diabetic autonomic neuropathy. Without adequate epinephrine stimulation, hepatic glycogenolysis and later hepatic and renal gluconeogenesis are impaired. Stimulation of lipolysis is also consequently blunted, reducing available FFAs and glycerol and maintaining reliance on circulating glucose. The inhibitory effect of epinephrine on skeletal muscle glucose uptake is lost, and hypoglycemia can be extended.
4. *Signs and symptoms*: Symptom responses become blunted together with reduced hormonal counter-regulatory responses (35). Reduced epinephrine levels are a factor, but reduced sympathetic neural outflow may also be implicated. Importantly, autonomic symptoms are initiated at progressively lower blood glucose levels, and, therefore, autonomic and neuroglycopenic symptom

thresholds become compressed, allowing less time to recognize and appropriately respond to a low blood glucose level before cognitive dysfunction ensues.

Failure of these protective mechanisms can lead to severe, unimpeded hypoglycemia. In cases of recurring episodes of hypoglycemia, the threshold for initiation of counter-regulatory hormone responses is reduced to a lower plasma glucose level, and hormone responses become blunted. A blunted epinephrine response increases the risk of iatrogenic hypoglycemia 25-fold (36). Patients also develop hypoglycemia unawareness, in which symptoms are delayed and blunted and may be unrecognizable to the individual. Hypoglycemia unawareness, affecting ~20%–25% of T1DM patients (37) and increasingly recognized in T2DM (38), elevates the risk of severe hypoglycemia 6-fold.

Collectively, the reduction of hormonal and symptom responses to recurring episodes of hypoglycemia (or other stressors that stimulate autonomic activation) is part of a disorder termed hypoglycemia-associated autonomic failure (HAAF) (39), the presence of which further increases the risk of severe hypoglycemia. HAAF develops independent of the presence of classic diabetic autonomic neuropathy and is not intrinsic to the diabetic state, as the syndrome can be induced in healthy nondiabetic individuals subjected to recurrent bouts of hyperinsulinemic hypoglycemia (40). Mild antecedent hypoglycemia (<70 mg/dL [3.9 mmol/L]) is sufficient to induce blunted glucagon and epinephrine responses to hypoglycemia on the following day. Deeper levels of hypoglycemia (60 and 52 mg/dL [3.3 and 2.9 mmol/L]) have more widespread effects, additionally reducing norepinephrine and GH levels as well as endogenous glucose production and lipolysis in response to next day hypoglycemia (41). Temporally, even very short periods of hypoglycemia (ie, 5–30 min) cause substantial blunting of hormonal responses to subsequent hypoglycemia (42). Related components of HAAF include exercise and sleep. Prolonged low-to-moderate endurance exercise blunts counter-regulatory responses to subsequent hypoglycemia (43), while, reciprocally, antecedent hypoglycemia blunts counter-regulatory responses to exercise (44). In either scenario, the patient is exposed to a greater risk of developing hypoglycemia. During sleep, counter-regulatory responses to and awareness of hypoglycemia are delayed and reduced (45), and prolonged nocturnal hypoglycemia is a common occurrence (46). Furthermore, nocturnal hypoglycemia blunts responses to next-day hypoglycemia (47). HAAF likely arises through multiple adaptive mechanisms, which are comprehensively reviewed elsewhere (39).

A number of interventions have been shown to rescue counter-regulatory responses to hypoglycemia at least partially. Firstly, strict avoidance of hypoglycemia by relaxing glycemic targets and educating patients about preventive strategies can help to recover hypoglycemia awareness and epinephrine responses (48). Experimental pharmacological interventions that enhance responses to hypoglycemia and/or minimize blunting effects of antecedent hypoglycemia include fluoxetine and sertraline (selective-serotonin reuptake inhibitors), naloxone (opioid receptor blocker), and diazoxide (ATP-sensitive K+ channel opener) (49).

Age Considerations

Compared with their younger counterparts, older people with diabetes are at increased risk of severe hypoglycemia, especially in cases of longer duration diabetes and limited residual insulin secretion (50). Although controversial, some data suggest that this may be a result of delayed initiation of hormonal responses and/or symptoms (lower blood glucose levels are required to stimulate counter-regulatory responses) (51) or reduced symptom scores in the face of a normal hormonal response (52,53). Reduced perception of milder hypoglycemia may occur with aging in general, as similar impairments were found in older individuals with and without T2DM (51). Regular education regarding symptom identification and treatment options is crucial in this population (54).

MANAGEMENT OF HYPOGLYCEMIA

Most cases of hypoglycemia in patients with diabetes are self-diagnosed and addressed at home, without intervention of a medical provider. Initial treatment generally consists of 15–20 grams of simple carbohydrate to ameliorate the symptoms of mild hypoglycemia

Table 25-2. Management of Mild, Self-Diagnosed, and Treated Hypoglycemia

1. Take 15–20 grams of carbohydrate:
• 3–4 glucose tablets *or* • 4 oz (1/2 cup) of fruit juice • 6 oz (1/2 can) of regular soda
2. Retest and wait 15 minutes
3. Recheck your blood sugar
4. Repeat if blood sugar still less than 80 mg/dL (4.4 mmol/L)

(Table 25-2, Figure 25-3). For a measured blood glucose of <50 mg/dL (2.8 mmol/L), 20–30 grams of carbohydrate should be considered. If the person is treated with an alpha-glucosidase inhibitor, only pure glucose gel or tablets should be taken, because this drug class inhibits absorption of other forms of carbohydrate. It is unknown how effective oral glucose supplementation is in the setting of delayed gastric emptying, for example, with gastroparesis or with medications that delay gastric emptying, such as glucagon-like peptide-1 (GLP-1) agonists, anticholinergics, and narcotics. Foods containing fats should not be ingested when treating for hypoglycemia, because fats delay absorption of glucose. Blood glucose should be measured 15 minutes after consuming carbohydrate, and additional carbohydrate should be ingested if hypoglycemia or hypoglycemic symptoms persist. Glucagon kits can be prescribed to patients with diabetes, and friends, family members, or coworkers can be trained to administer glucagon (1 mg) subcutaneously or intramuscularly, if the patient is unwilling or unable to ingest glucose orally. The effects of glucagon, which acts through stimulation of hepatic glycogenolysis, are delayed by approximately 10 minutes from time of injection and are only inducible in those with available glycogen stores. Of note, family members or responders should avoid sublingual placement

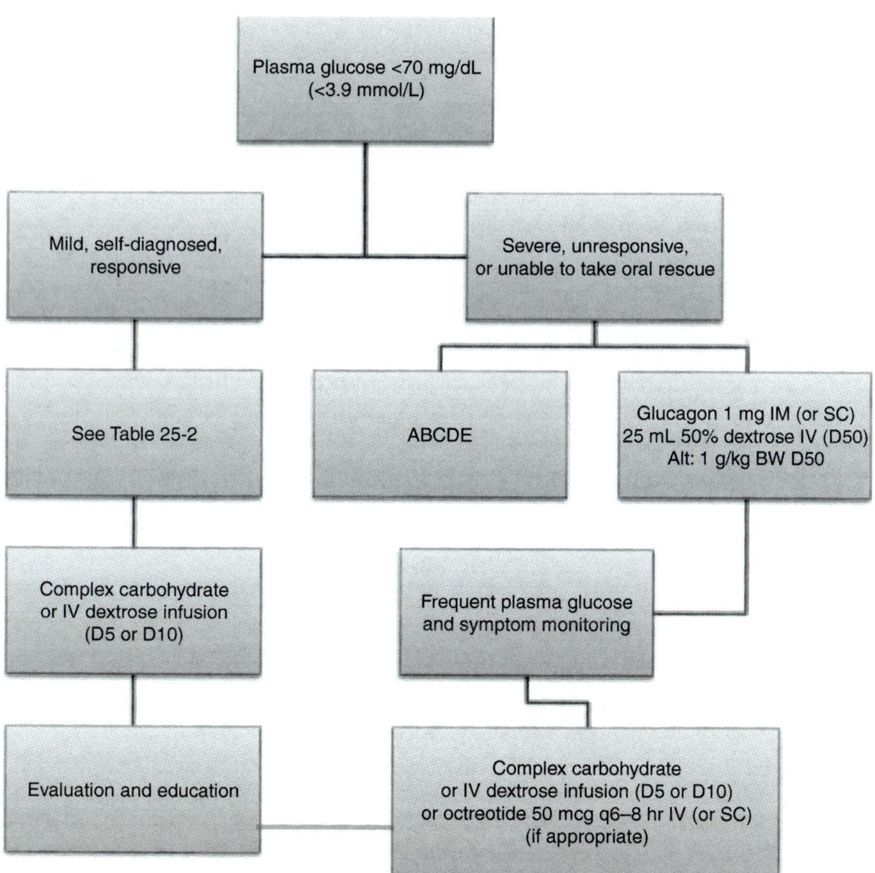

Figure 25-3. Algorithm for acute management of hypoglycemia.

of carbohydrates (ie, hard candy) in an unconscious or impaired individual because this can increase the risk for aspiration. After resolution of hypoglycemia, a full meal or complex snack should be consumed because an insulin depot may still be active and to restore glycogen stores. Pseudohypoglycemia in the setting of regimen intensification in an individual with previously uncontrolled glucoses should be treated with ~5 grams of carbohydrates to avoid overcorrection, and the individual should receive reassurance that he or she will adapt to improved glycemic control in about 3–4 weeks.

Severe hypoglycemia requiring assistance of a second or third party should be assessed and addressed in the hospital setting. Initial assessment and management should begin with the ABCDEs (airway, breathing, circulation, disability [ie, conscious level], and exposure [ie, examination and evaluation]). Consideration should always be given to other acute medical conditions that may mimic or coincide with hypoglycemia (eg, acute coronary syndrome, acute ischemic stroke, sepsis, and shock). However, rapid recognition of a low glucose is imperative because prolonged severe hypoglycemia can result in irreversible brain damage, cardiovascular strain, and death (23,55).

Patients hospitalized for hypoglycemia can be initially managed with intravenous (IV) infusion of 25 grams of 50% dextrose in water (D50) or 1 gram per kilogram of body weight D50. D50 is an irritant, and delivery through a large gauge port and vein, followed by a saline flush, is preferable. Alternatively, D20 (20% dextrose) or D10 (10% dextrose) are less irritating and can be administered via a peripheral vein in a proportionally larger volume.

As in self-treated patients, once euglycemia is attained, a meal or a snack including carbohydrate and protein should be ingested to prevent a recurrent episode of hypoglycemia. If oral intake is not an option, D5 or D10 can be infused to maintain euglycemia. Parenteral or enteric feeding may be considered in individuals to replenish glycogen stores as indicated. In cases of sulfonylurea-induced hypoglycemia, glucose administration can actually stimulate continued insulin secretion; 50–100 µg of the somatostatin analog octreotide, administered IV or SC every 8 hours, can be used to inhibit insulin secretion and prevent recurring hypoglycemia in this setting (56). Exogenous administration of long-acting insulin resulting in persistent hypoglycemia will require the administration of infused dextrose or continuous carbohydrate ingestion till the duration of insulin action is surpassed.

Individuals with malnutrition or suspected long-term alcohol use should receive thiamine (100 mg IV) to reduce the risk for Wernicke's encephalopathy (57). Due to reduced glycogen stores, these individuals may also benefit from enteral or parenteral feeding. When adrenal crisis is suspected, administration of IV saline solution and glucocorticoids with IV hydrocortisone 50–100 mg IV will provide glucocorticoid, mineralocorticoid, and vascular support (58). Hydrocortisone can be transitioned to oral therapy once the individual is stabilized.

In the case of suspected inborn errors of metabolism (Table 25-3), specific treatments may be indicated (59). For example, fructose elimination is the treatment for inherited fructose intolerance; carnitine supplementation and/or avoidance of fasting and maintenance of glucose levels during stress in mitochondrial fatty acid oxidation disorders; and avoidance of stress, frequent meals (especially overnight), and the use of uncooked starch supplementation in glycogen storage diseases.

Following resolution of hypoglycemia, blood glucose measurements should be repeated every 15–30 minutes for at least 2 hours, or longer depending on the etiology (3,4). Symptoms and signs of hypoglycemia should resolve once euglycemia is achieved and maintained. However, an alternative diagnosis (ie, stroke, delirium, drug overdose) should be considered if symptoms persist despite euglycemia.

ETIOLOGY

Once an individual and serum glucose have been stabilized, evaluation of the underlying etiology is imperative to reduce the risk of future episodes of hypoglycemia (Figure 25-3) and, in the case of nondiabetes-associated hypoglycemia, to ultimately treat the underlying condition (Table 25-4). The focus of investigation is markedly different in those individuals with diabetes as opposed to those with nondiabetes-associated hypoglycemia.

Table 25-3. Inborn Errors of Metabolism Causing Hypoglycemia (59)

Fasting hypoglycemia		
	Glycogen storage disorders	Types I, III, O, Fanconi-Bickel (GLUT 2)
	Defect in fatty acid oxidation	CPT1, VLCAD, MCAD, SCHAD, LCHAD, HMG-CoA synthase and lyase
	Gluconeogenesis	Fructose 1,6-bisphosphatase
Postprandial hypoglycemia		
	Noninsulinoma pancreatogenic hypoglycemia syndrome	Mutations in SUR1, Kir6.2, SCHAD, GDH, glucokinase, MCT1 (also associated with exercise-induced hypoglycemia), UCP2
	Congenital disorders of glycosylation	Types 1a, 1b, 1d
	Inherited fructose intolerance	
Rare (observed in children)		
	Biotin-responsive multiple carboxylase deficiency	
	Respiratory chain defects	
	Organic aciduria	

Abbreviations: CPT = carnitine palmitoyltransferase; GDH = glutamate dehydrogenase; GLUT 2 = glucose transporter 2; HMG = 3-hydroxy-3-methyl-glutary; LCHAD = long-chain 3 hydroxyacyl-CoA dehydrogenase; MCAD = medium-chain acyl-CoA dehydrogenase; MCT = monocarboxylate transporter; SCHAD = short-chain L-3-hydroxyacyl-CoA dehydrogenase; UCP = mitochondrial uncoupling protein; VLCAD = very long-chain acyl-CoA dehydrogenase.

Table 25-4. Etiologies and Possible Mechanisms of Hypoglycemia

Increased insulin	**Impaired gluconeogenesis/ glycogenolysis**	**Counter-regulatory failure**
• Exogenous insulin • Sulfonylurea • Meglitinides • Quinine • Trimethoprim-sulfamethoxazole • Alcohol • Insulinoma • Insulin or insulin receptor antibodies (autoimmune)	• Salicylates • Beta-adrenergic blockers • Hepatic failure • Renal failure • Alcohol	• Autonomic dysfunction • Exercise • Addison's disease • Pan-hypopituitarism • Growth hormone deficiency • Hypothyroidism
Increased insulin sensitivity	**Increased glucose utilization/ peripheral tissue uptake**	**Complex mechanisms**
• Exercise • Weight loss • Fasting	• Exercise • Sepsis	• Mesenchymal tumors (IGF-2) • Islet cell hyperplasia • Inborn errors of metabolism • Inherited enzyme defects
Beta-cell toxicity	**Decreased insulin clearance**	**Reactive hypoglycemia**
• Pentamidine	• Renal failure	• Idiopathic • Dumping syndrome

Abbreviations: IGF-2 = insulin-like growth factor 2.

Nonhospitalized Individuals

All outpatient encounters with individuals with diabetes should address hypoglycemia. Patients with diabetes (type 1 or type 2) with frequent and/or severe hypoglycemia that is treated outside of the hospital require extensive review of treatment regimen and adherence, timing and frequency of hypoglycemia, timing and frequency of hypoglycemia to medication administration (especially in those treated with insulin and insulin secretagogues or treatments that are in combination with either), new medications (such as indomethacin, nonselective beta blockers, and antibiotics like trimethoprim-sulfamethoxazole), and alcohol use. An individual should provide the glucose value at which he or she first feels hypoglycemic symptoms or signs. It is important to recognize that antihyperglycemic agents that are not routinely associated with hypoglycemia (ie, GLP-1 agonists, dipeptidyl-dipeptidase-4 [DPP-4] inhibitors, thiazolidinediones [TZD], acarbose, metformin, sodium-glucose cotransporter 2 [SGLT-2] inhibitors) may result in unanticipated hypoglycemic events when combined with insulin and/or sulfonylureas (60). A detailed exercise or weight-loss history can elucidate why particular patients may be more insulin-sensitive. Social situations like Ramadan fasting may necessitate temporary changes to an individual's diabetic regimen or the addition of a continuous glucose monitor (CGM) for improved glucose monitoring (61). Patients with T1DM may require additional education on carbohydrate counting and review of the often complex regimens that accompany insulin pump therapy. New or worsening neuropathy may be a red flag to indicate evaluation of autonomic dysfunction and hypoglycemic unawareness. Progressive renal disease may lead to decreased clearance of insulin or sulfonylureas and their metabolites (ie, glyburide [glibenclamide]) (62). An increased risk for adrenal insufficiency and thyroid disease may prompt appropriate evaluation in individuals with T1DM (63).

A number of large studies, including the ACCORD and the Veterans Affairs (VA) Diabetes Trial, have demonstrated that intensive glycemic control was associated with increased mortality and a higher frequency of hypoglycemia in individuals with type 2 diabetes (64,65). This should always prompt the provider to review and individualize treatment goals based on age and comorbidities while taking into account the established microvascular and macrovascular benefits of improved glycemic control (66). Implementation of flexible insulin regimens, increased frequency of self-monitoring of blood glucose (SMBG), and CGM should be considered, such as investigated in the Dose Adjustment for Normal Eating (DAFNE) trial (67). A switch to insulin pump therapy may be considered in individuals with T1DM or absolute insulin deficiency with frequent hypoglycemia. Use of insulin pump therapy has been shown to improve glycemic control while reducing the rate of hypoglycemia (68).

The dangerous condition of hypoglycemic unawareness is prevalent in patients with absolute insulin deficiency (T1DM or long-duration T2DM) (39) and can lead to a vicious cycle of hypoglycemia. There can be a substantial fear of nocturnal hypoglycemia and the associated "dead in bed" syndrome that precludes adequate treatment and achievement of glycemic goals (18). Review of basal regimens and bedtime glucose monitoring may be necessary (69). The use of CGM to alert individuals or close third-parties to a rapidly falling glucose and/or use of low glucose suspension thresholds on insulin pumps to automatically halt insulin delivery can reduce nocturnal hypoglycemia. In a recent study in T1DM patients using a low glucose suspend feature on the insulin pump, nocturnal hypoglycemia was reduced by 31.8% compared with controls (70). Sensor-augmented insulin pump therapy also reduces glycemic variability and achieves improved glycemic goals compared to multi-daily injections without an increased rate of hypoglycemia (71). Scrupulous avoidance of hypoglycemia by changing target glucoses and toleration of a higher threshold of average glucose for as little as 3 weeks can help improve symptom awareness to hypoglycemia in individuals with T1DM (39).

Exercise

Exercise is a significant component of the larger diabetes treatment plan. However, exercise-associated hypoglycemia can prevent individuals from embracing this beneficial intervention. Exercise-associated hypoglycemia can occur within minutes to several hours postexercise (72). Thus, patient education regarding the timing of exercise to insulin/secretagogue administration, carbohydrate ingestion, and frequent glucose monitoring before, during, and after exercise may be necessary to address this risk.

Alcohol

Alcohol consumption can block release of hepatic glucose stores, leading to hypoglycemia. Fasting, sustained physical exercise, malnutrition, and medication administration (ie, insulin or insulin secretagogues) are precipitating factors (73). Alcohol can cause hypoglycemia up to 24 hours after ingestion. Recommendations from the ADA include limited alcohol consumption, increased non-alcohol hydration (ie, water, tonic water), avoidance of using alcohol carbohydrates in carbohydrate counting, and maintaining carbohydrate intake while consuming alcohol. Increased frequency of SMBG may be necessary and should be performed prior to bedtime (3).

Other Activities

Specific recommendations should be provided to individuals at risk for hypoglycemia or those whom one is evaluating for hypoglycemia regarding driving and recreational activities like scuba diving. Driving restrictions have recently been relaxed in Europe and the United States for individuals with diabetes (74). However, individuals with diabetes should not drive if they have hypoglycemic unawareness or recent severe hypoglycemia (ie, within the last 12 months). They should receive regular diabetes education and evaluation. Prior to driving, SMBG should be checked and rechecked at 1–2 hour intervals. Individuals should wait at least 45 minutes to drive after blood glucose has returned to normal, and a fast-acting supply of carbohydrates should always be available.

Pregnancy

Maternal hypoglycemia during pregnancy is a risk factor for newborns small for gestational age, which in turn is associated with increased long-term risks such as development of diabetes, coronary artery disease, and hypertension (75). Postabsorptive blood glucose tends to decline in nondiabetic women during pregnancy by ~10 mg/dL (0.55 mmol/L), with a reported mean of 71 mg/dL (4.1 mmol/L) (76), although blood glucose measurements <70 mg/dL (3.9 mmol/L) are not abnormal. Therefore, recommendations for target premeal, postprandial, and average daily blood glucose levels in pregnant women with diabetes are 60–99 mg/dL (3.3–5.5 mmol/L), 100–129 mg/dL (5.6–7.1 mmol/L), and <110 mg/dL (6.0 mmol/L), respectively, with a target HbA1c <6.0% (77). Reports generally indicate that hormonal counter-regulatory responses to hypoglycemia are impaired during pregnancy (75), but risk of severe hypoglycemia is related to history of severe hypoglycemia, hypoglycemia unawareness, >10 years' diabetes duration, larger total daily dose of insulin, and HbA1c <6.5% (9,10). Recommendations for reducing the risk of hypoglycemia include educating pregnant women regarding recognizing and treating of hypoglycemia, SMBG, maintaining an available supply of carbohydrate snacks, and timing exercise, food consumption, and insulin dosing. Additionally, intensified glycemic control prior to pregnancy may help reduce risk, while relaxing glycemic targets is recommended for women reporting impaired awareness (75).

Hospitalized Individuals

The preceding discussion of the evaluation of hypoglycemia in the outpatient individual with diabetes should be a component of the assessment of the inpatient diabetic or nondiabetic individual with hypoglycemia. A detailed medication history is imperative. This should include the individual's outpatient diabetic regimen and whether this was continued, adjusted, and/or altered as an inpatient. Hypoglycemic events can be prevented with improved coordination of patient transfer within the hospital setting and at discharge. Insulin administration, especially with use of U-500 regular insulin, can identify incorrect prescriptions and administration errors (78,79). Hypoglycemia can occur when there is failure to recognize or adjust insulin regimens based on available blood glucose data. Continuation of prandial insulin or insulin secretagogue therapy in individuals who are not eating or have been placed on a dietary restriction should be identified and corrected, as should insulin therapy in patients in whom parenteral or enteral feeding is interrupted. There is a limited role for oral hypoglycemic agents in the inpatient setting (3). Concomitant malnourishment, renal or hepatic disease, sepsis, malignancy, and rapid withdrawal of glucocorticoid therapy may alter peripheral glucose uptake, gluconeogenesis and glycogenolysis, and medication clearance (80).

All hospitalized patients with diabetes benefit from a structured diabetes care plan, ideally supervised by specialists (81). As recommended by the ADA, glycemic goals should be tailored to the patient, surgical versus medical status, and level of acuity. Most ICU patients should aim for blood glucose levels from 140–180 mg/dL (7.8–10 mmol/L), and less-intensive patients should aim for premeal blood glucose levels <140 mg/dL (7.8 mmol/L) and random blood glucose levels <180 mg/dL (10 mmol/L). The use of IV insulin infusion in critically ill patients is the most effective method for controlling blood glucose (82). Validated written or computerized algorithms should be employed for adjustments to IV insulin infusion rate based on fluctuations in blood glucose (81). The Endocrine Society recommended that non-ICU patients benefit from structured basal and/or prandial/correction with rapid-acting insulin (83).

Nondiabetic Individuals

Nondiabetes-associated hypoglycemia is essentially a failure of endogenous glucose production to match high rates of glucose utilization. An extensive history, as well as physical and laboratory review, should be undertaken to identify drug-induced hypoglycemia, hormonal deficiencies, critical illness, and/or reactive hypoglycemia. Mechanisms of drug-induced hypoglycemia include exogenous hyperinsulinemia, impaired gluconeogenesis, and increased insulin secretion (84). By extension, trials off these offending agents should be attempted. Alcohol use or abuse should also be documented. Hormonal deficiencies such as adrenal insufficiency (primary, secondary, or postsurgical Cushing's disease patients) and hypopituitarism can lead to failure of glucose counter-regulation. A plasma cortisol at the time of hypoglycemia is not sufficient to diagnose adrenal insufficiency and should be followed by a formal short ACTH stimulation test (58). Hypothyroidism may be associated with abnormalities in the hypothalamic-pituitary-adrenal axis leading to hypoglycemia (85). Growth hormone deficiency is a rare cause of hypoglycemia. Sepsis can lead to increased glucose uptake whereas hepatic failure or severe malnutrition is associated with impaired gluconeogenesis and glycogenolysis. The kidney is responsible for 25%–50% of total gluconeogenesis, and individuals with advanced renal disease may present with hypoglycemia.

A childhood history of inherited metabolic disorders can also alert potential associations (ie, hereditary fructose intolerance or multiple endocrine neoplasia [MEN] syndromes) or the risk for polyglandular syndromes (ie, adrenal insufficiency, hypothyroidism). A number of inborn errors of metabolism can present with hypoglycemia (Table 25-3) (59). This is usually the result of impaired gluconeogenesis and inability to rely on ketone bodies for alternative fuel. Adult presentations of these disorders are usually less frequent and severe than the presentations observed in children. Hypoglycemia associated with encephalopathy, neurological defects, multiorgan involvement, and even death should raise one's suspicion of an inborn error of metabolism. Appropriate evaluation should include blood lactate, pyruvate, FFAs, glycerol, ketones, amino acid profile, carnitine, acylcarnitine, and a galactosemia screen. Urine tests should include organic acids and carnitine (59).

Postbariatric Surgery

With a history of reactive or postprandial hypoglycemia, documentation of recent bariatric or gastric surgery is helpful. Although as many as 30% of individuals in the postgastric bypass population may experience asymptomatic hypoglycemia, a small group are actually hospitalized (1%) (86). When the various types of gastric bypass surgery (restrictive vs malabsorptive) were evaluated, the rapid delivery of nutrients to the lower gut (by virtue of excluding the proximal gut) appears to be the critical element in the manifestation of severe hypoglycemia (87). The mechanism(s) by which this occurs remain poorly understood. Reactive hypoglycemia results in inappropriate hyperinsulinemia and GLP-1 release that usually occurs within 4 hours of an ingested mixed meal (88). The contribution of pancreatic islet nesidioblastosis, the contribution of GLP-1 action to beta-cell proliferation, and/or the association of postbariatric hypoglycemia with insulinoma are also reported (88,89). Mixed-meal testing (over 5 hours) can be supportive to the diagnosis (4), and treatment can include surgery (ie, partial pancreatectomy in the case of nesidioblastosis), dietary modifications (ie, long-acting carbohydrate sources or small frequent meals), and/or pharmaceutical treatment (ie, alpha-glucosidase inhibitor, calcium channel blockers, diazoxide, or somatostatin analogs such as octreotide or lanreotide).

In individuals without historical or physical findings that elucidate the etiology of hypoglycemia and who satisfy Whipple's triad, it is reasonable to perform diagnostic differentiation of endogenous and exogenous hyperinsulinemia from other causes. At the time of hypoglycemia, plasma glucose, insulin, C-peptide, proinsulin, beta-hydroxybutyrate, and an oral sulfonylurea screen that includes glinides should be obtained. Following the lab draw, administering glucagon IV and subsequent 30-minute plasma glucose can evaluate hepatic glycogen stores. Critical diagnostic values are plasma insulin of ≥3 mcgU/mL (18 pmol/L), C-peptide ≥0.6 ng/mL (0.2 nmol/L), and proinsulin of ≥5 pmol/L when the plasma glucose is <55 mg/dL (3 mmol/L). A beta-hydroxybutyrate level ≤2.7 mmol/L and an increase of at least 25 mg/dL (1.4 mmol/L) of plasma glucose after glucagon stimulation indicate normal glycogen stores. The patterns of specific laboratory findings and associated diagnoses can be found in "Evaluation and Management of Adult Hypoglycemic Disorders: An Endocrine Society Clinical Practice Guideline" (4). Obtaining insulin antibodies will identify those with insulin autoimmune hypoglycemia. Rarely, insulin receptor antibodies make a diagnosis (90). Treatment of autoimmune hypoglycemia with immunosuppressant therapy is variably effective, but the disease may be self-limiting. Nonislet cell tumors, such as large mesenchymal tumors or hepatocellular tumors, may secrete insulin-like growth factor 2 (IGF-2) or stimulate increased glucose utilization. Surgery, radiation, or chemotherapy can often resolve hypoglycemia in these cases, but medical therapy (as described previously) can be utilized.

Recreating certain circumstances may help in obtaining the laboratory evaluation, such as timing with early morning, fasting, or postprandial symptoms. Some patients can tolerate an overnight fast and others may require a formal 72-hour inpatient fast. Most patients with an insulinoma will meet diagnostic criteria in less than 72 hours (90). Detection of an insulinoma may be complicated. Because an insulin-sensitive individual, under high physiological insulinemia, can have a spuriously low venous plasma glucose, evaluation of insulinoma should be performed with a 72-hour fast rather than a 3-hour oral glucose tolerance test. They are often small (<1 cm), and negative imaging (CT, MRI, or transabdominal ultrasound) should not exclude the diagnosis. Selective arterial calcium injections or exploratory surgery may be necessary (92). Treatment of benign insulinoma is surgical resection.

Lastly, evaluation of an otherwise healthy individual with hypoglycemia requires some consideration of malicious or surreptitious abuse of insulin or insulin secretagogue therapy, or accidental inappropriate medication administration. This may be as simple as sending the oral sulfonylurea screen or close inspection of pills.

CONCLUSIONS

Acute hypoglycemia is a common endocrine emergency that requires prompt treatment and evaluation. Individuals with or without diabetes should be managed quickly with the same algorithm to avoid adverse morbidity and mortality. Most commonly seen in individuals with diabetes, an assessment of multiple factors, including regimen, comorbid conditions, and education, is necessary. The evaluation of individuals without diabetes is more complex and requires a careful history and potentially a laboratory evaluation to discern the underlying etiology. Ultimately, education is the key to prevention and early intervention.

ACKNOWLEDGMENTS

SND is a consultant to Sanofi.

REFERENCES

1. **Leese GP, Wang J, Broomhall J, et al.** Frequency of severe hypoglycemia requiring emergency treatment

in type 1 and type 2 diabetes: a population-based study of health service resource use. *Diabetes Care.* 2003;26:1176–1180.

2. **Hypoglycemia in the diabetes control and complications trial.** The diabetes control and complications trial research group. *Diabetes.* 1997;46:271–286.
3. Executive summary: standards of medical care in diabetes—2014. *Diabetes Care.* 2014;37(suppl 1):S5–S13.
4. **Cryer PE, Axelrod L, Grossman AB, et al.** *Evaluation and Management of Adult Hypoglycemic Disorders: an Endocrine Society Clinical Practice Guideline.* https://www.endocrine.org/~/media/endosociety/Files/Publications/Clinical%20Practice%20Guidelines/FINAL-Standalone-Hypo-Guideline.pdf.
5. **Seaquist ER, Anderson J, Childs B, et al.** Hypoglycemia and diabetes: a report of a workgroup of the American diabetes association and the Endocrine Society. *J Clin Endocrinol Metab.* 2013;98:1845–1859.
6. **Whipple A.** The surgical therapy of hyperinsulinism. *J Int Chir.* 1938;3:237–276.
7. **Miller ME, Bonds DE, Gerstein HC, et al.** The effects of baseline characteristics, glycaemia treatment approach, and glycated haemoglobin concentration on the risk of severe hypoglycaemia: post hoc epidemiological analysis of the ACCORD study. *BMJ.* 2010;340:b5444.
8. **Zoungas S, Patel A, Chalmers J, et al.** Severe hypoglycemia and risks of vascular events and death. *N Engl J Med.* 2010;363:1410–1418.
9. **Weinstock RS, Xing D, Maahs DM et al.** Severe hypoglycemia and diabetic ketoacidosis in adults with type 1 diabetes: results from the T1D Exchange Clinic Registry. *J Clin Endocrinol Metab.* 2013;98:3411–3419.
10. **Nielsen LR, Pedersen-Bjergaard U, Thorsteinsson B, Johansen M, Damm P, Mathiesen ER.** Hypoglycemia in pregnant women with type 1 diabetes: predictors and role of metabolic control. *Diabetes Care.* 2008;31:9–14.
11. **Mukherjee E, Carroll R, Matfin G.** Endocrine and metabolic emergencies: hypoglycaemia. *Ther Adv Endocrinol Metab.* 2011;2:81–93.
12. **Ginde AA, Espinola JA, Camargo CA Jr.** Trends and disparities in U.S. emergency department visits for hypoglycemia, 1993–2005. *Diabetes Care.* 2008;31:511–513.
13. **Lipska KJ, Wang Y, Ross JS, et al.** National trends in hospital admissions for hyperglycemia and hypoglycemia among Medicare beneficiaries, 1999–2010. *ADA.* 2013;Abstract 274-OR.
14. **Rhoads GG, Orsini LS, Crown W, Wang S, Getahun D, Zhang Q.** Contribution of hypoglycemia to medical care expenditures and short-term disability in employees with diabetes. *J Occup Environ Med.* 2005;47:447–452.
15. **Brod M, Christensen T, Thomsen TL, Bushnell DM.** The impact of non-severe hypoglycemic events on work productivity and diabetes management. *Value Health.* 2011;14:665–671.
16. **Awoniyi O, Rehman R, Dagogo-Jack S.** Hypoglycemia in patients with type 1 diabetes: epidemiology, pathogenesis, and prevention. *Curr Diab Rep.* 2013;13:669–678.
17. **Bailey CJ, Day C.** Hypoglycaemia: a limiting factor. *Brit J Diab Vasc Dis.* 2010;10:2–4.
18. **Gill GV, Woodward A, Casson IF, Weston PJ.** Cardiac arrhythmia and nocturnal hypoglycaemia in type 1 diabetes—the "dead in bed" syndrome revisited. *Diabetologia.* 2009;52:42–45.
19. **Robinson RT, Harris ND, Ireland RH, Macdonald IA, Heller SR.** Changes in cardiac repolarization during clinical episodes of nocturnal hypoglycaemia in adults with type 1 diabetes. *Diabetologia.* 2004;47:312–315.
20. **Lindstrom T, Jorfeldt L, Tegler L, Arnqvist HJ.** Hypoglycaemia and cardiac arrhythmias in patients with type 2 diabetes mellitus. *Diabet Med.* 1992;9:536–541.
21. **Razavi Nematollahi L, Kitabchi AE, Stentz FB, et al.** Proinflammatory cytokines in response to insulin-induced hypoglycemic stress in healthy subjects. *Metabolism.* 2009;58:443–448.
22. **Gogitidze Joy N, Hedrington MS, Briscoe VJ, Tate DB, Ertl AC, Davis SN.** Effects of acute hypoglycemia on inflammatory and pro-atherothrombotic biomarkers in individuals with type 1 diabetes and healthy individuals. *Diabetes Care.* 2010; 33:1529–1535.
23. **Wright RJ, Newby DE, Stirling D, Ludlam CA, Macdonald IA, Frier BM.** Effects of acute insulin-induced hypoglycemia on indices of inflammation: putative mechanism for aggravating vascular disease in diabetes. *Diabetes Care.* 2010;33:1591–1597.
24. **Gimenez M, Gilabert R, Monteagudo J, et al.** Repeated episodes of hypoglycemia as a potential aggravating factor for preclinical atherosclerosis in subjects with type 1 diabetes. *Diabetes Care.* 2011;34:198–203.
25. **Bonds DE, Miller ME, Bergenstal RM, et al.** The association between symptomatic, severe hypoglycaemia and mortality in type 2 diabetes: retrospective epidemiological analysis of the ACCORD study. *BMJ.* 2010;340:b4909.
26. **NICE-SUGAR Study Investigators, Finfer S, Liu B, et al.** Hypoglycemia and risk of death in critically ill patients. *N Engl J Med.* 2012;367:1108–1118.
27. **Sacks DB, Arnold M, Bakris GL, et al.** Guidelines and recommendations for laboratory analysis in the diagnosis and management of diabetes mellitus. *Clin Chem.* 2011;57:e1–e47.
28. **Sacks DB, Arnold M, Bakris GL, et al.** Position statement executive summary: guidelines and recommendations for laboratory analysis in the diagnosis and management of diabetes mellitus. *Diabetes Care.* 2011;34:1419–1423.
29. **Cryer PE, Davis SN, Shamoon H.** Hypoglycemia in diabetes. *Diabetes Care.* 2003;26:1902–1912.
30. **Aftab Guy D, Sandoval D, Richardson MA, Tate D, Davis SN.** Effects of glycemic control on target organ responses to epinephrine in type 1 diabetes. *Am J Physiol Endocrinol Metab.* 2005;289:E258–E265.
31. **Davis SN, Shavers C, Costa F.** Differential gender responses to hypoglycemia are due to alterations in CNS drive and not glycemic thresholds. *Am J Physiol Endocrinol Metab.* 2000;279:E1054–E1063.
32. **Davis SN, Fowler S, Costa F.** Hypoglycemic counterregulatory responses differ between men and women with type 1 diabetes. *Diabetes.* 2000;49:65–72.

33. **Sandoval DA, Ertl AC, Richardson MA, Tate DB, Davis SN.** Estrogen blunts neuroendocrine and metabolic responses to hypoglycemia. *Diabetes.* 2003;52: 1749–1755.
34. **Cryer PE, Gerich JE.** Relevance of glucose counterregulatory systems to patients with diabetes: critical roles of glucagon and epinephrine. *Diabetes Care.* 1983;6:95–99.
35. **Ryder RE, Owens DR, Hayes TM, Ghatei MA, Bloom SR.** Unawareness of hypoglycaemia and inadequate hypoglycaemic counterregulation: no causal relation with diabetic autonomic neuropathy. *BMJ.* 1990;301:783–787.
36. **White NH, Skor DA, Cryer PE, Levandoski LA, Bier DM, Santiago JV.** Identification of type I diabetic patients at increased risk for hypoglycemia during intensive therapy. *N Engl J Med.* 1983;308:485–491.
37. **Geddes J, Schopman JE, Zammitt NN, Frier BM.** Prevalence of impaired awareness of hypoglycaemia in adults with type 1 diabetes. *Diabet Med.* 2008;25:501–504.
38. **Schopman JE, Geddes J, Frier BM.** Prevalence of impaired awareness of hypoglycaemia and frequency of hypoglycaemia in insulin-treated type 2 diabetes. *Diabetes Res Clin Pract.* 2010;87:64–68.
39. **Cryer PE.** Mechanisms of hypoglycemia-associated autonomic failure in diabetes. *N Engl J Med.* 2013;369:362–372.
40. **Davis MR, Shamoon H.** Counterregulatory adaptation to recurrent hypoglycemia in normal humans. *J Clin Endocrinol Metab.* 1991;73:995–1001.
41. **Davis SN, Shavers C, Mosqueda-Garcia R, Costa F.** Effects of differing antecedent hypoglycemia on subsequent counterregulation in normal humans. *Diabetes.* 1997;46:1328–1335.
42. **Davis SN, Mann S, Galassetti P, et al.** Effects of differing durations of antecedent hypoglycemia on counterregulatory responses to subsequent hypoglycemia in normal humans. *Diabetes.* 2000;49: 1897–1903.
43. **Sandoval DA, Guy DL, Richardson MA, Ertl AC, Davis SN.** Effects of low and moderate antecedent exercise on counterregulatory responses to subsequent hypoglycemia in type 1 diabetes. *Diabetes.* 2004;53:1798–1806.
44. **Galassetti P, Tate D, Neill RA, Richardson A, Leu SY, Davis SN.** Effect of differing antecedent hypoglycemia on counterregulatory responses to exercise in type 1 diabetes. *Am J Physiol Endocrinol Metab.* 2006;290:E1109–E1117.
45. **Banarer S, Cryer PE.** Sleep-related hypoglycemia-associated autonomic failure in type 1 diabetes: reduced awakening from sleep during hypoglycemia. *Diabetes.* 2003;52(5):1195–1203.
46. **Juvenile Diabetes Research Foundation Continuous Glucose Monitoring Study Group.** Prolonged nocturnal hypoglycemia is common during 12 months of continuous glucose monitoring in children and adults with type 1 diabetes. *Diabetes Care.* 2010;33:1004–1008.
47. **Veneman T, Mitrakou A, Mokan M, Cryer P, Gerich J.** Induction of hypoglycemia unawareness by asymptomatic nocturnal hypoglycemia. *Diabetes.* 1993;42:1233–1237.
48. **Cranston I, Lomas J, Maran A, Macdonald I, Amiel SA.** Restoration of hypoglycaemia awareness in patients with long-duration insulin-dependent diabetes. *Lancet.* 1994;344:283–287.
49. **Briscoe VJ, Ertl AC, Tate DB, Davis SN.** Effects of the selective serotonin reuptake inhibitor fluoxetine on counterregulatory responses to hypoglycemia in individuals with type 1 diabetes. *Diabetes.* 2008;57:3315–3322.
50. **Amiel SA, Dixon T, Mann R, Jameson K.** Hypoglycaemia in type 2 diabetes. *Diabet Med.* 2008;25: 245–254.
51. **Meneilly GS, Cheung E, Tuokko H.** Altered responses to hypoglycemia of healthy elderly people. *J Clin Endocrinol Metab.* 1994;78:1341–1348.
52. **Brierley EJ, Broughton DL, James OF, Alberti KG.** Reduced awareness of hypoglycaemia in the elderly despite an intact counter-regulatory response. *QJM.* 1995;88:439–445.
53. **Bremer JP, Jauch-Chara K, Hallschmid M, Schmid S, Schultes B.** Hypoglycemia unawareness in older compared with middle-aged patients with type 2 diabetes. *Diabetes Care.* 2009;32:1513–1517.
54. **Kirkman MS, Briscoe VJ, Clark N, et al.** Diabetes in older adults. *Diabetes Care.* 2012;35:2650–2664.
55. **Graveling AJ, Frier BM.** Impaired awareness of hypoglycaemia: a review. *Diabetes Metab.* 2010;36 (suppl 3):S64–S74.
56. **Dougherty PP, Klein-Schwartz W.** Octreotide's role in the management of sulfonylurea-induced hypoglycemia. *J Med Toxicol.* 2010;6:199–206.
57. **Schabelman E, Kuo D.** Glucose before thiamine for Wernicke encephalopathy: a literature review. *J Emerg Med.* 2012;42:488–494.
58. **Falorni A, Minarelli V, Morelli S.** Therapy of adrenal insufficiency: an update. *Endocrine.* 2013;43: 514–528.
59. **Douillard C, Mention K, Dobbelaere D, Wemeau JL, Saudubray JM, Vantyghem MC.** Hypoglycaemia related to inherited metabolic diseases in adults. *Orphanet J Rare Dis.* 2012;7:26. doi:10.1186/1750-1172-7-26.
60. **Stein SA, Lamos EM, Davis SN.** A review of the efficacy and safety of oral antidiabetic drugs. *Expert Opin Drug Saf.* 2013;12:153–175.
61. **Khalil AB, Beshyah SA, Abu Awad SM, et al.** Ramadan fasting in diabetes patients on insulin pump therapy augmented by continuous glucose monitoring: an observational real-life study. *Diabetes Technol Ther.* 2012;14:813–818.
62. **Abe M, Okada K, Soma M.** Antidiabetic agents in patients with chronic kidney disease and end-stage renal disease on dialysis: metabolism and clinical practice. *Curr Drug Metab.* 2011;12:57–69.
63. **Hardy KJ, Burge MR, Boyle PJ, Scarpello JH.** A treatable cause of recurrent severe hypoglycemia. *Diabetes Care.* 1994;17:722–724.
64. **Action to Control Cardiovascular Risk in Diabetes Study Group, Gerstein HC, Miller ME, et al.** Effects of intensive glucose lowering in type 2 diabetes. *N Engl J Med.* 2008;358:2545–2559.

65. **Duckworth W, Abraira C, Moritz T, et al.** Glucose control and vascular complications in veterans with type 2 diabetes. *N Engl J Med.* 2009;360:129–139.
66. **Inzucchi SE, Bergenstal RM, Buse JB, et al.** Management of hyperglycemia in type 2 diabetes: a patient-centered approach. Position statement of the American Diabetes Association (ADA) and the European Association for the Study of Diabetes (EASD). *Diabetes Care.* 2012;35:1364–1379.
67. **Hopkins D, Lawrence I, Mansell P, et al.** Improved biomedical and psychological outcomes 1 year after structured education in flexible insulin therapy for people with type 1 diabetes: the U.K. DAFNE experience. *Diabetes Care.* 2012;35:1638–1642.
68. **Fatourechi MM, Kudva YC, Murad MH, Elamin MB, Tabini CC, Montori VM.** Hypoglycemia with intensive insulin therapy: a systematic review and meta-analyses of randomized trials of continuous subcutaneous insulin infusion versus multiple daily injections. *J Clin Endocrinol Metab.* 2009;94: 729–740.
69. **Gough SC.** A review of human and analogue insulin trials. *Diabetes Res Clin Pract.* 2007;77:1–15.
70. **Bergenstal RM, Klonoff DC, Garg SK, et al.** Threshold-based insulin-pump interruption for reduction of hypoglycemia. *N Engl J Med.* 2013;369:224–232.
71. **Bergenstal RM, Tamborlane WV, Ahmann A, et al.** Effectiveness of sensor-augmented insulin-pump therapy in type 1 diabetes. *N Engl J Med.* 2010;363: 311–320.
72. **MacDonald MJ.** Postexercise late-onset hypoglycemia in insulin-dependent diabetic patients. *Diabetes Care.* 1987;10(5):584–588.
73. **van de Wiel A.** Diabetes mellitus and alcohol. *Diabetes Metab Res Rev.* 2004;20:263–267.
74. **Inkster B, Frier BM.** Diabetes and driving. *Diabetes Obes Metab.* 2013;15:775–783.
75. **Blumer I, Hader E, Hadden DR, et al.** Diabetes and pregnancy: an Endocrine Society Clinical Practice Guideline. *J Clin Endocrinol Metab.* 2013;98: 4227–4249.
76. **Kitzmiller JL, Block JM, Brown FM, et al.** Managing preexisting diabetes for pregnancy: summary of evidence and consensus recommendations for care. *Diabetes Care.* 2008;31:1060–1079.
77. **Ringholm L, Pedersen-Bjergaard U, Thorsteinsson B, et al.** Impaired hormonal counterregulation to biochemical hypoglycaemia does not explain the high incidence of severe hypoglycaemia during pregnancy in women with type 1 diabetes. *Scand J Clin Lab Invest.* 2013;73:67–74.
78. **Dooley MJ, Wiseman M, McRae A, et al.** Reducing potentially fatal errors associated with high doses of insulin: a successful multifaceted multidisciplinary prevention strategy. *BMJ Qual Saf.* 2011;20: 637–644.
79. **Samaan KH, Dahlke M, Stover J.** Addressing safety concerns about U-500 insulin in a hospital setting. *Am J Health Syst Pharm.* 2011;68:63–68.
80. **Shrishrimal K, Hart P, Michota F.** Managing diabetes in hemodialysis patients: observations and recommendations. *Cleve Clin J Med.* 2009;76:649–655.
81. **Moghissi ES, Korytkowski MT, DiNardo M, et al.** American Association of Clinical Endocrinologists and American Diabetes Association consensus statement on inpatient glycemic control. *Diabetes Care.* 2009;32:1119–1131.
82. **Clement S, Braithwaite SS, Magee MF, et al.** Management of diabetes and hyperglycemia in hospitals. *Diabetes Care.* 2004;27:553–591.
83. **Umpierrez GE, Hellman R, Korytkowski MT, et al.** Management of hyperglycemia in hospitalized patients in non-critical care setting: an Endocrine Society Clinical Practice Guideline. *J Clin Endocrinol Metab.* 2012;97:16–38.
84. **Murad MH, Coto-Yglesias F, Wang AT, et al.** Clinical review: drug-induced hypoglycemia: a systematic review. *J Clin Endocrinol Metab.* 2009;94:741–745.
85. **Johnson EO, Kamilaris TC, Calogero AE, Konstandi M, Chrousos GP.** Effects of short- and long-duration hypothyroidism on function of the rat hypothalamic-pituitary-adrenal axis. *J Endocrinol Invest.* 2013;36:104–110.
86. **Marsk R, Jonas E, Rasmussen F, Naslund E.** Nationwide cohort study of post-gastric bypass hypoglycaemia including 5,040 patients undergoing surgery for obesity in 1986–2006 in Sweden. *Diabetologia.* 2010;53:2307–2311.
87. **Patti ME, Goldfine AB.** Hypoglycaemia following gastric bypass surgery—diabetes remission in the extreme? *Diabetologia.* 2010;53:2276–2279.
88. **Goldfine AB, Mun EC, Devine E, et al.** Patients with neuroglycopenia after gastric bypass surgery have exaggerated incretin and insulin secretory responses to a mixed meal. *J Clin Endocrinol Metab.* 2007;92:4678–4685.
89. **Carpenter T, Trautmann ME, Baron AD.** Hyperinsulinemic hypoglycemia with nesidioblastosis after gastric-bypass surgery. *N Engl J Med.* 2005;353:2192–2194; author reply 2192–2194.
90. **Basu A, Service FJ, Yu L, Heser D, Ferries LM, Eisenbarth G.** Insulin autoimmunity and hypoglycemia in seven white patients. *Endocr Pract.* 2005;11:97–103.
91. **Service FJ, O'Brien PC.** Increasing serum betahydroxybutyrate concentrations during the 72-hour fast: evidence against hyperinsulinemic hypoglycemia. *J Clin Endocrinol Metab.* 2005;90:4555–4558.
92. **Guettier JM, Kam A, Chang R, et al.** Localization of insulinomas to regions of the pancreas by intraarterial calcium stimulation: the NIH experience. *J Clin Endocrinol Metab.* 2009;94:1074–1080.

CHAPTER 26

Severe Hyperglycemia, Diabetic Ketoacidosis, and Hyperglycemic Hyperosmolar State

Ketan Dhatariya, Mark Savage, Mike Sampson, Glenn Matfin, and Adrian Scott

ABSTRACT

Emergency admissions due to hyperglycemia remain some of the most common and challenging metabolic conditions with which to deal. Diabetic ketoacidosis (DKA) and hyperglycemic hyperosmolar state (HHS) are biochemically different conditions that require different approaches to treatment. They often occur in different age groups, and there is a need for coordinated care from the multidisciplinary team to ensure the timely delivery of the correct treatments. Over the last few years, the management of these conditions has changed. With DKA, the use of bedside monitoring of plasma ketone levels now drives treatment. With HHS, the treatment now focuses on the use of fluid rehydration rather than insulin treatment as the means by which glucose lowering should be achieved, with insulin only being introduced when the rate of glucose lowering levels off.

This chapter, which is based largely on published guidelines from the United States and United Kingdom on the management of these conditions, highlights the recent changes in management, the differences between the guidelines, and the rationale for these changes.

INTRODUCTION

The hyperglycemic urgency, severe hyperglycemia, and emergencies, DKA and HHS are acute severe metabolic complications of uncontrolled diabetes mellitus (1). Severe hyperglycemia can escalate into the potentially fatal complications of DKA and HHS. Subsequently, these conditions demand immediate recognition and treatment.

Severe hyperglycemia is characterized by significant hyperglycemia (ie, glycosylated hemoglobin [HbA_{1c}] ≥10%; or fasting plasma glucose [FPG] >250 mg/dL [~14 mmol/L]; or random plasma glucose >300 mg/dL [16.7mmol/L]); or when symptomatic (eg, sudden persistent weight-loss, polyuria, and polydipsia) (2).

DKA is a complex disordered metabolic state characterized by severe hyperglycemia (ie, plasma glucose levels >250 mg/dL [~14 mmol/L]), ketonemia (ketosis), and metabolic acidosis (pH ≤7.3, serum bicarbonate <18 mEq/L [18 mmol/L]). The 2009 American Diabetes Association (ADA) Hyperglycemic Crises consensus guidelines further subdivide DKA into mild DKA (serum bicarbonate of 15 to 18 mEq/L [15 to 18 mmol/L], pH 7.25 to 7.30); moderate DKA (serum bicarbonate 10 to <15 mEq/L [10 to <15 mmol/L], pH 7.00 to 7.24): and severe DKA (serum bicarbonate <10 mEq/L [10 mmol/L], pH <7.00). More recently, the UK 2013 Joint British Diabetes Societies Inpatient (JBDS IP) group DKA guidelines have incorporated serum ketone levels (3-beta-hydroxybutyrate [βHBA]) into the definition of DKA (3). The measurement of βHBA for diagnosis and monitoring of DKA was also recommended in the 2011 ADA Diabetes Laboratory guidelines (4). The 2013 JBDS IP group DKA definition requires the combined presence of 3 biochemical abnormalities: ketonemia ≥3 mmol/L or significant ketonuria (≥2+ urine ketones on standard urine sticks); blood glucose >200 mg/dL (11.1 mmol/L) or known diabetes; and venous (or arterial) blood bicarbonate <15 mEq/L (15 mmol/L) and/or pH <7.3. DKA primarily affects persons with type 1 diabetes and may be an initial manifestation of previously undiagnosed type 1 diabetes (~25%) or may result from increased insulin requirements in existing patients during situations that increase the release of counter-regulatory hormones (ie, glucagon, cortisol, epinephrine, and growth hormone). When hyperglycemia initially presents in the presence of ketones or other signs of metabolic decompensation, the diagnosis of type 1 diabetes is generally straightforward (especially in children and adolescents). However, ketonemia can also be found in individuals with type 2 diabetes (ie, ketosis-prone hyperglycemia, especially in persons of African descent), with 5%–25% having DKA (5).

HHS is characterized by marked hyperglycemia (blood glucose levels >600 mg/dL [33.3 mmol/L]); hyperosmolarity (plasma osmolarity >320 mOsm/kg [320 mmol/kg]) and dehydration; the absence of ketoacidosis; and depression of the sensorium. The 2012 JBDS IP group HHS definition includes marked hyperglycemia (>540 mg/dL [30 mmol/L]); no significant ketonemia (<3 mmol/L); no acidosis (pH >7.3, bicarbonate >15 mEq/L [15 mmol/L]); hypovolemia; and osmolality usually >320 mOsmol/kg (320 mmol/kg). These guidelines also highlight that a mixed picture of HHS and DKA may occur. HHS is seen most frequently in persons with type 2 diabetes; however, approximately 20% of cases have no history of this diagnosis.

In the United States, the prevalence of DKA has risen while mortality has decreased. This is related to an improved understanding of the pathophysiology of DKA together with close monitoring and correction of electrolytes. More than one third of DKA hospitalizations are due to readmissions. Mortality rates have fallen significantly in the last 20 years from 7.96% to 0.67% (6,7). The mortality rate is still high in low-income countries and among nonhospitalized patients (8). This high mortality rate illustrates the necessity of early diagnosis and the implementation of effective prevention programs. The ready availability of insulin to all parts of the world should remain a priority. Cerebral edema remains the most common cause of mortality, particularly in young children and adolescents. The main causes of mortality in the adult population include severe hypokalemia (and related cardiac dysrhythmias), adult respiratory distress syndrome (ARDS), and comorbid states such as pneumonia, acute coronary syndromes (ACS), and sepsis (9). In comparison, HHS is rare but mortality attributed to HHS is considerably higher than that attributed to DKA, with recent mortality rates of 5%–20%. The prognosis of both conditions is substantially worsened at the extremes of age in the presence of coma, hypotension, and severe comorbidities.

PATHOPHYSIOLOGY

DKA usually occurs as a consequence of absolute or relative insulin deficiency that is accompanied by an increase in counterregulatory hormones (10). This type of hormonal imbalance enhances hepatic gluconeogenesis and glycogenolysis resulting in severe hyperglycemia. Enhanced lipolysis increases serum free fatty acids that are then metabolized as an alternative energy source in the process of ketogenesis (11). This results in accumulation of large quantities of ketone bodies and subsequent metabolic acidosis. Ketones include acetone, βHBA, and acetoacetate. The predominant ketone in DKA is βHBA.

There are several mechanisms responsible for fluid depletion in DKA. These include osmotic diuresis due to hyperglycemia, vomiting (commonly associated with DKA), and, eventually, inability to take in fluid due to a diminished level of consciousness. Electrolyte shifts and depletion are in part related to the osmotic diuresis. Hyperkalemia and hypokalemia need particular attention.

Unlike DKA, which is a condition most frequently associated with absolute insulin deficiency, in HHS there is sufficient insulin to prevent ketogenesis, but insufficient insulin to either prevent hepatic gluconeogenesis or cellular glucose uptake (12). If counter-regulatory hormone excess is also present (eg, concomitant illness), then this leads to a rise in blood glucose and a subsequent osmotic diuresis. If sufficient water is not available, this leads to dehydration and resultant impaired renal function. The high plasma glucose causes a raised serum osmolality. The impaired renal function then leads to a further inability to excrete glucose thus perpetuating the hyperglycemia osmotic diuresis, volume depletion, and dehydration (11). Alterations in mental status are common with serum osmolalities over 330 mOsmol/kg (330 mmol/kg).

ETIOLOGY

DKA and HHS can be precipitated by various conditions (which can be remembered easily by the letter **I**), including **I**nsulin deficiency (ie, diabetes presentation or failure to take enough insulin); **I**atrogenic (eg, glucocorticoids, thiazides, and atypical antipsychotic drugs); **I**nfection (the most common precipitating factor for both DKA and HHS); **I**nflammation (eg, acute pancreatitis, cholecystitis); **I**schemia or **I**nfarction (eg, ACS, stroke, bowel); and **I**ntoxication (eg, alcohol, cocaine).

Few studies have assessed factors associated with DKA in adults with type 1 diabetes. However, the T1D Exchange clinic registry at 70 US endocrinology centers recently performed a cross-sectional analysis that included 7,012 participants with type 1 diabetes (13). Higher frequencies of DKA were associated with lower socioeconomic status ($P < 0.001$), and higher HbA1c levels ($P < 0.001$) were associated with 21.0% of those with HbA1c ≥10.0% having an event in the past 12 months. Notably, the frequency was no higher in insulin pump users than injection users, an important finding because DKA is a potential risk with pump infusion site failure.

DIAGNOSTIC CONSIDERATIONS

The diagnostic criteria of severe hyperglycemia, DKA, and HHS are outlined in the introduction.

The initial laboratory evaluation of patients includes determination of plasma glucose, blood urea nitrogen (BUN, or urea), creatinine, electrolytes (with calculated anion gap), serum osmolality, serum and urinary ketones, urinalysis, baseline venous (or arterial) blood gases, complete (full) blood count with differential, and erythrocyte sedimentation rate (ESR) or C-reactive protein (CRP) (if indicated). An electrocardiogram (ECG), chest X-ray, and urine, sputum, and blood cultures should also be obtained. Other investigations are performed as warranted by the clinical situation (eg, cardiac troponins, serum lactate, appropriate imaging, toxicology, and drug screen).

Point-of-care ketone testing should be used to measure the plasma ketone concentrations (in particular, βHBA), because this is the direct marker of disease severity. The anion gap is calculated by subtracting the sum of chloride (Cl) and bicarbonate (HCO3) concentration from the uncorrected (see next paragraph) sodium (Na) concentration: (Na – [Cl + HCO3]). A normal anion gap is between 7 and 9 mEq/L (7–9 mmol/L) and an anion gap >10–12 mEq/L (10–12 mmol/L) indicates the presence of increased anion gap metabolic acidosis. Although arterial blood gas (ABG) is the most accurate method of assessing ventilation and acid-base status, venous blood gas (VBG) is preferred to ABG for bicarbonate and pH measurements because the differences in arterial and venous pH (eg, venous pH only 0.03 lower than arterial), bicarbonate, and potassium measurements are not great enough (in either direction) to alter management.

The admission serum sodium is usually low or normal despite water loss (renal and gut) because of an intracellular–extracellular fluid shift. To assess the severity of sodium and water deficit, serum sodium may be corrected by adding 1.6 mg/L (1.6 mmol/L) to the measured serum sodium for each 100 mg/dL (5.6 mmol/L) of glucose above 100 mg/dL (5.6 mmol/L) (14). Serum potassium levels may also be low, normal, or elevated, despite total body potassium depletion resulting from protracted polyuria and vomiting.

On admission, leukocytosis with cell counts in the 10,000–15,000 mm^3 range is the rule in DKA and is generally attributed to stress and may not be indicative of an infection. However, leukocytosis with cell counts

>25,000 mm^3 may designate infection, and appropriate evaluation is indicated.

Hyperamylasemia has been reported in 21%–79% of patients with DKA; however, there is little correlation between the presence, degree, or isoenzyme type of hyperamylasemia (eg, salivary amylase can also be increased in DKA) and the presence of gastrointestinal symptoms (nausea, vomiting, and abdominal pain) or pancreatic imaging studies. A serum lipase determination may be beneficial in the differential diagnosis of pancreatitis; however, lipase can also be elevated in DKA in the absence of pancreatitis.

Not all patients with ketoacidosis have DKA. Starvation ketosis and alcoholic ketoacidosis are distinguished by clinical history and by plasma glucose concentrations that range from mildly elevated (rarely >200 mg/dL [11.1 mmol/L]) to hypoglycemia. A clinical history of previous drug abuse and intoxication should be sought.

CLINICAL SIGNS AND FEATURES

The process of HHS usually evolves over several days to weeks, whereas the evolution of the acute DKA episode tends to be much shorter (typically <24 hr). For both DKA and HHS, the classical clinical picture includes a history of polyuria, polydipsia, weight loss, vomiting, dehydration, weakness, and mental status change. Physical findings may include increased rate and depth of respiration in DKA (ie, Kussmaul's breathing) with odor of acetone, tachycardia, and hypotension. Assessment of fluid status encompasses subjective observations (skin turgor, mucous membranes, and cerebral dysfunction), objective measurements (blood pressure, pulse, postural measurements, body weight), and laboratory measurements (serum sodium, serum osmolality, BUN, hematocrit, and urine osmolality). Severe hypovolemia may manifest as tachycardia (pulse >100 bpm) and/or hypotension (systolic blood pressure <100 mm Hg). Each has its limitations, particularly on initial assessment where previous comparator data may not be available.

Mental status can vary from full alertness to profound lethargy or coma, with the latter more frequent in HHS. Acute impairment in cognitive function may be associated with dehydration but is not specific to the condition and is not necessarily present. Alterations in mental status are common with serum osmolalities over 330 mOsmol/kg (330 mmol/kg). Focal neurological signs (hemianopia and hemiparesis), positive Babinski reflexes, aphasia, visual hallucinations, seizures (focal or generalized), and coma may also be features of HHS. As HHS more frequently occurs in older people, the neurological findings may be mistaken for a stroke.

Although infection is a common precipitating factor for both DKA and HHS, patients can be normothermic or even hypothermic primarily because of peripheral vasodilation. Nausea, vomiting, and diffuse abdominal pain are frequent in patients with DKA (>50%) but are uncommon in HHS. Further evaluation is necessary if this complaint does not resolve with resolution of dehydration and metabolic acidosis.

MANAGEMENT OF SEVERE HYPERGLYCEMIA, DIABETIC KETOACIDOSIS, AND HYPERGLYCEMIC HYPEROSMOLAR STATE

Successful treatment of severe hyperglycemia, DKA, and HHS requires correction of hyperglycemia, dehydration, and electrolyte imbalances; identification of comorbid precipitating events; and above all, frequent patient monitoring.

Acute Intervention

Once severe hyperglycemia, DKA, or HHS is recognized, the patient should be managed in an appropriate location. This could be in the outpatient setting (eg, rapid access clinic) for selected cases of severe hyperglycemia and mild DKA. However, the majority of patients will be hospitalized and managed in an emergency care setting such as an emergency department, acute medical unit (AMU), or equivalent, as well as more advanced step-up facilities such as a high dependency unit (HDU) or intensive care unit (ICU). As with all acute medical patients, prompt assessment and management of the ABCDEs should occur (ie, Airway, Breathing, Circulation, Disability [ie, conscious level], and Exposure [ie, examination]). Other markers of DKA and HHS severity should be assessed and recorded (Table 26-1).

Table 26-1. Markers of Severity in DKA (3) and HHS (21)

Marker of Severity	DKA (JBDS IP Group 2013)	HHS (JBDS IP Group 2012)
Mental status	GCS <12 or abnormal AVPU	GCS <12 or abnormal AVPU
Oxygen saturation	<92% on air (assuming normal baseline respiratory function)	<92% on air (assuming normal baseline respiratory function)
Venous/arterial pH	pH <7.1	pH <7.1
Potassium	Hypokalemia (<3.5 mEq/L [3.5 mmol/L]) or Hyperkalemia (>6 mEq/L [6 mmol/L])	Hypokalemia (<3.5 mEq/L [3.5 mmol/L]) or Hyperkalemia (>6 mEq/L [6 mmol/L])
Systolic blood pressure	<90 mm Hg	<90 mm Hg
Pulse	>100 or <60 bpm	>100 or <60 bpm
Urine output	<0.5 mL/kg/hr or other evidence of acute kidney injury	<0.5 mL/kg/hr or other evidence of acute kidney injury
Blood ketones	>6 mmol/L	>1 mmol/L
Bicarbonate level	<5 mEq/L (5 mmol/L)	
Anion gap	>16 mEq/L (16 mmol/L)	
Sodium		>160 mEq/L (160 mmol/L)
Osmolality		>350 mOsm/kg
Miscellaneous		Hypothermia Acute or serious comorbidity (eg, ACS, heart failure, or stroke)

After a diagnosis of DKA or HHS has been made, the presence of any of the markers above during the admission should prompt a swift senior review and/or indicate admission to a high-dependence unit (HDU) environment.
Abbreviations: DKA = diabetic ketoacidosis; HHS = hyperglycemic hyperosmolar state; GCS = Glasgow Coma Scale; AVPU = Alert, Voice, Pain, Unresponsive scale.

General Supportive Care

Supportive care includes inserting a large bore IV cannula and starting appropriate IV fluid resuscitation, electrolyte replacement, nutritional support, continuous cardiac monitoring, and pulse oximetry.

HYPERGLYCEMIA BUNDLE

Due to the increased risk of arterial and venous thromboembolism (VTE), all patients with DKA or HHS should receive low molecular weight heparin (LMWH) for the full duration of admission unless contraindicated. HHS (and some DKA) patients are also at high risk of pressure ulceration. An initial foot assessment should be undertaken and heel protectors applied in those with neuropathy, peripheral arterial disease (PAD), or lower limb deformity. The feet should be reexamined daily. Consider nasogastric (NG) tube with airway protection to prevent aspiration if Glasgow Coma Scale (GCS) is <12 or there is excessive vomiting. Consider urinary catheterization if the patient is incontinent, there is difficulty monitoring urine output (minimum urine output should be no less than 0.5 mL/kg/hr), or the patient is anuric (ie, has not passed urine by 60 min).

HYPERGLYCEMIA-SPECIFIC THERAPY

Severe Hyperglycemia

Health care providers are concerned by the risk of severe hyperglycemia during acute illness in persons with diabetes, especially those treated with insulin therapy. Prevention of hyperglycemia, and its management with a step-by-step procedure (generally referred to as "sick-day" rules) when it eventually occurs, is integral to diabetes management. Blood glucose levels normally increase during illness because of the release of stress hormones. Thus, sick-day rules should be initiated. The instructions include maintaining the usual food plan, noninsulin therapies, and/or insulin regimen whenever possible. Low-caloric fluid intake should be increased as appropriate. Persons with diabetes who experience nausea or vomiting should initiate the sick-day food plan. In patients treated with insulin, blood glucose and ketone (if available) monitoring should be carried out as recommended (eg, every 2 to 4 hours). If blood glucose is >250 mg/dL (~14 mmol/L) on 2 consecutive tests, persons with diabetes are recommended to contact their clinician due to the possible need to supplement their current insulin regimen with short- or rapid-acting insulin as necessary. The individual must be instructed to contact his or her health care provider when the blood glucose is persistently raised (eg, >300 mg/dL [16.6 mmol/L]) and/or he or she develops develop moderate to high ketonuria (ie, ≥2+ urine ketones) and/or increased serum ketones, where monitoring is available. DKA or HHS can occur in this setting, thus frequent contact is necessary between the clinician and the individual to prevent the situation from deteriorating further.

The most important consideration in the initial assessment of acute illness in persons with diabetes is whether the individual needs inpatient admission or can be safely managed in the community or outpatient setting (including review in a rapid-access clinic). The majority of these situations will be managed in the community or outpatient setting. However, this decision has to take into account various factors, including medical (eg, severity of metabolic decompensation, associated comorbidities, presence of confusion or impaired consciousness) and social issues (eg, whether the patient lives alone or has adequate family support, whether there are reliable communication channels between health care provider and person with diabetes and/or caregivers). Inpatient admission can be considered whenever there is (1) severe and prolonged hyperglycemia, (2) the presence of high ketones for more than 6 hours, (3) vomiting, diarrhea, and/or abdominal pain, (4) inadequate phone contact between the health care provider and person with diabetes and/or caregiver, or (5) at the discretion of the clinician and/or according to local practice guidelines.

DIABETIC KETOACIDOSIS AND HYPERGLYCEMIC HYPEROSMOLAR STATE

The 2009 ADA Hyperglycemic Crises consensus guideline protocols for the management of patients with DKA and HHS are summarized in Figure 26-1. The overall goals in treating DKA are to improve circulatory volume and tissue perfusion, decrease blood glucose, and correct the acidosis and electrolyte imbalances. These objectives usually are accomplished through the administration of low-dose insulin and IV fluid and electrolyte replacement solutions. An initial loading dose of short-acting or rapid-acting insulin is often given IV, followed by IV continuous insulin infusion (CII). Frequent laboratory tests are used to monitor blood glucose, venous pH, creatinine, and serum electrolyte levels and to guide fluid and electrolyte replacement. It is important to replace fluid and electrolytes and correct pH while bringing the blood glucose concentration to a normal level. Too rapid a drop in blood glucose may cause hypoglycemia. A sudden change in the osmolality of extracellular fluid can also occur when blood glucose levels are lowered too rapidly, and this can cause cerebral edema. Serum potassium levels often fall as acidosis is corrected and potassium moves from the extracellular into the intracellular compartment. Thus, it may be necessary to add potassium to the IV infusion. Identification and treatment of the underlying cause, such as infection, also are important.

During treatment of DKA, hyperglycemia is corrected faster than ketoacidosis. The mean duration of treatment until blood glucose is <250 mg/dL (~14 mmol/L) and ketoacidosis (pH >7.30; bicarbonate >18 mEq/L [18 mmol/L]) is corrected is 6 and 12 hours, respectively. Once the plasma glucose is <200 mg/dL (11.1 mmol/L), 5% dextrose should be added to replacement fluids to allow continued insulin administration until ketonemia is controlled, while at the same time avoiding hypoglycemia. For DKA occurring in individuals with type 2 diabetes (ie, ketosis-prone hyperglycemia), the initial management is similar to standard DKA (5).

In comparison, 2013 JBDS IP group DKA guidelines reflect 2 major recent developments: (a) a change in the way patients with DKA present clinically, and (b) development of rapid near-patient testing technology. Until recently there was no easily available assay for ketone bodies, hence, capillary glucose, venous pH, and bicarbonate were used to

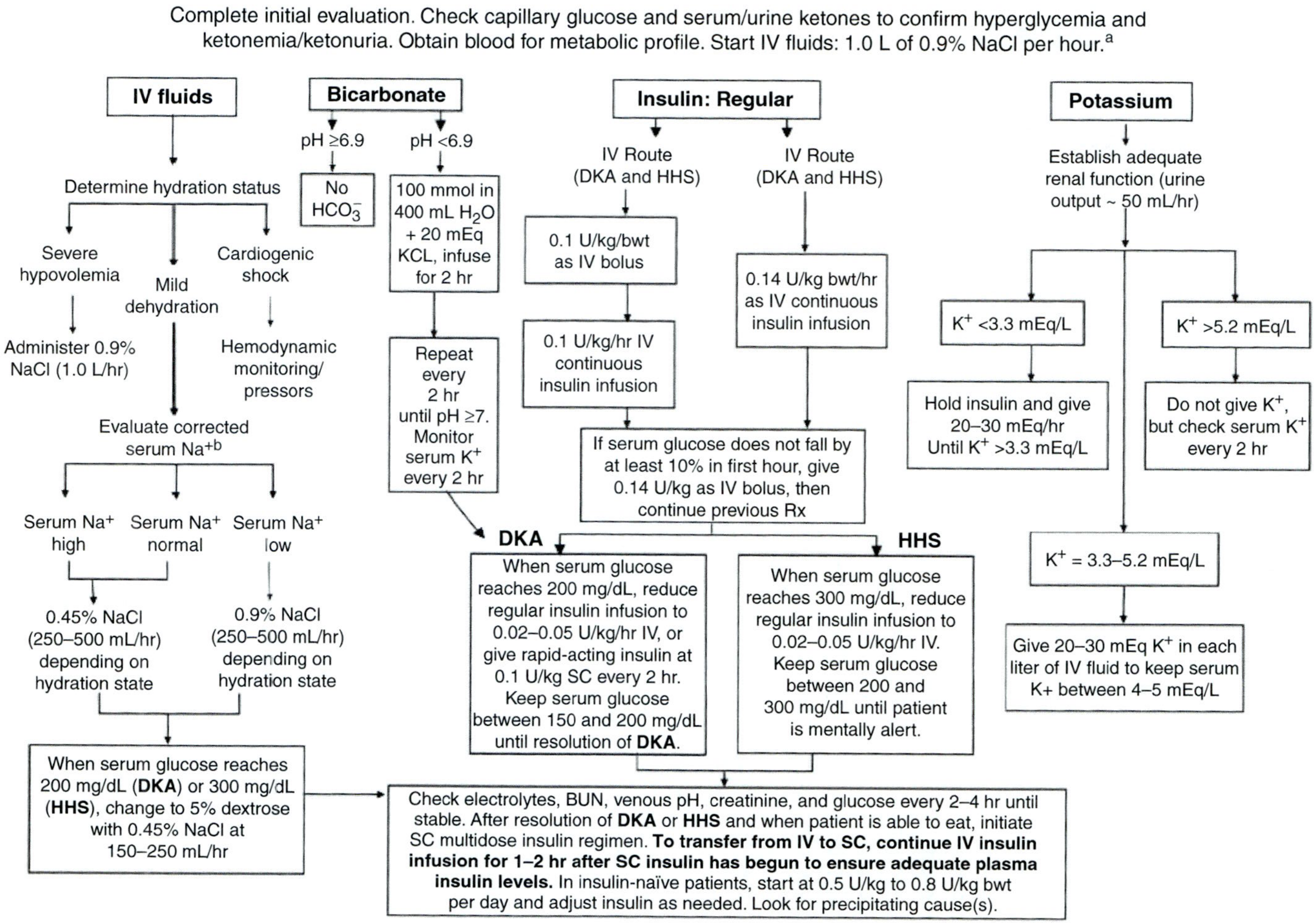

Figure 26-1. Protocol for management of adult patients with diabetic ketoacidosis (DKA) and hyperglycemic hyperosmolar state (HHS) (1). DKA diagnostic criteria: blood glucose 250 mg/dL (13.8 mmol/L), arterial pH 7.3, bicarbonate <15 mEq/L (15 mmol/L), and moderate ketonuria or ketonemia. HHS diagnostic criteria: serum glucose >600 mg/dL, arterial pH >7.3, serum bicarbonate >15 mEq/L, and minimal ketonuria and ketonemia. [a]15–20 mL/kg/hr; [b]serum Na should be corrected for hyperglycemia. (For each 100 mg/dL [5.6 mmol/L] > glucose 100 mg/dL [5.6 mmol/L], add 1.6 mEq/L [1.6 mmol/L] to sodium value for corrected serum value.) Copyright 2011 by the American Diabetes Association.

diagnose and monitor response to treatment in DKA. Near-patient testing for βHBA is now readily available for the monitoring of the abnormal metabolite, allowing for a shift away from using glucose levels to drive treatment decisions in the management of DKA.

Some of the major recommendations of the 2013 JBDS IP group DKA guidelines include the following:

1. Aim to treat the cause of the acidosis (ie, ketonemia). Subsequently, bedside ketone monitors should be used to measure βHBA, because this is the direct marker of disease severity. The resolution of DKA depends upon the suppression of ketonemia, and measurement of blood ketones now represents best practice in monitoring the response to treatment (15–18).
2. Insulin is given as a standard dose per kg until the ketones are cleared. A weight-based, fixed-rate IV insulin infusion (FRIII) via an infusion pump should be used. Fifty (50) units of short-acting insulin or rapid-acting insulin make up to 50 mL with 0.9% sodium chloride solution (resulting concentration of insulin is 1 unit per mL). The initial starting dose of a fixed dose per kg body weight (0.1 units per kg per hour [ie, 7 units per hour for a 70 kg individual]) enables rapid blood ketone clearance. The fixed rate may be adjusted if the metabolic targets are not met (ie, reduction of the blood ketone concentration by at least 0.5 mmol/L/hour; increase in venous bicarbonate concentrations by at least 3 mEq/L/hour [3 mmol/L/hour] or reduction in capillary blood glucose by at least 50 mg/dL/hour [3 mmol/L/hour]). The insulin infusion rate is increased by 1.0 unit/hr increments hourly until the ketones are falling at target rates. (Also check infusion set for leaks and connection problems.) There is no need to give a bolus dose of insulin as long as the CII is set up promptly. Only use a variable-rate IV insulin infusion (VRIII) with 10% dextrose when the blood glucose is <250 mg/dL (~14 mmol/L).
3. Subcutaneous injections of long-acting insulin should be continued if the patient is already using these agents. They provide background insulin when the CII is discontinued, and should avoid excess length of stay. This does not obviate the need for giving short-acting or rapid-acting insulin before discontinuing the CII. Most units experienced in managing DKA now also continue intermediate-acting insulin (NPH) if that is what the patient normally uses. The CII is thus a "top up" on the (inadequate) background insulin already circulating. Patients presenting with newly diagnosed type 1 diabetes should be given long-acting insulin (or NPH insulin, depending on local policy) at a dose of 0.25 units/kg subcutaneously once daily to mitigate against rebound ketosis when they are taken off the FRIII (19).
4. Use 0.9% sodium chloride solution for resuscitation, not colloid. If the systolic blood pressure (BP) is <90 mm Hg, consider causes other than fluid depletion, such as heart failure, sepsis, etc. Give 500 mL of 0.9% sodium chloride solution over 10–15 minutes, and repeat if necessary (ie, fluid challenge). If there has been no improvement in BP, call for urgent senior help. If the systolic BP is >90 mm Hg use the typical recommendations outlined in Table 26-2. More cautious fluid replacement should be considered in young people aged 18–25 years, the elderly, patients who are pregnant, and those with heart or renal failure (also consider HDU and/or central line). Reduce the rate of fluid replacement in the elderly/cardiac disease/mild-moderate DKA (eg, bicarbonate >10 mEq/L [10 mmol/l]). More rapid infusion increases risk of ARDS and cerebral edema.
5. Measure venous blood gas for pH, bicarbonate, and potassium at 60 minutes, 2 hours, and 2 hourly thereafter.

Table 26-2. Recommended Rate of Fluid Replacement in Diabetic Ketoacidosis[a]

Fluid	Volume
1 L 0.9% NaCl	1,000 mL over first hour
1 L 0.9% NaCl with KCl	1,000 mL over next 2 hr
1 L 0.9% NaCl with KCl	1,000 mL over next 2 hr
1 L 0.9% NaCl with KCl	1,000 mL over next 2 hr
1 L 0.9% NaCl with KCl	1,000 mL over next 4 hr
1 L 0.9% NaCl with KCl	1,000 mL over next 4 hr
Reassessment of cardiovascular status at 12 hr is mandatory; further fluid may be required.	

[a] *Assuming the individual has normal baseline cardiovascular reserve (3).*

Table 26-3. Recommended Rate of Potassium Replacement in DKA and HHS[a]

Potassium Level in First 24 hr (mEq/L [mmol/L])	Potassium Replacement in mEq/L (mmol/L) of Infusion Solution
>5.5	Nil
3.5–5.5	40 mEq/L (40 mmol/L)
<3.5	Senior review because additional potassium needs to be given

[a] *Assuming the individual has normal baseline renal function (3).*

6. Keep potassium between 4.5 and 5.5 mEq/L (4.5–5.5 mmol/L) (Table 26-3). Hypokalemia and hyperkalemia are life-threatening conditions and are common in DKA.
7. Avoid hypoglycemia. If the glucose falls below 250 mg/dL (~14.0 mmol/L), commence 10% dextrose given at 125 mL/hr alongside the 0.9% sodium chloride solution. This is to avoid hypoglycemia if the FRIII is still required to drive down the ketones and acidosis.
8. Bicarbonate should not generally be given because it may worsen intracellular acidosis, and it may precipitate cerebral edema, particularly in children and adolescents (20).
9. Hypophosphatemia and hypomagnesemia are common in DKA and HHS; routine replacement is not recommended, however, unless associated with significant malnutrition.
10. It is expected that by 24 hours the ketonemia (<0.6 mmol/L) and acidosis (venous bicarbonate >15 mEq/L [15 mmol/L]; venous pH >7.3) should have resolved. Continue IV fluids if the patient is not eating and drinking. If the patient is not eating and drinking and there is no ketonemia, move to a VRIII. Transfer to subcutaneous insulin if the patient is eating and drinking normally. Ensure that the subcutaneous insulin is started before the IV insulin is discontinued. Ideally give the subcutaneous short-acting or rapid-acting insulin at a meal, and discontinue IV insulin one hour later.
11. Where available, the diabetes inpatient team should ideally be involved as early as is practical after admission.

Unlike DKA, guidelines on the management of HHS in adults are uncommon and often there is little to differentiate them from the management of DKA. However, HHS is different from DKA and treatment requires a different approach. The person with HHS is often elderly, frequently with multiple comorbidities but always very sick. Even when specific hospital guidelines are available, adherence to and use of these is variable among inpatient teams. The major goals of treatment of HHS are to gradually and safely normalize the osmolality; replace fluid and electrolyte losses; and normalize blood glucose. Other goals include identifying and treating the underlying cause; preventing arterial or venous thrombosis; preventing other potential complications (eg, cerebral edema); and preventing foot ulceration.

Some of the major recommendations of the 2012 JBDS IP group HHS guidelines (21) include the following:

1. Measure or calculate osmolality (2× Na [mEq/L] + glucose [mg/dL)]/18 + BUN [mg/dL]/2.8); or (2× Na [mmol/L] + glucose [mmol/L] + urea [mmol/L]) frequently to monitor the response to treatment.
2. The goal of initial therapy is to expand the intra- and extravascular volume and to restore peripheral perfusion. The fluid replacement of choice is 0.9% sodium chloride. Measurement or calculation of osmolality should be undertaken every hour

initially and the rate of fluid replacement adjusted to ensure a positive fluid balance sufficient to promote a gradual decline in osmolality. Urinary fluid losses may be considerable due to osmotic diuresis, which may persist for hours as glucose concentrations slowly decrease. The fall in osmolality with lowering of blood glucose and shift of water into the intracellular space inevitably results in a rise in serum sodium. This is not necessarily an indication to give hypotonic solutions (so-called "isotonic" 0.9% sodium chloride is relatively hypotonic compared to the serum), especially if the person remains clinically hypovolemic. A rise in serum sodium concentration must be interpreted in the context of what is happening to tonicity (effective osmolality). Provided plasma glucose is declining at a safe rate—for example, no more than 90 mg/dL/hr (5 mmol/L/hr)—this will be accompanied by a rise in serum sodium, but a fall in osmolality. Serum sodium concentrations should be frequently monitored, and the concentration of sodium in fluids adjusted to promote a gradual decline in corrected serum sodium. An optimal rate of decline in serum sodium of 0.5 mEq/L (0.5 mmol/L) per hour has been recommended for hypernatremic dehydration (14). The rate of fall of plasma sodium should not exceed 10–12 mEq/L (10–12 mmol/L) per day. The aim of treatment should be to replace approximately 50% of estimated fluid loss within the first 12 hours and the remainder in the following 12 hours, although this will, in part, be determined by the initial severity, degree of renal impairment, and associated comorbidities, which may limit the speed of correction.

3. If significant ketonemia is present (βHBA >1 mmol/L), this indicates relative hypoinsulinemia, and insulin should be started at time zero. If significant ketonemia is not present (βHBA <1 mmol/L) insulin should not be started. Fluid replacement alone with 0.9% sodium chloride will result in a drop in blood glucose, and because most patients with HHS are insulin sensitive, there is a risk of lowering the osmolality precipitously. Insulin treatment prior to adequate fluid replacement may result in cardiovascular collapse as water moves out of the intravascular space, with a resulting decline in intravascular volume. Lack of appropriate decline in serum glucose with rehydration should prompt reassessment and evaluation of renal function. Insulin may be started at this point, or if already in place the infusion rate increased (increased by 1 unit/hr). The recommended insulin dose is an FRIII given at 0.05 units per kg per hour (eg, 4 units/hr in an 80-kg person). A fall of glucose at a rate of up to 90 mg/dL/hr (5 mmol/L/hr) is ideal.
4. Avoid hypoglycemia. A blood glucose target of between 180 and ~270 mg/dL (10 and 15 mmol/L) is a reasonable goal in the first 24 hours. If the blood glucose falls below 180 mg/dL (14 mmol/L), commence 5% or 10% dextrose at 125 mL/hr, and continue the 0.9% sodium chloride solution.
5. Potassium replacement: This is the same as DKA and the same principles can be applied using Table 26-3.
6. Complete normalization of electrolytes and osmolality may take up to 72 hours.
7. Assess for any complications of treatment (eg, fluid overload, cerebral edema, osmotic demyelination syndrome [eg, a deteriorating conscious level]).
8. Because of the increased risk of arterial and venous thromboembolism, all patients should receive prophylactic LMWH for the full duration of admission unless contraindicated. Consideration should be given to extending prophylaxis beyond the duration of admission in HHS patients deemed to be at high risk.
9. Discharge planning: Because many of these patients have multiple comorbidities, recovery will largely be

determined by their previous functional level and the underlying precipitant of HHS. IV insulin can usually be discontinued once they are eating and drinking, but their fluids may be required for longer if intake remains inadequate. Many patients may require conversion to subcutaneous insulin treatment. For patients with previously undiagnosed diabetes or who were well-controlled on oral agents, switching from insulin to the appropriate noninsulin therapy should be considered after a period of stability.

10. Where available, the diabetes inpatient team ideally should be involved as early as is practical after admission.

TREATMENT OF PRECIPITATING ILLNESS

For both DKA and HHS, consider any precipitating causes (especially sepsis) and treat appropriately.

CONCLUSIONS

Severe hyperglycemia, DKA, and HHS demand immediate recognition and treatment. However, prevention of these states is always preferred, and this requires appropriate education of patients, caregivers, and health care practitioners on an ongoing basis.

ACKNOWLEDGMENTS

KD is on the steering committee of the Joint British Diabetes Societies Inpatient Care Group and has been on the writing groups for several of the guidelines they have produced. His travel to these meetings was paid for by Diabetes UK. He has also been invited to speak at various local, regional, and national meetings in the United Kingdom. Travel to these meetings has been paid for by the organizers.

REFERENCES

1. **Kitabchi AE, Umpierrez GE, Miles JM, Fisher JN.** Hyperglycemic crises in adult patients with diabetes. *Diabetes Care.* 2009;32:1335–1343.
2. **Nathan DM, Buse JB, Davidson MB, et al.** Medical management of hyperglycemia in type 2 diabetes: a consensus algorithm for the initiation and adjustment of therapy: A consensus statement of the American Diabetes Association and the European Association for the Study of Diabetes. *Diabetes Care.* 2009;32:193–203.
3. **Dhatariya K, Savage M, Claydon A, et al.** Joint British Diabetes Societies Inpatient Care Group. The management of diabetic ketoacidosis in adults. 2010; http://www.diabetologists-abcd.org.uk/JBDS/JBDS_IP_DKA_Adults_Revised.pdf.
4. **Sacks DB, Arnold M, Bakris GL, et al.** Guidelines and recommendations for laboratory analysis in the diagnosis and management of diabetes mellitus. *Diabetes Care.* 2011;34:e61–e99.
5. **Smiley D, Chandra P, Umpierrez GE.** Update on diagnosis, pathogenesis and management of ketosis-prone Type 2 diabetes mellitus. *Diabetes Manag (Lond).* 2011;1:589–600.
6. **Lin SF, Lin JD, Huang YY.** Diabetic ketoacidosis: comparisons of patient characteristics, clinical presentations and outcomes today and 20 years ago. *Chang Gung Med J.* 2005;28:24–30.
7. **Wang J, Williams DE, Narayan KM, Geiss LS.** Declining death rates from hyperglycemic crisis among adults with diabetes, U.S., 1985–2002. *Diabetes Care.* 2006;29:2018–2022.
8. **Otieno CF, Kayima JK, Omonge EO, Oyoo GO.** Diabetic ketoacidosis: risk factors, mechanisms and management strategies in sub-Saharan Africa: a review. *E Afr Med J.* 2005;82:S197–S203.
9. **Hamblin PS, Topliss DJ, Chosich N, Lording DW, Stockigt JR.** Deaths associated with diabetic ketoacidosis and hyperosmolar coma. 1973–1988. *Med J Aust.* 1989;151:441–442.
10. **Matfin G.** Diabetes mellitus and the metabolic syndrome. In: Porth CM, Matfin G, eds. *Pathophysiology—Concepts of Altered Health States.* 8th ed. Philadelphia, PA: Lippincott Williams & Wilkins; 2008:1047–1077.
11. **English P, Williams G.** Hyperglycaemic crises and lactic acidosis in diabetes mellitus. *Postgrad Med J.* 2004;80:253–261.
12. **Barwell ND, McKay GA, Fisher M.** Drugs for diabetes: part 7 insulin. *Br J Cardiol.* 2011; 18:224–228.
13. **Weinstock RS, Xing D, Maahs DM, et al.** Severe hypoglycemia and diabetic ketoacidosis in adults with type 1 diabetes: results from the T1D Exchange Clinic Registry. *J Clin Endocrinol Metab.* 2013;98: 3411–3419.
14. **Verbalis JG, Goldsmith SR, Greenberg A, et al.** Diagnosis, evaluation, and treatment of hyponatremia: expert panel recommendations. *Am J Med.* 2013;126:S1–S42.
15. **Sheikh-Ali M, Karon BS, Basu A, et al.** Can serum beta-hydroxybutyrate be used to diagnose diabetic ketoacidosis? *Diabetes Care.* 2008;31: 643–647.
16. **Bektas F, Eray O, Sari R, Akbas H.** Point of care blood ketone testing of diabetic patients in the emergency department. *Endocr Res.* 2004;30:395–402.
17. **Khan AS, Talbot JA, Tieszen KL, Gardener EA, Gibson JM, New JP.** Evaluation of a bedside blood ketone sensor: the effects of acidosis, hyperglycaemia and acetoacetate on sensor performance. *Diabetic Med.* 2004;21:782–785.

18. **Wallace TM, Matthews DR.** Recent advances in the monitoring and management of diabetic ketoacidosis. *QJM.* 2004;97:773–780.
19. **Hsia E, Seggelke S, Gibbs J, et al.** Subcutaneous administration of glargine to diabetic patients receiving insulin infusion prevents rebound hyperglycemia. *J Clin Endocrinol Metab.* 2012;97:3132–3137.
20. **Chua HR, Schneider A, Bellomo R.** Bicarbonate in diabetic ketoacidosis—a systematic review. *Ann Intensive Care.* 2013;1:23.
21. **Scott A, Claydon A, Brennan G, et al.** The management of the hyperosmolar hyperglycaemic state (HHS) in adults with diabetes. The Joint British Diabetes Societies Inpatient Care Group. http://www.diabetologists-abcd.org.uk/JBDS/JBDS.htm. 2012.

CHAPTER 27

Short-Term Intensive Insulin Therapy in Persons with Newly Presenting Type 2 Diabetes Mellitus

Wen Xu, David Owens, and Jianpiang Weng

ABSTRACT

Type 2 diabetes mellitus (T2DM) is a complex metabolic disorder characterized by 2 major pathophysiological defects, namely, insulin resistance and pancreatic beta-cell dysfunction. However, the natural history of T2DM is primarily determined by the progressive deterioration of pancreatic beta-cell function, a pathological process that continues over time little influenced by current lifestyle and pharmacological interventions. In recent years, temporary administration of short-term intensive insulin therapy (STII) early in the course of T2DM has been a strategy of considerable interest to try to arrest or alter this natural history. In this chapter, we briefly discuss developments and clinical experience in the understanding of STII therapy of T2DM.

INTRODUCTION

Type 2 diabetes mellitus (T2DM) is a complex metabolic disorder, the pathophysiology of which is driven by 2 main coexisting defects, namely, target-cell resistance to the activity of insulin (insulin resistance) and relative insulin secretion insufficiency by the pancreatic beta-cell (beta-cell dysfunction) to overcome the insulin insensitivity. The relative contribution of these main defects varies among individuals. However, the natural history of T2DM is primarily determined by the progressive deterioration of pancreatic beta-cell function, a pathological process that continues over time little influenced by current lifestyle and pharmacological interventions. As a consequence, the typical clinical course of this disease consists of the sequential addition of antihyperglycemic preparations over time, followed ultimately by insulin therapy when functional beta-cell capacity deteriorates to the point at which glycemic control can no longer be achieved without exogenous insulin supplementation. At this point in the progressive course of T2DM, insulin therapy is generally continued indefinitely thereafter.

It is widely acknowledged that glycemic control in T2DM is suboptimal worldwide, and that evidence from several geographical areas demonstrates that glycosylated hemoglobin (HbA1c) is often high at the time of initial presentation (1,2). Among 1,256 newly diagnosed T2DM patients in 2 managed care databases in the United States, 66% had an HbA1c >7% in the 180 days prior to first medication, and nearly one quarter (23%) had an HbA1c ≥9.0% (1). In another population-based sample from Denmark of 1,136 newly diagnosed persons with T2DM (ie, single fasting whole blood glucose ≥126 mg/dL [7.0 mmol/L] or fasting plasma glucose [FPG] ≥144 mg/dL [8.0 mmol/L]) only 8.5% had an HbA1c ≤7.4% (2).

The importance of normalizing blood glucose early after diagnosis was firmly established by the United Kingdom Prospective Diabetes Study (UKPDS) (3), and as several recent reviews demonstrate, further supporting evidence continues to accrue (4,5). However, timely initiation of therapy alone is insufficient to ensure that the pathophysiological processes in T2DM are adequately interrupted. In recent years, temporary administration of short-term intensive insulin therapy (STII) early in the course of T2DM has been a strategy of considerable interest. STII therapy has been demonstrated to improve residual beta-cell function and thereby stabilize the disease process in its very early stages, proving to be of value in the treatment of newly presenting T2DM (6,7). Benefits of early intensive insulin therapy include marked reductions in glucose toxicity, as well as restoration of beta-cell responsiveness and insulin sensitivity, representing remission of the disease processes in many instances (7).

In the American Association of Clinical Endocrinologists (AACE) 2013 comprehensive disease management algorithm, insulin is recommended for T2DM patients presenting with symptoms and an HbA1c ≥9.0% (8). The Global Partnership for Effective Diabetes Management model also refers to the temporary use of insulin for newly diagnosed T2DM adults with HbA1c >9%, but fails to elaborate further, neither strongly endorsing or refuting the STII therapy concept (9). In addition, the American Diabetes Association (ADA)/European Association for the Study of Diabetes (EASD) consensus statement recommends initial insulin therapy as an option with HbA1c 8%–10% and definite consideration with HbA1c >10% (10). However, the ADA/EASD statement also mentions that it may be possible to taper off insulin once initial glucotoxicity is reversed and to consider transfer to other types of noninsulin therapies (10). Therefore, how to initiate insulin therapy in this situation, and how to select the follow-up treatment regimen after complete or partial discontinuation of insulin, still requires further exploration. In this chapter, we briefly discuss developments and clinical experience in the current understanding of STII therapy of T2DM.

CLINICAL EVIDENCE OF STII THERAPY IN NEWLY PRESENTING T2DM

There is a wide range of evidence currently available supporting the use of STII therapy in newly diagnosed T2DM. Our group has repeatedly shown that following STII therapy, many subjects are able to achieve and sustain prolonged remissions (periods of euglycemia) despite having discontinued all antihyperglycemic medications. In addition, numerous formal clinical studies have demonstrated that STII therapy (delivered via either continuous subcutaneous insulin infusion [CSII] or multiple daily injections [MDI]) can quickly normalize glycemic control, improve beta-cell function, and restore first-phase insulin secretion in newly diagnosed T2DM (7,11–14) (Table 27-1). STII therapy has also been favorably assessed in a recent meta-analysis (15) as well as in review articles, where it has either been the focus of the review (16) or been discussed along with other treatment options as a new therapeutic approach (5).

The largest and most robust clinical trial of STII therapy enrolled 382 newly diagnosed persons with T2DM at 9 centers in China and randomized them to either insulin (CSII or MDI) or oral antihyperglycemic therapy (7). Baseline assessments showed similar beta-cell function and insulin resistance in the 3 groups. Therapies were titrated to fasting and postprandial glucose targets after each of the 3 main meals and continued until normoglycemia was achieved for 2 consecutive weeks. Two days following cessation of treatment, the first-phase insulin secretion was increased in all 3 groups in response to intravenous glucose. Remission rates at 1 year were higher in the 2 insulin-treated groups (51.1% CSII, 44.9% MDI) than in the oral therapy group (26.7%). Furthermore, the increase in the first-phase insulin response was maintained at 1 year in the 2 insulin-treated groups, but declined in the group allocated to oral medication (Figure 27-1).

A meta-analysis including this trial and 6 other smaller trials of STII therapy, involving 839 participants, was performed (15). This meta-analysis further underscored the robustness of the evidence supporting STII therapy where 46% of patients were seen to remain in drug-free remission after 12 months. All but 1 study showed an improvement in beta-cell function, as assessed

Table 27-1. Characteristics of STII Studies Included in a Meta-Analysis (15)

	Year of Publication	Sample Size	Design	IIT Regimen	IIT Duration (days)	Baseline Mean Age (years)	Baseline Proportion of Men (%)	Baseline Mean BMI (kg/m²)	Baseline HbA1c (%)	Total Follow-up after IIT (months)	Evaluation of Glycemic Remission
Li Y et al (6)	2004	126	Interventional; one arm	CSII	14	48.6 (11.6)	61.9	25.1 (3.6)	10.0 (1.9)	24	Yes
Chen H et al (23)	2007	138	Interventional; one arm	CSII	14	45.8 (7.0)	62.3	25.4 (3.4)	11.9 (2.0)	0	No
Zhao Q et al (29)	2007	120	Interventional; one arm	CSII	14	47.0 (12.0)	83.3	24.0 (3.0)	Not available	0	No
Chen H et al (30)	2008	22	Randomized controlled trial; one arm long-term IIT; one arm on short-term IIT	MDI	14	58.7 (16.0)	77.3	27.7 (6.5)	11.7 (1.9)	0	No
Weng J et al (7)	2008	251	Randomized controlled trial; one arm on IIT	CSII and MDI	14	50.0 (10.5)	67.3	24.7 (2.8)	9.7 (2.3)	12	Yes
Chen A et al (28)	2012	118	Interventional; one arm	CSII	14–21	51.6 (10.2)	66.0	25.0 (3.0)	11.0 (2.1)	12	Yes
Liu L et al (21)	2012	64	Interventional; one arm	CSII	14	49.3 (9.5)	68.7	25.5 (3.5)	11.0 (1.8)	3	Yes

Data are mean (SD) unless otherwise stated.

Abbreviations: IIT = intensive insulin therapy; CSII = continuous subcutaneous insulin infusion; MDI = multiple daily injections; BMI = body mass index; HbA1c = glycated hemoglobin.

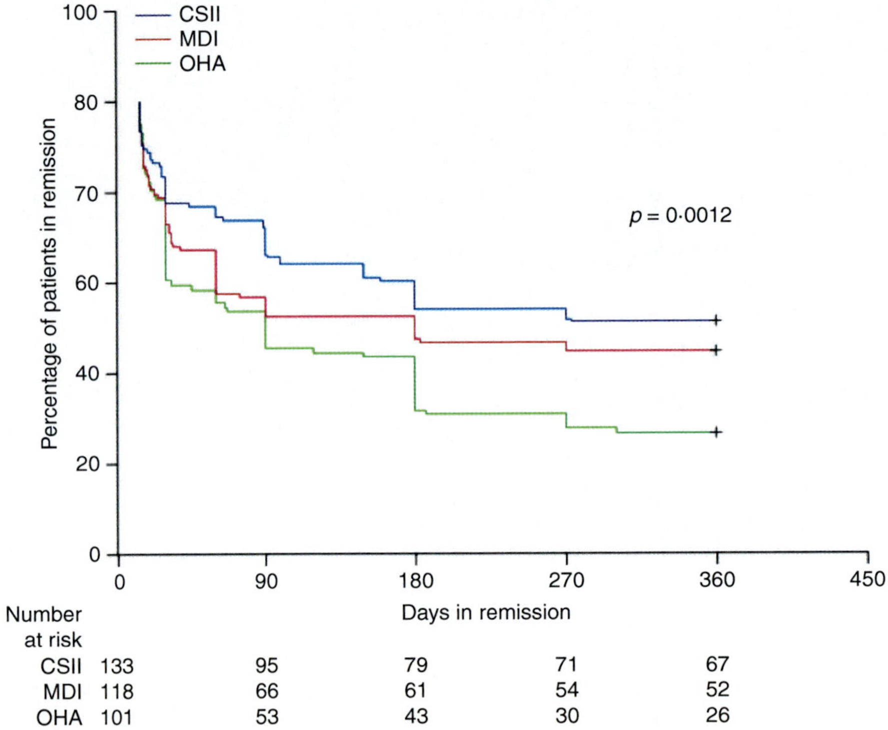

Figure 27-1. Percentage of patients with newly diagnosed type 2 diabetes treated with short-term continuous subcutaneous insulin infusion (CSII), multiple daily injections (MDI), and oral antihyperglycemic agents (OHA) in remission along with time (7).

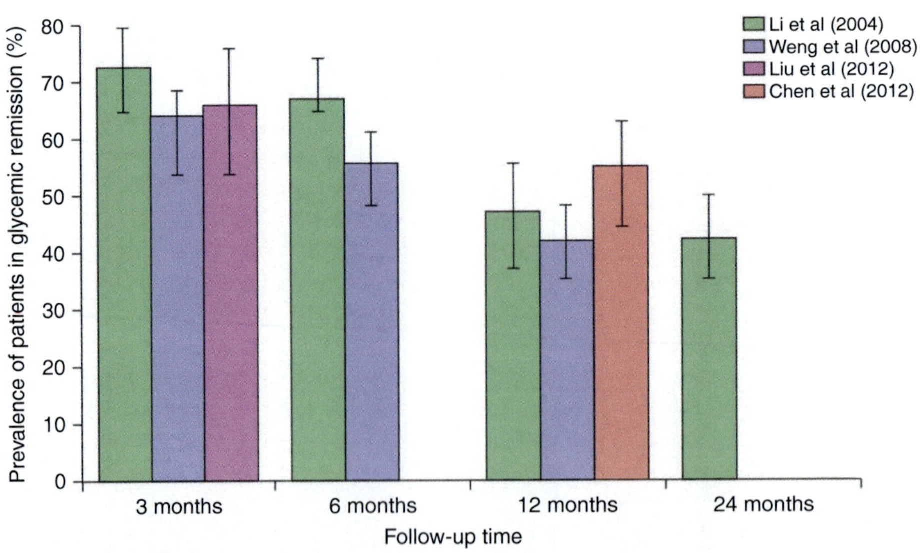

Figure 27-2. Prevalence of participants in drug-free glycemic remission during follow-up after short-term intensive insulin therapy, by study. Bars are 95% CIs (15).

by Homeostasis Model Assessment-Beta-cell function (HOMA-B), and all but 1 study showed a decrease in insulin resistance, as assessed by HOMA-Insulin Resistance (HOMA-IR). In the pooled data analysis, the proportion of patients in drug-free remission was 66.2% at 3 months, 58.9% at 6 months, 46.3% at 12 months, and 42.1% at 24 months (Figure 27-2).

Not all newly diagnosed T2DM subjects have experienced improved beta-cell function or achieved long-term remission following cessation of STII therapy (17), although any therapy that reduces glucotoxicity is likely to improve measures of pancreatic beta-cell response (18). Therefore, a critical requirement is to be able to identify those individuals most likely to achieve sustained preservation of beta-cells following STII by phenotypic characteristics and/or other biomarkers in order to personalize treatment approaches. Numerous predictors of long-term remission of hyperglycemia have been previously identified in clinical studies (15). Many of these predictors include markers of glycemic control. In the meta-analysis discussed previously, the presence at baseline of lower FPG and higher body mass index (BMI) were significantly associated with STII remission (19). Mechanistically, it is possible that once STII therapy is implemented, elimination of detrimental effects of glucotoxicity on existing beta-cell mass provides more capacity to improve endogenous insulin secretion. With respect to other specific characteristics and biomarkers, studies have indicated that improved beta-cell response and elimination of hyperglycemia can also be predicted by shorter diabetes duration (20), increased 1,5-anhydroglucitol (a validated short-term marker of glycemic control) (21), preserved late-phase insulin secretion (16), FPG (20,22), 2-hr postbreakfast plasma glucose (20) measured after cessation of STII treatment, and the presence of a higher HbA1c prior to STII therapy (19). The explanation for the latter finding is likely that persons with higher HbA1c at diagnosis may tend to have a greater residual beta-cell function that is masked by glucotoxicity.

As suggested previously, one problem with assessing the potential for remission in an individual with T2DM is that beta-cell function is influenced by a combination of factors that are potentially reversible with treatment (eg, glucotoxicity, lipotoxicity), as well as intrinsic functional deficits that are not improved by treatment (15). The relative contribution of these 2 sets of factors (reversible and irreversible) will vary within each person. This raises the question relating to the use of beta-cell function at baseline to predict remission. As has been shown in clinical trials, when beta-cell function is an outcome, it is important to first remove the confounding effect of having differential amounts of reversible components (15,16). Removing these confounding effects prior to randomization is essential if the mechanism of action by which STII therapy improves beta-cell function (beyond elimination of glucotoxicity, for example) is to be elucidated. Several other possible mechanisms have been proposed, including a decrease in tumor necrosis factor (TNF)-alpha, which may contribute to the positive effect of STII therapy on beta-cells (23). In another study, evidence implies that decreased visceral fat and increased skeletal muscle mass following insulin treatment may be associated with the observed improvements in beta-cell function (24).

CLINICAL PRACTICE OF STII THERAPY IN NEWLY PRESENTING T2DM

There is as yet no consensus about the most appropriate threshold (eg, HbA1c) for initiating STII treatment or about how long to maintain STII therapy after normalization of blood glucose. Due to the novelty of STII therapy and potential reservations among clinicians, it may be advisable to recommend STII therapy for those with an HbA1c >9.0% and FPG >200 mg/dL (11 mmol/L) (8,15). We believe it is important not to choose a lower HbA1c threshold in order not to cause concern to persons with T2DM or their health care providers. This may facilitate acceptance until more definitive evidence is available. A 2–3-week treatment course is adopted in most studies (15), although in a few studies, the duration has been prolonged to 3 months (12). With respect to optimal duration of treatment, future clinical studies are needed to examine time to failure of remission as it appears to vary according to the duration of STII therapy. Although the meta-analysis of STII therapy provides some guidance about time to failure, those data must be used cautiously, given that the studies were heterogeneous (15). Additionally, it would be important to know how long one can delay initiating STII therapy after diagnosis before the remission benefits are reduced.

The optimal treatment regimen following discontinuation of STII therapy also remains to be determined. Despite the benefits of a remission period free of drug therapy, it is possible that the optimal regimen would include some form of ongoing pharmacological treatment (in addition to lifestyle changes). To clarify this, one option would be to start with STII therapy and then to randomize the persons with T2DM to standard therapy or metformin or alternative noninsulin therapies (eg, incretin-based therapy, such as glucagon-like peptide-1 [GLP-1] agonists or dipeptidyl peptidase-4 [DPP-4] inhibitors) and compare time to remission failure. For example, in 1 trial currently in progress, all participants received a brief course of STII therapy to normalize blood glucose and then were randomized to either a GLP-1 agonist (ie, liraglutide) or placebo (Clinical Trials.Gov NCT01270789).

There is a substantial educational need among health care providers with respect to STII therapy, due to very limited clinical experience even among endocrinologists. However, health care practitioners should be aware that this is a viable option for certain groups of newly diagnosed persons with T2DM. A key difference, as well as potential advantage, which needs to be appreciated when using insulin early at the time of diagnosis of T2DM, is that the comparatively greater existing beta-cell mass should allow the use of lower insulin doses while still achieving the desired level of glucose control, with the added benefit of a low risk of hypoglycemia (because the residual beta-cells ultimately modulate the amount of endogenous insulin secreted, insulin secretion is inhibited in response to hypoglycemia). Indeed, with appropriate instructions on how to titrate and perform self-monitoring of blood glucose (SMBG), hypoglycemia can be largely avoided (15). Much, of course, depends on the competence of the health care team and the recipient's behavior and preconceptions about insulin therapy. Nevertheless, despite these considerations, it is quite feasible with experience to use STII therapy in an ambulatory setting.

Education in insulin initiation and intensification is also very important for clinicians and patients alike. Although reluctance to initiate insulin treatment in T2DM is well-described, other studies have shown that insulin administration issues become less of a concern once patients gain familiarity with insulin therapy and experience the clinical benefits (25). Indeed, several studies have now demonstrated that insulin can be well-accepted as initial therapy, particularly once patients are well-informed and understand the advantages (12,26,27). Positive attitudes have also been seen to correlate well with improved glycemic control (27). One study of 34 patients with insulin-naïve T2DM commenced a course of STII therapy for 4–8 weeks to determine eligibility for a clinical trial (26). Quality of life and treatment satisfaction were assessed at baseline and after completion of the STII. There were statistically significant improvements on the following items in the Medical Short-Form 36 (SF-36): physical functioning (P = 0.009), general health (P = 0.03), and mental health (P = 0.04). The Diabetes Quality of Life (DQOL) instrument also showed significant improvements in diabetes worry (P = 0.006) and treatment satisfaction (P = 0.007). In another study, insulin was used in conjunction with metformin in 63 newly diagnosed, treatment-naïve T2DM patients (12). Results indicated that 97% were satisfied with their insulin treatment. In another trial of newly diagnosed persons, insulin plus metformin were initiated for a 3-month lead-in period prior to randomization to further treatment of either continuing insulin plus metformin or triple oral therapy (metformin, pioglitazone, and glyburide [glibenclamide]) for 36 months (26). All of the subjects randomized to insulin were willing to continue, and there were no differences in treatment satisfaction between the 2 groups. In future clinical diabetes trials, STII therapy may be a useful prerandomization method of improving glycemic function (15). There is a real possibility that because the recipients will be satisfied with the results and clinical benefits that post-trial they may request to resume using insulin therapy, finding it much easier and better tolerated than expected.

From a practical perspective, there are some logistical issues that are potential barriers to achieving broader introduction and acceptance of the use of STII therapy. Endocrinologists, who may be the most comfortable at initiating this treatment regimen in T2DM, are usually managing patients well beyond the stage of being newly, or even recently, diagnosed except for maybe those presenting with a hyperglycemic emergency. By contrast, primary care physicians, who are more likely to make the initial diagnosis, are unlikely to initiate STII therapy themselves due to inadequate training and infrastructure (eg, lack of diabetes educators), and also limited consultation time with patients (especially in the ambulatory setting). There are also other logistical issues such as inadequate number and access to endocrinologists in many countries. From a public health standpoint, overall increasing numbers of persons with T2DM represent a huge challenge for diabetes management, especially as a significant proportion remain undiagnosed (eg, approximately 8 million out of a total of 25 million persons with T2DM in the United States are undiagnosed). If the diagnosis is undetected or significantly delayed, it may be that these persons are less likely to benefit from STII therapy due to the availability of insufficient residual beta-cell function. This problem is even more likely to be an issue in many low- and middle-income countries around the world due to limited public health infrastructure and robust access to insulin and monitoring tools. A better understanding of the cost-effectiveness of STII is clearly warranted. Other unique challenges include those individuals with T2DM who believe that insulin is only for the very severely ill and that using insulin represents a lifetime commitment. Another issue to be mindful of is that because the studies so far have been conducted predominantly in Asian populations, there is a perception that STII therapy is not applicable to other ethnic groups. However, a study conducted in multiple ethnic groups has recently addressed this issue (19).

CONCLUSIONS

STII therapy offers the possibility of preserving beta-cell function and inducing a long-term, drug-free period of remission in persons newly presenting with T2DM. It might be desirable to include STII therapy more explicitly in expert treatment guidelines. However, we appreciate that this represents a major paradigm shift in how the medical and nonmedical community interprets insulin therapy in the context of T2DM. The idea of using insulin as a way to alter the natural course of the disease is novel to both patients and health care providers alike. Because none of the current expert guidelines or diabetes management algorithms includes STII therapy as an option, clinicians may be reluctant to implement STII therapy, seeing it as a departure from typical practice. Thus, there is a need for further clinical evidence and appropriate education in order to gain broader acceptance and understanding of the role of STII therapy in the management of T2DM. Persons with T2DM, as well as their health care providers, tend to view insulin as an indicator of more advanced diabetes and treatment failure. Therefore, it will be very important to educate these groups as to why STII may be an appropriate option for the next stage of therapy after lifestyle modification in some newly presenting T2DM patients. It is important that STII therapy be considered an option at this early stage of the disease (when residual beta-cell mass is still present), when it may prove beneficial for some but not be adopted as the standard of care for all newly diagnosed patients with T2DM. Nevertheless, existing studies and clinical experience do indicate that this concept when implemented is very well-received by patients and clinicians alike, especially when they realize that insulin only needs to be used for a few weeks, and that STII therapy at that point in time does not necessarily commit them to continuing insulin therapy for the duration of their lives. However, several public health, clinical efficacy/effectiveness, and cost-effectiveness questions need to be better understood before widespread adoption of this novel treatment regimen can be more widely endorsed.

ACKNOWLEDGMENTS

This work was supported by the Changjiang Scholars Programme of China, the National Natural Science Funds for Distinguished Young Scholars (81025005), and the Program for Changjiang Scholars and Innovative Research Team in the University of Ministry of Education of China (985 project IRT0947). We are grateful to Sun Yat-sen University, the Third Affiliated Hospital of Sun Yat-sen University, and the Guangdong Provincial Key Laboratory of Diabetology for all of their support.

REFERENCES

1. **Brouwer ES, West SL, Kluckman M, et al.** Initial and subsequent therapy for newly diagnosed type 2 diabetes patients treated in primary care using data from a vendor-based electronic health record. *Pharmacoepidemiol Drug Saf.* 2012;21:920–928.

2. **Veloso AG, Siersma V, Heldgaard PE, de Fine Olivarius N.** Patients newly diagnosed with clinical type 2 diabetes mellitus but presenting with HbA1c within normal range: 19-year mortality and clinical outcomes. *Prim Care Diabetes.* 2013;7:33–38.
3. **Stratton IM, Adler AI, Neil HA, et al.** Association of glycaemia with macrovascular and microvascular complications of type 2 diabetes (UKPDS 35): prospective observational study. *BMJ.* 2000;321:405–412.
4. **Hanefeld M, Bramlage P.** Insulin use early in the course of type 2 diabetes mellitus: the ORIGIN trial. *Curr Diab Rep.* 2013;13:342–349.
5. **Owens DR.** Clinical evidence for the earlier initiation of insulin therapy in type 2 diabetes. *Diabetes Technol Ther.* 2013;15:776–785.
6. **Li Y, Xu W, Liao Z, et al.** Induction of long-term glycemic control in newly diagnosed type 2 diabetic patients is associated with improvement of beta-cell function. *Diabetes Care.* 2004;27:2597–2602.
7. **Weng J, Li Y, Xu W, et al.** Effect of intensive insulin therapy on beta-cell function and glycaemic control in patients with newly diagnosed type 2 diabetes: a multicenter randomised parallel-group trial. *Lancet.* 2008;371:1753–1760.
8. **Garber AJ, Abrahamson MJ, Barzilay JI, et al.** AACE comprehensive diabetes management algorithm 2013. *Endocr Pract.* 2013;19:327–336.
9. **Bailey CJ, Aschner P, Del Prato S, Lasalle J, Ji L, Matthaei S.** Global Partnership for Effective Diabetes Management. Individualized glycaemic targets and pharmacotherapy in type 2 diabetes. *Diab Vasc Dis Res.* 2013;10:397–409.
10. **Inzucchi SE, Bergenstal RM, Buse JB, et al.** Management of hyperglycemia in type 2 diabetes: a patient-centered approach: position statement of the American Diabetes Association (ADA) and the European Association for the Study of Diabetes (EASD). *Diabetes Care.* 2012;35:1364–1379. Erratum in *Diabetes Care.* 2013;36:490.
11. **Ilkova H, Glaser B, Tunçkale A, Bagriaçik N, Cerasi E.** Induction of long-term glycemic control in newly diagnosed type 2 diabetic patients by transient intensive insulin treatment. *Diabetes Care.* 1997;20: 1353–1356.
12. **Lingvay I, Kaloyanova PF, Adams-Huet B, Salinas K, Raskin P.** Insulin as initial therapy in type 2 diabetes: effective, safe, and well accepted. *J Investig Med.* 2007;55:62–68.
13. **Chon S, Oh S, Kim SW, Kim JW, Kim YS, Woo JT.** The effect of early insulin therapy on pancreatic β-cell function and long-term glycemic control in newly diagnosed type 2 diabetic patients. *Korean J Intern Med.* 2010;25:273–281.
14. **Retnakaran R, Qi Y, Opsteen C, Vivero E, Zinman B.** Initial short-term intensive insulin therapy as a strategy for evaluating the preservation of beta-cell function with oral antidiabetic medications: a pilot study with sitagliptin. *Diabetes Obes Metab.* 2010;12:909–915.
15. **Kramer CK, Zinman B, Retnakaran R.** Short-term intensive insulin therapy in type 2 diabetes mellitus: a systematic review and meta-analysis. *Lancet Diabetes Endocrinol.* 2013
16. **Xu W, Weng J.** Current role of short-term intensive insulin strategies in newly diagnosed type 2 diabetes. *J Diabetes.* 2013;5:268–274.
17. **Retnakaran R, Yakubovich N, Qi Y, Opsteen C, Zinman B.** The response to short-term intensive insulin therapy in type 2 diabetes. *Diabetes Obes Metab.* 2010;12:65–71.
18. **Chiasson JL.** Early insulin use in type 2 diabetes: what are the cons? *Diabetes Care.* 2009;32(suppl 2):S270–S274.
19. **Kramer CK, Choi H, Zinman B, Retnakaran R.** Determinants of reversibility of beta-cell dysfunction in response to short-term intensive insulin therapy in patients with early type 2 diabetes. *Diabetes.* 2013;62(suppl 1):A243.
20. **Xu W, Li YB, Deng WP, Hao YT, Weng JP.** Remission of hyperglycemia following intensive insulin therapy in newly diagnosed type 2 diabetic patients: a long-term follow-up study. *Chin Med J (Engl).* 2009;122:2554–2559.
21. **Liu L, Wan X, Liu J, Huang Z, Cao X, Li Y.** Increased 1,5-anhydroglucitol predicts glycemic remission in patients with newly diagnosed type 2 diabetes treated with short-term intensive insulin therapy. *Diabetes Technol Ther.* 2012;14:756–761.
22. **Liu J, Liu J, Fang D, et al.** Fasting plasma glucose after intensive insulin therapy predicted long-term glycemic control in newly diagnosed type 2 diabetic patients. *Endocr J.* 2013;60:725–732.
23. **Chen H, Ren A, Hu S, Mo W, Xin X, Jia W.** The significance of tumor necrosis factor-alpha in newly diagnosed type 2 diabetic patients by transient intensive insulin treatment. *Diabetes Res Clin Pract.* 2007;75:327–332.
24. **Son JW, Jeong HK, Lee SS, et al.** The effect of early intensive insulin therapy on body fat distribution and β-cell function in newly diagnosed type 2 diabetes [published online ahead of print January 3, 2013] *Endocr Res.*
25. **Casciano R, Malangone E, Ramachandran A, Gagliardino JJ.** A quantitative assessment of patient barriers to insulin. *Int J ClinPract.* 2011;65:408–414.
26. **Lingvay I, Legendre JL, Kaloyanova PF, Zhang S, Adams-Huet B, Raskin P.** Insulin-based versus triple oral therapy for newly diagnosed type 2 diabetes: which is better? *Diabetes Care.* 2009;32:1789–1795.
27. **Opsteen C, Qi Y, Zinman B, Retnakaran R.** Effect of short-term intensive insulin therapy on quality of life in type 2 diabetes. *J Eval Clin Pract.* 2012;18:256–261.
28. **Chen A, Huang Z, Wan X, et al.** Attitudes toward diabetes affect maintenance of drug-free remission in patients with newly diagnosed type 2 diabetes after short-term continuous subcutaneous insulin infusion treatment. *Diabetes Care.* 2012;35:474–481.
29. **Zhao QB, Wang HF, Sun CF, Ma AQ, Cui CC.** Effect of short-term intensive treatment with insulin pump on beta cell function and the mechanism of oxidative stress in newly diagnosed type 2 diabetic patients [in Chinese]. *Nan Fang Yi Ke Da Xue Xue Bao.* 2007;27:1878–1879.
30. **Chen HS, Wu TE, Jap TS, Hsiao LC, Lee SH, Lin HD.** Beneficial effects of insulin on glycemic control and beta-cell function in newly diagnosed type 2 diabetes with severe hyperglycemia after short-term intensive insulin therapy. *Diabetes Care.* 2008;31:1927–1932.

CHAPTER 28

Management of Hyperglycemia and Diabetes in Noncritical Care Settings

Guillermo E Umpierrez and Susan Braithwaite

ABSTRACT

Extensive observational data and prospective randomized trials in hospitalized patients indicate a strong association between hyperglycemia and poor clinical outcome, such as increased mortality, morbidity, length of stay, infections, and overall number of complications. This association is well documented not only with glycemic status upon admission but also for the mean glucose level during the hospital stay. Cross-sectional studies have shown that the risk of complications and mortality relates to the severity of hyperglycemia, with a higher risk observed in patients without a history of diabetes (new onset and stress-induced hyperglycemia) compared to those with a known diagnosis of diabetes. In addition, numerous studies have also shown that complication rates decrease when blood glucose levels are controlled during the hospital stay. This chapter reviews the risks associated with hyperglycemia in different clinical situations in noncritical care patients and outlines practical protocols for the management of hyperglycemia in patients admitted to general medicine and surgery services.

INTRODUCTION

Extensive observational data and prospective randomized trials in hospitalized patients indicate a strong association between hyperglycemia and poor clinical outcome, such as increased mortality, morbidity, length of stay, infections, and overall number of complications (1,2). This association is well-documented not only with glycemic status upon admission but also for the mean glucose level during the hospital stay (3–5). Cross-sectional studies have shown that the risk of complications and mortality relates to the severity of hyperglycemia, with a higher risk observed in patients without a history of diabetes (new onset and stress-induced hyperglycemia) compared to those with a known diagnosis of diabetes. In addition, numerous studies have also shown that complication rates decrease when blood glucose levels are controlled during the hospital stay. This chapter reviews the risks associated with hyperglycemia in different clinical situations in noncritical care patients and outlines practical protocols for the management of hyperglycemia in patients with stress hyperglycemia and in patients with diabetes admitted to general medicine and surgery services.

PREVALENCE OF HYPERGLYCEMIA IN NONCRITICAL CARE SETTINGS

Diabetes is the seventh leading cause of death (6,7) and is the fourth leading comorbid condition among hospital discharges in the

United States (8). Adults with diabetes are hospitalized substantially more frequently than persons without diabetes (9). Approximately 1 in 4 patients admitted to the hospital has a known diagnosis of diabetes (2,10). Observational studies have reported a prevalence of hyperglycemia ranging from 32% to 38% in community hospitals (2,11,12), 41% of patients with acute coronary syndromes (13), 44% of patients with heart failure (13), and 80% of patients after cardiac surgery (14,15).

STRESS HYPERGLYCEMIA

The Endocrine Society (16), American Association of Clinical Endocrinologists (AACE), and American Diabetes Association (ADA) (17) define stress hyperglycemia or hospital-related hyperglycemia as any blood glucose concentration >140 mg/dL (7.8 mmol/L) without evidence of previous diabetes and a hemoglobin A1C (HbA1c) <6.5% (Table 28-1). Although stress hyperglycemia typically resolves as the acute illness or surgical stress abates (18), it is important to identify and track patients because 40%–60% of patients admitted with new or stress-related hyperglycemia had confirmed diabetes at 1 year (19). Until recently, clinical guidelines recommended that all patients with stress hyperglycemia should be tested with an oral glucose tolerance test (OGTT) shortly after discharge to assess glucose tolerance (20). More recently, the use of A1C is recommended over OGTT as the preferred diagnostic testing in hospitalized patients with hyperglycemia (16,17). Measurement of an A1C during periods of hospitalization provides the opportunity to differentiate patients with stress hyperglycemia from those with diabetes who were previously undiagnosed, as well as to identify patients with known diabetes who would benefit from intensification of their glycemic management. However, it is important to emphasize that A1C testing in the hospital has significant limitations in the presence of hemoglobinopathies, recent transfusion, severe hepatic or liver disease, and iron deficiency anemia (21,22).

The literature about stress hyperglycemia in noncritical illness is smaller than that concerning its role among critically ill patients. In a systematic review of 54 stroke studies accompanying a single-site study, it was shown that higher admission glucose was associated with less favorable outcome and more symptomatic intracranial hemorrhage; the adjusted odds ratio (95% CI) per 18 mg/dL (1 mmol/L) increase in the adjusted glucose level was 0.92 (0.90–0.94) for favorable outcome, and 1.09 (1.04–1.14) for symptomatic intracranial hemorrhage (23). A study of general hospital admissions reported that patients with newly recognized hyperglycemia had a longer length of hospital stay and higher admission rate to an intensive care unit (ICU), and were less likely to be discharged to home, frequently requiring transfer to a transitional care unit or nursing home facility (2). A study of perioperative hyperglycemia after noncardiac general surgery showed that the risk of death increased in proportion to perioperative glucose levels; however, this association was significant only for patients without a history of diabetes ($P = 0.008$) compared with patients with known diabetes ($P = 0.748$) (24).

Stress hyperglycemia may occur during acute stress through multiple mechanisms, including treatment interventions, patient predisposition, and neuroendocrine derangements that are introduced by illness. Acute illness raises levels of counter-regulatory hormones such as glucagon, epinephrine, cortisol, and growth hormone. The counter-regulatory response results in a number of alterations in carbohydrate metabolism, including insulin resistance, increased hepatic glucose production, impaired peripheral glucose utilization, and relative insulin deficiency (25). Epinephrine stimulates glucagon secretion and inhibits insulin release by pancreatic beta-cells (26). High cortisol levels increase hepatic glucose production and stimulate protein catabolism and increased gluconeogenesis (27,28). Thus, stress adversely affects multiple biological processes resulting in diminished insulin action, and if the pancreas is unable to compensate by increasing insulin production, the end result is the appearance of hyperglycemia.

The development of hyperglycemia also leads to generation of reaction oxygen species and elevated cardiovascular inflammatory markers (29–32). It also increases proinflammatory cytokines such as tumor necrosis factor-alpha (TNF-α), interleukin (IL)-6, and IL-1, which

Table 28-1. The Endocrine Society Recommendations for Inpatient Management of Hyperglycemia and Diabetes in Non-ICU Settings (16)

- For patients who have diabetes admitted to the hospital, diabetes should be clearly identified in the medical record.
- Glucose monitoring with orders for correction insulin should be initiated for patients who are not known to be diabetic but receive therapy associated with a high risk for hyperglycemia.
- Nondiabetic subjects with hyperglycemia should have an A1C level measured to diagnose diabetes. Similarly, patients with diabetes should have A1C level determined if the results of testing in the previous 2 to 3 months are not available.
- Goals for blood glucose levels:
  - *Noncritically ill patients:* Fasting and premeal blood glucose levels should be <140 mg/dL (7.8 mmol/L), and random glucose levels should be <180 mg/dL (10.0 mmol/L).
- Use of scheduled basal and prandial insulin is recommended for treatment of hyperglycemia.
  - Basal insulin using intermediate- or long-acting insulin.
  - Prandial doses should be appropriately timed in relation to meals and should be adjusted according to point-of-care glucose levels.
  - Correction or supplementary insulin may be used in addition to scheduled insulin to correct premeal hyperglycemia.
- Episodes of hypoglycemia should be tracked. A plan for treating hypoglycemia should be established for each patient.
- A diabetes education plan should be developed for each patient.

ultimately alter the immune system. Increasing evidence suggests that TNF-α mediates insulin resistance by interfering with insulin receptor signaling (33,34) or synthesis and/or translocation of the glucose transporter GLUT-4 to the plasma membrane (35), which may lead to insulin resistance in peripheral tissues.

HYPERGLYCEMIA IN PERSONS WITH DIABETES IN NONCRITICAL CARE SETTINGS

Hyperglycemia in noncritically ill patients admitted to general medicine and surgery services is associated with increased risk of infections and complications (2,36). In a prospective study of 2,471 patients admitted for community-acquired pneumonia (37), the mortality rate was 13% in those with admission glucose levels >200 mg/dL (11 mmol/L) and 9% in those with admission levels ≤200 mg/dL (11 mmol/L). The group with the higher admission levels also had a higher rate of in-hospital complications (29% vs 22%). In a retrospective study of 348 patients with acute exacerbation of chronic obstructive pulmonary disease and respiratory tract infection, the relative risk of death was 2.1 in those with a blood glucose of 126–160 mg/dL (7–8.9 mmol/L), and 3.4 for those with a blood glucose of >162 mg/dL (9.0 mmol/L) compared to patients with a blood glucose of 108 mg/dL (6.0 mmol/L) (38). Furthermore, each 18 mg/dL (1 mmol/L) increase in blood glucose was associated with a 15% increase in the risk of an adverse clinical outcome (defined as death or length of stay of >9 days).

In general surgery patients, the development of hyperglycemia is also associated with increased risk for adverse outcomes. Patients with glucose levels of 110–200 mg/dL (5.6–11.1 mmol/L) and those with glucose levels of >200 mg/dL (11.1 mmol/L) had, respectively, 1.7-fold and 2.1-fold increased mortality compared to those with glucose levels <110 mg/dL (5.6 mmol/L). In another study, patients with glucose levels ≥220 mg/dL (12.2 mmol/L) on the first postoperative day had a rate of infection 2.7 times higher than those who had serum glucose levels <220 mg/dL (12.2 mmol/L). Another study in general surgery (39) showed an increase of postoperative infection rate by 30% for every 40 mg/dL (2.2 mmol/L) rise in postoperative blood glucose level >110 mg/dL (5.6 mmol/L). Similarly, several recent studies and a recent meta-analysis in general noncardiac surgery have reported an association between perioperative hyperglycemia and the postoperative infection rates in patients with diabetes (24,40,41).

STRATEGIES FOR THE MANAGEMENT OF INPATIENT HYPERGLYCEMIA

The Endocrine Society, AACE, and ADA guidelines on inpatient glycemic control recommend targeting a glucose level <140 mg/dL

(7.8 mmol/L) before meals and random glucose levels <180 mg/dL (10.0) for the majority of non-ICU patients (16,17). The American College of Physicians recommends blood glucose levels <11.1 mmol/L (200 mg/dL) for most patients in non-ICU settings (42).

All hospitals should have protocols that are in line with current guidelines for identifying and managing hyperglycemia (Figure 28-1). These protocols should be simple and user friendly, identify patients who require initiation or modification of insulin therapy, address requirements for insulin infusion, and determine the consultation and educational needs of patients. When a patient with known diabetes is admitted to the hospital, it is important to avoid common errors that may result in hyperglycemia. The most obvious of these errors is neglecting to continue treatment of the patient's diabetes while addressing other acute issues. Another common error is failure to modify outpatient treatment regimens to account for the changes in glucose control that occur during hospitalization. Finally, withholding therapy of high blood glucose levels because of fear of hypoglycemia should not be accepted.

Insulin is the treatment of choice for hyperglycemia in the hospital setting. To meet the daily insulin requirements, subcutaneous (SC) insulin regimens should cover the patient's basal requirements and nutritional needs. In addition, correction-dose or supplemental insulin should be available to address episodes of hyperglycemia. Basal insulin requirements may be met with once-daily administration of a long-acting insulin analog (glargine or detemir) or with twice-daily administration of the intermediate-acting neutral protamine Hagedorn (NPH) insulin. Rapid-acting insulin analogs (lispro, aspart, or glulisine) or short-acting regular human insulin may be used to meet nutritional needs and to provide correctional insulin coverage. Monotherapy consisting of SC short-acting insulin based on a sliding scale is ineffective and is not recommended in patients with diabetes.

The starting insulin dose can be selected based on a patient's body weight and administered within a daily range of 0.3 to 0.5 units per kg (Figure 28-2). Patients with adequate oral intake should receive a basal bolus regimen divided half as basal and half as prandial insulin. Patients with inadequate oral intake or who will be kept NPO (nil per oral) should receive basal insulin (0.15–0.25 units/kg/day) without scheduled prandial insulin. Rapid-acting insulin analogs or short-acting insulin is given to provide correctional insulin coverage for glucose >140–180 mg/dL (7.8–10 mmol/L). The recent RABBIT Surgery trial, a randomized multicenter study, compared the efficacy and safety of improving glucose control with basal bolus insulin as compared to sliding scale insulin (SSI) in patients with type 2 diabetes undergoing general surgery (43). Study outcomes included differences in daily blood glucose levels and a composite of postoperative complications, including wound infection,

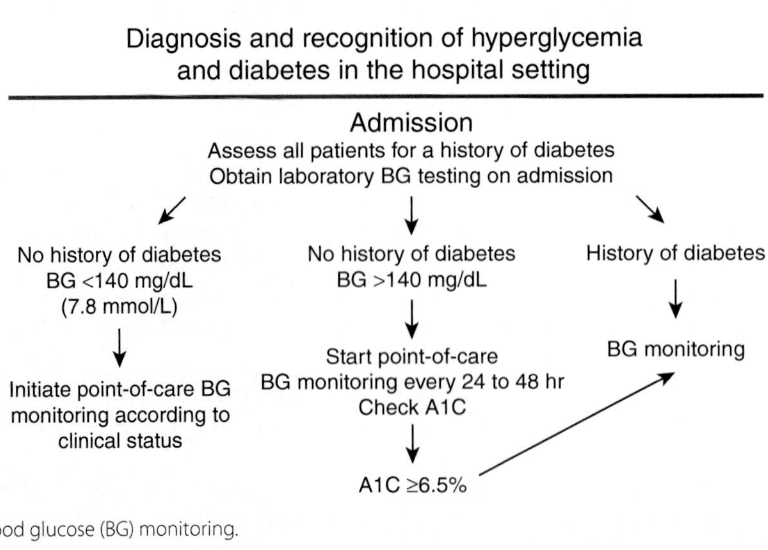

Figure 28-1. Blood glucose (BG) monitoring.

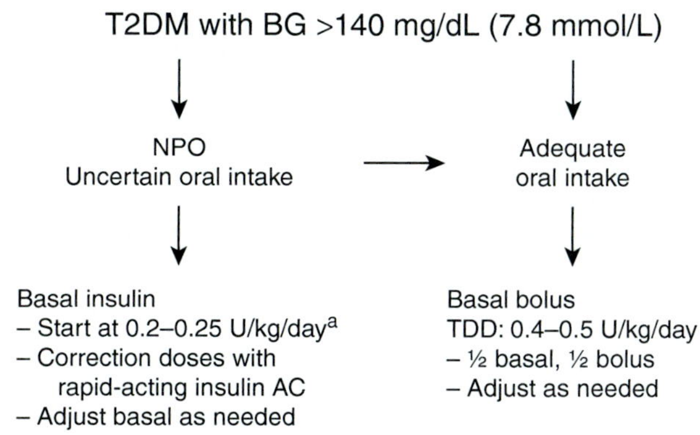

Figure 28-2. Initial insulin treatment in non-ICU medical and surgical settings. BG target: fasting and premeal glucose concentration between 100 mg/dL and 140 mg/dL. [a] Reduced TDD to 0.15 U/kg/day if age >70 years or creatinine ≥2.0 mg/dL. AC = premeals; BG = blood glucose; TDD = total daily dose; T2DM = type 2 diabetes.

pneumonia, respiratory failure, acute renal failure, and bacteremia. Patients were randomized to receive basal bolus regimen with glargine and glulisine at a starting dose of 0.5 unit/kg/day or SSI given 4 times/day. The basal bolus regimen resulted in significant improvement in glucose control and in a reduction in the frequency of the composite outcome. The results of this trial indicate that treatment with glargine once daily plus rapid-acting insulin before meals improves glucose control and reduces hospital complications compared to SSI in general surgery patients with type 2 diabetes.

The recently reported Basal Plus trial (44) recruited 375 patients with type 2 diabetes treated with diet, oral antidiabetic agents, or low-dose insulin (≤0.4 unit/kg/day) to receive a basal bolus regimen with glargine once daily and glulisine before meals, a basal plus regimen with glargine once daily and supplemental doses of glulisine for correction of hyperglycemia (>140 mg/dL [7.8 mmol/L]) per sliding scale, and SSI. This trial reported that the basal plus resulted in similar improvement in glycemic control and in the frequency of hypoglycemia compared to a standard basal bolus regimen. In addition, treatment with basal bolus and basal plus resulted in fewer treatment failures than treatment with SSI. Thus, in insulin-naïve patients or in those receiving low-dose insulin on admission (less than 0.4 unit/kg/day), as well as patients with reduced oral intake, the use of a basal plus regimen is an effective alternative to basal bolus. If needed, patients with persistent hyperglycemia or with regular caloric intake could be moved up to a basal bolus regimen.

Hospital Use of Oral Antidiabetic Agents in Noncritical Care Settings

In general, the use of oral antidiabetic agents is not recommended because of the lack of safety and efficacy in the inpatient setting (45,46). There are major limitations to the use of most oral antidiabetic agents, including the slow onset of action, which may not allow rapid dose adjustment to meet the changing needs of the acutely ill patient, and risk of hypoglycemia with insulin secretagogues. Sulfonylureas may increase the risk of hypoglycemia in the hospitalized patient with poor appetite or ordered dietary restrictions. In addition to inhibiting ATP-sensitive potassium channels, sulfonylurea therapy may inhibit ischemic preconditioning leading to worsening cardiac and cerebral ischemia (47,48). A large number of patients have one or more contraindications to the use of metformin upon admission (49,50), including acute congestive heart failure, renal or liver dysfunction, or hypoperfusion, which may increase the risk of lactic acidosis (51). Finally, the use of thiazolidinediones is limited because they can increase intravascular volume and may precipitate or worsen congestive heart failure and peripheral edema (50,52–54).

A recent randomized 2-center open label pilot trial determined differences in glycemic control between treatment with sitagliptin alone or in combination with basal insulin in general medicine and surgery patients with type 2 diabetes (55). In this pilot study, general medicine and surgery patients with a blood glucose between 140 mg/dL and 400 mg/dL

(7.8–22.2 mmol/L) treated with diet, oral antidiabetic drugs, or low-dose insulin (≤0.4 units/kg/day) were randomized to sitagliptin once daily, sitagliptin and basal insulin, or basal bolus insulin. All groups received correction doses of lispro before meals and bedtime for blood glucose >140 mg/dL (7.8 mmol/L). Patients in the sitagliptin group received a single daily dose of 50–100 mg based on kidney function. Sitagliptin was well-tolerated, and in those with mild-to-moderate hyperglycemia (<180 mg/dL [10 mmol/L]), the use of sitagliptin plus supplemental (correction doses) or in combination with basal insulin resulted in no significant differences in mean daily blood glucose, frequency of hypoglycemia, or in the number of treatment failures compared to basal bolus regimen. These preliminary results suggest that treatment with sitagliptin alone or in combination with basal insulin is safe and may represent an alternative for the management of hyperglycemia in some patients with type 2 diabetes. These encouraging results need to be confirmed in larger randomized controlled trials. The role of incretin-based therapies generally in the inpatient setting has been a source of controversy and requires further exploration (56).

Hypoglycemia and Hospital Outcomes

Although intensive insulin therapy is the standard of care in hospitals, it also can be the source of errors and poor outcome. An analysis of medication errors between 2006 and 2008 revealed that insulin was the drug with the greatest number of medication errors in hospitals (57). Several meta-analyses (mainly in ICU settings) demonstrated that the risk ratio for occurrence of hypoglycemic events with intensive insulin therapy versus conventional glycemic control in critically ill patients was on average 6-fold and 7.7-fold increased, with some studies showing a risk ratio >10 (15,58). Hypoglycemia has been associated with adverse cardiovascular outcomes, such as prolonged QT intervals, ischemic electrocardiogram changes/angina, arrhythmias, sudden death, and increased inflammation (59,60).

The evidence regarding a link between hypoglycemia and increased risk of mortality is varied, with 2 recent studies reporting that hypoglycemia (blood glucose <70 mg/dL [4 mmol/L]) was independently associated with increased mortality risk in critically ill and ICU patients independent of their diabetes status (61,62). In contrast, a recent meta-analysis evaluating clinical studies in hospitalized patients, including those in the ICU, found a small reduction in mortality in hospitalized patients, whereas no impact on ICU mortality was reported (63).

Insulin-induced hypoglycemia has been associated with increases in C-reactive protein and proinflammatory cytokines (TNF-α, IL-1β, IL-6, and IL-8), markers of lipid peroxidation, reactive oxygen species, and leukocytosis (64,65). In addition, acute hypoglycemia creates a prothrombotic environment, with increased levels of vasoconstrictors, platelet aggregation, endothelial dysfunction and vasoconstriction, and abnormal cardiac repolarization, as well as catecholamine-induced cardiovascular changes, such as increased heart rate, angina, and myocardial infarctions, all contributing to increased mortality (64,66).

Glycemic Variability

Mortality in the critical care setting has been linked to the glycemic variability experienced by individual patients, and in some studies the association of variability with mortality has been demonstrable independent of hyperglycemia or hypoglycemia. Outside of the ICU, there is relatively less information on the potential importance of glycemic variability to outcomes. Our understanding of glycemic variability is limited by the lack of patient-level data in some studies, lack of consensus on definition or metrics for glycemic variability, and reliance upon sporadic point-of-care testing from observational studies. Experimental evidence for an effect of variability upon oxidative stress, endothelial dysfunction, and cellular apoptosis suggests that vascular injury could be a plausible explanation for the impact of glycemic variability upon patient outcomes. In a single-center retrospective study of 748 patients having discharge diagnosis of congestive heart failure, the median glycemic lability index was higher in nonsurvivors than in survivors (18.1 vs 6.82, $P = 0.0003$) (67). In a prospective study of 276 medical and surgical patients receiving total parenteral nutrition (TPN), glycemic variability was significantly higher in deceased patients than nondeceased patients (SD: 48 ± 25 vs 34 ± 18 mg/dL, and delta change: 75 ± 39 vs 51 ± 29 mg/dL, both $P < 0.01$) (68). In a retrospective study of 935 admissions to the general medicine or surgery services involving 620 patients at a single US Veterans Affairs center, the risk of death within 90 days increased by 10% with each 10 mg/dL (0.55 mmol/L) increment in SD of glucose (risk ratio [RR] 1.10 [95% CI 1.04–1.16], $P < 0.001$) and by 21% with each 10–percentage-point increment in CV of glucose (RR 1.21 [1.07–1.35], $P = 0.002$) (69).

Recommendations after Hospital Discharge

Few studies have focused on the optimal management of hyperglycemia after hospital discharge. Although insulin is used for most patients with diabetes in the hospital, many patients do not require insulin after discharge. The recent Endocrine Society inpatient guidelines for the management of non-ICU patients with diabetes (16) recommended that patients with diabetes and hyperglycemia should have an A1C measured to assess preadmission glycemic control and to tailor treatment regimen at discharge. Patients with acceptable diabetes control could be discharged on their prehospitalization treatment regimen (noninsulin agents and/or insulin therapy) if there were no contraindications to therapy. Patients with suboptimal control should have intensification of therapy, either by addition or increase in noninsulin agents, addition of basal insulin, or a more complex insulin regimen as warranted by their admission glucose control. Our preliminary experience indicates that measurement of A1C on admission is useful in assessing metabolic control on admission and to guide treatment regimen at the time of hospital discharge in patients with type 2 diabetes. Patients admitted with an A1C <7% can be discharged on the same preadmission diabetes therapy (noninsulin agents or insulin). Those with A1C between 7% and 9% can be discharged on noninsulin agents plus basal insulin at 50% to 80% of the hospital basal insulin, and patients with A1C >9% should be discharged on basal bolus insulin or in the combination of metformin plus basal insulin at 80% of hospital dose.

CONCLUSIONS

Hyperglycemia is a common finding in noncritically ill patients with and without diabetes. Observational and randomized controlled studies indicate that improvement in glycemic control results in lower rates of hospital complications and mortality. Implementing a standardized subcutaneous insulin order set promoting the use of scheduled basal and nutritional insulin therapy is a key intervention in the inpatient management of diabetes.

ACKNOWLEDGMENTS

GU is supported in part by research grants from the American Diabetes Association (1-14-LLY-36) and PHS Grant UL1 RR025008 from the Clinical and Translational Science Award program, National Institutes of Health, National Center for Research Resources. He has received research grant support to Emory University from Sanofi, Novo Nordisk, Merck, and Boehringer Ingelheim. He has also received an honorarium for participating in advisory/consultant meetings from Sanofi, Novo Nordisk, Boehringer Ingelheim, Regeneron, and Merck.

REFERENCES

1. **Furnary AP, Wu Y, Bookin SO.** Effect of hyperglycemia and continuous intravenous insulin infusions on outcomes of cardiac surgical procedures: the Portland Diabetic Project. *Endocr Pract.* 2004;10(suppl 2):21–33.
2. **Umpierrez GE, Isaacs SD, Bazargan N, You X, Thaler LM, Kitabchi AE.** Hyperglycemia: an independent marker of in-hospital mortality in patients with undiagnosed diabetes. *J Clin Endocrinol Metab.* 2002;87:978–982.
3. **Falciglia M, Freyberg RW, Almenoff PL, D'Alessio DA, Render ML.** Hyperglycemia-related mortality in critically ill patients varies with admission diagnosis. *Crit Care Med.* 2009;37:3001–3009.
4. **Krinsley JS.** Association between hyperglycemia and increased hospital mortality in a heterogeneous population of critically ill patients. *Mayo Clin Proc.* 2003;78:1471–1478.
5. **Furnary AP, Zerr KJ, Grunkemeier GL, Starr A.** Continuous intravenous insulin infusion reduces the incidence of deep sternal wound infection in diabetic patients after cardiac surgical procedures. *Ann Thorac Surg.* 1999;67:352–360; discussion 360–352.
6. **Xu J, Kochanek KD, Murphy SL, Tejada-Vera B.** Deaths: final data for 2007. *National Vital Statistics Reports.* 2010;58.

7. **Centers for Disease Control and Prevention.** *National Diabetes Fact Sheet: National Estimates and General Information on Diabetes and Prediabetes in the United States, 2011*. Atlanta, GA: U.S. Department of Health and Human Services, Centers for Disease Control and Prevention; 2011.
8. **Elixhauser A YK, Steiner C, Bierman AS.** Hospitalization in the United States, 1997. Rockville, MD: Agency for Healthcare Research and Quality; 2000. HCUP Fact Book No. 1; AHRQ Publication No. 00-0031.
9. **Harris MI.** Medical care for patients with diabetes. Epidemiologic aspects. *Ann Intern Med.* 1996;124:117–122.
10. **Jiang HJ, Stryer D, Friedman B, Andrews R.** Multiple hospitalizations for patients with diabetes. *Diabetes Care.* 2003;26:1421–1426.
11. **Cook CB, Kongable GL, Potter DJ, et al.** Inpatient glucose control: a glycemic survey of 126 U.S. hospitals. *J Hosp Med.* 2009;4:E7–E14.
12. **Levetan CS, Passaro M, Jablonski K, Kass M, Ratner RE.** Unrecognized diabetes among hospitalized patients. *Diabetes Care.* 1998;21:246–249.
13. **Kosiborod M, Inzucchi SE, Spertus JA, et al.** Elevated admission glucose and mortality in elderly patients hospitalized with heart failure. *Circulation.* 2009;119:1899–1907.
14. **Schmeltz LR, DeSantis AJ, Thiyagarajan V, et al.** Reduction of surgical mortality and morbidity in diabetic patients undergoing cardiac surgery with a combined intravenous and subcutaneous insulin glucose management strategy. *Diabetes Care.* 2007;30:823–828.
15. **van den Berghe G, Wouters P, Weekers F, et al.** Intensive insulin therapy in the critically ill patients. *N Engl J Med.* 2001;345:1359–1367.
16. **Umpierrez GE, Hellman R, Korytkowski MT, et al.** Management of hyperglycemia in hospitalized patients in non-critical care setting: an Endocrine Society Clinical Practice Guideline. *J Clin Endocrinol Metab.* 2012;97:16–38.
17. **Moghissi ES, Korytkowski MT, DiNardo M, et al.** American Association of Clinical Endocrinologists and American Diabetes Association consensus statement on inpatient glycemic control. *Diabetes Care.* 2009;32:1119–1131.
18. **Dungan KM, Braithwaite SS, Preiser JC.** Stress hyperglycaemia. *Lancet.* 2009;373:1798–1807.
19. **Greci LS, Kailasam M, Malkani S, et al.** Utility of HbA(1c) levels for diabetes case finding in hospitalized patients with hyperglycemia. *Diabetes Care.* 2003;26:1064–1068.
20. **Garber AJ, Moghissi ES, Bransome ED Jr, et al.** American College of Endocrinology position statement on inpatient diabetes and metabolic control. *Endocr Pract.* 2004;10(suppl 2):4–9.
21. **Saudek CD, Derr RL, Kalyani RR.** Assessing glycemia in diabetes using self-monitoring blood glucose and hemoglobin A1c. *JAMA.* 2006;295:1688–1697.
22. **International Expert Committee.** International Expert Committee report on the role of the A1C assay in the diagnosis of diabetes. *Diabetes Care.* 2009;32:1327–1334.
23. **Desilles JP, Meseguer E, Labreuche J, et al.** Diabetes mellitus, admission glucose, and outcomes after stroke thrombolysis: a registry and systematic review. *Stroke.* 2013;44:1915–1923.
24. **Frisch A, Chandra P, Smiley D, et al.** Prevalence and clinical outcome of hyperglycemia in the perioperative period in noncardiac surgery. *Diabetes Care.* 2010;33:1783–1788.
25. **Farrokhi F, Smiley D, Umpierrez GE.** Glycemic control in non-diabetic critically ill patients. *Best Pract Res Clin Endocrinol Metab.* 2011;25:813–824.
26. **Scherpereel PA, Tavernier B.** Perioperative care of diabetic patients. *Eur J Anaesthesiol.* 2001;18:277–294.
27. **Chan TM.** The permissive effects of glucocorticoid on hepatic gluconeogenesis. Glucagon stimulation of glucose-suppressed gluconeogenesis and inhibition of 6-phosphofructo-1-kinase in hepatocytes from fasted rats. *J Biol Chem.* 1984;259:7426–7432.
28. **McMahon M, Gerich J, Rizza R.** Effects of glucocorticoids on carbohydrate metabolism. *Diabetes Metab Rev.* 1988;4:17–30.
29. **Esposito K, Nappo F, Marfella R, et al.** Inflammatory cytokine concentrations are acutely increased by hyperglycemia in humans: role of oxidative stress. *Circulation.* 2002;106:2067–2072.
30. **Stentz FB, Umpierrez GE, Cuervo R, Kitabchi AE.** Proinflammatory cytokines, markers of cardiovascular risks, oxidative stress, and lipid peroxidation in patients with hyperglycemic crises. *Diabetes.* 2004;53:2079–2086.
31. **Umpierrez GE, Kitabchi AE.** ICU care for patients with diabetes. *Current Opin Endocrinol* 2004;11:75–81.
32. **Lang CH, Dobrescu C, Bagby GJ.** Tumor necrosis factor impairs insulin action on peripheral glucose disposal and hepatic glucose output. *Endocrinology.* 1992;130:43–52.
33. **Fan J, Li YH, Wojnar MM, Lang CH.** Endotoxin-induced alterations in insulin-stimulated phosphorylation of insulin receptor, IRS-1, and MAP kinase in skeletal muscle. *Shock.* 1996;6:164–170.
34. **del Aguila LF, Claffey KP, Kirwan JP.** TNF-alpha impairs insulin signaling and insulin stimulation of glucose uptake in C2C12 muscle cells. *Am J Physiol.* 1999;276:E849–E855.
35. **Robinson LE, van Soeren MH.** Insulin resistance and hyperglycemia in critical illness: role of insulin in glycemic control. *AACN Clin Issues.* 2004;15:45–62.
36. **Montori VM, Bistrian BR, McMahon MM.** Hyperglycemia in acutely ill patients. *JAMA.* 2002;288:2167–2169.
37. **McAlister FA, Majumdar SR, Blitz S, et al.** The relation between hyperglycemia and outcomes in 2,471 patients admitted to the hospital with community-acquired pneumonia. *Diabetes Care.* 2005;28:810–815.
38. **Baker EH, Janaway CH, Philips BJ, et al.** Hyperglycaemia is associated with poor outcomes in patients admitted to hospital with acute exacerbations of chronic obstructive pulmonary disease. *Thorax.* 2006;61:284–289.
39. **Ramos M, Khalpey Z, Lipsitz S, et al.** Relationship of perioperative hyperglycemia and postoperative infections in patients who undergo general and vascular surgery. *Ann Surg.* 2008;248:585–591.

40. **Kwon S, Thompson R, Dellinger P, et al.** Importance of perioperative glycemic control in general surgery: a report from the Surgical Care and Outcomes Assessment Program. *Ann Surg.* 2013;257:8–14.
41. **Murad MH, Coburn JA, Coto-Yglesias F, et al.** Glycemic control in non-critically ill hospitalized patients: a systematic review and meta-analysis. *J Clin Endocrinol Metab.* 2012;97:49–58.
42. **Qaseem A, Chou R, Humphrey L, Shekelle P, for the Clinical Guidelines Committee of the American College of Physicians.** Inpatient Glycemic Control: Best Practice Advice from the Clinical Guidelines Committee of the American College of Physicians [published online May 23, 2013]. *Am J Med Qual.* 2014;29:95–98.
43. **Umpierrez E, Smiley D, Jacobs S, et al.** Randomized study of basal bolus insulin therapy in the inpatient management of patients with type 2 diabetes undergoing general surgery (RABBIT 2 Surgery). *Diabetes Care.* 2013;36(11):3430–3435.
44. **Umpierrez GE, Smiley D, Hermayer K, et al.** Randomized study comparing a basal bolus with a basal plus correction insulin regimen for the hospital management of medical and surgical patients with type 2 diabetes: Basal Plus Trial. *Diabetes Care.* 2013; 36(8):2169–2174.
45. **Clement S, Braithwaite SS, Magee MF, et al.** Management of diabetes and hyperglycemia in hospitals. *Diabetes Care.* 2004;27:553–597.
46. **Levetan CS, Magee MF.** Hospital management of diabetes. *Endocrinol Metab Clin North Am.* 2000;29:745–770.
47. **Terzic A, Jahangir A, Kurachi Y.** Cardiac ATP-sensitive K+ channels: regulation by intracellular nucleotides and K+ channel-opening drugs. *Am J Physiol.* 1995;269:C525–C545.
48. **Tomai F, Crea F, Gaspardone A, et al.** Ischemic preconditioning during coronary angioplasty is prevented by glibenclamide, a selective ATP-sensitive K+ channel blocker. *Circulation.* 1994; 90:700–705.
49. **Horlen C, Malone R, Bryant B, et al.** Frequency of inappropriate metformin prescriptions. *JAMA.* 2002;287:2504–2505.
50. **Calabrese AT, Coley KC, DaPos SV, Swanson D, Rao RH.** Evaluation of prescribing practices: risk of lactic acidosis with metformin therapy. *Arch Intern Med.* 2002;162:434–437.
51. **Pasquel FJ, Klein R, Adigweme A, et al.** Metformin-associated lactic acidosis [published online December 10, 2013]. *Am J Med Sci.*
52. **Delea TE, Edelsberg JS, Hagiwara M, Oster G, Phillips LS.** Use of thiazolidinediones and risk of heart failure in people with type 2 diabetes: a retrospective cohort study: response to Karter et al. *Diabetes Care.* 2004;27:852–853.
53. **Delea TE, Edelsberg JS, Hagiwara M, Oster G, Phillips LS.** Use of thiazolidinediones and risk of heart failure in people with type 2 diabetes: a retrospective cohort study. *Diabetes Care.* 2003;26:2983–2989.
54. **Nesto RW, Bell D, Bonow RO, et al.** Thiazolidinedione use, fluid retention, and congestive heart failure: a consensus statement from the American Heart Association and American Diabetes Association. *Diabetes Care.* 2004;27:256–263.
55. **Umpierrez GE, Gianchandani R, Smiley D, et al.** Safety and efficacy of sitagliptin therapy for the inpatient management of general medicine and surgery patients with type 2 diabetes: a pilot, randomized, controlled study. *Diabetes Care.* 2013;36:3430–3435.
56. **Umpierrez GE, Korytkowski M.** Is incretin-based therapy ready for the care of hospitalized patients with type 2 diabetes? *Diabetes Care.* 2013;36:2112–2117.
57. **Classen DC, Jaser L, Budnitz DS.** Adverse drug events among hospitalized Medicare patients: epidemiology and national estimates from a new approach to surveillance. *Jt Comm J Qual Patient Saf.* 2010;36(1):12–21.
58. **Marik PE, Preiser JC.** Toward understanding tight glycemic control in the ICU: a systematic review and metaanalysis. *Chest.* 2010;137:544–551.
59. **Gill GV, Woodward A, Casson IF, Weston PJ.** Cardiac arrhythmia and nocturnal hypoglycaemia in type 1 diabetes–the 'dead in bed' syndrome revisited. *Diabetologia.* 2009;52:42–45.
60. **Desouza C, Salazar H, Cheong B, Murgo J, Fonseca V.** Association of hypoglycemia and cardiac ischemia: a study based on continuous monitoring. *Diabetes Care.* 2003;26:1485–1489.
61. **Krinsley JS, Egi M, Kiss A, et al.** Diabetic status and the relation of the three domains of glycemic control to mortality in critically ill patients: an international multicenter cohort study. *Crit Care.* 2013; 17:R37.
62. **Sechterberger MK, Bosman RJ, Oudemans-van Straaten HM, et al.** The effect of diabetes mellitus on the association between measures of glycaemic control and intensive care unit mortality: a retrospective cohort study. *Crit Care.* 2013;17:R52.
63. **Jacobi J, Bircher N, Krinsley J, et al.** Guidelines for the use of an insulin infusion for the management of hyperglycemia in critically ill patients. *Crit Care Med.* 2012;40:3251–3276.
64. **Desouza CV, Bolli GB, Fonseca V.** Hypoglycemia, diabetes, and cardiovascular events. *Diabetes Care.* 2010;33:1389–1394.
65. **Razavi Nematollahi L, Kitabchi AE, Stentz FB, et al.** Proinflammatory cytokines in response to insulin-induced hypoglycemic stress in healthy subjects. *Metabolism.* 2009;58:443–448.
66. **Rana OA, Byrne CD, Greaves K.** Intensive glucose control and hypoglycaemia: a new cardiovascular risk factor? [published online May 22, 2013). *Heart.* doi: 10.1136/heartjnl-2013-303871.
67. **Dungan KM, Binkley P, Nagaraja HN, Schuster D, Osei K.** The effect of glycaemic control and glycaemic variability on mortality in patients hospitalized with congestive heart failure. *Diabetes Metab Res Rev.* 2011;27:85–93.
68. **Farrokhi F, Chandra P, Smiley D, et al.** Glucose variability is an independent predictor of mortality in hospitalized patients treated with total parenteral nutrition. *Endocr Pract.* 2014;20:41–45.
69. **Mendez CE, Mok KT, Ata A, et al.** Increased glycemic variability is independently associated with length of stay and mortality in noncritically ill hospitalized patients. *Diabetes Care.* 2013;36: 4091–4097.

CHAPTER 29

Management of Insulin Pumps in Hospitalized Patients

Curtiss B Cook

ABSTRACT

Continuous subcutaneous insulin infusion (CSII) therapy (also known as insulin pump therapy) is employed to treat patients with diabetes mellitus. Although most frequently seen in the outpatient setting, insulin pump technology is now encountered by clinicians in various other clinical scenarios not originally intended for CSII use. This chapter summarizes guidelines for CSII use in the hospital and reviews available published data on their use in the inpatient setting.

INTRODUCTION

Continuous subcutaneous insulin infusion (CSII) therapy (also known as insulin pump therapy) is employed to treat patients with diabetes mellitus. An estimated 400,000 patients in the United States use CSII to manage their hyperglycemia (1). Although most frequently seen in the outpatient setting, insulin pump technology is now encountered by clinicians in various other clinical scenarios not originally intended for use. Consequently, health care professionals are being confronted with how to manage CSII therapy in these situations. One such situation is when the patient on CSII requires hospitalization.

Information on the number of hospitalizations associated with diabetes is available; however, there are no data on hospital discharges among CSII users (2). Nonetheless, many patients on insulin pumps are likely hospitalized for reasons other than their diabetes, and some of these CSII patients are actually doing very well on their technology. On the other hand, the hospital environment limits many of the choices the patients can make regarding their diabetes care and can induce a sense of frustration when the patient has to transfer his diabetes self-management to hospital staff who may be less knowledgeable about diabetes than the patient. Empowering patients to make decisions in areas where they have demonstrated competency could alleviate some of that distress and make them more involved in their care without jeopardizing their outcome.

Inpatient self-management of CSII can be defined as a process whereby patients, in collaboration with the hospital staff and if not contraindicated, are provided a choice to remain on their insulin pump. Some institutions have published guidelines on inpatient CSII self-management (3–6). Recent reports confirm that with proper patient selection, individuals treated with insulin pumps can successfully transition their treatment from the outpatient to the inpatient environment (6–10).

Given the potential safety issues associated with self-management of CSII in the hospital, the lack of familiarity of inpatient practitioners with the technology, and the ensuing angst on the part of hospital staff when such patients are encountered, a process for insulin pump self-management should be clearly described in an institutional policy (11–13). This chapter summarizes guidelines for use of CSII in the hospital and reviews available published data on their use in the inpatient setting.

POTENTIAL INPATIENT SCENARIOS INVOLVING CSII THERAPY

Inpatient practitioners may encounter 4 possible scenarios when someone on an outpatient CSII program is admitted to the hospital. First, the clinical situation may permit ongoing self-management of the CSII program from admission to discharge without interruption in therapy. Second, the patient's status may necessitate early disconnection from the device. The pump may or may not be restarted prior to discharge depending on the clinical course. Third, CSII self-management may continue for a period of time, but may have to be discontinued due to a changing clinical status. Last, the patient may be admitted to the hospital and may not participate with self-management of the CSII program at all throughout his or her hospitalization. This last scenario may either occur because of the patient's clinical status, or because the institution simply does not permit CSII therapy. Regardless of the reasons, if CSII therapy is discontinued for other than a short period of time (eg, for a radiological procedure), then insulin treatment should be substituted with a multiple daily injections (MDI) program or intravenous (IV) continuous insulin infusion (CII) depending on the clinical circumstances. Hospitals that do not allow CSII therapy should have a formal process in place to transfer the patient to MDI or CII as needed.

GENERAL CONSIDERATIONS

CSII users represent only a small subset of patients with diabetes in the hospital. Therefore, it is assumed that institutional guidelines for CSII self-management exist within a larger framework of already established policies and procedures for inpatient diabetes care that also includes recognition and treatment of hypoglycemia, point-of-care glucose testing, and subcutaneous or IV insulin administration. Institutional guidelines and procedures for inpatient insulin pump use should have 3 general components: (1) contraindications for CSII self-management within the hospital; (2) an agreement signed by the patient detailing the conditions for CSII use in the hospital; and (3) procedures to guide the hospital staff in managing the insulin pump after admission. Patients selected for inpatient self-management should already be on a CSII program as outpatients. Patients initially can continue the rates of basal and dose of meal-time insulin in a manner similar to their outpatient practice. However, changes in the pump settings during the hospitalization may be appropriate based on the patient's glycemic status and ongoing clinical situation. Carbohydrate counting can be one method for the meal-time insulin doses. The process involving CSII self-management in the hospital requires ongoing evaluation to ascertain its continued safety and efficacy. The transition to an alternate insulin regimen should take place whenever safety parameters set in place for the patient seem to be at risk of being breached by the patient's CSII management.

CONTRAINDICATIONS TO INPATIENT CSII SELF-MANAGEMENT

The proper selection of patients for this protocol is the critical first step in ensuring its success (Table 29-1). The service managing the patient's diabetes should be the one deciding whether CSII therapy is suitable for that individual. Anything that impairs the patient's ability to self-manage CSII therapy, such as altered sensorium, should prompt a change to an alternative insulin therapy. The author's institution does permit a family member to assist with managing the patient's insulin pump if the patient cannot, contingent upon that person being available to come to the bedside 24 hours a day. Changes in the patient's clinical status that are deemed to be posing a major stress on glycemic control (eg, liver failure, renal failure, frequent hypoglycemic events, or severe hyperglycemia) or otherwise place the patient at risk (eg, suicidal tendencies) should lead to reconsideration of CSII self-management. Hyperglycemia during critical illness or due to diabetic ketoacidosis (DKA)/hyperglycemic hyperosmolar state (HHS) is best managed with CII until the episode is resolved. Discontinuation of therapy is recommended if the patient does

Table 29-1. Suggested Contraindications for CSII Self-Management in the Hospital

Patient with altered state of consciousness
Presence of diabetic ketoacidosis/hyperglycemic hyperosmolar state at admission
Critically ill patient requiring intensive care or other major stresses on glycemic control
Patient at risk for suicide
Inability of the patient to participate in CSII management, or inability of the patient to identify a family member who is knowledgeable and competent with the insulin pump function who can remain at the bedside to assist with pump management
Patient's refusal to agree with conditions of CSII self-management
Other circumstances identified by the physician primarily responsible for the individual's care in the hospital

Abbreviations: CSII = continuous subcutaneous insulin infusion.

Table 29-2. Elements Suggested for Inclusion in Any Hospital-Based CSII Self-Management Patient Agreement Form

Change the infusion set every 48–72 hr or as needed
Provide own nonmedication insulin pump supplies
Show staff basal rates and bolus amounts[a]
Agree to let staff perform point-of-care glucose testing
Report signs of low blood sugar to the staff
Report any pump problems
Understanding that a family member may assist with the operation of the insulin infusion pump on condition that they remain in the hospital during my entire hospital stay
The pump may be discontinued and a different insulin delivery given for any of the following: Doctor's order Changes in judgment Changes in level of awareness or consciousness Any X-ray procedure Other reasons deemed necessary by medical staff

Abbreviations: CSII = continuous subcutaneous insulin infusion.
[a]Recorded on a flow sheet kept at bedside (see reference 7 for sample agreement and flow sheet).

not wish to cooperate with the hospital staff, or otherwise does not meet the requirements as detailed in the patient agreement form.

PATIENT AGREEMENT

To assure safety and optimal medical care during hospital-based CSII management, patients should recognize and acknowledge their responsibility in the process. At the author's institution this is achieved via an agreement that the patient, or a patient representative, reviews and signs. There are some basic elements that should be considered for inclusion in any such agreement (Table 29-2).

The patient should already be accustomed to changing the catheter infusion set every 48 to 72 hours, and this requirement should be no different in the hospital setting. Additionally, it is unlikely that inpatient formularies are going to stock supplies for the various CSII devices on the market, and patients should, therefore, agree to have their own on hand. In some cases, the patient's brand of insulin may not be on the hospital formulary, and the patient will either have to provide his or her own or agree to the hospital substitution. Many patients have point-of-care glucose measurement technology that communicates directly with the pump. Nonetheless, because hospitals have standardized technology that often communicates with their laboratory information system for purposes of tracking and quality control, the patient should still agree to let staff perform measurements. Daily communication with the staff on blood glucose readings, pump parameters, and insulin boluses is essential. The patient (or a proxy) should keep track of basal rates and mealtime boluses. A bedside flow sheet that the patient can complete is a convenient way to track glucose levels, basal rates, and bolus amounts, and allows a quick review whenever staff members visit the patient's bedside. The patient should agree to report any issues with pump function or hypoglycemia to the staff. Finally, the patient should be made aware that there may be circumstances when it is best to terminate CSII self-management and disconnect the pump.

ADMISSION/POSTADMISSION PROCEDURES

A diabetes history should be obtained by the physician and nonphysician hospital staff who are performing the admission, and use of CSII therapy should be documented in the medical record (Figure 29-1). The type of insulin used and the insulin pump parameters (basal rates, bolus amounts, insulin carbohydrate ratios, correction factors) are documented. Contraindications to CSII self-management are assessed, and if none are present, the patient can be offered the option of continuing insulin pump therapy in the hospital. If CSII therapy is contraindicated, then the device should be disconnected and an alternative insulin therapy ordered. For noncritically ill patients a combination of long-acting or intermediate-acting insulin combined with a short- or rapid-acting insulin given with meals is most effective to control hyperglycemia, supplemented by correction doses for high glucose values when needed (14).

If both patient and staff find no contraindications to CSII self-management, the agreement

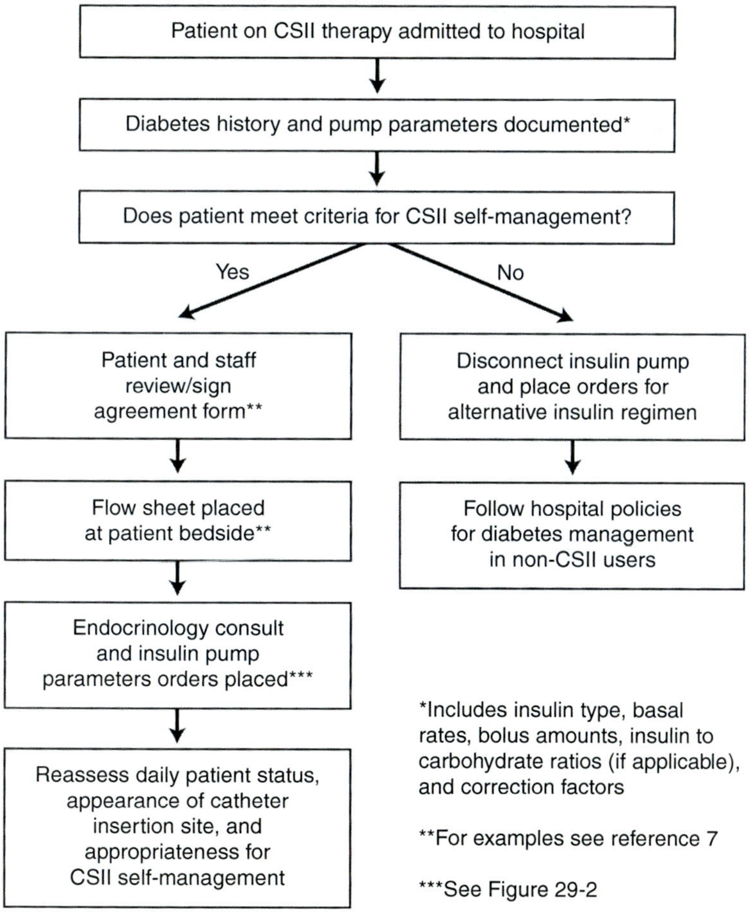

Figure 29-1. Care process model outlining steps to transition a patient on outpatient continuous subcutaneous insulin infusion (CSII) therapy to the hospital. The model assumes that other diabetes care policies (eg, recognition and management of hypoglycemia, point-of-care glucose testing, insulin administration) are already in place.

is reviewed and signed by the patient and countersigned by one of the hospital staff, the flow sheet is placed at the bedside, and the corresponding orders are placed (see Figure 29-2 for an example of a CSII electronic order set). If access to one is available, an endocrinologist should be consulted to provide support to the patient and inpatient staff. Daily assessment and engagement with the patient is needed, including examination of the insulin pump catheter site and the flow sheet, to identify problems and establish any changes in the patient's status that might warrant cessation of CSII self-management.

PRACTICAL EXPERIENCE WITH INPATIENT CSII SELF-MANAGEMENT

Safety data on inpatient CSII use and effectiveness in controlling hyperglycemia are limited, but suggest that in properly selected patients, successful transition from outpatient to inpatient insulin pump therapy is possible. Noschese and colleagues examined glycemic and safety data in 50 consecutive CSII-treated patients admitted to their hospital between 2004 and 2006 (6). Only 2 minor events were noted (1 pump malfunction and 1 catheter infusion site problem). Patient satisfaction with

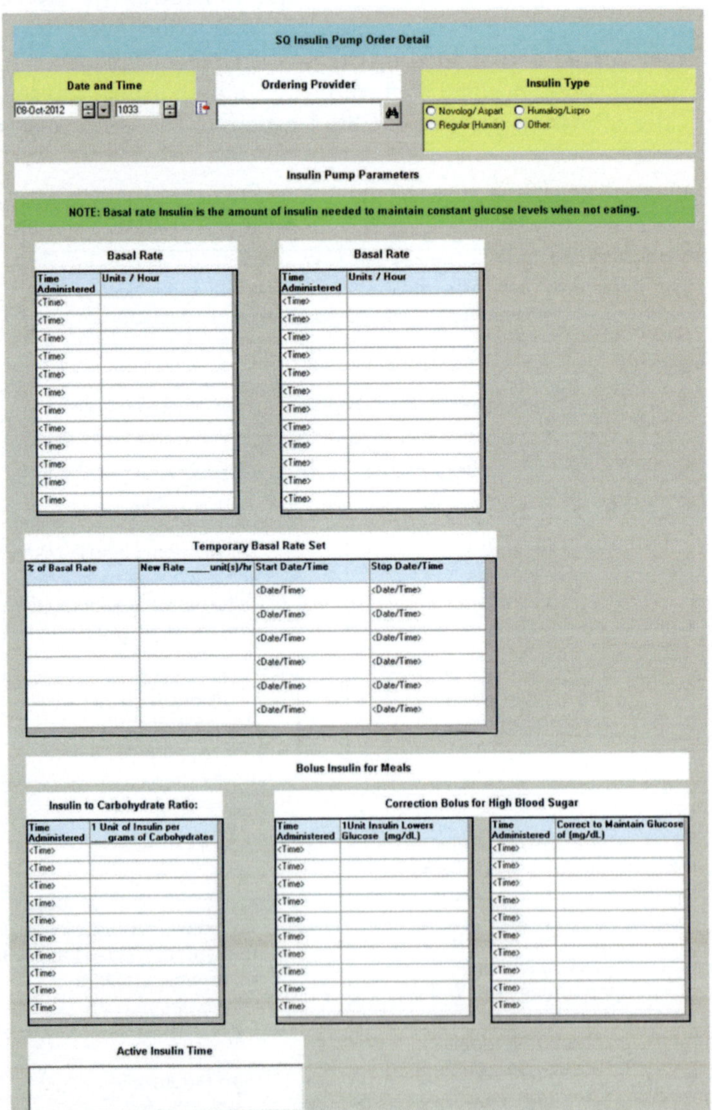
SQ Insulin Pump Order Detail

Date and Time: 08-Oct-2012 1033

Ordering Provider

Insulin Type: Novolog/ Aspart; Humalog/Lispro; Regular (Human); Other

Insulin Pump Parameters

NOTE: Basal rate Insulin is the amount of insulin needed to maintain constant glucose levels when not eating.

Basal Rate

Time Administered	Units / Hour
<Time>	
<Time>	
<Time>	
<Time>	
<Time>	
<Time>	
<Time>	
<Time>	
<Time>	
<Time>	
<Time>	
<Time>	

Basal Rate

Time Administered	Units / Hour
<Time>	
<Time>	
<Time>	
<Time>	
<Time>	
<Time>	
<Time>	
<Time>	
<Time>	
<Time>	
<Time>	
<Time>	

Temporary Basal Rate Set

% of Basal Rate	New Rate ____unit(s)/hr	Start Date/Time	Stop Date/Time
		<Date/Time>	<Date/Time>
		<Date/Time>	<Date/Time>
		<Date/Time>	<Date/Time>
		<Date/Time>	<Date/Time>
		<Date/Time>	<Date/Time>
		<Date/Time>	<Date/Time>

Bolus Insulin for Meals

Insulin to Carbohydrate Ratio:

Time Administered	1 Unit of Insulin per ___ grams of Carbohydrates
<Time>	
<Time>	
<Time>	
<Time>	
<Time>	
<Time>	
<Time>	
<Time>	
<Time>	
<Time>	

Correction Bolus for High Blood Sugar

Time Administered	1Unit Insulin Lowers Glucose (mg/dL)	Time Administered	Correct to Maintain Glucose of (mg/dL)
<Time>		<Time>	
<Time>		<Time>	
<Time>		<Time>	
<Time>		<Time>	
<Time>		<Time>	
<Time>		<Time>	
<Time>		<Time>	
<Time>		<Time>	
<Time>		<Time>	
<Time>		<Time>	

Active Insulin Time

Figure 29-2. Sample format for electronic ordering of inpatient parameters for use of continuous subcutaneous insulin infusion (CSII) therapy. Reproduced with permission from Wilson RD, Bailey M, Boyle ME, et al. *J Diabetes Sci Technol.* 2013;7:1547–1560.

their inpatient pump experience was generally high (6).

In sequential publications with ever increasing sample sizes, the author has been reporting on his institution's experience with transitioning insulin pump users from their outpatient-based therapy to the hospital setting, detailing compliance with required procedures, evaluating glycemic control, and assessing safety among those patients conducting inpatient CSII self-management. The most recent analysis comprising 136 patients totaling 253 hospitalizations between 2006 and 2011 is the largest reported series to date (7–10). By the time of this last assessment, 3 subsets of patients were identified. The "pump on" group (164/253 or 65%) comprised hospitalized patients who met criteria for CSII self-management and continued until discharge. "Pump off" patients (38/253 or 15%) did not meet the conditions for inpatient CSII use and had therapy discontinued at admission and remained off even at the time of discharge. "Intermittent pump" cases (50/253 or 20%) were either those cases whose CSII therapy was continued at admission but then stopped during their hospitalization because of changing clinical circumstances, or patients whose CSII was stopped at admission but then restarted when their clinical status improved and they satisfied institutional criteria for use of the devices. Thus, most cases were able to complete CSII self-management throughout their hospital course (10).

In addition, it was found that compliance with necessary procedures (eg, placing appropriate orders, completion of patient agreement and endocrinology consult) was high. Mean point-of-care glucose was not significantly different between cases who remained on CSII and those for whom it was discontinued ($P > 0.1$), but episodes of severe hyperglycemia (>300 mg/dL [16.7 mmol/L]) and hypoglycemia (<40 mg/dL [2.2 mmol/L]) were significantly less common among individuals who continued to perform CSII self-management. In this entire case series, only 1 adverse event occurred when an infusion catheter kinked, resulting in correctable nonfatal hyperglycemia that was recognized and corrected. No pump site infections, mechanical pump failures, or episodes of DKA were observed among patients remaining on therapy (10).

LIMITATIONS OF GUIDELINES

The guidelines outlined here are geared toward transitioning noncritical adults from outpatient to inpatient CSII use and are not intended for the hospitalized pediatric population or patients in labor and delivery. There has been some interest in the literature about allowing use in the hospitalized pediatric population, but no data on safety of the devices in this population are available (15). Furthermore, these guidelines do not apply to application of CSII therapy to patients not on treatment as outpatients as a means to control inpatient hyperglycemia (16,17). Data are emerging indicating perioperative insulin pump use is also safe (18,19), but this scenario is best addressed through development of a separate care process (20).

CONCLUSIONS

Individuals whose diabetes is managed via CSII may require hospitalization. Although these are low frequency events in comparison to the total number of hospitalizations, they are high visibility when they are admitted. Available data suggest that, in properly selected patients and with appropriate guidelines in place, most patients on outpatient CSII therapy can safely transition treatment to the hospital setting. A key factor in minimizing errors and adverse events in these situations is a collaborative relationship between the patient and hospital staff. In addition, adequate education of all stakeholders regarding insulin pumps is warranted.

ACKNOWLEDGMENTS

The author has nothing to disclose.

REFERENCES

1. **Anonymous.** Research and markets: US insulin delivery devices market: an analysis. *Business Wire.* http://www.businesswire.com/news/home/20110825005874/en/Research-Markets-Insulin-Delivery-Devices-Market-Analysis.
2. **Centers for Disease Control and Prevention.** Hospitalizations for diabetes as any-listed diagnosis. http://www.cdc.gov/diabetes/statistics/dmany/fig1.htm.
3. **Lee SW, Im RM, Magbual R.** Current perspectives on the use of continuous subcutaneous insulin infusion in the acute care setting and overview of therapy. *Crit Care Nurs Q.* 2004;27:172–184.

4. **Cook CB, Boyle ME, Cisar NS, et al.** Use of continuous subcutaneous insulin infusion (insulin pump) therapy in the hospital setting: proposed guidelines and outcome measures. *Diabetes Educator.* 2005;31:849–857.
5. **Dalton MF, Klipfel L, Carmichael K.** Safety issues: use of continuous subcutaneous insulin infusion (CSII) pumps in hospitalized patients. *Hospital Pharmacy.* 2006;41:956–969.
6. **Noschese ML, DiNardo MM, Dohini AC, et al.** Patient outcomes after implementation of a protocol for inpatient insulin pump therapy. *Endocr Pract.* 2009;15:415–424.
7. **Leonhardi BJ, Boyle ME, Beer KA, et al.** Use of continuous subcutaneous insulin infusion (insulin pump) therapy in the hospital setting: A follow-up analysis. *J Diabetes Sci Technol.* 2008;2:948–962.
8. **Bailon RM, Partlow BJ, Miller-Cage V, et al.** Continuous subcutaneous insulin infusion (insulin pump) therapy can be safely used in the hospital in select patients. *Endocr Pract.* 2009;15:24–29.
9. **Nassar AA, Partlow BJ, Boyle ME, Castro JC, Bourgeois PB, Cook CB.** Outpatient to inpatient transition of insulin pump therapy: successes and continuing challenges. *J Diabetes Sci Technol.* 2010;4:863–872.
10. **Cook CB, Beer KA, Seifert KM, Boyle ME, Mackey P, Castro JC.** Transitioning insulin pump therapy from the outpatient to the inpatient setting: a review of 6 years' experience with 253 cases. *J Diabetes Sci Technol.* 2012;6:995–1002.
11. **Cook CB, McNaughton D, Braddy C, et al.** Management of inpatient hyperglycemia: assessing perceptions and barriers to care among resident physicians. *Endocr Pract.* 2007;13:117–125.
12. **Cook CB, Jameson KA, Hartsell ZC, et al.** Beliefs about hospital diabetes and perceived barriers to glucose management among inpatient midlevel practitioners. *Diabetes Educ.* 2008;34:75–83.
13. **Cheekati V, Osburne RC, Jameson KA, Cook CB.** Perceptions of resident physicians about management of inpatient hyperglycemia in an urban hospital. *J Hosp Med.* 2009;4:E1–E8.
14. **Umpierrez GE, Hellman R, Korytkowski MT, et al.** Management of hyperglycemia in hospitalized patients in non-critical care setting: an Endocrine Society Clinical Practice Guideline. *J Clin Endocrinol Metab.* 2012;97:16–38.
15. **Einis SB, Mednis GN, Rogers JE, Walton DA.** A program to train inpatient pediatric nurses in insulin pump use. *Am J Nurs.* 2011;111:51–55.
16. **Lee I-T, Liau Y-J, Lee W-J, Huang C-N, Sheu W H-H.** Continuous subcutaneous insulin infusion providing better glycemic control and quality of life in type 2 diabetic subjects hospitalized for marked hyperglycemia. *J Eval Clin Pract.* 2010;16:202–205.
17. **Bodur HA, Saygil F, Saygil S, Doganay LH, Yesil S.** Continuous infusion of subcutaneous compared to intravenous insulin for tight glycaemic control in medical intensive care unit patients. *Anaesth Intensive Care.* 2008;36:52–527.
18. **Boyle ME, Seifert KM, Beer KA, et al.** Insulin pump therapy in the perioperative period: a review of care after implementation of institutional guidelines. *J Diabetes Sci Technol.* 2012;6:1016–1021.
19. **Corney SM, Dukatz T, Rosenblat S, et al.** Comparison of insulin pump therapy (continuous subcutaneous insulin infusion) to alternative methods for perioperative glycemic management in patients with planned postoperative admissions. *J Diabetes Sci Technol.* 2012;6:1003–1015.
20. **Boyle ME, Seifert KM, Beer KA, et al.** Guidelines for application of continuous subcutaneous insulin infusion (insulin pump) therapy in the perioperative period. *J Diabetes Sci Technol.* 2012;6: 184–190.

CHAPTER 30

Management of U-500 Insulin in Hospitalized Patients

Osama Hamdy, Martin J Abrahamson, and Alissa R Segal

ABSTRACT

U-500 human (regular) insulin is 5 times more concentrated than U-100 insulin. U-500 insulin is used in persons with diabetes who have high insulin requirements. Due to the lack of a specific U-500 insulin syringe, patients will often express their insulin doses using unit measurements on the U-100 insulin or tuberculin (TB) syringes, which often leads to errors in dosing. This brief chapter provides a guide for the safe ordering, storage, dispensing, and administration of U-500 insulin in hospital settings.

INTRODUCTION

U-500 human (regular) insulin became commercially available in 1997. Its use is primarily for obese patients with type 2 diabetes and severe insulin resistance requiring >200 units of insulin daily (1–5). Early studies supported the concept of an inverse relationship between insulin concentration and insulin absorption. In obese patients, U-500 insulin has an onset of action in 30–45 minutes with a lower peak effect compared with U-100 human regular insulin; a peak pharmacodynamic action occurs at 7–8.5 hours, and a duration of action is 11.5 hours (6). Thus, U-500 insulin has both a bolus effect with similar onset and slightly delayed peak effect compared with U-100 human regular insulin and a basal effect with a duration of the "tail" expected to be considerably longer with higher doses than those typically used in practice.

The Food and Drug Administration (FDA) Adverse Event Reporting System (AERS) showed that U-500 insulin administration and dispensing errors were the most common (82% of cases), with hypoglycemia occurring in 36.3% of cases (7). There were few reported cases involving U-500 insulin associated with fatal outcomes. For these reasons, clinicians and patients alike must be diligent with U-500 dose adjustments and frequent self-monitoring of blood glucose (SMBG) to minimize adverse events (8). It is anticipated that this situation will become even more complex with the approval of other concentrated insulin formulations currently in advanced development.

USE OF U-500 INSULIN IN HOSPITALIZED PATIENTS

Patients admitted to the hospital may have been already treated with U-500 insulin or initiated on U-500 insulin during their hospital stay. To avoid errors in U-500 insulin dosing or administration, many hospitals implemented strict policies in dispensing and administering U-500 insulin (9,10). The following is a summary of the inpatient use of U-500 insulin.

1. Ordering
   - Patients who are appropriate for U-500 insulin therapy include those requiring large doses of insulin, defined as ≥200 units/day or ≥2 units/kg, who are

unable to achieve adequate glycemic control, despite individualized management while adhering to a prescribed U-100 insulin regimen.

- U-500 insulin is used in place of intermediate or long-acting insulin and should not be used as sliding scale insulin.
- Dose adjustments should be made for NPO (nil per oral) patients and should be written as separate one-time orders.
- Continuation of an outpatient regimen of U-500 insulin may be done if the following criteria are met:
    - o The patient's specific outpatient regimen (including dose, route, and frequency) is verified prior to ordering (see Table 30-1).
    - o The order includes insulin type, concentration, dose, route, and frequency. The units of insulin must be expressed using the total number of units and not the syringe markings.

2. Pharmacist's verification
    - The hospital pharmacist should verify the specific scheduled outpatient regimen (including dose, route, and frequency) with the patient using the U-500 insulin patient assessment tool (see Table 30-1).
    - Verify with the patient whether he/she uses an insulin U-100 syringe or a tuberculin (TB) syringe to administer U-500 insulin.
    - Ask the patient to demonstrate how he/she uses U-500 insulin.
    - Inform the patient that only a TB syringe will be used to administer the medication during their inpatient stay.
    - Refer to Table 30-2 for information on how to determine U-500 insulin dosing if either TB syringes or U-100 syringes are used.
    - U-500 insulin storage:
        - o U-500 insulin vials should be stored in a bin clearly labeled "High-Risk." The bin should bear

Table 30-1. Regular U-500 Insulin Patient Home Regimen[a]

Patient/care provider verbalized and demonstrated measuring to the marks described for each dose below:

	Patient uses **TUBERCULIN SYRINGE** at home {reports measuring dose in volume (mL)}		Patient uses **U-100 INSULIN SYRINGE** at home {reports unit marking measured on an insulin syringe}
Dose measured using a TB syringe	☐ **Breakfast dose: Take at:** ________ **AM/PM**	**Dose measured using a U-100 insulin syringe**	☐ **Breakfast dose: Take at:** ________ **AM/PM**
	500 X ____ mL =		5 X ____ unit marking on a **U-100 INSULIN SYRINGE** =
	☐ units **U-500 regular insulin**		☐ units **U-500 regular insulin**
	☐ **Lunch dose: Take at:** ________ **AM/PM**		☐ **Lunch dose: Take at:** ________ **AM/PM**
	500 X ____ mL =		5 X ____ unit marking on a **U-100 INSULIN SYRINGE** =
	☐ units **U-500 regular insulin**		☐ units **U-500 regular insulin a**
	☐ **Dinner dose: Take at:** ________ **AM/PM**		☐ **Dinner dose: Take at:** ________ **AM/PM**
	500 X ____ mL =		5 X ____ unit marking on a **U-100 INSULIN SYRINGE** =
	☐ units **U-500 regular insulin**		☐ units **U-500 regular insulin**
	☐ **Bedtime dose: Take at:** ________ **AM/PM**		☐ **Bedtime dose: Take at:** ________ **AM/PM**
	500 X ____ mL =		5 X ____ unit marking on a U-100 INSULIN **SYRINGE** =
	☐ units **U-500 regular insulin**		☐ units **U-500 regular insulin**

Practitioner's name (print): ______________________________

Practitioner's name (signature): ______________________ **Date/time:** ________

[a]*Place in the patient's medical record.*

Table 30-2. Dose Conversion Table for U-500 Insulin Doses Using Syringe Markings

U-500 Insulin Dose (actual units)	U-100 Syringe (units markings)	Tuberculin Syringe (volume in mL)
25	5	0.05
50	10	0.1
75	15	0.15
100	20	0.2
125	25	0.25
150	30	0.3
175	35	0.35
200	40	0.4
225	45	0.45
250	50	0.5
275	55	0.55
300	60	0.6
325	65	0.65
350	70	0.7
375	75	0.75
400	80	0.8
425	85	0.85
450	90	0.9
475	95	0.95
500	100	1
Actual units	Divide by 5	Divide by 500

Dose (actual units)/5 = unit markings on U-100 insulin syringe; dose (actual units)/500 = milliliter markings on a tuberculin syringe.

a "High Risk" warning sticker as well as a laminated notification card labeled "For Sterile Products Area Use Only."
   - o Storage outside the pharmacy is not advised. Multidose vials should not be dispensed to the floor.

3. Preparation and dispensing
   - All U-500 insulin doses should be prepared by the pharmacy in ready-to-administer syringes.
   - All doses should be prepared in a 1-mL TB safety needle syringe only.
   - Prepared syringes should not have any overfill and the syringes should contain the needle.
   - Consistent use of a TB syringe with U-500 insulin is recommended, with total doses expressed in terms of both units and volume (eg, 200 units [0.4 mL]).
   - Each syringe should be given a 24-hour expiration date.
   - Each syringe should be dispensed with a High-Risk medication sticker.
   - To ensure timely availability of U-500 insulin syringes, the pharmacy should deliver the drug to the patient care unit at least 2 hours prior to the scheduled time of administration.
   - The pharmacists should modify due times in the dosing schedule.
4. Administration
   - U-500 insulin is administered 2–4 times per day. Administration needs to be timed with regard to meals and is generally given 30 minutes before meals. Doses are generally divided equally or 40/30/30. May add additional bedtime dose (small amount) to correct fasting hyperglycemia (eg, 30/30/30/10).
   - NPO patients: It is advisable not to hold dose but anticipate dose reductions (a common dose reduction is 50%). Treating clinician must write ×1 order for change in dose. Clinician should notify pharmacy with planned or unplanned NPO status.
   - Prior to administration of the first dose of U-500 regular insulin, a pharmacist-to-nurse communication should occur.
     - o The pharmacist and registered nurse (RN) caring for the patient should review the clinician order, U-500 insulin dose, route, and frequency. Emphasis should be on the U-500 insulin dose conversion and the use of a TB syringe.
   - Prior to each administration of U-500 regular insulin, 2 RNs must perform an independent double-check that is documented.
   - Once components of the ordered medication are verified to be correct, the RN may administer the dose subcutaneously.
   - Nurses should not be permitted to alter the amount of U-500 insulin to be administered in a prepared syringe (eg, a nurse obtained a syringe from pharmacy containing 80 units

of U-500 insulin to be administered and the prescriber gives a verbal order to administer 60 units instead).

- Any changes to a patient's regimen must be reordered by the prescriber, and a new syringe with the appropriate dose must be prepared and dispensed by pharmacy.
- Nurse-to-nurse communication should occur at each shift change.
- Any changes to the scheduled administration times must be communicated to the pharmacist.

5. Discharge instructions
   - The discharge prescriptions should be written in actual dose units and include patient's instructions using UNIT markings (U-100 insulin syringe) or VOLUME markings (TB syringe) as appropriate.

     Example:
     Regular U-500 insulin
     200 units subcutaneously TID
     Patient instructions: Draw to 40-unit marking on a U-100 insulin syringe (or 0.4 mL on a tuberculin syringe), and take 30 minutes before breakfast, lunch, and dinner.
   - A prescription should be written for glucagon.
6. Education
   - Refer to Table 30-3 for information on U-500 insulin.
   - Nursing and pharmacy should coordinate to educate the patient receiving U-500 insulin during the patient's hospital stay and prior to discharge. The following points should be reviewed:
     - Purpose of U-500 insulin
     - Differencesbetweenregular U-500 regular insulin and U-100 regular insulin
     - Discharge dose, route, and frequency of U-500 insulin
     - Clarification of the syringe type used to draw up and administer the U-500 insulin (TB syringe vs U-100 insulin syringe)
     - Appropriate use of U-500 insulin when the patient experiences

Table 30-3. Key Educational Points on U-500 Insulin for Nurses and Pharmacists

Background information	• U-500 insulin use is increasing for the management of patients demonstrating severe insulin resistance. • Patients who are appropriate for U-500 insulin therapy include those requiring large doses of insulin, defined as ≥200 units/day or ≥2 units/kg, who are unable to achieve adequate glycemic control, despite individualized management while adhering to a prescribed U-100 insulin regimen
Safety and patient risk	• U-500 regular insulin is a highly concentrated form of regular insulin **FIVE times more concentrated than traditional U-100 regular insulin**. • U-500 regular insulin is **NOT** interchangeable on a unit-to unit ratio with U-100 regular insulin. • Currently, no U-500 insulin syringes are manufactured. • Patients may report their dose in terms of "units" using a U-100 syringe (which may not accurately indicate the U-500 dose) or in terms of "volume" milliliters/mL using a tuberculin/TB syringe. This creates confusion and a risk for error. The table below illustrates comparisons of some U-500 doses based on the syringe the patient uses.

U-500 Dose (units)	U-100 Syringe Marking (units)	TB Syringe Volume (mL)
25	5	0.05
50	10	0.1
100	20	0.2

Onset, duration, and appropriate use of U-500 insulin	• U-500 insulin's onset of action is 30 minutes, but its duration of action ranges from 6.5 to 10 hr. • U-500 insulin is commonly administered 2 or 3 times daily; may be occasionally prescribed 4 times a day. • Patients using U-500 insulin are not using any other long-acting insulin so missing a dose may risk severe hyperglycemia. • U-500 insulin is not used for sliding scale/correction doses. • U-500 insulin is only administered by subcutaneous route (IV, IM routes are **NOT** permitted).

illness or anticipated prolonged periods without eating
  - o Risks of hypoglycemia and how to treat
  - o Storage of U-500 insulin
  - o Use of glucagon for hypoglycemic events.

HYPOGLYCEMIA

- Hypoglycemia when using U-500 insulin can be prolonged and severe. Teach patients the signs and symptoms of hypoglycemia and the importance of testing their blood glucose. Hypoglycemia can occur suddenly and symptoms include sweating, dizziness, tremors, hunger, slurred speech, anxiety, and headache.
- Deep secondary hypoglycemia reactions may develop 18–24 hours after the original injection. Consequently, patients should be carefully observed, and prompt treatment of recurrent reactions should be initiated with 15–30 g of carbohydrates orally (eg, as 4–8 oz of fruit juice, 6–12 oz of regular soft drink, or 3 to 6 glucose tablets) if the patient is sufficiently alert; otherwise, intramuscular glucagon injection or intravenous glucose should be administered.
- Patients on insulin therapy should keep an in-date glucagon emergency kit in case of severe hypoglycemia episodes. Before treating a patient, the signs and symptoms of severe hypoglycemia should be confirmed by a blood glucose meter if safe to do so (expected SMBG concentration of <70 mg/dL [3.9 mmol/L]). Family members or other individuals close to the patient should be instructed on the appropriate use of glucagon.

OTHER SAFETY ISSUES

- Remind patients that switching to U-500 insulin will only manage hyperglycemia; underlying reasons leading to obesity and insulin resistance must still be assessed and addressed appropriately with lifestyle changes—caloric reduction and exercise program or be referred for bariatric surgery.
- It is important for patients with diabetes to carry medical alert identification.
- The best places to give insulin are the abdomen, upper arms, and thighs. It is important to remember to rotate the injections between these injection sites.

COST CONSIDERATIONS

U-500 insulin is supplied in a 20-mL vial (containing 10,000 units) and has a considerably higher cost per vial compared with U-100 insulins (10-mL vials, 1,000 units). However, given the concentrated nature of this insulin, the cost on a per-unit basis is substantially less than other currently available insulin products on the market. Improving glycemic control over time, potentially reducing long-term diabetes complications in this population of difficult-to-manage patients, may lead to the greatest cost savings of U-500 insulin use, though this has not been studied in prospective, randomized clinical trials.

ACKNOWLEDGMENTS

The author has nothing to disclose.

REFERENCES

1. **Ballani P, Tran MT, Navar MD, et al.** Clinical experience with U-500 regular insulin in obese, markedly insulin-resistant type 2 diabetic patients. *Diabetes Care.* 2006;29:2504–2505.
2. **Cochran E, Musso C, Gorden P.** The use of U-500 in patients with extreme insulin resistance. *Diabetes Care.* 2005;28:1240–1244.
3. **Larsen J, Goldner W.** Approach to the hospitalized patient with severe insulin resistance. *J Clin Endocrinol Metab.* 2011;96:2652–2662.
4. **Garg R, Johnston V, McNally PG, et al.** U-500 insulin: why, when, and how to use in clinical practice. *Diabetes Metab Res Rev.* 2007;23:265–268.
5. **Reutrakul S, Wroblewski K, Brown RL.** Clinical use of U-500 regular insulin: review and meta-analysis. *J Diabetes Sci Technol.* 2012;6:412–420.
6. **de la Peña A, Riddle M, Morrow LA, et al.** Pharmacokinetics and pharmacodynamics of high-dose human regular U-500 insulin versus human regular U-100 insulin in healthy obese subjects. *Diabetes Care.* 2011;34:2496–2501.
7. **Food and Drug Administration.** Potential signals of serious risks/new safety information identified from the Adverse Event Reporting System (AERS) between January–March 2008. www.fda.gov/Drugs/Guidance

ComplianceRegulatoryInformation/Surveillance/AdverseDrug Effects/ucm085914.htm.

8. **Segal AR, Brunner JE, Burch FT, Jackson JA.** Use of concentrated insulin human regular (U-500) for patients with diabetes. *Am J Health Syst Pharm.* 2010;67:1526–1535.
9. **Hellman R.** A systems approach to reducing errors in insulin therapy in the inpatient setting. *Endocr Pract.* 2004;10(suppl 2):100–108.
10. **Cohen MR, Smetzer JL.** ISMP medication error report analysis: insulin concentrate U-500. *Hosp Pharm.* 2007;42:887.

CHAPTER 31

Emergent Perioperative Hyperglycemia Management

Ketan Dhatariya and Glenn Matfin

ABSTRACT

Persons with diabetes require surgical procedures at a higher rate and have longer hospital stays than those without diabetes. Approximately 5% of persons with diabetes will require emergency surgery over their lifetime. The actual perioperative glycemic treatment recommendations for a given patient should be individualized based on factors such as current glycemic control, type of diabetes, nature and extent of surgical procedure, and antecedent diabetes therapy. The management goal is to optimize metabolic control through close monitoring, adequate fluid and caloric repletion, and judicious use of insulin.

INTRODUCTION

Persons with diabetes require surgical procedures at a higher rate and have longer hospital stays than those without diabetes (1). In particular, diabetes patients admitted for general and orthopedic surgery have some of the longest overall lengths of hospital stay (2). The presence of diabetes and/or hyperglycemia in surgical patients also leads to increased morbidity and mortality, with perioperative mortality rates up to 50% higher than the nondiabetes population (3). The reasons for these adverse outcomes are multifactorial but include failure to identify patients with diabetes and/or hyperglycemia (4); multiple comorbidities, including microvascular and macrovascular complications (5–8); complex polypharmacy and insulin prescribing errors (9); increased perioperative and postoperative infections (3); associated hypoglycemia and hyperglycemia (3); a lack of or inadequate institutional guidelines for management of inpatient diabetes and/or hyperglycemia (3,10); and inadequate knowledge of diabetes and hyperglycemia management among staff delivering care (4).

Several studies have shown that high preoperative and perioperative glucose and glycosylated hemoglobin (HbA1c) levels lead to poor surgical outcomes. These findings occur in both elective and emergency surgery and include various types of surgery, including spinal, vascular, colorectal, cardiac, trauma-related, mastectomy, foot and ankle, neurosurgery, and hepatobiliary surgery. Adverse outcomes related to increased morbidity and mortality include increased wound infection rates, urinary tract infections, admission to and time in intensive care and development of acute kidney injury or acute coronary syndromes. However, there are data to show that the outcomes of persons with diabetes may not be different—or may indeed be better—than those without diabetes if the diagnosis is known prior to surgery (11,12). The reasons for this are unknown, and may be due to increased vigilance surrounding glucose control given to those with a diagnosis of diabetes.

In view of these findings, elective surgery with acceptable glycemic control (eg, HbA1c <8.5% and ambient glycemic levels within acceptable range) and no evidence of diabetes-related acute decompensation (eg, diabetic ketoacidosis [DKA], hyperglycemic hyperosmolar state [HHS], or electrolyte disturbance) would be the preferred option for diabetes patients requiring surgery (13). However, approximately 5% of persons with diabetes will require emergency surgery over their lifetime (14). Emergency surgery is performed on patients who have an acute condition that threatens life, limb, or the integrity of a body structure. Some emergency operations are time critical and need to be performed immediately (day or night). Emergency surgical care comprises 40%–50% of the workload of most surgical specialties, and can result in additional complications, higher mortality (25%), increased costs, and disruption to elective surgery planning and implementation. By definition, the timing of these emergencies cannot be predicted, and appropriate surgical care must not be unduly delayed. Nonetheless, particular care must be taken in persons with diabetes who are being considered for emergency surgery to exclude DKA and other conditions (eg, vomiting related to undiagnosed or poorly controlled gastroparesis or glucagon-like peptide-1 [GLP-1] agonist adverse effect) that may be mistaken for surgical emergencies. Many patients with DKA and prominent abdominal symptoms have undergone needless surgical exploration for a nonexistent acute abdominal emergency (14).

APPROACHES TO MANAGEMENT

The actual perioperative glycemic treatment recommendations for a given patient should be individualized based on factors such as current glycemic control, type of diabetes, nature and extent of surgical procedure, and antecedent diabetes therapy (15,16). Unfortunately, many patients who require emergency surgery will have suboptimal glycemic control. However, this is not necessarily a contraindication to the timely performance of potentially life-saving surgery. An intravenous (IV) access should be secured, and immediate blood specimens should be sent for glucose, electrolyte, and acid-base assessment. Gross derangements of volume and electrolytes (eg, hypokalemia, hypernatremia) should be corrected. Surgery should be delayed, whenever feasible, in patients with DKA, so that the underlying acid-base disorder can be corrected or, at least, ameliorated. Patients with HHS are markedly dehydrated and should be restored to good volume and improved metabolic status before surgery. For those having emergency surgery, aiming for a pragmatic blood glucose of between 110 and 180 mg/dL (6–10 mmol/L) should be the target. Blood glucose should be monitored at least hourly during the procedure and in the immediate postoperative period using an appropriate point-of-care measure to allow early detection of any alterations in metabolic control. On January 1, 2014, the US Centers for Medicare & Medicaid Services (CMS) introduced a surgical care improvement project (SCIP) quality measure for cardiovascular surgery patients (eg, coronary artery bypass grafting [CABG]), including those undergoing emergency surgery. This quality measure is designed to identify patients with controlled postoperative glucose levels ≤180 mg/dL (10 mmol/L) in the specified time frame (18 and 24 hours after anesthesia end-time). The intention is to trigger earlier insulin therapy (eg, when glucose >160 mg/dL [8.9 mmol/L]) in order to prevent the occurrence of hyperglycemia (ie, >180 mg/dL [10 mmol/L]) or initiate corrective insulin therapy if this level is exceeded to reduce the well-recognized postoperative glucose-related complications in these patients (eg, deep sternal wound infections). All patients receiving insulin before admission require insulin during the perioperative period (17). In the emergency setting, this is best achieved with an IV continuous insulin infusion (CII, also known as variable rate intravenous insulin infusion [VRIII]) using an effective and safe protocol (16). Other patients not previously on insulin therapy should be reviewed on an individualized basis to determine appropriate therapy. Patients not expected to miss more than 1 meal (ie, short starvation period) might be candidates for alternative glucose-lowering therapies without the need for CII (VRIII) (13). In comparison, patients expected to miss more than 1 meal should generally have a CII (VRIII). However, if blood glucose concentration rises above 180 mg/dL (10 mmol/L), a CII

(VRIII) should be commenced and continued until the patient is eating and drinking. CII (VRIII) is often poorly managed in the perioperative setting and thus requires explicit guidelines, including how to transition from IV to subcutaneous insulin or noninsulin therapies. Other important factors include optimizing and maintaining volume status, electrolyte balance, avoidance of pressure damage to the feet during surgery, and prevention and optimal treatment of hypoglycemia. Early involvement of the critical care and diabetes specialist teams is recommended in the management of any high-risk surgical patient with diabetes and/or hyperglycemia.

CONCLUSIONS

A wealth of evidence shows that poor preoperative, perioperative, and postoperative glycemic control is associated with poor surgical outcomes. Despite the lack of robust data to confirm this, most clinicians agree that controlling glucose levels to an acceptable range is likely to reduce the risk of developing complications. The management goal is to optimize metabolic control through close monitoring, adequate fluid and caloric repletion, and judicious use of insulin.The management of perioperative glucose control in the emergency setting usually requires the use of a CII (VRIII). However, any opportunities that arise to optimize glycemic control preoperatively (especially to allow stabilization of patients with diabetes-related crises) should be taken.

ACKNOWLEDGMENTS

KD is on the steering committee of the Joint British Diabetes Societies Inpatient Care Group and has been on the writing groups for several of the guidelines they have produced. His travel to these meetings was paid for by Diabetes UK. He has also been invited to speak at various local, regional, and national meetings in the United Kingdom. Travel to these meetings has been paid for by the organizers.

REFERENCES

1. **Daultrey H, Gooday C, Dhatariya K.** Increased length of inpatient stay and poor clinical coding: audit of patients with diabetes. *J R Soc Med Sh Rep.* 2011;2:83.
2. **Sampson MJ, Dozio N, Ferguson B, Dhatariya K.** Total and excess bed occupancy by age, speciality and insulin use for nearly one million diabetes patients discharged from all English Acute Hospitals. *Diabetes Res Clin Pract.* 2007;77:92–98.
3. **Frisch A, Chandra P, Smiley D, et al.** Prevalence and clinical outcome of hyperglycemia in the perioperative period in noncardiac surgery. *Diabetes Care.* 2010;33:1783–1788.
4. **Rayman G.** Inpatient audit. Diabetes Update. http://www.diabetes.org.uk/upload/Professionals/publications/Comment_Inpatient%20audit_new.pdf.
5. **Cullinane M, Gray AJ, Hargraves CM, Lansdown M, Martin IC, Schubert M.** Who Operates When? II. The 2003 report of the national confidential enquiry into perioperative deaths. http://www.ncepod.org.uk/pdf/2003/03full.pdf.
6. **O'Brien MM, Gonzales R, Shroyer AL, et al.** Modest serum creatinine elevation affects adverse outcome after general surgery. *Kidney Int.* 2010;62:585–592.
7. **Lee TH, Marcantonia ER, Mangione EJ, et al.** Derivation and prospective validation of a simple index for prediction of cardiac risk of major noncardiac surgery. *Circulation.* 1999;100:1043–1049.
8. **Gordois A, Scuffham P, Shearer A, Oglesby A, Tobian JA.** The health care costs of diabetic peripheral neuropathy in the U.S. *Diabetes Care,* 2003;26: 1790–1795.
9. **National Patient Safety Agency.** Insulin safety. Reducing harm associated with the unsafe use of insulin products. http://patientsafety.health.org.uk/sites/default/files/resources/tackling_insulin_safety.pdf.
10. **Sampson MJ, Brennan C, Dhatariya K, Jones C, Walden E.** A national survey of in-patient diabetes services in the United Kingdom. *Diabetic Med.* 2007;24:643–649.
11. **Kwon S, Thompson R, Dellinger P, Yanez D, Farrohki E, Flum D.** Importance of perioperative glycemic control in general surgery: A report from the surgical care and outcomes assessment program. *Ann Surg.* 2013;257:8–14.
12. **Fortington LV, Geertzen JH, van Netten JJ, Postema K, Rommers GM, Dijkstra PU.** Short and long term mortality rates after a lower limb amputation. *Eur J Vasc Endovasc Surg.* 2013;46:124–131.
13. **Dhatariya K, Levy K, Kilvert A, et al for the Joint British Diabetes Societies.** Diabetes UK Position Statements and Care Recommendations. NHS Diabetes guideline for the perioperative management of the adult patient with diabetes. *Diabetic Medicine.* 2012; 29:420–433.
14. **Dagogo-Jack S, Alberti K.** Management of diabetes mellitus in surgical patients. *Diabetes Spectr.* 2002;15:44–48.
15. **Umpierrez GE, Hellman R, Korytkowski MT, et al.** Management of hyperglycemia in hospitalized patients in non-critical care setting: an Endocrine Society Clinical Practice Guideline. *J Clin Endocrinol Metab.* 2012;97:16–38.
16. **Standards of medical care in diabetes—2014.** *Diabetes Care.* 2014;37 (suppl 1):S14–S80.
17. **Dobri GA, Lansong MC.** How should we manage insulin therapy before surgery? *Cleve Clin.* 2013;80:702–704.

CHAPTER 32

Management of Hyperglycemia Related to Parenteral and Enteral Nutrition

M Molly McMahon and John M Miles

ABSTRACT

Hyperglycemia is a frequent occurrence in adult hospitalized patients who receive nutrition support. Both hyperglycemia and hypoglycemia are associated with adverse outcomes in persons with diabetes as well as those without diabetes. This chapter reviews indications for initiating nutrition support, estimation of daily caloric needs (and avoidance of overfeeding), proposed glucose goal ranges, nutrition program design, and unique glucose control strategies during nutrition support.

INTRODUCTION

Hyperglycemia is a frequent occurrence in adult hospitalized patients who receive nutrition support (1). Both hyperglycemia and hypoglycemia (the latter resulting from attempts to correct hyperglycemia) are associated with adverse outcomes in persons with diabetes as well as those without diabetes. No clinical trials have been specifically designed to determine the effect of different blood glucose targets on clinical outcomes in adult hospitalized patients receiving nutrition support. This chapter reviews indications for initiating nutrition support, estimation of daily caloric needs (and avoidance of overfeeding), proposed glucose goal ranges, nutrition program design, and unique glucose control strategies during nutrition support.

INDICATIONS FOR NUTRITION SUPPORT

In general, the nutrition assessment, indications for nutrition support, and estimate of nutrition requirements for critically ill patients with hyperglycemia are similar to those of nondiabetic patients. The need for nutrition support in malnutrition is a reflection of the timing and extent of recent (previous 3 to 6 months) unintentional weight loss, the degree of depletion of energy stores (in turn dependent on baseline energy stores or body mass index [BMI]), the presence or absence of clinical markers of stress, and the anticipated time that the patient will be unable to safely meet nutritional requirements orally (2). There is no gold standard for assessing nutrition status, and the accuracy of nutrition assessment methods as a true marker of nutrition status has never been validated. Studies that have demonstrated a beneficial influence of nutrition support on clinical outcome have provided nutrition for a minimum of 1 week. Because there is no evidence that shorter duration nutrition support provides benefit, Society of Critical Care Medicine (SCCM) and American Society for Parenteral and Enteral Nutrition (ASPEN) joint guidelines state that parenteral nutrition (PN) should not be given unless the anticipated need is for ≥7 days (3). Enteral nutrition, rather than

PN, should be used in patients with a functioning gastrointestinal tract.

ESTIMATION OF DAILY CALORIC NEEDS: AVOIDANCE OF OVERFEEDING

Common causes of hyperglycemia in hospitalized patients include overfeeding, infection, and medications. Dextrose content and calories from all sources (nutrition, dextrose-containing crystalloid, medications, and dialysis) should be considered when developing nutrition programs. Intravenous (IV) fluids may contain dextrose, IV medications may be compounded with dextrose-containing solutions, and some medications provide calories in other forms. For instance, propofol is an anesthetic agent that is formulated in a 10% fat emulsion, and its administration may necessitate a decrease or complete elimination of IV fat from a parenteral nutrition regimen. In addition, both peritoneal dialysis (dextrose) and renal replacement therapy (dextrose plus citrate) can be a source of significant additional calories.

Therefore, avoidance of overfeeding is a goal when providing nutrition to this group of patients. The daily caloric requirement of patients can be estimated by using a predictive formula such as the Harris–Benedict equation or Mifflin-St. Jeor equation, or be measured by indirect calorimetry. The premise that sick hospitalized patients have elevated energy requirements, especially when stressed by surgery, trauma, or sepsis, is no longer supported. Substantial variability in energy expenditure among studies in patients with comparable severity of illness has been reported and may be due to errors in indirect calorimetry measurement. A review of the literature has shown that the majority of hospitalized patients have surprisingly normal energy expenditure, in the range of 100%–120% of estimated basal energy expenditure (Harris–Benedict equation) (4).

GLUCOSE GOALS DURING NUTRITION SUPPORT

Most national societies (American Association of Clinical Endocrinologists [AACE], the American Diabetes Association [ADA] [5], and the Endocrine Society [6]) recommend that the target blood glucose concentration in the critically ill adult should be 140–180 mg/dL (7.8–10 mmol/L). No randomized controlled trials have been conducted in non-ICU patients. No clinical trials have been specifically designed to determine the effect of different blood glucose targets on clinical outcomes in adult hospitalized patients receiving nutrition support. We endorse the glucose goal of 140–180 mg/dL (7.8–10 mmol/L), as discussed in the ASPEN Clinical Guideline (7).

Program Design Principles and Strategies for Achieving Glucose Control (Table 32-1)

During parenteral nutrition. It is our practice to provide calories equal to 100%–120% of estimated basal energy expenditure (Harris–Benedict equation) to patients with a normal BMI. Permissive underfeeding is recommended for patients who are overweight or obese, especially in those with hyperglycemia or hypertriglyceridemia. We recommend 1.0 to 1.5 grams of protein per kilogram body weight (~20%–25% of total calories), providing protein at the higher end of the spectrum for more stressed patients (Table 32-2). Intravenous fat is administered as 20% to 30% of the total daily caloric content. After determining the amount of protein and fat, the patient's remaining daily caloric needs are provided as carbohydrate. Although approximately two thirds of American adults are obese or overweight, data about how to feed obese patients are limited. We and others advocate permissive hypocaloric feeding (eg, 75% of actual basal energy requirements), whereas still others base

Table 32-1. Principles for Nutrition Support Program Design

Determine indication for nutrition support.
Choose route: enteral or parenteral nutrition.
Design program: estimate calorie, protein, lipid (if PN), and carbohydrate needs (if PN).
Determine volume of program.
If enteral nutrition is selected, determine gastric feeding or small bowel feeding: - Gastric feeding can be provided by intermittent (gravity) administration. - Jejunal feeding should be provided by continuous (12–24-hr) feeding.

Table 32-2. Guidelines for the Estimation of Daily Caloric, Protein, and Fat Requirements in Hospitalized Adult Patients

Calories[a]	Basal calories to HB plus 20%, using the Harris–Benedict (HB) equation
Protein[b]	1.0 to 1.5 g/kg of body weight
Fat	20% to 30% of total calories

1. Harris–Benedict equation:

   Men: 66.5 + (13.8 × wt, kg) + (5.0 × ht, cm) – (6.8 × age, yr)

   Women: 655 + (9.6 × wt, kg) + (1.8 × ht, cm) – (4.7 × age, yr)

2. Indirect calorimetric measurement of daily caloric needs may be useful in the following groups of patients: severely stressed patients (eg, closed head injury, multiple trauma, severe burn), nutritionally supported patients in whom weaning from mechanical ventilation is difficult, or in patients requiring home parenteral nutrition.

[a] *If patient has BMI ≥25 and <30, provide basal HB calories; if patient has BMI ≥30, provide 75% HB using the obese weight.*
[b] *The guidelines for protein assume normal hepatic and renal function.*

calories on an adjusted body weight. Higher amounts of protein (up to 25%–30% of estimated basal energy needs) should be used with hypocaloric feeding in order to avoid worsening nitrogen balance.

Glucose management issues unique to PN for patient with diabetes mellitus or hyperglycemia.

- A glucose level should be measured before initiation of PN. We avoid overfeeding and limit PN dextrose to 150 to 200 grams on the first day of nutrition support.
- We recommend measuring glucose levels in all patients the first and second morning following initiation of PN. The frequency of subsequent monitoring should be individualized. For patients with established diabetes or significant hyperglycemia, we initially measure glucose levels 2 to 4 times per day until glucose values are stable. Subsequently, glucose levels are checked twice daily.
- The majority of diabetic patients require insulin coverage when dextrose is infused. For patients previously treated with insulin or oral diabetic agents or patients with 2 consecutive glucose values greater than 150 mg/dL (8.3 mmol/L), generally we initially add 0.1 units of short-acting (regular) insulin per gram of dextrose (eg, 20 units/liter of D 20% [200 g/L]). In our experience, this ratio of insulin to dextrose is unlikely to cause hypoglycemia and thus minimizes the need to waste a bag of PN. If the patient has significant renal disease, we initially add 0.05 units per gram. This approach automatically implies a proportional change in PN insulin when PN dextrose content is increased or decreased.
- If PN is discontinued, it is important to remember that the PN insulin also will be stopped. The advantage of this approach is that the infusion of dextrose and insulin are linked; if the infusion is interrupted for any reason, the administration of insulin is also stopped.
- If needed, supplemental subcutaneous (SC) short-acting insulin or IV insulin infusion is administered according to an algorithm (discussed in earlier chapters).
- If over a 24-hour period glucose values consistently exceed the desired goal range, we increase the PN insulin each day by 0.05 units of short-acting insulin per gram of dextrose to a maximum of 0.2 units of insulin per gram of dextrose.
- At this point, reassessment of caloric provision is indicated. Permissive underfeeding should be considered.
- PN dextrose content should not be increased until the glucose values of the previous 24-hour period are in the goal range.
- If the patient develops hypoglycemia, refer to Table 32-3. The ADA and Endocrine Society Workgroup on Hypoglycemia (8) and the AACE and ADA

Table 32-3. Treatment of Hypoglycemia in Hospitalized Adult Patients Receiving Insulin or Oral Antidiabetic Agents

This protocol applies to the following situations:

- Symptoms of hypoglycemia present (eg, shaking, sweating, hunger, weakness, anxiousness, confusion, slurred speech, lack of coordination).
- Glucose less than 60 mg/dL (3.3 mmol/L), regardless of whether the patient is symptomatic.
- In areas where nurses perform glucose point-of-care (POC) testing, obtain POC prior to starting treatment for hypoglycemia.
- In areas where nurses do not perform glucose POC testing, treat hypoglycemia without waiting to check glucose level.

Treatment

If patient is able to swallow safely and has a functioning gastrointestinal tract, provide oral administration of carbohydrate in 1 of the following forms: For patients on alpha-glucosidase inhibitors (ie, acarbose or miglitol), oral glucose (eg, glucose oral gel) must be used.

- 4 ounces (1/2 cup) of fruit juice. Do not use orange juice if patient has renal failure.
- 5 sugar packets dissolved in 4 ounces (1/2 cup) of water.
- Glucose tablets 16 grams (4 tablets, 4 grams each).
- Glucose oral gel (eg, Glutose 15) 15 grams (1 tube).

If the patient has a functioning feeding tube, administer 1 of the following via the feeding tube:

- 4 ounces (1/2 cup) of fruit juice (not orange juice or other juice with pulp).
- 5 sugar packets dissolved in 4 ounces (1/2 cup) of water.

If the patient is not able to take oral feeding safely, does not have a functioning gastrointestinal tract or feeding tube, is NPO (nil per oral), or does not respond to 2 consecutive oral or feeding tube glucose treatments for hypoglycemia:

- If IV access is available, administer D50W 25 mL (12.5 grams) IV.
- If no IV access is present, administer glucagon 1 mg subcutaneously. Glucagon may only be given once.

Following treatment with glucagon a source of glucose should be started to maintain blood glucose level (eg, patient should eat oral carbohydrates if allowed or prescriber should be contacted to consider starting fluids containing dextrose).

Monitoring

- Obtain a glucose point-of-care test 15 minutes after initial treatment in areas that perform POC testing.
- Repeat treatment and glucose point-of-care tests at 15-minute intervals until the glucose is greater than 80 mg/dL (4.4 mmol/L) for nonpregnant patients or greater than 60 mg/dL (3.3 mmol/L) for pregnant patients.

Consensus Statement on Inpatient Glycemic Control define hypoglycemia as any blood glucose <70 mg/dL (<3.9 mmol/L) (5). Ideally, because of imprecision of point-of-care (POC) glucose measurements, hypoglycemia should be confirmed with a laboratory-based analytical method.

- A substantial (~50%) reduction of insulin in the subsequent PN admixture is generally indicated, unless concurrent subcutaneous insulin administration contributed to the episode of hypoglycemia. This approach should decrease the incidence of subsequent hypoglycemia.
- The incidence of symptomatic hypoglycemia after sudden discontinuation of continuous PN is uncommon if satisfactory glucose control has been achieved (ie, glucose levels <160 mg/dL [8.9 mmol/L]).

Lipid management issues unique to PN. A number of studies suggest that administration of IV fat emulsions (IVFEs) is responsible for the increased infection rates commonly observed with PN use, and some suggest this occurs because of impairment of immune function (9). It is not known whether hypertriglyceridemia, a common occurrence in PN-fed patients and exacerbated by administration of IVFEs, is a factor in impaired immune function. Nonetheless, it is our practice to check a triglyceride level 1 to 2 days postinitiation of an IVFE. If triglyceride values are >300 mg/dL (3.4 mmol/L), the IVFE dose should be reduced or stopped and a hypocaloric regimen should usually be employed, because isocaloric fat-free feeding can lead to worsening of hypertriglyceridemia.

During enteral nutrition. Calorie and protein goals are the same as outlined previously. The availability of enteral formulas with lower carbohydrate and higher monounsaturated fat content (compared to standard formulas commonly used in clinical settings), and with or without added fiber, has prompted studies examining the effects of these formulas on glycemic control. Most trials are short-term or single-meal studies, use oral nutrition supplements, or were conducted in long-term care facilities or rehabilitation or other outpatient settings, limiting their application to hospitalized patients requiring enteral nutrition. The trials that evaluated disease-specific formulas in patients requiring long-term nutrition support used glycemic or lipid control as their primary outcomes, as they were not sufficiently powered to detect differences in morbidity and/or mortality (10,11). The impact on glycemic and lipid control was inconclusive. We do not recommend routine use of these formulas, but instead advise careful avoidance of overfeeding.

Diabetes mellitus can affect the entire gastrointestinal tract. Significant diabetic gastroparesis is often present in patients with longstanding type 1 diabetes. The diagnosis should be suspected from the patient's history, and requires exclusion of other factors capable of slowing gut motility. Demonstration of delayed gastric emptying establishes the diagnosis of gastroparesis. Accurate diagnosis of diabetic gastroparesis is important, because it avoids erroneous attribution of gastrointestinal symptoms to tube feeding or to other factors capable of slowing gut motility. Most patients with diabetic gastroparesis intolerant of gastric feedings are able to tolerate iso-osmolar jejunal tube feedings when initiated at a low rate and advanced slowly. Parenteral nutrition should be used only if patients fail a reasonable trial of tube feeding.

Glucose management unique to enteral nutrition for patient with diabetes mellitus or hyperglycemia.

- Tube feeding can be administered into the stomach or the small bowel. Tube feeding in the stomach can be continuous or intermittent. Often, continuous feeding is used in critically ill patients, and intermittent (gravity) feeding is used in medically stable patients. By contrast, jejunal feeding should always be continuous (nocturnal or 24-hr infusion). The format of the feeding regimen has a major impact on the design of insulin management programs.
- Glucose goals prior to intermittent (gravity) or continuous (12–24-hr) tube feedings are similar to those described earlier.
- Increases in the tube feeding infusion rate should be avoided until adequate glucose control has been achieved by appropriate insulin management.
- For patients with hyperglycemia without prior diagnosis of diabetes and no prior use of insulin or oral diabetic agents, initially we recommend treatment with short-acting insulin until tube feeding is well-tolerated. This minimizes the risk of hypoglycemia, which may result from continued SC absorption of intermediate-acting NPH insulin following unexpected discontinuation of tube feeding because of tube feeding intolerance. Once the tube feeding infusion rate has reached 30–40 mL/hr, the use of intermediate-acting insulin is generally safe.
- Gravity administration: The glucose concentration should be checked immediately before each feeding and no sooner than 4 hours after the end of the prior feeding. Thus, feedings should be spaced a minimum of 4 hours apart. Although some patients receiving gravity feedings can be managed with once-or twice-daily intermediate-acting insulin alone, others will need combined intermediate and short-acting insulin therapy.
- Continuous feeding over 12 hours: We generally use this form for patients on home tube feeding. Most patients will require only a once-daily administration of intermediate-acting insulin (alone or combined with a short-acting insulin preparation) prior to the onset of tube feeding.
- Continuous feeding over 24 hours: Scheduled administration of intermediate-acting insulin, usually given every 8 hours, may be required. We prefer use of intermediate-acting rather than long-acting insulin. If the feeding tube is removed or dislodged, the potential for prolonged hypoglycemia is greater if long-acting insulin is used. Also, reliance on intermediate insulin requires a more frequent dose-adjustment (than use of long-acting insulin) resulting in

the potential for more rapid achievement of glucose control.

- For hospitalized diabetic subjects treated with once-or twice-daily SC intermediate-acting insulin (with or without short-acting insulin), we begin by providing one half of the patient's total preadmission morning insulin as a morning intermediate-acting insulin SC dose. Similarly, one half of the patient's total preadmission evening insulin may be provided as an evening intermediate-acting insulin SC dose.
- For patients with type 1 diabetes treated with long-acting insulin for basal insulin needs, we generally continue their long-acting SC insulin at the preadmission dose. We adhere to a rapid-acting SC insulin algorithm for management of hyperglycemia above the patient's glucose goal range.
- An insulin infusion should be initiated for severe hyperglycemia or if glucose goals cannot be achieved with SC insulin. At this point, reassessment of caloric provision also is indicated. Permissive underfeeding should be considered.
- For patients on tube feeding, the most common cause of hypoglycemia is unexpected discontinuation of tube feedings. Refer to Table 32-3 for treatment guidelines.

CONCLUSIONS

In summary, the need for nutrition support requires an assessment of the patient's nutrient intake, body fat and protein stores, severity of illness, and anticipated duration of inadequate volitional oral intake. When possible, enteral rather than parenteral feeding should be used in patients requiring nutrition support. Hyperglycemia is common in patients receiving nutrition support. No clinical trials have been specifically designed to determine the effect of different blood glucose targets on clinical outcomes in adult hospitalized patients receiving nutrition support. We recommend a glucose goal of 140–180 mg/dL (7.8–10 mmol/L). Approaches to minimize hyperglycemia and hypoglycemia are needed in this patient population.

ACKNOWLEDGMENTS

The authors have nothing to disclose.

REFERENCES

1. **Cook CB, Kongable GL, Potter DJ, et al.** Inpatient glucose control: a glycemic survey of 126 U.S. hospitals. *J Hosp Med.* 2009;4:E7–E14.
2. **McMahon M.** Parenteral nutrition. In: Goldman I, Ausiello D, eds. *Cecil Textbook of Medicine.* Philadelphia, PA: W.B. Saunders Company;2004: 1322–1326.
3. **McClave SA, Martindale RG, Vanek VW, et al.** ASPEN Board of Directors and American College of Critical Care Medicine. Guidelines for the Provision and Assessment of Nutrition Support Therapy in the Adult Critically Ill Patient: Society of Critical Care Medicine (SCCM) and American Society for Parenteral and Enteral Nutrition (A.S.P.E.N.). *JPEN J Parenter Enteral Nutr.* 2009;33:277–316.
4. **Miles JM.** Energy expenditure in hospitalized patients: implications for nutritional support. *Mayo Clin Proc.* 2006;81:809–816.
5. **Moghissi ES, Koroytkowski MT, Dinardo M, et al.** American Association of Clinical Endocrinologists Association consensus statement on inpatient glycemic control. *Diabetes Care.* 2009;32:1119–1131.
6. **Umpierrez GE, Hellman R, Koroytkowski MT, et al.** Management of hyperglycemia in hospitalized patients in non-critical care setting: an Endocrine Society Clinical Practice Guideline. *J Clin Endocrinol Metab.* 2012;97:16–38.
7. **McMahon MM, Nystrom E, Braunschweigh C, et al.** American Society for Parenteral and Enteral Nutrition (A.S.P.E.N.) Board of Directors. A.S.P.E.N. Clinical Guidelines: Nutrition support of adult patients with hyperglycemia. *JPEN J Parenter Enteral Nutr.* 2013;37:23–36.
8. **Seaquist ER, Anderson J, Childs B, et al.** Hypoglycemia and diabetes: a report of a workgroup of the American Diabetes Association and the Endocrine Society. *J Clin Endocrinol Metab.* 2013;98: 1845–1859.
9. **Miles JM.** Intravenous fat emulsions in nutrition support. *Curr Opin Gastroenterol.* 1991;7:306–311.
10. **Leon-Sanz M, Garcia-Luna PP, Sanz-Paris A, et al.** Glycemic and lipid control in hospitalized type 2 diabetic patients: evaluation of 2 enteral nutrition formulas (low carbohydrate-high monounsaturated fat vs. high carbohydrate). *JPEN J Parenter Enteral Nutr.* 2005;29:21–29.
11. **Mesejo A, Acosta JA, Ortega C, et al.** Comparison of a high-protein disease-specific enteral formula with a high-protein enteral formula in hyperglycemic critically ill patients. *Clin Nutr.* 2003;22:296–305.

CHAPTER 33

Management of Hyperglycemia in Hospitalized Patients with Renal Insufficiency or Glucocorticoid-Induced Diabetes

David Baldwin

INTRODUCTION

Hyperglycemia is commonly encountered in hospitalized patients receiving pharmacological doses of glucocorticoids; many such patients have a known history of diabetes, some have previously undiagnosed diabetes, and some have normal glucose tolerance prior to glucocorticoid therapy. The latter two groups can be delineated with glycosylated hemoglobin (HbA1C) measurement. Virtually all patients with diabetes will experience significant worsening of glycemic control during treatment with glucocorticoids and will require specific approaches to insulin dosing for successful blood glucose control.

Chronic renal failure is also frequently encountered in hospitalized patients with diabetes and is an important risk factor for hypoglycemia if these patients are treated with sulfonylureas and/or insulin. Common reasons include decreased insulin clearance, reduced gluconeogenesis, gastroparesis, hypoglycemic unawareness, and decreased food intake due to poor appetite or lack of timely access to food. Current guidelines recommend avoiding noninsulin agents in this setting and using subcutaneous basal (background) and prandial (mealtime) insulin. Patients with diabetes and renal failure are known to have decreased insulin requirements, and a specific approach for insulin dosing in this population of hospitalized patients is needed to minimize the incidence of hypoglycemia.

Current literature on glucocorticoid-induced hyperglycemia and the use of insulin in renal failure is reviewed, and management guidelines are offered for each of these 2 special populations of hospitalized patients.

GLUCOCORTICOID THERAPY IN DIABETES

It is well known that glucocorticoid therapy may provoke hyperglycemia, new onset type 2 diabetes and will invariably worsen hyperglycemia in patients with preexisting diabetes (1–4). The mechanism is increased insulin resistance in the face of inadequate insulin secretion. Known risk factors for the development of glucocorticoid-induced diabetes include age, body mass index, presence of impaired fasting glucose/glucose tolerance, and higher doses of glucocorticoid. In one observational study, 11% of general medical inpatients received ≥40 mg/day of prednisone or the equivalent for at least 2 days (5). Of these, 64% had blood glucose >200 mg/dL (11.1 mmol/L). Glucocorticoid treated patients with hyperglycemia have a significantly longer length of hospital stay after adjustment for comorbidities. In our experience, the tendency for high-risk outpatients to develop new glucocorticoid-induced hyperglycemia is often not anticipated, and these patients can require hospitalization for intravenous (IV) hydration and initiation of insulin therapy that could have been prevented.

Table 33-1. Glucocorticoids Commonly Used in Hospitalized Patients

Name	IV Dosing	PO Dosing	Relative Potency (mg)	Duration of Metabolic Effect (hr)	Typical Dosing (mg/day)
Hydrocortisone	Yes	Yes	20	8	20–200
Prednisone (Prednisolone)	No	Yes	6	16	5–100
Methylprednisolone	Yes	Yes	5	16	50–1,000
Dexamethasone	Yes	Yes	0.5–0.75	24	2–24

Table 33-1 shows properties of commonly used glucocorticoids.

One common use of glucocorticoids in the hospital setting is the treatment of acute exacerbations of chronic obstructive pulmonary disease (AECOPD). A 2005 *Cochrane Review* found that treatment of AECOPD with oral glucocorticoids was associated with an increased risk of developing hyperglycemia (odds ratio [OR] 5.48, 95% CI 1.58 to 18.96) (6). When inpatients with AECOPD treated with glucocorticoids were studied, the risk of death increased by 10% (95% CI 0–22) per 18 mg/dL (1 mmol/L) increase in blood glucose (P = 0.055) after adjustment for age, sex, and previous diagnosis of diabetes mellitus (7). Chakrabarti et al reported that patients with AECOPD have a worse outcome if blood glucose is >126 mg/dL (7 mmol/L) in the first 24 hours after admission (8). Continuous glucose monitoring (CGM) in patients with AECOPD who received prednisolone daily at 0800 found that hyperglycemia is predominantly in the afternoon and evening with near normal AM glucose levels (9). Pharmacodynamic data for prednisolone show a duration of 16–18 hours, and this fits with what we commonly see clinically (10).

Glucocorticoids are a common component of chemotherapy regimens, many of which are administered in the hospital setting. In a recent prospective study, patients who developed hyperglycemia on hyper-CVAD chemotherapy were randomized to an intensive insulin regimen of glargine and aspart or conventional therapy (glycemic control managed at the discretion of the clinician) (11). The target glucose values of the intensive group were fasting glucose less than 120 mg/dL (6.7 mmol/L) and postprandial glucose less than 180 mg/dL (10 mmol/L). Over the span of a mean of 8 hospitalizations, mean glucose levels were significantly lower in the intensive insulin arm than the conventional treatment arm, although the conventional treatment group mean blood glucose levels for each cycle of chemotherapy were also well-controlled (usually <150 mg/dL [8.3 mmol/L]). The trial was terminated early for its failure to show a difference in overall survival, rates of complete remission, complete remission duration, progression-free survival, infectious complications, hospitalizations, and intensive care unit (ICU) admissions. Another recent study compared a sliding scale insulin approach with a basal-bolus insulin regimen (ie, detemir and aspart) in hyperglycemic patients receiving dexamethasone for hematological malignancies. The results showed that the sliding scale regimen, which delivered less insulin, resulted in an increase in mean daily blood glucose of 128 mg/dL (7.1 mmol/L) compared with a decrease in mean blood glucose of 52 mg/dL (2.9 mmol/L) in the basal-bolus group (P < 0.001) (12). In addition, 3 patients in the sliding scale group (n = 28) developed diabetic ketoacidosis (DKA) or hyperglycemic hyperosmolar state (HHS) during dexamethasone therapy.

Glucocorticoids are commonly used in hospitalized solid organ and bone marrow transplant recipients either as part of immunosuppression induction or for treatment of acute rejection or graft-versus-host disease. A retrospective study found that survival after bone marrow transplant was decreased in patients whose blood glucose values were less than 60 mg/dL (3.3 mmol/L) or greater than 200 mg/dL (11.1 mmol/L) (13). A dedicated glucose management team utilizing IV and subcutaneous insulin delivery can be highly successful at keeping the mean blood glucose ~160 mg/dL (8.9 mmol/L) despite high doses of glucocorticoids typically given after solid organ transplants (14). Table 33-2 summarizes

Table 33-2. Practical Aspects to Hyperglycemia Management During Glucocorticoid Treatment

1. Patients with glucocorticoid-induced hyperglycemia or patients with type 2 diabetes who begin glucocorticoids will almost always require insulin treatment. All oral antidiabetes agents or GLP-1 agonists (monotherapy or in combination) are generally ineffective.
2. Sulfonylureas are especially problematic in patients receiving prednisone every morning, because blood glucose levels will be very high in the afternoon and evening but will be very low overnight as the duration of all sulfonylureas outlasts that of once-daily prednisone. Chronic once-daily prednisone >10 mg/day also predictably will suppress endogenous cortisol production, therefore, increasing the risk for fasting AM hypoglycemia if glucose-lowering agents are active after midnight.
3. Monitoring of blood glucose premeals and at bedtime is critical to safe titration of insulin therapy. Postmeal testing is not recommended. All hospitalized patients who begin treatment with glucocorticoids should have blood glucose monitored and insulin therapy initiated if blood glucose levels exceed 180 mg/dL (10 mmol/L).
4. All patients with glucocorticoid-induced or glucocorticoid-worsened hyperglycemia should be treated with both basal insulin and multiple injections of mealtime insulin.
5. The choice of basal insulin depends on the duration of action of the glucocorticoid and its dosing interval.
6. Patients with glucocorticoid-induced hyperglycemia being treated in a critical care unit should be managed with an IV continuous insulin infusion (CII) with hourly blood glucose measurements and insulin dose titration.
7. Once-daily long-acting insulin (eg, glargine or detemir) or twice-daily intermediate-acting insulin (NPH) coupled with rapid-acting insulin with meals is appropriate for patients receiving dexamethasone or twice-daily methylprednisolone/prednisone. If patients are insulin naïve, begin with long-acting insulin 0.3 units/kg/day or NPH 0.2 units/kg BID and rapid-acting insulin 0.1 units/kg/meal. All patients will require 2–3 times daily dose titration, and many patients will require dramatic up-titrations such as 50%–100% per day in order to bring blood glucose levels back under 200 mg/dL (11.1 mmol/L).
8. Patients receiving once-daily methylprednisolone or prednisone will have an increase in blood glucose only lasting 16–20 hours. Thus, long-acting insulin is best avoided to protect from fasting hypoglycemia. NPH given once daily at the same time as the dose of prednisone along with mealtime dosing of rapid-acting insulin is usually the optimal approach.
9. Patients with type 1 diabetes who have glucocorticoid worsening of glucose control should remain on their usual insulin regimen with up-titration of doses as needed. As a general rule, patients with type 1 diabetes will be less susceptible to glucocorticoid-induced worsening of glucose control than patients with type 2 diabetes.
10. Premixed insulins (such as 70/30 or 75/25) are generally not useful because of their inherent inflexibility for dosing.
11. Because glucocorticoid dosing in hospitalized patients frequently changes from day to day, close attention to daily insulin dose titration is mandatory, as is paying close attention to enteral or parenteral carbohydrate intake.

Abbreviations: GLP-1 = glucagon-like peptide-1; NPH = neutral protamine Hagedorn.

practical suggestions for successful management of diabetes in the setting of glucocorticoid therapy.

DIABETES, HYPOGLYCEMIA, AND CHRONIC KIDNEY DISEASE

Diabetes is the leading cause of chronic kidney disease (CKD; also known as chronic renal failure), and the combination of renal failure and diabetes is commonly encountered in clinical practice. Development of CKD is characterized by a progression from stage 1 to 5 (Table 33-3). In patients with diabetes and end-stage renal disease (ESRD), there is a significant correlation between HbA1C and survival; increased mortality is associated with either HbA1C <7% or >8% as compared with 7%–8% (15–17). The finding of an increased mortality associated with HbA1C <6%–7% is particularly important in light of the increased incidence of hypoglycemia in renal failure patients. In a study of hypoglycemia among 243,222 patients cared for by the US Veterans Health Administration, the rate

Table 33-3. Stages of Chronic Kidney Disease

Stage	Estimated GFR (eGFR)	Clinical Severity
1	>90 mL/min	Minimal
2	60–89 mL/min	Mild
3A	45–59 mL/min	Moderate
3B	30–44 mL/min	
4	15–29 mL/min	Severe
5	<15 mL/min or Renal replacement therapy (transplant or dialysis)	ESRD

Abbreviations: eGFR = estimated glomerular filtration rate; GFR = glomerular filtration rate; ESRD, end-stage renal disease.

Table 33-4. Therapeutic Agents for Type 2 Diabetes Mellitus in Chronic Kidney Disease

Class/Name	Usual Dosing Range	Safe in Renal Failure?	Dose Modification for Renal Failure
Sulfonylureas			
Glyburide	1.25–10 mg/day	No	Not advised
Glipizide	2.5–20 mg/day	With caution	Limit to stages 1–3 only
Glimepiride	1–8 mg/day	With caution	Limit to stages 1–3 only
Glinides			
Repaglinide	0.5–2 mg with meals	With caution	Limit to stages 1–3 only
Nateglinide	80–160 mg with meals	Yes	
Metformin	500–2,000 mg/day	With caution	Full dose in stages 1–2 50% reduced dose in stage 3 Avoid in stages 4–5
Pioglitazone	15–45 mg/day	Yes	
DPP-4 inhibitors			
Sitagliptin	100 mg/day	Yes	Full dose in stages 1–2 50 mg/day in stage 3 25 mg/day in stages 4–5
Saxagliptin	5 mg/day	Yes	Full dose in stages 1–3 2.5 mg/day in stages 4–5
Linagliptin	5 mg/day	Yes	Full dose
Alogliptin	25 mg/day	Yes	Full dose in stages 1–2 12.5 mg/day in stage 3 6.25 mg/day in stages 4–5
GLP-1 agonists			
Exenatide	10 mcg BID	With caution	Full dose in stages 1–3 Avoid in stages 4–5
Liraglutide	1.8 mg/day	With caution	Full dose in stages 1–3 Avoid in stages 4–5
Alpha-glucosidase inhibitors			
Acarbose	25–50 mg with meals	Yes	Full dose
Miglitol	25–50 mg with meals	With caution	Limit to stages 1–3 only
SGLT-2 inhibitor			
Canagliflozin	300 mg/day	With caution	Full dose in stages 1–2 100 mg/day if eGFR 45–60 mL/min Avoid if eGFR <45 mL/min
Dapagliflozin	10 mg/day	With caution	Full dose in stages 1–2 Avoid if eGFR <60 mL/min

Abbreviations: DPP-4 = dipeptidyl peptidase-4; eGFR = estimated glomerular filtration rate; GLP-1 = glucagon-like peptide-1; SGLT-2 = sodium-glucose cotransporter 2.

of blood glucose <70 mg/dL (3.9 mmol/L) was 10.72 per 100 patient-months in patients with diabetes and estimated glomerular filtration rate (eGFR) <60 mL/min per 1.73 m^2 as compared with 5.33 per 100 patient-months in patients with diabetes and normal renal function after adjustment for age, race, and other comorbidities (18). Approximately 57% of 2,040,206 glucose measurements collected in this database were from patients during hospitalization. Mortality within 1 day of the hypoglycemic episode was increased in all patients with CKD, OR 1.85 for blood glucose 60–69 mg/dL (3.3–3.8 mmol/L), OR 4.10 for blood glucose 50–59 mg/dL (2.8–3.2), and OR 6.09 for blood glucose <50 mg/dL (2.8 mmol/L) (all $P < 0.0001$). Thus hypoglycemia is a potential threat to inpatients with diabetes and renal failure. Table 33-4 shows currently available noninsulin therapies for type 2 diabetes and their safety in various stages of CKD. Metformin is not recommended for inpatients

Table 33-5. Improving the Safety of Insulin Therapy in Patients with Chronic Renal Failure

1. Elderly patients may have a substantial decrease in eGFR despite having a mild elevation in serum creatinine. Always incorporate eGFR into dosing of noninsulin therapies and into weight-based initiation of insulin dosing.
2. 0.5–0.6 units/kg/day is a commonly recommended total daily dose for initiation of inpatient insulin therapy, 50% long-acting insulin and 50% rapid-acting insulin split into 3 meals.
3. Reduce the total daily insulin dose to 0.25 units/kg/day, 50% long-acting insulin and 50% rapid-acting, in patients with eGFR <45 mL/min in order to reduce the frequency of hypoglycemia.
4. If intermediate-acting NPH insulin is used in patients with ESRD, once daily AM dosing will usually suffice; PM dosing increases the risk of next AM hypoglycemia and is usually not needed.
5. Hypoglycemia in insulin-treated patients occurs most frequently between 0200 and 0700 hours, a time window largely regulated by the dose of long-acting insulin.
a. Decrease the dose of basal insulin every day by at least 20% if the 0600 blood glucose level is <100 mg/dL (5.6 mmol/L). b. Increase the dose of basal insulin every day by at least 20% if the 0600 blood glucose level is >200 mg/dL (11.1 mmol/L). c. Avoid the temptation to give "correction" doses of rapid-acting insulin at bedtime if the blood glucose is elevated. The most common outcome is 0700 hypoglycemia. d. Reduce the dose of basal insulin by 25% on hemodialysis days in ESRD.
6. Titrate doses of rapid-acting insulin up or down by 20% if prelunch, predinner, or bedtime blood glucose levels are below 100 mg/dL (5.6 mmol/L) or above 200 mg/dL (11.1 mmol/L). All hospitalized patients treated with insulin must have a blood glucose level >100 mg/dL (5.6 mmol/L) before going to sleep for the night. Recheck a 0200 blood glucose level on all patients with bedtime blood glucose <100 mg/dL (5.6 mmol/L).
7. 20-minute postmeal dosing of rapid-acting insulin and last minute reduction or holding of mealtime insulin when meal ingestion is poor or absent are successful strategies to reduce postprandial hypoglycemia.
8. Discharge recommendations for patients with ESRD and type 2 diabetes: the role of inpatient HbA1C
a. When HbA1C is <8% in a type 2 diabetes patient with ESRD, stop sulfonylurea therapy because of the increased risk of hypoglycemia. b. When HbA1C is <7% in a type 2 diabetes patient with ESRD, stop rapid-acting insulin. c. When HbA1C is <6% in a type 2 diabetes patient with ESRD, stop all antidiabetic therapy. d. When HbA1C is >8% and antidiabetic therapy is needed, DPP-4 inhibitors, pioglitazone (watch for fluid-retention), or low-dose long-acting insulin are the safest choices.

Abbreviations: eGFR = estimated glomerular filtration rate; ESRD = end-stage renal disease; NPH = neutral protamine Hagedorn.

because of possible fluctuations in renal function during an acute hospital admission. All 3 commonly used sulfonylureas (ie, glyburide [glibenclamide], glipizide, and glimepiride) are known to accumulate in CKD and thus are not an ideal class of therapy for patients with stage 4–5 renal failure (19). This is especially true in the hospital setting where the timing of meals is frequently disrupted. There have been no studies of glinides or glucagon-like peptide-1 (GLP-1) agonists in the hospital setting, although dipeptidyl peptidase-4 (DPP-4) inhibitors showed efficacy and safety in a pilot study of patients with mild-to-moderately severe type 2 diabetes (20).

INSULIN CLEARANCE IN RENAL FAILURE

Multiple alterations in insulin and glucose metabolism occur in chronic renal failure. Because endogenous insulin is secreted via the portal vein, the liver metabolizes ~50% of insulin in the first pass. The kidney plays a secondary role in the metabolism of endogenous insulin but will clear ~65% of insulin reaching it. In contrast, however, exogenous insulin is absorbed systemically, and thus the kidney plays a primary role in the metabolism of injected therapeutic insulin (21). After GFR <20 mL/min, renal clearance of insulin is dramatically reduced (22). Other factors in ESRD that mitigate diabetes and increase the risk for hypoglycemia include decreased renal gluconeogenesis, anorexia, weight loss, and protein malnutrition.

When patients with diabetes are followed from the onset of overt nephropathy to ESRD, insulin requirements decrease by 38% from 0.72 units/kg/day to 0.45 units/kg/day in type 1 diabetes and by 51% from 0.68 units/kg/day to 0.33 units/kg/day in type 2 diabetes (23). Many patients with type 2 diabetes progress to needing no therapy for hyperglycemia after developing ESRD, a phenomenon known as "burnt out" type 2 diabetes (24).

There are significant changes in insulin sensitivity and glycemic control in patients with type 2 diabetes and ESRD when these parameters were compared before and after a hemodialysis treatment. CGM in 19 subjects found that mean blood glucose was 226 ± 101 mg/dL (12.5 ± 5.6 mmol/L) in the 24 hours prior to dialysis but dropped to 176 ± 68 mg/dL (9.8 ± 3.8 mmol/L) in the 24 hours after dialysis (25). Asymptomatic hypoglycemia was more common after dialysis. A study using the euglycemic clamp technique demonstrated a 25% reduction in basal insulin requirements on the day after dialysis as compared with the day before dialysis, with no difference in mealtime insulin needs (26).

A recent study evaluated insulin glargine and glulisine in noncritically ill hospitalized subjects with type 2 diabetes and chronic renal failure (mean eGFR 31 mL/min) (27). Some 107 subjects not yet requiring dialysis were randomized to a total daily insulin dose of 0.5 units/kg versus 0.25 units/kg. Fifty percent of the total dose was given daily as insulin glargine, and subjects who were eating also received one sixth of the total dose as insulin glulisine with each meal. Doses were titrated daily, based on premeal and bedtime blood glucose measurements. Mean HbA1C on admission was 8%, and 76% of patients were treated with insulin prior to admission. Mean blood glucose was the same for both insulin dose groups on day 1 (196 ± 62 mg/dL [10.9 ± 3.4 mmol/L]) and decreased to mean 174 ± 49 mg/dL (9.7 ± 2.7 mmol/L) in both groups on subsequent days. Although the glucose lowering effect of the different insulin doses did not differ, there was a 50% reduction in the frequency of hypoglycemia in the lower dose group. Table 33-5 summarizes practical suggestions for successful management of diabetes in patients with chronic renal failure.

How should these studies impact the care of patients with diabetes and CKD during hospitalization? HbA1C should be measured in all inpatients with hyperglycemia or a history of diabetes if a recent result is not available (28). Patient diabetes treatment regimens should be adjusted at the time of hospital discharge if the HbA1C is either too low (<7%) or too high (>8%). Many dialysis patients with diabetes, treated with insulin or a sulfonylurea, will have inpatient HbA1C <7%. It is important to recognize that these patients have significant risks for hypoglycemia and increased mortality, and their insulin regimen should be incrementally "down-titrated" (or sulfonylurea ideally discontinued) at the time of hospital discharge. Blood glucose patterns and insulin doses during the hospital stay are usually informative as to which components of an insulin regimen should be modified.

ACKNOWLEDGMENTS

DB has received a research grant from Novo Nordisk.

REFERENCES

1. **Gurwitz JH, Bohn RL, Glynn RJ, Monane M, Mogun H, Avorn J.** Glucocorticoids and the risk for initiation of hypoglycemic therapy. *Arch Intern Med.* 1994;154:97–101.
2. **Gulliford MC, Charlton J, Latinovic R.** Risk of diabetes associated with prescribed glucocorticoids in a large population. *Diabetes Care.* 2006:29:2728–2729.
3. **Clore JN, Thurby-Hay L.** Glucocorticoid-induced hyperglycemia. *Endocr Pract.* 2009;15:469–474.
4. **Braithwaite SS, Barr WG, Rahman A, Quddusi S.** Managing diabetes during glucocorticoid therapy. How to avoid metabolic emergencies. *Postgrad Med.* 1998;104:163–166.
5. **Donihi AC, Raval D, Saul M, Korytkowski MT, DeVita MA.** Prevalence and predictors of corticosteroid-related hyperglycemia in hospitalized patients. *Endocr Pract.* 2006;12:358–362.
6. **Wood-Baker RR, Gibson PG, Hannay M, Walters EH, Walters JA.** Systemic corticosteroids for acute exacerbations of chronic obstructive pulmonary disease. *Cochrane Database Syst Rev.* 2005;(1):CD001288.
7. **Baker EH, Janaway CH, Philips BJ, et al.** Hyperglycaemia is associated with poor outcomes in patients admitted to hospital with acute exacerbations of chronic obstructive pulmonary disease. *Thorax.* 2006;61:284–289.
8. **Chakrabarti B, Angus RM, Agarwal S, Lane S, Calverley PM.** Hyperglycaemia as a predictor of outcome during non-invasive ventilation in decompensated COPD. *Thorax.* 2009;64:857–862.
9. **Burt MG, Roberts GW, Aguilar-Loza NR, Frith P, Stranks SN.** Continuous monitoring of circadian glycemic patterns in patients receiving prednisolone for COPD. *J Clin Endocrinol Metab.* 2011;96: 1789–1796.
10. **Magee MH, Blum RA, Lates CD, Jusko WJ.** Prednisolone pharmacokinetics and pharmacodynamics in relation to sex and race. *J Clin Pharmacol.* 2001;41:1180–1194.

11. **Vu K, Busaidy N, Cabanillas ME, et al.** A randomized controlled trial of an intensive insulin regimen in patients with hyperglycemic acute lymphoblastic leukemia. *Clin Lymphoma Myeloma Leuk.* 2012;12: 355–362.
12. **Gosmanov AR, Goorha S, Stelts S, Peng L, Umpierrez GE.** Management of hyperglycemia in diabetic patients with hematologic malignancies during dexamethasone therapy. *Endocrine Pract.* 2013;19: 231–235.
13. **Pidala J, Kim J, Kharfan-Dabaja AM, et al.** Dysglycemia following glucocorticoid therapy for acute graft-versus-host disease adversely affects transplantation outcomes. *Biol Blood Marrow Transplant.* 2011;17:239–248.
14. **Wallia A, Parikh ND, O'Shea-Mahler E, et al.** Glycemic control by a glucose management service and infection rates after liver transplantation. *Endocr Pract.* 2011;17:546–551.
15. **Ricks J, Molnar MZ, Kovesdy CP, et al.** Glycemic control and cardiovascular mortality in hemodialysis patients with diabetes: a 6-year cohort study. *Diabetes.* 2012;61:708–715.
16. **Shurraw S, Hemmelgarn B, Lin M, et al.** Association between glycemic control and adverse outcomes in people with diabetes mellitus and chronic kidney disease: a population-based cohort study. *Arch Intern Med.* 2011;171:1920–1927.
17. **Kalantar-Zadeh K.** A critical evaluation of glycated protein parameters in advanced nephropathy: a matter of life or death: A1C remains the gold standard outcome predictor in diabetic dialysis patients. *Diabetes Care.* 2012:35:1625–1628.
18. **Moen MF, Zhan M, Hsu VD, et al.** Frequency of hypoglycemia and its significance in chronic kidney disease. *Clin J Am Soc Nephrol.* 2009;4:1121–1127.
19. **Holstein A, Hammer C, Hahn M, Kulamadayil NS, Kovacs P.** Severe sulfonylurea-induced hypoglycemia: a problem of uncritical prescription and deficiencies of diabetes care in geriatric patients. *Expert Opin Drug Saf.* 2010;9:675–681.
20. **Umpierrez GE, Gianchandani R, Smiley A, et al.** Safety and efficacy of sitagliptin therapy for the inpatient management of general medicine and surgery patients with type 2 diabetes: a pilot randomized controlled trial [published online July 22, 2013]. *Diabetes Care.*
21. **Iglesias P, Díez JJ.** Insulin therapy in renal disease. *Diabetes Obes Metab.* 2008;10:811–823.
22. **Mak RH.** Impact of end-stage renal disease and dialysis on glycemic control. *Semin Dial.* 2000;13:4–8.
23. **Biesenbach G, Raml A, Schmekal B, Eichbauer-Sturm G.** Decreased insulin requirement in relation to GFR in nephropathic Type 1 and insulin-treated Type 2 diabetic patients. *Diabet Med.* 2003;20:642–645.
24. **Park J, Lertdumrongluk P, Molnar MZ, Kovesdy CP, Kalantar-Zadeh K.** Glycemic control in diabetic dialysis patients and the burnt-out diabetes phenomenon. *Curr Diab Rep.* 2012;12:432–439.
25. **Kazempour-Ardebili S, Lecamwasam VL, Dassanyake T, et al.** Assessing glycemic control in maintenance hemodialysis patients with type 2 diabetes. *Diabetes Care.* 2009;32:1137–1142.
26. **Sobngwi E, Enoru S, Ashuntantang G, et al.** Day-to-day variation of insulin requirements of patients with type 2 diabetes and end-stage renal disease undergoing maintenance hemodialysis. *Diabetes Care.* 2010;33:1409–1412.
27. **Baldwin D, Zander J, Munoz C, et al.** A randomized trial of two weight-based doses of insulin glargine and glulisine in hospitalized subjects with type 2 diabetes and renal insufficiency. *Diabetes Care.* 2012;35: 1970–1974.
28. **Umpierrez GE, Hellman R, Korytkowski MT, et al.** Management of hyperglycemia in hospitalized patients in non-critical care setting: an Endocrine Society Clinical Practice Guideline. *J Clin Endocrinol Metab.* 2012;97:16–38.

CHAPTER 34

Diabetic Foot Infections

Karim Gariani, Ilker Uçkay, and Benjamin A Lipsky

ABSTRACT

Complications related to diabetes, particularly peripheral neuropathy and peripheral arterial disease (PAD), can lead to potentially serious foot problems, such as ulcers or Charcot neuropathic-osteoarthropathy (CN). Foot ulcers often become infected, and these can present urgent problems requiring rapid and appropriate medical and surgical interventions. We will review key concepts of diabetic foot infections and their management and discuss the related problems of PAD and acute CN.

INTRODUCTION

Foot problems are among the most common and feared complications of diabetes mellitus and are now the leading diabetes-related cause of hospitalization, as well as the major cause of lower extremity amputations. The most common foot complication is skin ulceration, which is usually secondary to diabetes-related peripheral neuropathy (with loss of protective sensation) and less often related to peripheral arterial disease (PAD). The lifetime risk of a person with diabetes developing a foot ulcer is estimated at 25%, with an annual incidence of 3% to 10% (1,2).

About half of diabetic foot ulcers (DFU) are clinically infected at presentation, and these wounds are at substantially increased risk of various adverse outcomes. Infection is usually the final precipitating cause of lower extremity amputations, the risk of which is 23 times higher in persons with diabetes than those without (3). Over 85% of lower extremity amputations in persons with diabetes are preceded by foot ulceration (4). These amputations are associated with a 5-year survival rate of only 50% (5). Another serious, but less common, complication of diabetic neuropathy is Charcot neuropathic-osteoarthropathy (CN), which can lead to foot deformities and ulceration. Understanding the management of these severe diabetic foot complications is key, because most foot infections are preventable, or at least treatable.

CLASSIFICATION AND DIAGNOSIS

Over the past 2 decades, several schemes for classification of the most common diabetic foot complications have been published. In 2004, guidelines specifically devoted to diabetic foot infections (DFIs), including an infection-related classification scheme, were published by multidisciplinary panels of experts from the Infectious Diseases Society of America (IDSA) and the International Working Group on the Diabetic Foot (IWGDF); each of these was updated in 2012 (6,7). These guidelines have been widely cited, and specific components have been validated in several studies. The scheme for defining infection and classifying its severity is shown in Table 34-1. The updated IDSA guidelines provide answers to 10 key questions (Table 34-2), along with the evidence supporting the recommendations and a grading of the quality and strength of the recommendations. A key feature is that DFIs are defined by the presence of clinical

Table 34-1. IDSA/IWGDF Diabetic Foot Infection Severity Classification Scheme (6)

Clinical Description	IDSA	IWGDF
Wound without purulence or any manifestations of inflammation	Uninfected	1
≥2 manifestations of inflammation (purulence or erythema, pain, tenderness, warmth, or induration); any cellulitis or erythema extends ≤2 cm around ulcer, and infection is limited to skin or superficial subcutaneous tissues; no local complications or systemic illness	Mild	2
Infection in patient who is systemically well & metabolically stable but has ≥2 cm of cellulitis; lymphangitis; spread beneath fascia; deep tissue abscess; gangrene; muscle, tendon, joint, or bone involvement	Moderate	3
Patient who demonstrates signs of SIRS manifested by ≥2 of the following: • Temperature >38°C (100.4°F) or <36°C (96.8°F) • Heart rate >90 bpm • Respiratory rate >20 breaths/minute or $PaCO_2$ <32 mm Hg • White blood cell count >12×10^9/L or <4×10^9/L or ≥10% immature cells (bands)	Severe	4
Systemic toxicity may also present with anorexia, chills, hypotension, confusion, vomiting, acidosis, hyperglycemia, and/or azotemia; the presence of critical limb ischemia may increase the level of severity		

Abbreviations: IDSA = Infectious Diseases Society of America; IWGDF = International Working Group on the Diabetic Foot; SIRS = systemic inflammatory response syndrome.

Table 34-2. The 10 Key Questions Posed and Answered in the IDSA DFI Guidelines (6)

1. **In which diabetic patients with a foot wound should I suspect infection, and how should I classify it?**
   Every foot wound in a diabetic patient should be considered as possibly infected, particularly if the patient is at high risk due to the presence of peripheral neuropathy or arterial disease.
   The classifications by the IDSA/IWGDF (Table 34-1) define and rate the severity of infection.
2. **How should I assess a patient presenting with a DFI?**
   Clinicians should assess the patient at 3 different levels: first the patient as a whole, then the affected limb, and finally the wound. Assess for neuropathy, vasculopathy and infection.
3. **When and from whom should I request a consultation for a patient with a DFI?**
   Outpatients and inpatients with a DFI should benefit from a multidisciplinary team. If not available, the clinicians in charge of the patient should attempt to coordinate obtaining and deploying the advice of all the specialists required.
4. **Which patients with a diabetic foot infection should I hospitalize, and what criteria should they meet before I discharge them?**
   Hospitalization should be considered in case of severe infection, moderate infection with complications (eg, peripheral artery disease), and for those who cannot or would not comply with an outpatient treatment regimen.
5. **When and how should I obtain specimen(s) for culture from a patient with a diabetic foot wound?**
   Only for wounds presenting evidence of infection. Clinicians should obtain appropriate specimens for aerobic and anaerobic culture. The samples should be taken before starting empirical antibiotic therapy. After careful cleaning and wound debridement, obtain the sample from deep tissue by biopsy or curettage or by aspiration of purulent secretions, if at all possible.
6. **How should I initially select, and when should I modify, an antibiotic regimen for a DFI?**
   Select an empiric regimen based on the likeliest pathogens and known local antibiotic sensitivity patterns, and consider modifying it based on the clinical response to treatment and the results of culture and sensitivity tests.
7. **When should I consider imaging studies to evaluate a DFI, and which should I select?**
   Order plain radiographs for all patients with a new DFI to look for bony abnormalities, soft tissue gas, or radio- opaque foreign bodies. Advanced imaging tests may be needed in some instances such as magnetic resonance imaging (MRI), single-photon emission CT (SPECT)/CT and positron-emission tomography (PET).
8. **How should I diagnose and treat osteomyelitis of the foot in a patient with diabetes?**
   In any infected, deep, or large foot ulcer, particularly if the lesion is chronic or overlies a bony prominence, consider the possibility of osteomyelitis. When a definitive diagnosis of osteomyelitis is required clinicians should obtain a bone specimen for microbiological and histopathological evaluation. Treating osteomyelitis almost always requires antibiotic therapy, which may be effective alone but is often combined with at least some surgical resection of necrotic and infected bone.

(Continued)

Table 34-2. The 10 Key Questions Posed and Answered in the IDSA DFI Guidelines (6) (Continued)

9. In which patients with a DFI should I consider surgical intervention, and what type of procedure may be appropriate?
Many DFIs require some type of surgical procedure, and a surgeon should evaluate most moderate, and all severe (especially potentially limb-threatening; see Table 34-3) DFIs, if possible. Emergency amputation is rarely needed except in life-threatening infections or with extensive tissue necrosis. An elective amputation may be appropriate in several situations, such as irreversible loss of limb function, recurrence of the wound despite adequate preventive management, or the need for an unacceptably prolonged or intensive hospital management.

10. What types of wound care techniques and dressings are appropriate for diabetic foot wounds?
Adequate management of a wound should include proper cleansing, followed by debridement of callus and necrotic tissue and pressure off-loading.

Abbreviations: IDSA = Infectious Diseases Society of America; DFI = diabetic foot infection; IWGDF = International Working Group on the Diabetic Foot.

signs and symptoms of inflammation (ie, redness, warmth, swelling, pain, or tenderness) or purulent secretions, rather than by the results of wound cultures.

MANAGEMENT OF DIABETIC FOOT INFECTIONS

Evaluation

Clinicians assessing a patient presenting with a DFI should consider the problem at 3 levels: the whole patient, the affected limb, and finally, the wound. The clinician should measure the vital signs, palpate for pedal pulses, check for peripheral neuropathy, and debride and probe any open wounds. Special attention should be paid to detecting crepitus, bullae, new onset tenderness or anesthesia, rapidly advancing cellulitis, or gangrenous tissue (Table 34-3 and Figure 34-1). The presence of any of these findings should prompt rapid consultation with an experienced foot surgeon. In addition to basic hematology and blood chemistry tests, virtually all patients with a foot wound should have a plain radiograph of the foot to look for the presence of gas, a foreign body, or bone lesions. Where clinical circumstances or the findings on plain X-ray suggest a more sensitive or specific imaging test is needed, magnetic resonance imaging (MRI) is generally best (8).

Classifying the severity of a DFI is important as it helps determine which patients may require hospitalization and broad-spectrum, intravenous (IV) antibiotic therapy, which is usually required for severe infections but rarely for mild (or many moderate) infections. DFIs also may require inpatient management when they are associated with critical limb ischemia, have not responded

Table 34-3. Signs of a Possibly Imminently Limb-Threatening Infection[a]

- Evidence of systemic inflammatory response syndrome
- Rapid progression of infection
- Extensive necrosis or gangrene
- Crepitus on examination or tissue gas on imaging
- Extensive ecchymoses or petechiae
- Bullae, especially hemorrhagic
- New onset wound anesthesia
- Pain out of proportion to clinical findings
- Recent loss of neurological function
- Critical limb ischemia
- Extensive soft tissue loss
- Extensive bony destruction, especially midfoot/hindfoot
- Failure of infection to improve with appropriate therapy

In clinical settings where advanced health care is not available, even lesser degrees of infection severity may make an infection limb-threatening.

[a] *From IDSA Guidelines 2012 (6), with some examples demonstrated in Figure 34-1.*

to outpatient therapy, or when social or psychological issues do not allow management in the outpatient setting. A severe DFI requires rapid evaluation (especially for vascular status), attention to any metabolic disorders, and consideration of appropriate surgical procedures. Similarly, the presence of a deep soft tissue abscess or osteomyelitis also requires surgical evaluation.

Multidisciplinary Teams and Clinical Pathways

Early and continued care by a multidisciplinary team has been repeatedly shown to likely be associated with better outcomes in inpatient, as well as outpatient, settings, and to reduce the likelihood of major lower extremity amputation. This team can be composed of various specialists with an interest in foot wounds, including infectious disease experts, surgeons, podiatrists, diabetologists, and nurses. The key criterion for team membership is less the specific specialty of the members than their expertise and interest (9,10). Multidisciplinary teams meeting together at the bedside may be optimal, but when this is not possible teams may be set up to communicate by telemedicine, teleconference, or e-mail (10). Several recent DFI guidelines address the critical role of multidisciplinary teams, which have, unfortunately, largely been established only in large hospitals in resource-rich countries (6,11,12). However, even in resource-rich countries the existence and appropriate referral to multidisciplinary foot teams may be deficient. For example, in the UK 2012 Inpatient Diabetes Audit, 31% of hospitals provided no inpatient podiatry service. In addition, despite nearly half of diabetes-specific admissions being due to foot disease, more than one third were not referred to a multidisciplinary foot team, in defiance of national guidance.

Antibiotic Therapy

Clinically uninfected wounds do not need to be cultured, as there is no evidence that treating colonization with antibiotics will improve wound healing or prevent infection. Infected wounds, however, virtually always require antibiotic therapy. Obtaining a tissue sample for culture from any clinically infected wound,

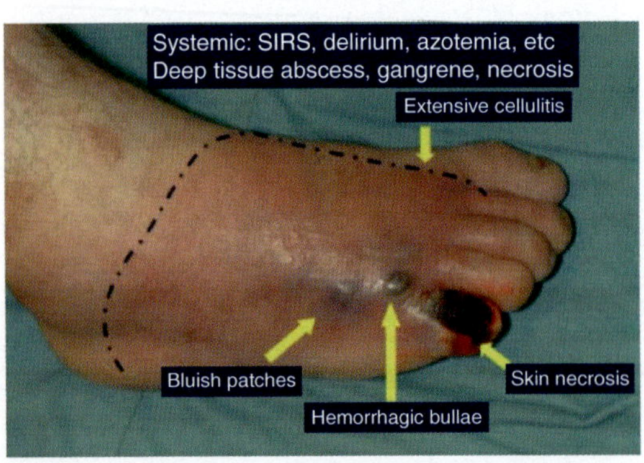

Figure 34-1. Diabetic foot infection with rapidly spreading soft tissue infection demonstrating characteristics of a serious soft tissue infection requiring urgent surgical exploration.

preferably before initiating empirical antibiotic therapy, is a crucial step toward ensuring an appropriate agent is selected. Wound specimens should be taken only after careful cleaning and debriding. Specimens of deep tissue obtained by biopsy or curettage, or aspirations of purulent secretions are more apt to grow the true pathogens and less likely to yield colonizing microorganisms. Swabs should be avoided (6). Blood cultures are rarely positive, except in patients with evidence of systemic sepsis.

The choice of empiric antibiotic(s) should be based on the severity of the infection, consideration of the most likely pathogens, and knowledge of their probable antibiotic susceptibility pattern (Table 34-4). Additional considerations include whether or not the patient has had any recent antibiotic therapy, if he has any allergies or comorbidities, which agents have been shown to be effective in DFI, cost and convenience of the drugs, and any formulary restrictions. Suggested guidance on selecting antibiotic therapy is shown in Table 34-5. For a patient with a mild or moderate DFI, who has not had any prior recent antibiotic treatment, empirically selecting an oral agent targeting only aerobic gram-positive cocci (especially *Staphylococcus aureus*) is usually sufficient. When the infection is chronic, or the patient has been treated with antimicrobials, aerobic gram-negative organisms often join the gram-positives. In cases of severe infection empirical antibiotic therapy should be administrated parenterally and should be broad-spectrum, covering staphylococci, streptococci, and commonly reported gram-negatives. Obligate anaerobes are almost always part of a mixed infection and usually one accompanied by gangrene or ischemia.

Initial empiric antibiotic choices may need to be adapted based on the results of culture and sensitivity tests. If the patient is clinically responding, it may not be necessary to cover all isolates, especially relatively avirulent organisms (eg, coagulase-negative staphylococci or enterococci) isolated from a suboptimal wound specimen. The clinician should attempt to narrow unnecessarily broad-spectrum therapy whenever possible and consider switching from parenteral to oral therapy when the patient's general clinical condition and wound infection have improved. Antibiotic therapy

Table 34-4. Factors That May Influence the Choice of an Antibiotic Regimen for Diabetic Foot Infections (Specific Agents, Route of Administration, and Duration of Therapy)[a]

Infection-related
– Clinical severity of the infection (Table 34-1)
– History of antibiotic therapy within previous 3 months
– Presence of bone infection (presumed or proven)
Pathogen-related
– Likelihood of nongram-positive cocci etiological agent(s)
– History of colonization or infection with MDROs
– Local rates of antibiotic resistance
Patient-related
– Allergies to antibiotics
– Impaired immunological status
– Patient treatment preferences
– Renal or hepatic insufficiency
– Impaired gastrointestinal absorption
– Arterial insufficiency in affected limb
– Exposure to environment with high risk of MDROs or unusual pathogens
Drug-related
– Safety profile (frequency and severity of adverse effects)
– Drug interaction potential
– Frequency of dosing
– Formulary availability/restrictions
– Cost considerations (acquisition and administration)
– Approval for indication
– Likelihood of inducing *Clostridium difficile* disease or antibiotic resistance
– Published efficacy data

Abbreviations: MDRO = multidrug resistant organism.
[a] From IWGDF Guidelines 2012 (7).

need only be given until resolution of the infectious signs and symptoms and not prolonged until the complete healing of the wound. The usual duration needed for soft tissue infection is 1 to 3 weeks.

Surgical Interventions

Surgical procedures are needed for most severe infections and for many moderate and some mild infections. These may range from minor bedside debridement or incision and drainage, performed at the bedside or in the clinic, to major operative procedures (eg, drainage of abscess, bone resection) that are done in the operating theater. Surgery should not be delayed in cases of life- or limb-threatening infections, such as extensive soft tissue necrosis or gas gangrene. Consider a surgical exploration when there are systemic signs of infection that are not responding, or there is local evidence suggesting a deep infection. All wounds require daily inspection and some will need serial debridement. If conservative surgical management has not resolved the infection, or has left the patient with a nonfunctional foot, or if there is recurrence of the ulcers despite appropriate preventive treatment, an elective amputation may be the best option. Efforts should be made to make the amputation at as low an anatomical level as possible. Patients with evidence of limb ischemia should undergo vascular evaluation; if blood flow is inadequate (based on transcutaneous oxygen measurements or other appropriate studies) consider early revascularization by open surgery or an endovascular approach (13).

Additional Care

Antibiotics and surgery are necessary, but not sufficient, to cure DFI. Concomitant with these specific treatments clinicians must also manage metabolic disorders (principally hyperglycemia) and comorbidities, such as cardiovascular disease or kidney failure (Figure 34-2). Wounds should be covered with properly selected dressings (largely dependent on whether they are predominantly dry or exudative), and any pressure on the wound must be adequately off-loaded (10). Effective off-loading is also an important aspect of the successful clinical management of DFU. The total contact cast (TCC) and other nonremovable devices are most effective because they avoid the problem of patient nonadherence to using the device. Contraindications to using a TCC are acute infection, limb ischemia, deep ulcers, and draining wounds. Uncomplicated plantar ulcers should heal in 6 to 8 weeks with adequate off-loading (14). Hyperbaric oxygen (HBO) therapy is defined as the inhalation of 100% oxygen at pressures greater than sea level. HBO has been shown to improve formation of granulation tissue, improve leukocyte function, stimulate angiogenesis, and promote vasoconstriction that reduces edema (15,16). Although HBO has been used as an adjunct

Table 34-5. Suggested Empiric Antibiotic Recommendations Based on Clinical Severity for Diabetic Foot Infections

Infection Severity	Probable Pathogens(s)	Antibiotic Agent	Comments
Mild (usually treated with oral agent[s])	MSSA; *Streptococcus* spp.	Dicloxacillin	Requires QID dosing; narrow spectrum; inexpensive
		Clindamycin	Usually active against community-associated MRSA but check macrolide sensitivity and consider ordering a "D-test" before using for MRSA; inhibits protein synthesis of some bacterial toxins
		Cephalexin	Requires QID dosing; inexpensive
		Levofloxacin	Once daily dosing; suboptimal against *S. aureus*
		Amoxicillin/clavulanate	Relatively broad-spectrum oral agent that includes anaerobic coverage
	MRSA	Doxycycline	Active against many MRSA and some gram-negatives; uncertain against *Streptococcus* spp.
		Trimethoprim/ sulfamethoxazole	Active against many MRSA and some gram-negatives; uncertain against streptococci
Moderate (may be treated with oral or initial parenteral agent[s]) or severe (usually treated with parenteral agent[s])	MSSA; *Streptococcus* spp.; Enterobacteriaceae; obligate anaerobes	Levofloxacin	Once a day dosing; suboptimal against *S. aureus*
		Cefoxitin	Second-generation cephalosporin with anaerobic coverage
		Ceftriaxone	Once daily dosing; third-generation cephalosporin
		Ampicillin/sulbactam	Adequate if low suspicion of *Pseudomonas aeruginosa*
		Moxifloxacin	Once-daily oral dosing; relatively broad spectrum, including most obligate anaerobic organisms
		Ertapenem	Once-daily dosing; relatively broad spectrum, including anaerobes, but not active against *P. aeruginosa*
		Tigecycline	Active against MRSA; spectrum may be excessively broad; high rates of nausea and vomiting and increased mortality warning; nonequivalent to ertapenem + vancomycin in 1 randomized clinical trial
		Levofloxacin or ciprofloxacin with clindamycin	Limited evidence supporting clindamycin for severe *S. aureus* infections; PO & IV formulations for both drugs
		Imipenem-cilastatin	Very broad spectrum (but not only against MRSA); use only when this is required; consider when ESBL-producing pathogens suspected
	MRSA	Linezolid	Expensive; increased risk of toxicities when used more than 2 weeks
		Daptomycin	Once-daily dosing; requires serial monitoring of CPK
		Vancomycin	Vancomycin MICs for MRSA gradually increasing
	Pseudomonas aeruginosa	Piperacillin/tazobactam	TID/QID dosing; useful for broad-spectrum coverage; *P. aeruginosa* is an uncommon pathogen in DFI except in special circumstances
	MRSA, Enterobacteriaceae, *Pseudomonas*, and obligate anaerobes	Vancomycin plus 1 of the following: ceftazidime, cefepime, piperacillin-tazobactam, aztreonam, or a carbapenem	Very broad-spectrum coverage; usually only used for empiric therapy of severe infection; consider addition of obligate anaerobes coverage if ceftazidime, cefepime, or aztreonam selected

Abbreviations: MIC = minimum inhibitory concentration; MRSA = methicillin-resistant S. aureus; *MSSA = methicillin-sensitive* S. aureus; *ESBL = extended spectrum beta-lactamase; CPK = creatine phosphokinase.*

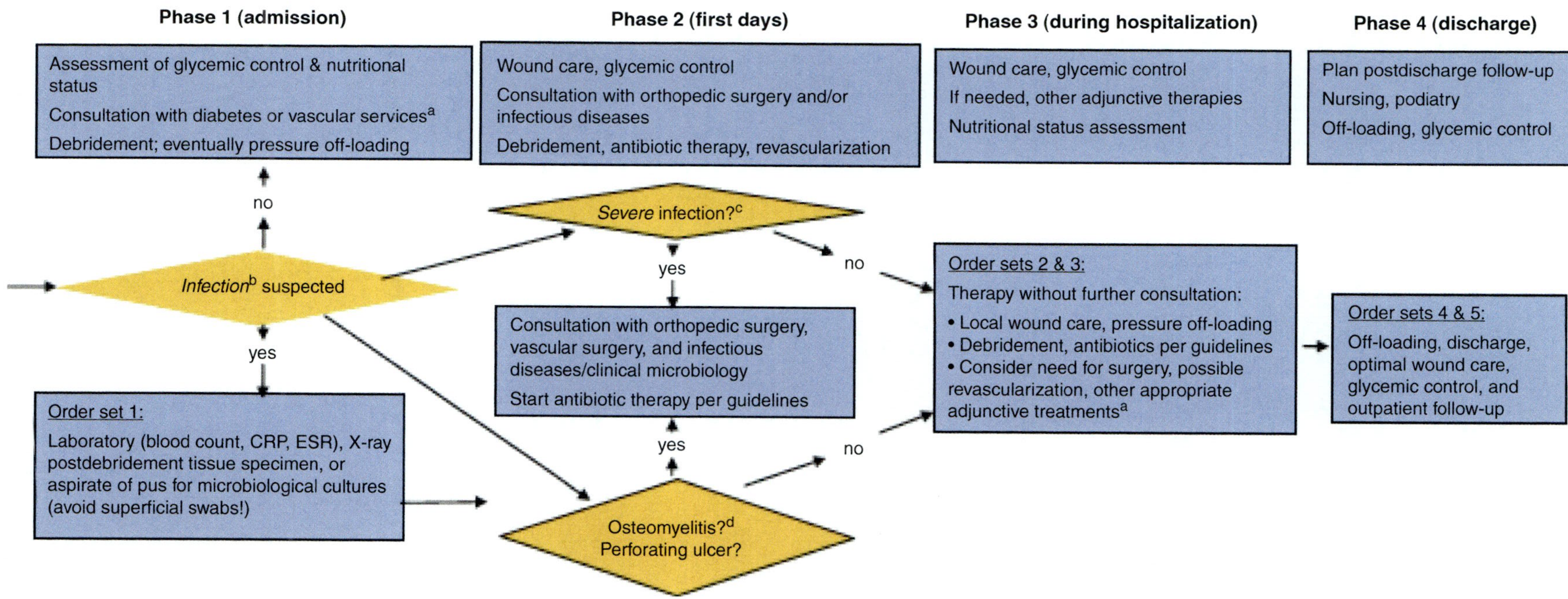

[a] Ankle-brachial index; $TcPO_2$ only if amputation planned
[b] Pus, local warmth, redness, induration, pain/tenderness
[c] Hypotension, chills, fever, necrotizing fasciitis, extensive gangrene, leukocytosis, blood cultures (2 pairs)
[d] Palpable or visible bone, characteristic lesions on X-ray or MRI; osteomyelitis does not always need surgery or antibiotic treatment

Figure 34-2. Suggested scheme for management of patients with diabetic foot wounds.

for healing DFU for decades, and despite many clinical trials, its efficacy remains a matter of debate (17–19). A Cochrane systematic review concluded that HBO led to an increased rate of ulcer healing at short-term follow-up (6 weeks) but not longer-term follow-up (1 year) and did not appear to reduce the major amputation rate (20). Because the function of leukocytes may be altered in patients with diabetes, administering granulocyte-colony stimulating factor (G-CSF) has been evaluated for DFI in several studies. A recent Cochrane review reported on studies of the effects of administering various types of adjunctive G-CSF compared with a placebo or no growth factor in patients with DFI. It concluded there was no evidence of increased rates of infection cure or wound healing with adjunctive G-CSF, but there was a reduced need for surgical procedures, especially amputations, and a reduced length of hospital stay (21).

OSTEOMYELITIS

Osteomyelitis is apparent at presentation in about 20% of cases of all DFI, but in over 60% of severe infections. Its clinical manifestations can vary depending on the site involved, the extent of the infection, the causative pathogen(s), the involvement of soft tissue, and the vascular status. Suspect osteomyelitis in a patient with an infected, large, or deep wound, particularly if the ulcer is chronic, or if there is a swollen, erythematous ("sausage") toe. The probe-to-bone test is a valuable diagnostic tool when correctly performed (with a sterile blunt metal probe, after wound debridement) and interpreted (based on the likelihood of osteomyelitis). For patients with a low pretest probability of osteomyelitis a negative test substantially reduces the likelihood of osteomyelitis (22). When the pretest probability of osteomyelitis is high, a positive test has a high predictive value for osteomyelitis (23).

Imaging for osteomyelitis generally begins with plain X-rays, but these have a relatively low sensitivity (for acute infection) and specificity. The main issue is differentiating osteomyelitis from noninfectious CN (Table 34-6) (24). Serial plain films over time may be useful for diagnosis and follow-up. Computed tomography (CT) scans or nuclear medicine imaging (eg, with ^{99tm}TC-methylene diphosphonate) is more sensitive but relatively nonspecific (25). Among the advanced imaging tests, MRI is currently the best technique, not only for the diagnosis of bone infection but also to appreciate deep soft tissue or sinus tract involvement. The few available studies of newer procedures such as single-photon emission CT (SPECT)/CT and positron-emission tomography (PET) combined with MRI suggest they may be more accurate than MRI alone (8).

The generally accepted criterion standard for diagnosing osteomyelitis remains obtaining a specimen of bone (either at surgery or percutaneously) for the combination of microbiological culture and histopathological evaluation (26,27). This approach is not always needed, but is particularly useful when there is diagnostic uncertainty, uninterpretable cultures, or a nonresponse to empirical antibiotic therapy. Osteomyelitis is generally treated with antibiotic therapy, either alone or combined with surgery to removed necrotic and infected bone. The duration of antibiotic therapy for osteomyelitis remains controversial, but depends on whether or not necrotic bone has been resected, and probably does not need to exceed 4 to 6 weeks (28). A trial of antibiotic therapy alone can be undertaken in selected cases; several retrospective studies (29,30) and 1 recent prospective study show a remission rate of 60% to 70% (31). Surgical resection may allow a reduced hospital stay, a shorter duration of antibiotic treatment, and higher remission rates, but can be associated with operative and postoperative complications.

NECROTIZING FASCIITIS

Necrotizing fasciitis (NF) is a life-threatening, rapidly progressive, invasive soft tissue infection involving subcutaneous fat and deep fascia layers (2,32). The rapid tissue necrosis often leads to systemic sepsis, toxic-shock like syndrome, and multi-organ failure. The mortality of NF is reported to be 15% to 30%. NF in diabetic patients is usually polymicrobial and most often involves both aerobic organisms (especially streptococci, staphylococci, Enterobacteriaceae) and obligate anaerobes (usually *Bacteroides* species, peptostreptococci). Less commonly, infection may be monomicrobial, usually with β-hemolytic streptococci or

Table 34-6. Characteristic Features of Osteomyelitis and Charcot Neuropathic-Osteoarthropathy on Plain X-Ray and MRI (24)

Plain Radiographs[a]	
Osteomyelitis	Charcot neuropathic-osteoarthropathy
➤ Periosteal reaction or elevation ➤ Loss of cortex with bony erosion ➤ Focal loss of trabecular pattern or marrow radiolucency ➤ New bone formation ➤ Bone sclerosis with or without erosion ➤ Sequestrum: devitalized bone with radiodense appearance that has become separated from normal bone ➤ Involucrum: a layer of new bone growth outside existing bone resulting from the stripping off of the periosteum and new bone growing from the periosteum ➤ Cloacae: opening in involucrum or cortex through which sequestra or granulation tissue may be discharged	➤ Nonspecific changes: ✓ Periosteal reaction ✓ Traumatic fractures ✓ Bone destruction ✓ Joint fragmentation and dislocation
MRI[a]	
Osteomyelitis	Charcot neuropathic-osteoarthropathy
➤ Low focal signal intensity on T1-weighted images ➤ High focal signal on T2-weighted images ➤ High bone marrow signal in short tau inversion recovery sequences ➤ Less specific or secondary changes: ✓ Cortical disruption ✓ Adjacent cutaneous ulcer ✓ Soft tissue mass ✓ Sinus tract formation ✓ Adjacent soft tissue inflammation or edema	➤ Altered bone marrow signal manifested by low signal intensity in the subchondral bone on both T1- and T2-weighted images ➤ Signal intensity abnormalities demonstrated by osteosclerosis and cyst-like lesion ➤ Cortical fragmentation ➤ Joint deformity or subluxation ➤ Bone marrow edema pattern: tends to be periarticular and subchondral ➤ Predominant midfoot involvement ➤ Deformity common along with bony debris ➤ Overlying skin usually intact but may be edematous

[a] *For both modalities, bony changes are often accompanied by contiguous soft tissue swelling.*

staphylococci (33). Gas gangrene is a less common separate entity that is usually caused by *Clostridium* species.

NF typically begins as an area of inflamed, swollen skin, with or without a history of recent local trauma. Although diagnosis in the early stages may be difficult, it is important to differentiate more common skin infections, such as erysipelas, cellulitis, or soft tissue abscess, from the more dangerous NF. In NF, pain may be disproportionately severe compared to the limited visible extent of infection. Conversely, as infection progresses there may be new onset local anesthesia, presumably related to necrosis of nerve fibers. NF can be accompanied by fever and crepitus, but spontaneous drainage and pus are usually not present. As the infection progresses, bullae, petechiae, ecchymoses, purplish coloration, and skin lesions resembling deep burns may develop. NF can involve almost any part of the body, including the foot in cases with preexisting ulcers. Scoring systems using clinical findings and blood tests, as well as CT, may aid in suspected NF, but direct examination of the involved tissues is usually necessary to make a definitive diagnosis (33).

Using multivariable analysis, 1 study of patients with NF found that the presence of diabetes was associated with a significantly increased risk of amputation, as were other selected underlying conditions and evidence of cutaneous gangrene on admission (34). Similarly, factors found to be associated with significantly increased mortality include underlying conditions, advanced or very young age, or evidence of sepsis (34).

Treatment of NF requires rapid fluid and electrolyte corrections, hemodynamic stabilization, support for failing organ systems, and appropriate parenteral antibiotic therapy. Several different regimens of antibiotics have been recommended, and the choice may be institution dependent. In general, consider broad-spectrum agents, such as piperacillin-tazobactam, or carbapenems, often with concomitant clindamycin, or vancomycin if methicillin-resistant *Staphylococcus aureus* (MRSA) is suspected. In addition, early aggressive surgical debridement (often repeated to ensure all necrotic tissue has been removed) is usually necessary. Delayed or inadequate operative debridement may be associated with increased mortality rates. In a few cases, an experienced surgeon may decide that urgent ablative surgery may not be needed; in such cases, frequent, careful follow-up is mandatory. Various adjunctive treatments, including HBO and IV immunoglobulin, have been used but their efficacy is unclear.

CHARCOT NEUROPATHIC-OSTEOARTHROPATHY

CN is a noninfectious condition affecting bone, joints, and soft tissues of the foot and ankle. The exact pathogenesis remains unclear, but available evidence suggests that it is caused by a combination of peripheral neuropathy, PAD, unrecognized or untreated injury, and continued repetitive trauma (35,36). In addition, other potential contributory factors include reduced bone density, nonenzymatic collagen glycation, and excessive local inflammation accompanied by increases in various cytokines (eg, tumor necrosis factor-alpha, interleukin-1 beta) (37).

In the acute phase a Charcot foot is erythematous, indurated, and painful and may be mistaken for gout, deep venous thrombosis, cellulitis, or a sprain (36). In the chronic phase CN is associated with subluxations and fractures, especially of the midfoot (Lisfranc injury), causing substantial deformity. The estimated prevalence of CN among persons with diabetes is 7.5% with an incidence of about 0.2%, but the true figure is probably higher because many cases remain undiagnosed (38,39). CN is indirectly a potentially limb- (and even life-) threatening condition because the resultant foot deformities lead to high pressures, recurrent ulcerations, and potentially to lower extremity amputation (40).

CN can be classified by anatomical localization, clinical stage, or natural history. Pain is often minimal or absent, due to the sensory neuropathy, and pedal pulses are usually present (37). Plain radiographs are the first-line imaging method, but they can be normal for up to 3 weeks after the start of the acute episode. Typical early radiographical findings include subtle fractures and dislocations, while in later stages features such as "pencil in cup" deformity of the metatarsophalangeal joints or talocalcaneal dislocation are common (41). In the absence of characteristic findings, MRI can provide a noninvasive and sensitive diagnostic tool in the evaluation of soft tissue and bone marrow abnormalities (42–44). Nuclear medicine studies, such as 3-phase bone scans with technetium-99m (^{99m} Tc), provide an alternative technique when MRI is unavailable or contraindicated (45). As with osteomyelitis, bone scans have a high sensitivity for early CN but lack specificity.

The management of active CN consists mainly of immediate pressure off-loading, optimally with a TCC (46), which should be replaced after ~3 days, then changed every week to permit examination of the foot. Casting is usually needed for 3 to 6 months, or until there is a resolution of the swelling and warmth and evidence of healing on X-rays or MRI. After resolution of the acute episode the most appropriate type of device will depend on the level of deformities. For patients with a minor foot deformity, prefabricated footwear with extra depth and a stiff rocker bottom walking sole is appropriate, while for moderate deformity, consider a custom-made shoe associated with custom-molded, full contact insoles. In situations with severe foot deformities or ankle involvement, a removable Charcot Restraint Orthotic Walker (CROW) is useful. Close monitoring is also required after an acute episode for all stages (47).

In cases of CN refractory to off-loading and immobilization, or when ulcers fail to heal, surgical treatment is generally beneficial to prevent severe deformity or joint instability. It is preferable to delay the surgery after the acute phase of CN to avoid the risk of secondary infection or mechanical failure. In cases where a bony prominence leads to ulcers that cannot be accommodated with prosthetics or orthotics, exostectomy is usually required. When there is abnormal plantar pressure distribution, consider an Achilles tendon lengthening or gastrocnemius tendon reduction to decrease forefoot pressure and improve alignment of the ankle and hindfoot to the midfoot and forefoot. In cases of recurrent ulcers, arthrodesis may be helpful. If these procedures fail to stabilize the foot an amputation may be required.

Various medical therapies, such as bisphosphonates, have been tried for the management of acute CN. In some studies bisphosphonate treatment has reduced skin temperature and bone turnover, but the long-term efficacy, particularly for preventing the occurrence of ulcerations and deformities, remains unclear (48). Early identification and management of acute CN is necessary to avoid the rapid progression toward permanent foot deformation and its associated devastating complications.

PERIPHERAL ARTERIAL DISEASE (PAD)

PAD is present in about half of patients with a DFU and is an independent risk factor for limb loss in diabetes (49). Identifying PAD can be challenging in these patients as the signs and the symptoms may be masked (or mimicked) by coexisting distal symmetrical polyneuropathy. All patients presenting with a foot ulcer should undergo at least a basic evaluation of the vascular status of the lower extremities. This should include a history (specifically targeting claudication, rest pain, and any previous vascular assessments) and palpation of pedal (dorsalis pedis and posterior tibial) pulses. Patients without palpable pedal pulses or with clinical signs of ischemia should be evaluated with a hand-held Doppler device to assess for the presence of pulses, identify their waveforms (mono-, bi-, or triphasic), and measure ankle brachial index (ABI). If these examinations are inconclusive, consider measuring the transcutaneous pressure of oxygen ($TcPO_2$) or toe-brachial index (TBI) (50). An ABI <0.6, a $TcPO_2$ <50 mm Hg, or toe pressure <55 mm Hg suggest clinically significant ischemia, with a low probability of wound healing (51).

A vascular surgeon or angiologist should assess patients with signs, symptoms, or Doppler evidence of clinically significant PAD. Among radiological evaluations of PAD, most consider intra-arterial digital subtraction angiography optimal because of its high spatial resolution. Although it allows concomitant endovascular therapy during the procedure, it can provoke contrast-induced nephropathy, allergic reactions, or severe hematomas. Color Doppler ultrasound (CDUS) is a relatively inexpensive and noninvasive technique but requires specialized knowledge, and its reliability is dependent on operator expertise. It can be useful as the basis for initial clinical decisions but needs to be performed in conjunction with other radiological procedures, such as contrast-enhanced magnetic resonance angiography (CE-MRA), CT angiography (CTA), or intra-arterial digital subtraction angiography. CE-MRA is a minimally invasive, highly sensitive procedure associated with limited risk of nephrotoxicity (by use of paramagnetic contrast agents) and no exposure to radiation. The disadvantages, in addition to the usual contraindications for MRI, are the possibility of artifacts, if there have been previous stent implantations, and limited spatial resolution (52). CTA has similar diagnostic accuracy to CE-MRA, and is a rapid and relatively noninvasive procedure with better spatial resolution than CE-MRA. However, it is less useful in the presence of severely calcified arteries, exposes the patient to radiation, and can cause contrast-induced nephropathy (53).

The decision on when to revascularize a patient with an ulcerated foot remains complex. Considerations should include the probability of wound healing without revascularization compared with the potential benefits and risks of a revascularization procedure. Patients with good skin perfusion ($TcPO_2$ >50 mm Hg), relatively mild PAD (ABI ≥0.6), and a small wound can usually be treated initially by optimal wound care and a 6-week period of observation. Patients who present with more severe PAD, especially if associated with a foot infection and large ulceration, usually benefit from early revascularization. The clinician must then choose between open bypass surgery and endovascular interventions. Although there are several published cases series using each procedure, there are no randomized controlled clinical trials comparing the 2 techniques in patients with ischemic DFU. Available data and systematic reviews suggest the outcomes are similar, and there is insufficient evidence to recommend one method of revascularization over another (54). Selecting a treatment strategy relies on issues such as the extent and the site of the disease, the patient's associated comorbidities, and the preferences and skills of the available operators.

CONCLUSIONS

Foot ulcerations complicated by infection are a major and growing problem for patients with diabetes. These disorders largely result from peripheral neuropathy and PAD and are associated with severe consequences if they are not properly managed. DFI is often an epiphenomenon, reflecting poor glycemic control, and is associated with increased morbidity and mortality. Many of the studies published in past decades have allowed experts to develop robust recommendations and guidelines for management of DFI and CN. Perhaps the most important task to undertake now is to develop a multidisciplinary team infrastructure that permits optimal care for these complications with appropriate ongoing education of patients and health care providers about the importance of prevention and early recognition of diabetes-related foot problems (9,55).

ACKNOWLEDGMENTS

The authors have nothing to disclose.

REFERENCES

1. **Singh N, Armstrong DG, Lipsky BA.** Preventing foot ulcers in patients with diabetes. *JAMA.* 2005;12;293:217–228.
2. **Reiber GE, Vileikyte L, Boyko EJ, et al.** Causal pathways for incident lower-extremity ulcers in patients with diabetes from two settings. *Diabetes Care.* 1999;22:157–162.
3. **National diabetes audit executive summary 2011–12.** The NHS Information Centre 2012. http://www.hscic.gov.uk/nda.
4. **Pecoraro RE, Reiber GE, Burgess EM.** Pathways to diabetic limb amputation. Basis for prevention. *Diabetes Care.* 1990;13:513–521.
5. **Morbach S, Furchert H, Gröblinghoff U, et al.** Long-term prognosis of diabetic foot patients and their limbs: amputation and death over the course of a decade. *Diabetes Care.* 2012;35:2021–2027.
6. **Lipsky BA, Berendt AR, Cornia PB, et al.** 2012 Infectious Diseases Society of America Clinical Practice Guideline for the diagnosis and treatment of diabetic foot infections. *Clin Infect Dis.* 2012;54:e132–e173.
7. **Lipsky BA, Peters EJ, Senneville E, et al.** Expert opinion on the management of infections in the diabetic foot. *Diabetes Metab Res Rev.* 2012;28(suppl 1):163–178.
8. **Israel O, Sconfienza LM, Lipsky BA.** Diagnosing diabetic foot infection: the role of imaging and a proposed flow chart for assessment. *Q J Nucl Med Mol Imaging.* 2013;57:1–13.
9. **Wukich DK, Armstrong DG, Attinger CE, et al.** Inpatient management of diabetic foot disorders: a clinical guide. *Diabetes Care.* 2013;36:2862–2871.
10. **Armstrong DG, Bharara M, White M, et al.** The impact and outcomes of establishing an integrated interdisciplinary surgical team to care for the diabetic foot. *Diabetes Metab Res Rev.* 2012;28:514–518.
11. **Lazzarini PA, O'Rourke SR, Russell AW, Derhy PH, Kamp MC.** Standardising practices improves clinical diabetic foot management: the Queensland Diabetic Foot Innovation Project, 2006–09. *Aust Health Rev.* 2012;36:8–15.
12. **Nather A, Siok Bee C, Keng Lin W, et al.** Value of team approach combined with clinical pathway for diabetic foot problems: a clinical evaluation. *Diabet Foot Ankle.* 2010;1:1–5.
13. **Setacci C, Sirignano P, Mazzitelli G, et al.** Diabetic foot: surgical approach in emergency. *Int J Vasc Med.* 2013;2013:296169.
14. **Cavanagh PR, Bus SA.** Off-loading the diabetic foot for ulcer prevention and healing. *J Vasc Surg.* 2010;52(suppl 3):37S–43S.
15. **Hunt TK, Pai MP.** The effect of varying ambient oxygen tensions on wound metabolism and collagen synthesis. *Surg Gynecol Obstet.* 1972;135:561–567.
16. **Hunt TK, Linsey M, Grislis H, Sonne M, Jawetz E.** The effect of differing ambient oxygen tensions on wound infection. *Ann Surg.* 1975;181:35–39.
17. **Liu R, Li L, Yang M, Boden G, Yang G.** Systematic review of the effectiveness of the hyperbaric oxygenation therapy in the management of chronic diabetic foot ulcers. *Mayo Clin Proc.* 2013;88:166–175.
18. **Margolis DJ, Gupta J, Hoffstad O, et al.** Lack of effectiveness of hyperbaric oxygen therapy for the treatment of diabetic foot ulcer and the prevention of amputation: a cohort study. *Diabetes Care.* 2013;36:1961–1966.
19. **Berendt AR.** Counterpoint: hyperbaric oxygen for diabetic foot wounds is not effective. *Clin Infect Dis.* 2006;15;43:193–198.
20. **Kranke P, Bennet MH, Martyn-St James M, Schnabel A, Debus SE.** Hyperbaric oxygen therapy for chronic wounds. *Cochrane Database Syst Rev.* 2012;4:CD004123.
21. **Cruciani M, Lipsky BA, Mengoli C, de Lalla F.** Granulocyte-colony stimulating factors as adjunctive therapy for diabetic foot infections. *Cochrane Database Syst Rev.* 2013;17:8.
22. **Butalia S, Palda VA, Sargeant RJ, Detsky AS, Mourad O.** Does this patient with diabetes have osteomyelitis of the lower extremity? *JAMA.* 2008;20;299:806–813.
23. **Aragón-Sánchez J, Lipsky BA, Lázaro-Martínez JL.** Diagnosing diabetic foot osteomyelitis: is the combination of probe-to-bone test and plain radiography sufficient for high-risk inpatients? *Diabet Med.* 2011;28:191–194.
24. **Ertugrul BM, Lipsky BA, Sayk O.** Osteomyelitis or Charcot neuro-osteoarthropathy? Differentiating these disorders in diabetic patients with a foot problem. *Diabet Foot Ankle.* 2013;5:4.
25. **Uçkay I, Gariani K, Pataky Z, Lipsky BA.** Diabetic foot infections: state-of-the-art. *Diabetes Obes Metab.* 2014;16(4):305–316.

26. **Hatzenbuehler J, Pulling TJ.** Diagnosis and management of osteomyelitis. *Am Fam Physician.* 2011;84:1027–1033.
27. **Berendt AR, Peters EJ, Bakker K, et al.** Diabetic foot osteomyelitis: a progress report on diagnosis and a systematic review of treatment. *Diabetes Metab Res Rev* 2008;24(suppl 1):S145–S161.
28. **Lazzarini L, Lipsky BA, Mader JT.** Antibiotic treatment of osteomyelitis: what have we learned from 30 years of clinical trials? *Int J Infect Dis.* 2005;9:127–138.
29. **Pittet D, Wyssa B, Herter-Clavel C, Kursteiner K, Vaucher J, Lew PD.** Outcome of diabetic foot infections treated conservatively: a retrospective cohort study with long-term follow-up. *Arch Intern Med.* 1999;159:851–856.
30. **Jeffcoate WJ, Lipsky BA.** Controversies in diagnosing and managing osteomyelitis of the foot in diabetes. *Clin Infect Dis.* 2004;39(suppl 2):S115–S122.
31. **Lázaro-Martínez J, Aragón-Sánchez J, García-Morales E.** Antibiotics versus conservative surgery for treating diabetic foot osteomyelitis. A randomized comparative trial. *Diabetes Care.* 2014;37(3):789–795.
32. **Jallali NJ.** Necrotising fasciitis: its aetiology, diagnosis and management. *Wound Care.* 2003;12:297–300.
33. **Ustin JA, Malangoni MA.** Necrotizing soft-tissue infections. *Crit Care Med.* 2011;39:2156–2162.
34. **Dworkin MS, Westercamp MD, Park L, McIntyre A.** The epidemiology of necrotizing fasciitis including factors associated with death and amputation. *Epidemiol Infect.* 2009;137:1609–1614.
35. **Rogers LC, Frykberg RG, Armstrong DG, et al.** The Charcot foot in diabetes. *Diabetes Care.* 2011;34:2123–2129.
36. **Wukich DK, Sung W, Wipf SA, Armstrong DG.** The consequence of complacency: managing the effects of unrecognized Charcot feet. *Diabet Med.* 2011;28:195–198.
37. **Papanas N, Maltezos E.** Etiology, pathophysiology and classifications of the diabetic Charcot foot. *Diabet Foot Ankle.* 2013;May 21:4.
38. **Rathur RM, Boulton HAM.** Recent advances in the diagnosis and management of diabetic neuropathy. *J Bone Joint Surg Br.* 2005;87-B:1605–1610.
39. **Gouveri E, Papanas N.** Charcot osteoarthropathy in diabetes: a brief review with an emphasis on clinical practice. *World J Diabetes.* 2011;2:59–65.
40. **van Baal J, Hubbard R, Game F, Jeffcoate W.** Mortality associated with acute Charcot foot and neuropathic foot ulceration. *Diabetes Care.* 2010;33:1086–1089.
41. **Rajbhandari SM, Jenkins RC, Davies C, Tesfaye S.** Charcot neuroarthropathy in diabetes mellitus. *Diabetologia.* 2002;45:1085–1096.
42. **Kapoor A, Page S, Lavalley M, Gale DR, Felson DT.** Magnetic resonance imaging for diagnosing foot osteomyelitis: a meta-analysis. *Arch Intern Med.* 2007;167:125–132.
43. **Zampa V, Bargellini I, Rizzo L, et al.** Role of dynamic MRI in follow-up of acute Charcot foot in patients with diabetes mellitus. *Skeletal Radiol.* 2011;40:991–999.
44. **Schlossbauer T, Mioc T, Sommerey S, Kessler SB, Reiser MF, Pfeifer KJ.** Magnetic resonance imaging in early stage Charcot arthropathy—coorelation of imaging findings and clinical symptoms. *Eur J Med Res.* 2008;13:409–414.
45. **Prandini N, Beretta F.** Nuclear medicine imaging of diabetic foot. In: Lazzeri E, Signore A, Erba PA, et al, eds. *Radionuclide Imaging of Infection and Inflammation.* New York: Springer; 2013: 253–269.
46. **Van der Ven A, Chapman CB, Bowker JH.** Charcot neuroarthropathy of the foot and ankle. *J Am Acad Orthop Surg.* 2009;17:562–571.
47. **Milne TE, Rogers JR, Kinnear EW.** Developing an evidence-based clinical pathway for the assessment, diagnosis and management of acute Charcot neuroarthropathy: a systematic review. *J Foot Ankle Res.* 2013;6:30.
48. **Richard JL, Almasri M, Schuldiner S.** Treatment of acute Charcot foot with bisphosphonates: a systematic review of the literature. *Diabetologia.* 2012;55:1258–1264.
49. **Prompers L, Huijberts M, Apelqvist J, et al.** High prevalence of ischaemia, infection and serious comorbidity in patients with diabetic foot disease in Europe. Baseline results from the Eurodiale study. *Diabetologia.* 2007;50:18–25.
50. **Schaper NC, Andros G, Apelqvist J, et al.** Diagnosis and treatment of peripheral arterial disease in diabetic patients with a foot ulcer. A progress report of the International Working Group on the Diabetic Foot. *Diabetes Metab Res Rev.* 2012;28(suppl 1):218–224.
51. **Kalani M, Brismar K, Fagrell B, Ostergren J, Jörneskog G.** Transcutaneous oxygen tension and toe blood pressure as predictors for outcome of diabetic foot ulcers. *Diabetes Care.* 1999;22:147–151.
52. **Koelemay MJ, Lijmer JG, Stoker J, Legemate DA, Bossuyt PM.** Magnetic resonance angiography for the evaluation of lower extremity arterial disease: a meta-analysis. *JAMA.* 2001;285:1338–1345.
53. **Met R, Bipat S, Legemate DA, Reekers JA, Koelemay MJ.** Diagnostic performance of computed tomography angiography in peripheral arterial disease: a systematic review and meta-analysis. *JAMA.* 2009;301:415–424.
54. **Hinchliffe RJ, Andros G, Apelqvist J, et al.** A systematic review of the effectiveness of revascularization of the ulcerated foot in patients with diabetes and peripheral arterial disease. *Diabetes Metab Res Rev.* 2012;28(suppl 1):179–217.
55. **Darbellay P, Uçkay I, Dominguez D, et al.** Diabetic foot infection: a multidisciplinary approach. *Rev Med Suisse.* 2011;7:894–897.

CHAPTER 35

Emergent Diabetes Management in Pregnancy

Natasha Kasid and Florence Brown

ABSTRACT

Despite goals targeting near normal glycemia in pregnancies complicated by preexisting or newly diagnosed diabetes, pregnant women with diabetes may present with urgent challenges. Suboptimal outpatient glycemic control in the woman who presents with a newly diagnosed unplanned pregnancy, extremes of blood glucose levels as with diabetic ketoacidosis (DKA) and severe hypoglycemia, iatrogenic hyperglycemia from treatment with glucocorticoids to promote fetal lung maturity, and rapidly changing insulin requirements during the peripartum period presents unique and emergent challenges to the health care provider. The pathophysiology, effects on the mother and fetus, and management of these diabetes-related emergencies are briefly discussed.

INTRODUCTION

Despite goals targeting near normal glycemia in pregnancies complicated by preexisting and newly diagnosed diabetes, pregnant women with diabetes may present with urgent challenges. Suboptimal outpatient diabetes control in the woman who presents with a newly diagnosed unplanned pregnancy, extremes of blood glucose levels as with diabetic ketoacidosis (DKA) and severe hypoglycemia, iatrogenic hyperglycemia from treatment with glucocorticoids to promote fetal lung maturity, and rapidly changing insulin requirements during the peripartum period presents unique and emergent challenges to the health care provider. When any of these conditions occur, it is important to normalize glycemic control as quickly and safely as possible to avoid potential maternal, fetal, and neonatal complications. DKA due to underlying illness or suboptimal adherence or insulin pump catheter occlusion may occur at lower blood glucose levels in the ketosis-prone state of pregnancy. Severe hypoglycemia is more likely to occur in the setting of targeting near normal glycemia. Marked hyperglycemia is also seen in instances of inpatient glucocorticoid administration and requires insulin adjustment and close monitoring. Finally, in the postpartum period, insulin requirements markedly decrease as insulin resistance resolves after delivery of the placenta and a period of increased insulin sensitivity ensues. The pathophysiology, effects on the mother and fetus and management of these diabetes-related emergencies are briefly discussed.

SUBOPTIMAL OUTPATIENT DIABETES CONTROL DURING PREGNANCY

Ideally, the patient with preexisting diabetes should be evaluated preconception by a multidisciplinary team with a special focus on glycemic control and self-management skills, meal planning, physical activity, the status of diabetes-related complications, concurrent and past medical and obstetrical conditions, and contraception and medication use. The preconception hemoglobin A1c (A1C) target should be <7% if this can be achieved safely (1). The Diabetes Control and Complications Trial (DCCT), which compared intensive glycemic control to conventional care in individuals with type 1 diabetes and included women who became pregnant during the study, noted rates of congenital malformations of 1% in the intensive group versus 7% in the conventionally treated group when mean first trimester A1C levels (+/−1 SD) were 7.4% (+/−1.3%) versus 8.1% (+/−1.7%), respectively (2). However, Suhonen et al (3) found a 3-fold relative risk even when the A1C was only slightly raised (5.6%–6.8%). After pooling data from 7 cohort studies involving almost 2,000 patients, Guerin et al (4) developed a tool for estimating absolute risk of major or minor congenital malformation according to periconception A1C with absolute risk of 3% when the A1C is 6%–7%, 6% when the A1C is 9.0%, and up to 8%–20% when the A1C is greater than 10%. Numerous studies of preconception care with attainment of target A1C goals prior to conception demonstrate reduced risks of birth defects. A more detailed discussion of preconception care (and other aspects of management) has recently been reviewed in the 2013 Diabetes and Pregnancy Endocrine Society Clinical Practice Guidelines (5).

During pregnancy, optimal glycemic goals are premeal, bedtime, and overnight glucose 60–99 mg/dL (3.3–5.5 mmol/L), peak postprandial glucose 100–129 mg/dL (5.6–7.2 mmol/L), mean daily glucose <110 mg/dL (6 mmol/L), and A1C <6.0% with avoidance of significant hypoglycemia (6). Adverse pregnancy, fetal, and neonatal outcomes are associated with poor control of diabetes during pregnancy, including preeclampsia (7), spontaneous and indicated preterm delivery, macrosomia or large for gestational age (LGA), neonatal hypoglycemia, respiratory distress syndrome, hypertrophic cardiomyopathy, shoulder dystocia, and hyperbilirubinemia (8). Thus, rapid improvement of glycemic control and lowering of the A1C are necessary in pregnancies complicated by poorly controlled diabetes. However, rapid correction of hyperglycemia may also exacerbate or precipitate retinopathy (9). Therefore, evaluation of retinopathy and other complications of diabetes need to be closely monitored (5,6).

For patients treated with noninsulin agents for preexisting type 2 diabetes, it is important to discontinue these and transition to basal and bolus insulin regimens without compromising glycemic control. Intermediate-acting (NPH) and short-acting insulin has traditionally been the gold standard to treat diabetes during pregnancy. However, some insulin analogs have been shown to be safe and effective in pregnancy. Compared with NPH, the long-acting insulin analog detemir has been shown to achieve noninferior metabolic control (10). Fetal and perinatal outcomes, including preterm delivery <37 weeks, small for gestational age (SGA), LGA, macrosomia, neonatal hypoglycemia, congenital malformations, and live births and fetal losses, were similar except for longer gestational age in the detemir group (11). Recently, the Food and Drug Administration (FDA) has designated detemir as pregnancy category B. There have been no randomized controlled clinical trials of insulin glargine in pregnancy, although results of various observational studies do not find an increase in adverse maternal or neonatal events with glargine use (12). Glargine does have increased affinity for the insulin growth factor-1 (IGF-1) receptor, which plays a role in fetal development. The long-term risks of glargine use in pregnancy are not known. The FDA lists insulin glargine as category C for use in pregnancy. For patients who present to their first prenatal visit using glargine as long-acting basal insulin, we recommend switching to a 3 times daily NPH or twice daily detemir dosing schedule. However, the 2013 Diabetes and Pregnancy Endocrine Society Clinical Practice Guidelines suggest that if insulin glargine is successfully used before conception, it could be continued during pregnancy after discussion and documentation about the risk-benefit of this approach (5). The rapid-acting insulins, lispro and aspart, are widely used in nonpregnant individuals because they better mimic physiological insulin release with meals compared with short-acting insulin. Both lispro and aspart are FDA category B in pregnancy. Aspart and lispro are widely used in pregnancy and have been recommended by the 2013 Diabetes and Pregnancy Endocrine Society Clinical Practice Guidelines (5). There are no reports of glulisine in pregnancy, so it is not recommended.

When transitioning patients with type 2 diabetes from noninsulin therapies to insulin, one can initially estimate total daily insulin requirements based on 0.7–1.0 units/kg of body weight (6). Insulin requirements (units/kg/day) and total insulin requirements (units/day) peak in week 9, nadir in week 16, and peak again in week 37 (13). Over the course of pregnancy there is a greater increase in bolus (400%) compared with basal (50%) insulin requirements (14). From 30 weeks gestation to delivery, insulin requirements are variable and less pronounced than other weeks of pregnancy with about 40% of women demonstrating a 15% rise, 10% of women having a 15% fall in requirements, and the rest not having a significant change (15).

The American Diabetes Association (ADA) recommends persons with diabetes should be aware of sick-day rules, and in the setting of illness or unexplained or persistent glucose >200 mg/dL (11.1 mmol/L), it is recommended to check for presence of urine or serum ketones and to contact medical professionals if positive (16).

In patients who have poor outpatient glycemic control, it is important to assess any underlying cultural, financial, or personal stressors impairing their ability to manage their diabetes adequately. It will be important to provide a consultation with a registered dietician. Patients should keep daily food and self-monitoring of blood glucose (SMBG) records. Carbohydrates should be 40%–45% of total daily calories with 15–30 grams at breakfast, 45 grams at lunch and dinner, and 15–30 grams for a bedtime snack. In addition, patients should have 14 grams of fiber/1,000 kcal per day and 1.1 grams of protein per kg/day. In general, 30%–40% of total calories should come from fat with <10% of fat intake from saturated fat. To avoid hypoglycemia, patients should have consistent mealtimes and accessibility to snacks. They should also be encouraged to participate in daily exercise as tolerated. Patients will benefit from a multidisciplinary team approach for optimal management (5,6,16,17).

DIABETIC KETOACIDOSIS

The prevalence of DKA in pregnancy has decreased from 16.7% noted in 1960 to 1.2% more recently due to intensive insulin therapies and improved SMBG (18). As is the case with nonpregnant individuals, reduced insulin availability or action and increased insulin counterregulatory hormones causing hyperglycemia, ketosis, metabolic acidosis, and dehydration contribute to the pathophysiology of DKA (19). DKA occurs at lower glucose levels in pregnancy. In one series, 4 of 11 patients presented in DKA with blood glucose <200 mg/dL (11.1 mmol/L) (20). Several factors contribute to the occurrence of DKA in the setting of near euglycemia in pregnancy, including an increased flux of glucose from the maternal circulation to the fetus and placenta, possibly by means of an increase in the glucose transporter GLUT-1, the accelerated starvation state of pregnancy contributing to ketonuria, and a lowered renal threshold for glucose leading to enhanced glycosuria due to reduced tubular reabsorption capacity (21). In addition, higher progesterone levels in pregnancy induce a respiratory alkalosis that results in a compensatory metabolic acidosis, which reduces buffering capacity. DKA can precipitate under conditions of infection, new onset of type 1 or occasionally type 2 diabetes (ketosis-prone hyperglycemia) occurring in pregnancy, insulin omission, insulin pump malfunction or catheter occlusion, glucocorticoid use to induce fetal lung maturity, and the use of terbutaline (to prevent preterm labor) (18,19).

While maternal mortality rate has been estimated at 5%–15%, fetal mortality rate is estimated at 9%–35% (22). Maternal complications of DKA are similar in nonpregnant women. Fetal complications, including mortality, may be due to fetal acidosis and hypoxemia due to reduced uterine blood flow. Hypokalemia may cause fetal cardiac arrest. Hypophosphatemia may lead to reduced red blood cell 2,3-diphosphoglycerate and reduced oxygen delivery to the fetus. On fetal heart rate tracings, one may see poor heart rate variability and late decelerations (22). However, these findings are not indications for delivery as they may reverse with appropriate DKA management (18). Maternal morbidity may be worsened if there is premature intervention at this time for transient fetal distress. The objective should be to stabilize the mother before a decision to deliver is taken.

Prompt evaluation for DKA should occur in the setting of nausea, vomiting, abdominal discomfort, limited oral intake, or fever and hyperglycemia (6,19). DKA is diagnosed and managed as in nonpregnant adults and is comprehensively reviewed elsewhere (23,24). It is important to determine the underlying cause of DKA, including any potential infectious source, with urinalysis or chest X-ray and consider antibiotic administration (22). Catheter occlusion in the setting of insulin pump use can also precipitate DKA. When hyperglycemia is unexplained, persistent, or associated with positive ketones in the setting of insulin pump use, it is important for patients to treat themselves immediately with a subcutaneous injection by syringe, change the insulin infusion set, perform other insulin pump "troubleshooting" as needed, and contact their provider to assess the need for further evaluation and treatment with intravenous insulin infusion in an acute care setting such as an emergency room or obstetrical triage unit.

HYPOGLYCEMIA

Hypoglycemia is more common in pregnancy than in nonpregnant individuals with type 1 diabetes (25,26). Precipitating factors for hypoglycemia are multifactorial and include lowered glucose targets in pregnancy, abrupt changes in activity such as during or after exercise, overestimation of carbohydrate content in a meal, frequent insulin administration of high glucose correction doses (ie, stacking of insulin), excessive basal insulin, or excessive insulin provided by the correction factor or insulin-to-carbohydrate ratio (27). Early studies suggested impaired glucose counterregulation in pregnancy contributing to pathophysiology, but more recent studies do not demonstrate a role for deficient counterregulation (28). The nausea and vomiting seen in pregnancy has been suggested to contribute to hypoglycemia (25); however, it does not appear to be a major factor for severe hypoglycemia. Severe hypoglycemia, defined as an episode of low blood glucose requiring assistance from another person, is frequent in pregnancy, occurring in up to 45% of patients with type 1 diabetes (27). Severe hypoglycemia is most common in the first trimester of pregnancy, and contributing risk factor, include a history of hypoglycemia in the 4 months prior to gestation, reduced hypoglycemia awareness, history of diabetes >10 years, a higher insulin dose in unit/kg/day, and A1C ≤6.5% in the first trimester (25).

Hypoglycemia does not appear to increase the risk of birth defects or fetal death, or alter fetal heart rate, breathing, body movement, umbilical artery Doppler waveforms, or child intelligence. Although rare, severe maternal hypoglycemia with altered mental status could, nonetheless, result in involvement in motor vehicle or other accident, coma, or death (27), which would be catastrophic for both mother and fetus. Frequent SMBG and maintaining a detailed log of carbohydrate, meal insulin, and correction insulin are required to identify the above causes of hypoglycemia and make appropriate adjustments to the insulin plan. Particular attention should be given to checking glucose levels before and after meals, around exercise, and always before driving. In patients with hypoglycemic unawareness, it may be beneficial to raise glucose targets. Women should be comfortable assessing and managing hypoglycemia. They are advised to take in 15 grams of glucose (eg, 8-oz cup of milk, 4 oz of juice, or 3–4 glucose tablets) during mild hypoglycemia (50–70 mg/dL [2.8–4 mmol/L]) and 30 grams (ie, 1 cup of orange juice or 7–8 glucose tablets) if glucose <50 mg/dL (2.8 mmol/L), and recheck blood glucose every 15 minutes until glucose >70 mg/dL (4 mmol/L) (6). In the setting of inability to swallow, the patient's family should be counseled on how to administer 1 mg of glucagon subcutaneously and seek immediate medical assistance (16,26).

Hypothetically, continuous glucose monitoring (CGM) systems might be expected to reduce the prevalence of hypoglycemia in pregnancy. However, in a randomized control trial assessing intermittent CGM use in addition to SMBG, it did not improve glycemic control or reduce hypoglycemic events (28).

MANAGEMENT OF GLUCOCORTICOID-INDUCED HYPERGLYCEMIA

Pregnant women with diabetes are at increased risk for preterm labor. Preterm labor has been noted to occur in 22%–45% of patients with type 1 diabetes (29). Antenatal administration of corticosteroids is given to pregnant women at 24–34 weeks gestation if preterm delivery is anticipated or after 34 weeks gestation if there are signs of impaired fetal lung maturity (30). One should anticipate steroid-induced hyperglycemia in the setting of glucocorticoid administration for development of fetal lung maturity.

There are limited data on the insulin requirements needed during pregnancy in the setting of 2-day betamethasone administration of 12 mg IM repeated after 24 hours. Mathiesen et al (31) tested an algorithm that potentially can guide insulin dosing in this setting. The insulin algorithm that was used increased the baseline pre-betamethasone insulin doses by 27%, 45%, 40%, 31%, and 11% on days 1 through 5, respectively, after the initial betamethasone dosing. Providers can use this published algorithm as a general suggestion of incremental insulin requirements, but due to the small sample size we recommend close inpatient monitoring and insulin adjustment to keep in line with the recommended antepartum glucose goals. Future studies designed to fine-tune this algorithm to develop practice guidelines would be beneficial.

DIABETES IN LABOR AND POSTPARTUM CARE

Based on data from Curet et al (32), we have targeted antepartum blood glucoses of 80–110 mg/dL (4.4–6.0 mmol/L) at our institution using an intravenous (IV) insulin and dextrose infusion protocol. Recently, Ryan and Al-Agha (33) reviewed 24 studies of insulin management in labor and delivery and found an inverse relationship between maternal glucose during labor and the incidence of neonatal hypoglycemia. Using IV short-acting regular insulin +/– dextrose solution, they recommend targeting a minimum glucose of 72 mg/dL (4 mmol/L) to an upper range of 108 to 126 mg/dL (6–7 mmol/L), with the upper goal of 108 mg/dL (6 mmol/L) being commonly used in their practice. Hourly blood glucose testing should be performed antepartum and after delivery until the patient is eating. In the immediate postpartum period, insulin sensitivity is maximal and there is a sharp decline in insulin requirements to as much as 50% of the preconception dose followed by a gradual return to preconception dosing. We establish a postpartum insulin plan that is approximately 50% of the preconception insulin regimen several weeks in advance of the expected due date in order to adequately prepare our patients and clinical colleagues for this marked change. If an insulin infusion was used to maintain normoglycemia during labor, the insulin infusion should be overlapped by 1 hour after initiation of the patient's short- or rapid-acting insulin—or by 2 hours if initiating the patient's long-acting insulin—in the postpartum period to allow for adequate coverage during the transition.

ACKNOWLEDGMENTS

The authors have nothing to disclose.

REFERENCES

1. **Mahmud M, Mazza D.** Preconception care of women with diabetes: a review of current guideline recommendations. *BMC Women's Health.* 2010;10:5. doi:10.1186/1472-6874-10-5
2. **DCCT trial group.** Pregnancy outcomes in the Diabetes Control and Complications Trial. *Am J Obstet Gynecol.* 1996;174(4):1343–1353.
3. **Suhonen L, Hiilesmaa V, Teramo K.** Glycaemic control during early pregnancy and fetal malformations in women with type I diabetes mellitus. *Diabetologia.* 2000;43(1):79–82.
4. **Guerin A, Nisenbaum R, Ray JG.** Use of maternal GHb concentration to estimate the risk of congenital anomalies in the offspring of women with prepregnancy diabetes. *Diabetes Care.* 2007;30(7):1920–1925.
5. **Blumer I, Hader E, Hadden DR, et al.** Diabetes and pregnancy: an endocrine society clinical practice guideline. *J Clin Endocrinol Metab.* 2013;98: 4227–4249.
6. **Kitzmiller J, BlockJl, Brown FM, et al.** Managing preexisting diabetes for pregnancy. *Diabetes Care.* 2008;31:1060–1079.
7. **Cohen AL, Wenger JB, James-Todd T, et al.** The association of circulating angiogenic factors and HbA1c with the risk of preeclampsia in women with preexisting diabetes. *Hypertens Pregnancy.*2014;33(1):81–92 [published online ahead of print December 19, 2013]. doi: 10.3109/10641955.2013.837175.
8. **Evers IM, de Valk HW, Visser GH.** Risk of complications of pregnancy in women with type 1 diabetes: nationwide prospective study in the Netherlands. *BMJ.* 2004;328(7445):915.
9. **Chew EY, Mills JL, Metzger BE, et al.** Metabolic control and progression of retinopathy. The Diabetes in Early Pregnancy Study. National Institute of Child Health and Human Development Diabetes in Early Pregnancy Study. *Diabetes Care.* 1995;18(5):631–637.

10. **Mathiesen E, Hod M, Ivanisevic M, et al.** Maternal efficacy and safety outcomes in a randomized, controlled trial comparing insulin detemir with NPH insulin in 310 pregnant women with type 1 diabetes. *Diabetes Care.* 2012;35:2012–2017.
11. **Hod M, Mathiesen ER, Jovanovič L, et al.** A randomized trial comparing perinatal outcomes using insulin detemir or neutral protamine Hagedorn in type 1 diabetes. *J Matern Fetal Neonatal Med.* 2014;27(1): 7–13.
12. **Pollex E, Moretti ME, Koren G, Feig DS.** Safety of insulin glargine use in pregnancy: a systematic review and meta-analysis. *Ann Pharmacother.* 2011;45(1): 9–16.
13. **García-Patterson A, Gich I, Amini SB, Catalano PM, de Leiva A, Corcoy R.** Insulin requirements throughout pregnancy in women with type 1 diabetes mellitus: three changes of direction. *Diabetologia.* 2010;53(3):446–451.
14. **Mathiesen JM, Secher AL, Ringholm L, et al.** Changes in basal rates and bolus calculator settings in insulin pumps during pregnancy in women with type 1 diabetes. *J Matern Fetal Neonatal Med.* Sep 27, 2013. [Epub ahead of print]
15. **Achong N, Callaway L, d'Emden M, McIntyre HD, Lust K, Barrett HL.** Insulin requirements in late pregnancy in women with type 1 diabetes mellitus: a retrospective review. *Diabetes Res Clin Pract.* 2012;98(3):414–421.
16. **American Diabetes Association.** Standards of Medical Care in Diabetes—2014. *Diabetes Care.* 2014;37(1):S11–S66.
17. **Joslin Diabetes Center.** Guideline for Detection and Management of Diabetes in Pregnancy. http://www.joslin.org/bin_from_cms/Preg_guideline_5_10_11_(2)-0615-11.pdf.
18. **Schneider MB, Umpierrez GE, Ramsey RD, Mabie WC, Bennett KA.** Pregnancy complicated by diabetes ketoacidosis: maternal and fetal outcomes. *Diabetes Care.* 2003;26:958–959.
19. **de Veciana M.** Diabetes ketoacidosis in pregnancy. *Semin Perinatol.* 2013;37:267–273.
20. **Cullen MT, Reece EA, Homko CJ, Sivan E.** The changing presentations of diabetic ketoacidosis during pregnancy. *Am J Perinatol.* 1996;13(7):449–451.
21. **Guo RX, Yang LZ, Li LX, Zhao XP.** Diabetic ketoacidosis in pregnancy tends to occur at lower blood glucose levels: case-control study and a case report of euglycemic diabetic ketoacidosis in pregnancy. *J Obstet Gynaecol Res.* 2008;34(3): 324–330.
22. **Carroll MA, Yeomans ER.** Diabetic ketoacidosis in pregnancy. *Crit Care Med.* 2005;33(suppl 10): S347–S353.
23. **Dhatariya K, Savage M, Claydon A, et al.** Joint British Diabetes Societies Inpatient Care Group. The management of diabetic ketoacidosis in adults. 2nd ed. Update: September 2013. http://www.diabetologistsabcd.org.uk/JBDS/JBDS_IP_DKA_Adults_Revised.pdf. 2013.
24. **Kitabchi AE, Umpierrez GE, Miles JM, Fisher JN.** Hyperglycemic crises in adult patients with diabetes. *Diabetes Care.* 2009;32(7):1335–1343.
25. **Evers IM, ter Braak EW, de Valk HW, van Der Schoot B, Janssen N, Visser GH.** Risk indicators predictive for severe hypoglycemia during the first trimester of type 1 diabetic pregnancy. *Diabetes Care.* 2002;25(3):554–559.
26. **Seaquist ER, Anderson J, Childs B, et al.** Hypoglycemia and diabetes: a report of a workgroup of the American Diabetes Association and the Endocrine Society. *J Clin Endocrinol Metab.* 2013;98:1845–1859.
27. **Ringholm L, Pedersen-Bjergaard U, Thorsteinsson B, Damm P, Mathiesen ER.** Hypoglycaemia during pregnancy in women with Type 1 diabetes. *Diabet Med.* 2012;29:558–566.
28. **Secher AL, Ringholm L, Andersen HU, Damm P, Mathiesen ER.** The effect of real-time continuous glucose monitoring in pregnant women with diabetes: a randomized controlled trial. *Diabetes Care.* 2013;36(7):1877–1883.
29. **Lepercq J, Coste J, Theau A, Dubois-Laforgue D, Timsit J.** Factors associated with preterm delivery in women with Type 1 diabetes. *Diabetes Care.* 2004;27:2824–2828.
30. **Miracle X, Di Renzo GC, Stark A, Fanaroff A, Carbonell-Estrany X, Saling E.** Coordinators of World Association of Perinatal Medicine Prematurity Working Group. Guideline for the use of antenatal corticosteroids for fetal maturation. *J Perinat Med.* 2008;36(3):191–196.
31. **Mathiesen ER, Christensen AL, Hellmuth E, Hornnes P, Stage E, Damm P.** Insulin dose during glucocorticoid treatment for fetal lung maturation in diabetic pregnancy: test of an algorithm. *Acta Obstet Gynecol Scand.* 2002;81:835–839.
32. **Curet LB, Izquierdo LA, Gilson GJ, Schneider JM, Perelman R, Converse J.** Relative effects of antepartum and intrapartum maternal blood glucose levels on incidence of neonatal hypoglycemia. *J Perinatol.* 1997;17(2):113–115.
33. **Ryan EA, Al-Agha R.** Glucose control during labor and delivery. *Curr Diab Rep.* 2014;14(1):450.

SECTION X

Sodium Disorders

SECTION INTRODUCTION

Emergent Management of Sodium Disorders

Daniel G Bichet

With this section describing hyper- and hyponatremic emergencies we can reflect how much new epidemiological, clinical, and basic data have been obtained on this subject since the detailed observations and adage coined by Tomas Berl in 1990: "Treating hyponatremia: damned if we do and damned if we don't" (1).

There is a renewed interest in hyper/hyponatremic disorders stemming from (1) basic studies on thirst and vasopressin secretion; (2) large epidemiological studies all demonstrating increased odds ratio to die if you are hyper/hyponatremic; (3) powerful new therapeutic agents to increase water excretion; and (4) clinical recommendations to decrease or increase plasma sodium intended to improve clinical status and never to induce osmotic demyelination syndrome (ODS).

THIRST, CENTRAL AND PERIPHERAL OSMORECEPTORS, DENDRITIC RELEASE OF VASOPRESSIN IN PARAVENTRICULAR NUCLEI, AND INCREASED RENAL SYMPATHETIC OUTFLOW

Thirst, which is deficient in adipsic hypernatremia and not suppressed enough in hyponatremic, euvolemic, or hypervolemic states, is a fascinating homeostatic "emotion": It is an impelling urge to drink water or aqueous fluids (2). The lamina terminalis region of the brain contains neuronal osmoreceptors thought to increase their blood-oxygen-level dependent (BOLD) signal as measured by magnetic resonance imaging in healthy humans, under conditions of stimulation of thirst by an infusion of hypertonic saline (3). Magnocellular cells of the supraoptic and paraventricular nucleus (SON and PVN) are also osmosensitive, but they require input by glutamatergic afferents from the lamina terminalis to respond fully to osmotic challenges. Lamina terminalis osmoreceptors and magnocellular cells producing vasopressin express stretch inactivated transient receptor potential-vanilloid type-receptors (TRPV1) conferring "perfect" osmoreceptor sensing to these cells (4). Because the lamina terminalis neurons lie outside the blood-brain barrier, they can integrate endocrine signals borne by circulating hormones like angiotensin II, relaxin, and atrial natriuretic peptide. Angiotensin II blood concentration, which is elevated in hyponatremic patients with heart failure and cirrhosis, confers an osmoregulatory gain because it amplifies osmosensory transduction (5). The osmoregulatory function of these brain osmoreceptors is complemented by peripheral neuronal receptors recently identified on neuronal terminals around the portal vein, sensing its osmolality, with hepatic afferents and relays to the magnocellular PVN (6).

New data also demonstrate that during disturbances of fluid and electrolyte homeostasis, activation of magnocellular neurosecretory and presympathetic neurons in the PVN results in the concerted systemic release of the hormone vasopressin, along with an increase in renal sympathetic outflow, respectively, acting together to restore fluid/electrolyte balance (7). Here vasopressin is released locally by dendrites (8) in the PVN and stimulates neighboring presynaptic neurons bearing V1 receptors. Son et al suggested a possible link between neurohumoral activation with high vasopressin and sympathetic outflow and the high morbidity and mortality observed in hypertension and heart failure (7). I would go further and suggest that increased morbidity and mortality may be observed in all the clinical states with vasopressin stimulation. Thus, in both hyper/hyponatremic states increases in central vasopressin may induce a sympathetic drive with excess morbidity and mortality, possibly independent of other confounding factors like the severity of the underlying disease.

RELATIONSHIP BETWEEN HOSPITAL ADMISSION SERUM SODIUM AND INPATIENT MORTALITY

In a study by Wald, analyzing 97,472 hospitalizations during a 7-year period, there was a progressive increase in mortality as soon as plasma sodium was lower or higher than 140 mEq/L (140 mmol/L), indicating that a plasma sodium from 138 to 142 mEq/L (138–142 mmol/L) could be the operational definition of normonatremia. It remains unclear, however, whether biochemical correction of hyper/hyponatremia will confer improved patients outcomes (9).

VAPTANS OR UREA TO INCREASE WATER EXCRETION

The nonpeptide vasopressin V2 receptor antagonist tolvaptan has been shown to improve plasma sodium in patients with the syndrome of inappropriate antidiuretic hormone (SIADH) secretion or in hyponatremic patients with heart failure or cirrhosis (10). However, patients with activating mutations of the *AVPR2* gene R137L/C have hyponatremia that could not be reversed with tolvaptan (11). By contrast, tolvaptan completely silenced the constitutive activity of another activating mutation F229V (12). Of interest, hyponatremic patients bearing the R137L/C mutations have been successfully treated with oral urea (13). Medicinal urea is often prescribed in Europe (14) but rarely in North America. The molecular weight of urea is 60, therefore 60 g of urea corresponds to 1,000 mmol. If 60 g of urea is ingested and if the urine osmolality of a patient with the SIADH secretion is 500 mOsm, urea will "drag" 2 L of water into the urine. One can use different urine osmolalities and different loads of urea and calculate the expected water excretion (15).

DO NOT INDUCE OSMOTIC DEMYLINATION DURING THE TREATMENT OF HYPONATREMIA!

This is well emphasized by authors on both hypernatremia and hyponatremia. I teach my junior doctors to fear a rapid increase in plasma sodium in the middle of the night or during a change of staff in the emergency department, and I involve the nurses in charge of hyponatremic patients, explaining the necessity not to increase the plasma sodium by more than 6 mEq/L (6 mmol/L) the first day. The "rule of sixes" is easy to remember: "six-a-day" makes sense for safety and "six in six hours" for severe symptoms (Figure X-1) (16). An increase of 8 mEq/L (8 mmol/L) every 24 hours thereafter until a plasma sodium concentration of 130 mEq/L (130 mmol/L) is attained is recommended. The expected changes in plasma sodium should be written as orders in the patient's chart and the responsible clinician in charge should be immediatey called if the measured changes in plasma sodium are outside the safe range. Of note is that Stern is now recommending to manage patients who present with serum sodium concentrations lower or equal to 120 mEq/L (120 mmol/L) with a combination of desmopressin and hypertonic saline in

- A 6 mEq/L (6 mmol/L) increase every 24 hours is an appropriate and safe therapeutic target, even in patients with profound hyponatremia (allowing room for a 2 mEq/L [2 mmol/L] unintentional overshoot)
- This translates to an easy-to-remember "rule of sixes" to define correction goals:
  - For all patients with chronic hyponatremia, the correction goal is 6 mEq/L (6 mmol/L) during the initial 24 hours
  - For those with severe symptoms (eg, seizure, severe delirium, and unresponsiveness), the goal is preloaded in the first 6 hours, postponing subsequent efforts to increase serum sodium level until the next day.

Figure X-1. Treating profound hyponatremia: a strategy for controlled correction (16).

order to "clamp" the desired increase in plasma sodium irrespective of a spontaneous correction of the antidiuretic state (17). Also, prevention of ODS could be achieved with infusions of 5% dextrose (D5W) and DDAVP for an overcorrected plasma sodium (18).

ACKNOWLEDGMENTS

The author has nothing to disclose.

REFERENCES

1. **Berl T.** Treating hyponatremia: damned if we do and damned if we don't. *Kidney Int.* 1990;37:1006–1018.
2. **McKinley MJ.** Thirst. In: Berntson GG, Cacioppo JT, eds. *Handbook of Neuroscience for the Behavioral Sciences.* Vol 2. Hoboken, NJ: John Wiley and Sons; 2009:680–709.
3. **Bourque CW.** Central mechanisms of osmosensation and systemic osmoregulation. *Nat Rev Neurosci.* 2008;9:519–531.
4. **Ciura S, Liedtke W, Bourque CW.** Hypertonicity sensing in organum vasculosum lamina terminalis neurons: a mechanical process involving TRPV1 but not TRPV4. *J Neurosci.* 2011;31:14669–14676.
5. **Zhang Z, Bourque CW.** Amplification of transducer gain by angiotensin II-mediated enhancement of cortical actin density in osmosensory neurons. *J Neurosci.* 2008;28:9536–9544.
6. **Lechner SG, Markworth S, Poole K, et al.** The molecular and cellular identity of peripheral osmoreceptors. *Neuron.* 2011;69:332–344.
7. **Son SJ, Filosa JA, Potapenko ES, et al.** Dendritic peptide release mediates interpopulation crosstalk between neurosecretory and preautonomic networks. *Neuron.* 2013;78:1036–1049.
8. **Ludwig M, Leng G.** Dendritic peptide release and peptide-dependent behaviours. *Nat Rev Neurosci.* 2006;7:126–136.
9. **Wald R, Jaber BL, Price LL, Upadhyay A, Madias NE.** Impact of hospital-associated hyponatremia on selected outcomes. *Arch Intern Med.* 2010;170:294–302.
10. **Schrier RW, Gross P, Gheorghiade M, et al.** Tolvaptan, a selective oral vasopressin V2-receptor antagonist, for hyponatremia. *N Engl J Med.* 2006;355:2099–2112.
11. **Decaux G, Vandergheynst F, Bouko Y, Parma J, Vassart G, Vilain C.** Nephrogenic syndrome of inappropriate antidiuresis in adults: high phenotypic variability in men and women from a large pedigree. *J Am Soc Nephrol.* 2007;18:606–612.
12. **Carpentier E, Greenbaum LA, Rochdi D, et al.** Identification and characterization of an activating F229V substitution in the V2 vasopressin receptor in an infant with NSIAD. *J Am Soc Nephrol.* 2012;23: 1635–1640.
13. **Huang EA, Feldman BJ, Schwartz ID, Geller DH, Rosenthal SM, Gitelman SE.** Oral urea for the treatment of chronic syndrome of inappropriate antidiuresis in children. *J Pediatr.* 2006;148:128–131.
14. **Soupart A, Coffernils M, Couturier B, Gankam-Kengne F, Decaux G.** Efficacy and tolerance of urea compared with vaptans for long-term treatment of patients with SIADH. *Clin J Am Soc Nephrol.* 2012;7:742–747.
15. **Bichet DG.** What is the role of vaptans in routine clinical nephrology? *Clin J Am Soc Nephrol.* 2012;7: 700–703.
16. **Sterns RH, Hix JK, Silver S.** Treating profound hyponatremia: a strategy for controlled correction. *Am J Kidney Dis.* 2010;56:774–779.
17. **Sood L, Sterns RH, Hix JK, Silver SM, Chen L.** Hypertonic saline and desmopressin: a simple strategy for safe correction of severe hyponatremia. *Am J Kidney Dis.* 2013;61:571–578.
18. **Sterns RH, Hix JK.** Overcorrection of hyponatremia is a medical emergency. *Kidney Int.* 2009;76: 587–589.

CHAPTER 36

Emergency Management of Acute and Chronic Hypernatremia

Mark J Hannon and Christopher J Thompson

ABSTRACT

Hypernatremia is a common condition in emergency medicine; it is associated with high morbidity, and in many conditions is a predictor of excess mortality. The majority of cases of hypernatremia arise secondary to inadequate water intake, often exacerbated by comorbid acute illnesses and excess fluid loss. Diabetes insipidus (DI), which results in inappropriate hypotonic polyuria, rarely causes hypernatremia, because the intact thirst mechanism generates sufficient drinking to replace renal water losses. However, if DI is associated with adipsia, diminished consciousness levels, or vomiting, severe hypernatremia may occur. In this chapter, we will outline the various causes of acute hypernatremia and the correct management of this important condition.

INTRODUCTION

Hypernatremia is rare in noncritically ill hospital inpatients, but is a much more common finding in seriously ill patients, the elderly, and in children (1). Hypernatremia has a significant impact on patient morbidity and mortality if the correct management is not promptly initiated (2). In addition, in the emergency department, hypernatremia has been reported to be more common than hyponatremia; in a retrospective review of 3,182 patients presenting to this setting, 13% had hypernatremia, compared with 4% who had hyponatremia (3). In subsequent studies of the entire hospital population similar figures were found, and hypernatremia was also found to be strongly predictive of mortality (4). Hypernatremia in adults is almost always due to water depletion rather than excessive sodium intake. Elderly subjects are more vulnerable to the development of hypernatremia, because osmotically stimulated thirst is attenuated, leading to reduced fluid intake (5). Many elderly patients in long-term care institutions exhibit permanent hypernatremia, through a combination of cognitive impairment, age-related attenuation of thirst, and reduced mobility (6).

Diabetes insipidus is characterized by inadequate urinary concentration due to inadequate secretion or action of the neurohypophyseal hormone, vasopressin. In most patients, fluid intake compensates for renal water losses, such that plasma sodium concentrations are normal. In ambulatory patients with DI, hyponatremia due to overtreatment with desmopressin is relatively common, but hypernatremia is exceptionally rare, unless the patient has associated adipsia. However, during acute illness precipitating presentation to emergency care, hypernatremia is much more common in all patients with DI, particularly if vomiting and/or diarrhea cause the combination of excess fluid losses and difficulty in absorbing desmopressin.

Hypernatremia is associated with cellular shrinkage due to osmotic movement of water from the intracellular to the extracellular space. Clinical features of hypernatremia are predominantly a consequence of shrinkage of brain cells, and include lethargy, drowsiness, and altered mental status, progressing to seizures, coma, and death if left untreated (7). The cornerstone of management of hypernatremia is immediate administration of hypo-osmolar fluids, usually intravenously.

In this chapter, we will discuss the physiological control of water balance, the main pathologies affecting this system, and the differential diagnosis and management of hypernatremia.

THE PHYSIOLOGICAL CONTROL OF WATER BALANCE

Plasma osmolality in healthy men varies by only 1%–2% in physiological conditions where there is free access to water. This precise regulation of plasma osmolality is maintained by the homeostatic process of osmoregulation.

Changes in plasma osmolality are detected by specialized osmoreceptor cells in the anterior hypothalamus (Figure 36-1). Changes in plasma osmolality cause these hypothalamic nuclei to depolarize, sending neural signals, via the nucleus medianus, to the supraoptic and paraventricular nuclei. Elevation in plasma osmolality causes depolarization of these nuclei, leading to increased synthesis of vasopressin (AVP), and secretion of vasopressin from the posterior pituitary.

If plasma concentrations are lowered by excessive ingestion of hypotonic fluid to below 280–285 mOsm/kg, secretion of vasopressin is suppressed, and plasma concentrations of the hormone are undetectable, leading to hypotonic polyuria (8). The increase in free water clearance allows plasma osmolality to rise into the normal range. If plasma osmolality rises, due to dehydration, there is an increase in plasma concentrations of vasopressin, in proportion to the rise in plasma osmolality. The action of vasopressin, to concentrate the urine and allow reabsorption of water, restores plasma osmolality to normal. This homeostatic process occurs continuously to maintain plasma osmolality within a narrow reference range, as shown in Figure 36-2. The relationship between plasma vasopressin concentration and urine osmolality is shown in Figure 36-3.

Although physiological control of vasopressin secretion and thirst is almost entirely osmotic, the switch off of both is nonosmotic and is triggered by the act of drinking. In studies of healthy men who have been rendered hyperosmolar, drinking is associated with an immediate fall in plasma vasopressin and thirst, before any changes in plasma osmolality can be measured (9). The fall in plasma vasopressin following fluid intake is very rapid and

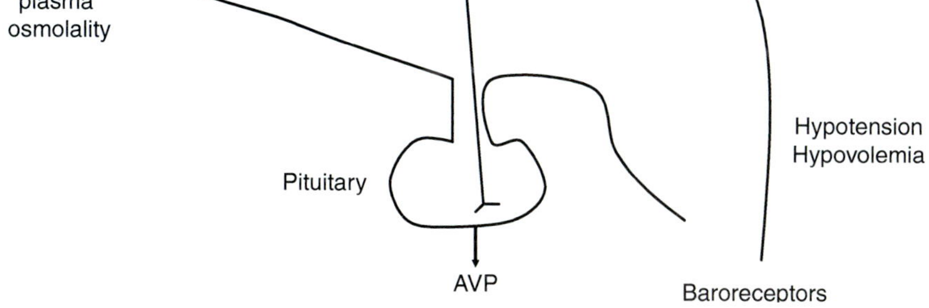

Figure 36-1. Factors governing vasopressin secretion. CVO = circumventricular organ (site of osmoreceptors); SON = supraoptic nuclei; PVN = paraventricular nuclei.

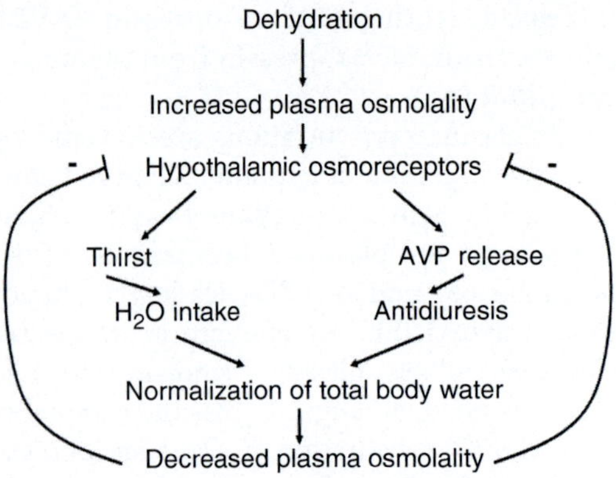

Figure 36-2. The regulation of plasma osmolality.

suggests that a neuroendocrine reflex, stimulated by oropharyngeal distension, switches off vasopressin secretion.

CAUSES OF HYPERNATREMIA

The large number of potential causes of hypernatremia in the inpatient setting can be divided into 5 major groups:

1. Decreased water intake
2. Excess water losses with inadequate replacement
3. Redistribution of intracellular water to the extracellular space
4. Excess salt intake
5. Hyperaldosteronism

The causes of hypernatremia contained in each group are summarized in Table 36-1, and several of these etiologies will now be discussed in more detail.

Decreased Water Intake

Healthy individuals are vulnerable to the development of hypernatremia in circumstances where water intake cannot replace water excretion. Diminished water intake most often occurs in the setting of decreased cognitive awareness, but it can reflect the presence of genuine adipsia. There are 4 distinct clinical patterns of adipsia (9):

1. Type A adipsia: This is characterized by an upward resetting of the osmotic thresholds for both thirst and vasopressin release, and is also termed "essential hypernatremia." The patient's osmotic threshold is often over 300 mOsm/kg; however, once plasma osmolality exceeds the elevated set-point, thirst is stimulated and vasopressin is secreted with the result that severe hypernatremia is

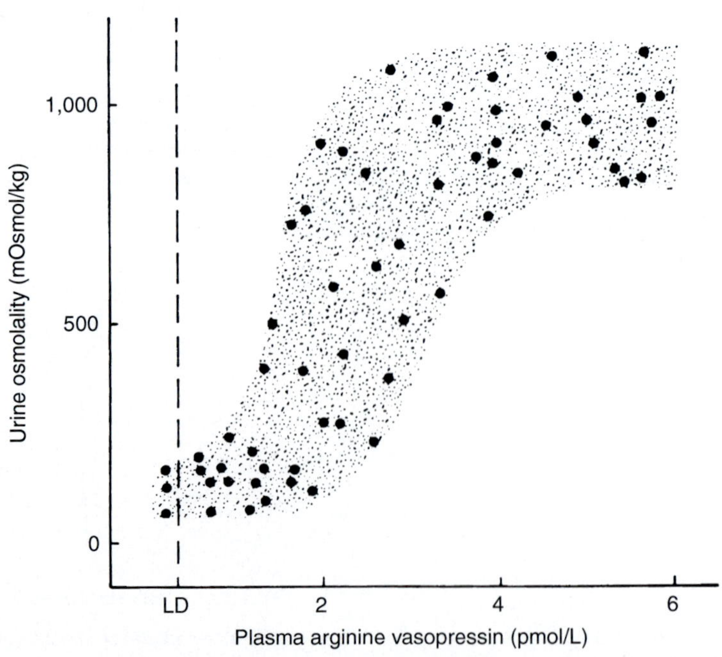

Figure 36-3. The relationship between plasma vasopressin concentration and urine osmolality.

Table 36-1. Causes of Hypernatremia

Decreased water intake	Aging Impaired cognition Inadequate access to fluids Adipsia Essential hypernatremia
Excess water losses with inadequate replacement	Gastrointestinal losses Fever/hyperventilation Tubing and drains Intraoperative losses Diuretics DKA/HHS Mannitol DI Demeclocycline, vaptans
Redistribution of intracellular water to the extracellular space	Exercise Seizures
Excess salt intake	Salt/seawater ingestion Intravenous bicarbonate administration
Hyperaldosteronism	Conn's syndrome Cushing's syndrome Carbenoxolone/licorice ingestion

often avoided (10,11). Usually, therefore, the only biochemical abnormality is mild chronic hypernatremia.

2. Type B adipsia: This results from subnormal thirst and vasopressin responses to osmotic stimuli, due to malfunction of the hypothalamic osmoreceptors. Because baroreceptor function is intact, there is often vigorous AVP secretion in response to hypotension. If the patient, therefore, becomes so blood volume depleted due to hypernatremic dehydration that the baroreceptors are unloaded, the subsequent nonosmotic vasopressin secretion to a certain extent protects the patient from extreme hypernatremia. This condition is also rare and generally associated with other congenital anomalies (12).
3. Type C adipsia: Although rare, this is the most common and severe form of adipsia (9), with complete absence of thirst and osmotically stimulated vasopressin secretion. It is most commonly seen after clipping of anterior communicating artery aneurysms, following subarachnoid hemorrhage (13); the vascular supply to the osmoreceptors is derived from small arteries arising from the anterior communicating artery, and it is assumed that these vessels may be damaged during aneurysm clipping. The osmoregulatory defect is almost always permanent. Extensive hypothalamic surgery for craniopharyngioma (13), or, rarely, pituitary macroadenoma (14), has also been reported to cause adipsia. In adipsia secondary to clipping of the anterior communicating artery, there is a pure osmoreceptor defect. Thus, these patients can produce vasopressin in response to nonosmotic stimuli such as nausea and hypotension, but not in response to hyperosmolarity (15). In patients who have destructive surgery to the pituitary, all secretory function is lost, and no vasopressin can be produced under any circumstances (15); in this situation hypernatremia can be severe. The combination of absent thirst and an inability to produce vasopressin in response to appropriate stimuli is termed adipsic diabetes insipidus (ADI).
4. Type D adipsia: This extremely rare form of adipsia manifests as pure thirst-absence with no defect in vasopressin secretion, with only 1 case reported to date (16).

Excess Water Losses with Inadequate Replacement

Excess water loss can result in hypernatremic dehydration if the patient is unable to consume adequate fluid to replace his or her losses. Diabetes insipidus (DI) may be central or nephrogenic, and will also result in inappropriate renal water loss. A full list of causes of DI is shown in Table 36-2. The majority of patients with DI are able to maintain a normal plasma sodium even in the absence of treatment, because their intact thirst mechanism allows them to maintain a sufficient fluid intake to compensate for excessive urinary losses (17). However, if their thirst sensation is impaired, for example through the presence of a comorbid condition such as a head injury, hypernatremia will rapidly develop. Hypernatremia appears to be more common in nephrogenic diabetes insipidus (NDI) due to lithium administration rather than cranial diabetes insipidus (CDI);

Table 36-2. Causes of Diabetes Insipidus

Cranial DI	
Congenital	Hereditary (X-linked or AD) DIDMOAD
Acquired	Pituitary surgery Tumors (craniopharyngioma, germinoma, pinealoma, metastases) Traumatic brain injury Granuloma (TB, sarcoid, histiocytosis X) Infections (encephalitis, meningitis) Vascular disorders (Sheehan's syndrome, aneurysms, subarachnoid hemorrhage, gastrointestinal bleed) Hypophysitis (autoimmune, lymphocytic) Idiopathic Pregnancy
Nephrogenic DI	
Congenital	Hereditary (X-linked recessive or AD)
Acquired	Chronic kidney disease (polycystic kidneys, obstructive uropathy) Metabolic disease (hypercalcemia, hypokalemia) Drugs (lithium, demeclocycline) Osmotic diuresis (glucose, mannitol) Amyloidosis Myelomatosis

Abbreviations: AD = autosomal-dominant; DIDMOAD = DI, diabetes mellitus, optic atrophy, and deafness; TB = tuberculosis.

the reasons for this are unclear (18). However, bipolar disorder is associated with cognitive impairment that may reduce patients' ability to drink appropriate volumes of water, resulting in hypernatremia (19); lithium itself does not have a major effect on cognition (31). In the extremely rare condition of adipsic DI, the patient has both a vasopressin secretory defect and an impaired thirst mechanism, commonly resulting in hypernatremia (13).

Demeclocycline is a tetracycline derivative that is utilized in the treatment of the syndrome of inappropriate antidiuresis (SIAD) because it causes NDI in about 60% of patients for whom it is prescribed. However, the induced vasopressin resistance is not predictable and some patients may become markedly symptomatic, occasionally developing hypernatremia if access to water is compromised. Lithium therapy also causes NDI in 30% of patients (13), and an even larger proportion of patients have attenuation of maximal urine concentrating ability (15). This effect is usually (16) but not always reversible upon stopping the medication. More recently, a new class of medications known as the vaptans, or selective vasopressin receptor antagonists, have been used in the management of SIAD; these rarely cause hypernatremia when used to treat SIAD (19,20) but may lead to profound water loss if given to those who are already volume depleted but erroneously diagnosed with euvolemic hyponatremia (21,22).

Hyperaldosteronism

Sodium and potassium excretion is regulated at the level of the kidney by the mineralocorticoid hormone aldosterone. Excess aldosterone production due to an adrenal adenoma (Conn's syndrome) or bilateral adrenal hyperplasia may lead to excessive potassium loss and sodium retention (23), resulting in mild chronic hypernatremia. However, only 40% of those with excess aldosterone production have any electrolyte imbalance, usually hypokalemia rather than hypernatremia (24). Chronic mild volume expansion also leads to upward resetting of the osmostat such that patients with mild hypernatremia due to hyperaldosteronism do not drink large volumes of fluid to normalize their sodium levels (25). Thus, although patients with aldosterone excess may have a mild chronic hypernatremia (usually between 143 and 147 mEq/L [143–147 mmol/L]), it does not usually lead to adverse clinical events (23).

Excess glucocorticoid production due to Cushing's syndrome may also cause hypernatremia. However, this is rare and only occurs when grossly elevated plasma glucocorticoid concentrations overwhelm the enzyme 11-beta-hydroxysteroid dehydrogenase type 2, which normally converts cortisol to inactive cortisone at the level of the mineralocorticoid receptor, such that cortisol activates the mineralocorticoid receptor. This is particularly seen in those with Cushing's syndrome due to ectopic ACTH secretion (26). Licorice and carbenoxolone may cause hypertension, hypernatremia, and hypokalemia, also via inhibition of 11-beta-hydroxysteroid dehydrogenase type 2, producing apparent mineralocorticoid excess, despite normal plasma aldosterone concentrations (27,28).

CONSEQUENCES OF HYPERNATREMIA

Hypernatremia has multiple adverse effects, predominantly due to the movement of water from cells to the extracellular space, leading to cell shrinkage (1,29). One of the most common and feared effects is free water shift leading to brain shrinkage, which may cause vascular rupture and permanent cognitive deficits (7). Cerebral demyelination has also been reported in severe hypernatremia (30), particularly in liver disease (31). Hypernatremia also leads to muscle weakness (32), impaired glucose utilization and insulin function (33) that may lead to hyperglycemia in the critically ill (34), an increase in venous thromboembolism risk (35), and decreased left ventricular contractility (1). The cellular shrinkage induced by hypernatremia can have catabolic effects and induce proinflammatory cytokine responses (36), which may impair lactate clearance (37). In addition, severe hypernatremia has been reported to cause rhabdomyolysis and consequent acute kidney injury (38).

In the intensive care setting, even mild hypernatremia has been shown to double mortality (39). Hypernatremia due to DI has been linked with excess mortality following both traumatic brain injury (40) and subarachnoid hemorrhage (41), and patients with adipsic DI due to surgery for craniopharyngioma have an extremely high mortality (13), due to multiple pathologies, including obesity, obstructive sleep apnea, and venous thromboembolism. Cardiovascular and thromboembolic events are particularly common in those with hypernatremia due to the hyperglycemic hyperosmolar state (HHS) (42). Hypernatremia has also been associated with a doubling of mortality and prolonged length of stay in the intensive care unit following cardiac surgery (43).

Although hypernatremia is common in the emergency department, a recent Swiss study showed that no corrective action was taken in 18% of those with hypernatremia on presentation, even though 35% had acute, severe, symptomatic hypernatremia (44). Understanding the disorders that cause hypernatremia is essential to enable prompt, correct management. It is extremely important to note that the severity of symptoms is strongly influenced by the rapidity of the development of hypernatremia—those with acute hypernatremia are at far higher risk than those with chronic hypernatremia (1,29). We will now discuss the management of acute and chronic of hypernatremia.

MANAGEMENT OF ACUTE HYPERNATREMIA

The majority of cases of acute hypernatremia seen in acute general medical inpatients are simply due to water depletion, usually precipitated by an intercurrent illness, exacerbated by poor thirst response. Before hypernatremia is corrected, assessment should be made to determine whether the hypernatremia is acute (occurring in the previous 48 hr) or chronic. When hypernatremia is documented to be acute or when severe symptoms are present (such as seizures, coma, or focal neurological deficit), immediate treatment is indicated. This is because compensatory mechanisms such as the intracerebral movement of organic solutes will not yet have begun, and the patient will likely be acutely decompensated due to the hypernatremia; therefore, the rate of correction can reach a maximum of 1 mmol/L/hr to a maximum of 10 to 12 mEq/L/day (10–12 mmol/L/day). If hypernatremia is chronic and only slightly symptomatic, correction then should take place gradually as cerebral edema may develop if correction is over rapid; a maximum correction rate of 6 to 8 mEq/L/day (6–8 mmol/L/day) should be applied (7,45).

When a patient with hypernatremia is hypotensive, treatment should start with isotonic intravenous (IV) fluids (either crystalloids or colloids) because they restore hemodynamic stability faster than hypotonic fluids and are still hypotonic relative to the hypernatremic, hyperosmolar patient (7). In all other settings, hypernatremia can be treated with hypotonic fluids administered either orally or intravenously; patients who are acutely unwell may have difficulty in consuming large volumes of oral fluids, and so we recommend IV administration of either 0.45% saline or 5% dextrose hypotonic solutions. The patient's total body water deficit can be calculated prior to commencing the infusion using the following formula: 0.6 × lean body weight × ([serum sodium (mEq/L [mmol/L])/140] – 1).

The volume and rate of fluid replacement needed to achieve a certain rate of decline in plasma sodium concentration can be calculated using the Adrogue-Madias formula (7); however, these calculations are not always accurate (46). We would, therefore, advise frequent monitoring of the patient's sodium level every 2 to 4 hours, depending on the severity of hypernatremia and the rapidity of correction required, with concomitant clinical evaluation (45).

Patients who develop severe hypernatremic dehydration have an increased hematocrit and are at risk, therefore, of producing thrombotic complications due to the hypercoagulable state. This is well-recognized in HHS, and we have also reported pulmonary thromboembolism during severe hypernatremia in adipsic DI (13). For this reason we recommend the use of prophylactic anticoagulation with heparin in patients with vascular disease, in the elderly, and in very severe dehydration. Although there is very little evidence base to support this practice, prophylactic short-term anticoagulation in at-risk patients seems sensible.

Hypernatremia caused by volume depletion due to diabetic ketoacidosis (DKA) or HHS may worsen if there is over-rapid correction of hyperglycemia (47,48). It is important, therefore, to monitor for the development of hypernatremia during the correction of severe hyperglycemia, particularly in the management of HHS.

If DI is present, then desmopressin treatment and the previously mentioned volume status correction need to be immediately instigated. Acute CDI is often seen in neurosurgical patients; the majority of cases are transient, so our practice is to administer a single parenteral (subcutaneous or intramuscular) dose of DDAVP (synthetic, long-lasting vasopressin), which is active for 6 to 12 hours, and re-treat only if there is development of further symptoms (49). Regular DDAVP is only prescribed if there is persistent polyuria for more than 48 hours (49). Withdrawal of DDAVP prior to discharge from the hospital is helpful in identifying those patients who have recovered secretion of endogenous vasopressin.

MANAGEMENT OF CHRONIC HYPERNATREMIA

Elderly patients in long-term care are at risk of developing chronic hypernatremia, which may worsen during acute illness. The importance of adequate fluid intake should be emphasized to the patient's caregivers. Any nonspecific decline in the patient's cognition or the development of intercurrent illness should prompt urgent electrolyte measurement.

The intact thirst mechanism generally prevents hypernatremic dehydration in DI in the outpatient setting. The treatment of choice for CDI is DDAVP, which can be administered as an intranasal spray, or, more often, orally, in 2 to 3 daily doses (50). The main complication is dilutional hyponatremia, and in our experience less than 3% of plasma sodium concentrations in ambulatory patients with DI are in the hypernatremic range (unpublished data).

NDI due to an acquired metabolic problem is best managed by addressing the underlying cause and maintaining adequate hydration while function recovers. For those patients with congenital NDI, or in whom the acquired defect is irreversible, a number of additional measures, including thiazide diuretics (25 mg hydrochlorothiazide every 24 hr); prostaglandin inhibitors such as nonsteroidal anti-inflammatory drugs (200 mg ibuprofen every 24 hr); and dietary salt restriction, can be used. All probably work through a combination of reducing glomerular filtration rate and interference with the diluting capacity of the distal nephron. Occasionally, DDAVP can produce some benefit (50).

The diagnosis of adipsic DI presents a management dilemma, because severe hypernatremia is a particular hazard. Management requires regular DDAVP; fixed fluid intakes, which may vary with climatic conditions; and regular review for measurement of plasma sodium. Associated hypothalamic abnormalities are often seen with ADI, including hypothalamic obesity and seizure disorders (13). Episodes of dehydration are often complicated by thrombotic complications, including pulmonary thromboembolism. Many patients die prematurely, due to postsurgical complications, electrolyte abnormalities, or sleep apnea. The main management points are summarized in Table 36-3.

The use of demeclocycline for the treatment of SIAD can cause NDI in up to 60% of patients for whom it is prescribed (21). Although there is no reliable way to predict those who will develop NDI, the presence of an intact thirst mechanism will prevent the development of hypernatremia unless an intercurrent illness supervenes. Although the vaptan

Table 36-3. Management of Adipsic Diabetes Insipidus

Inpatient management initially to determine correct fluid intake and desmopressin dose to ensure eunatremia
Daily weights
Fixed daily fluid intake—approximately 2 L/day (depending on weight, climatic conditions, and exercise levels), with extra fluid repletion if patient is below his/her eunatremic weight
Regular clinic review and plasma sodium measurement
Low molecular weight heparin during periods of hypernatremia dehydration
Screen for sleep apnea
Formal diet and exercise programs
Clinician awareness of heightened risk of poikilothermia and hypothalamic seizures

class of medications rarely causes hypernatremia in patients with SIAD (20), these medications have the potential to cause severe hypernatremia if used erroneously in patients with hypovolemic hyponatremia. Given that clinical assessment of blood volume status is difficult (51), vaptans should only be prescribed by those with expertise in this field (21,51).

CONCLUSIONS

Hypernatremia is common in the emergency setting, and it is associated with significant morbidity and mortality, primarily caused by cell shrinkage due to extracellular movement of water. Acute hypernatremia usually occurs due to inadequate water intake and/or excessive water loss, leading to inappropriate plasma hyperosmolality. It is often seen in elderly patients with insensible fluid losses and/or a comorbid condition that further affects cognition and thirst. In a small number of cases, hypernatremia develops in patients with DI, who develop intercurrent illnesses such as gastroenteritis.

The mainstay of management of acute hypernatremia is rehydration with 0.45% saline or 5% dextrose, used for their high free water content when compared with isotonic saline. However, if the patient is hemodynamically unstable, isotonic saline should be used initially. Acute symptomatic hypernatremia may be corrected relatively rapidly; the rate of correction can reach a maximum of 1 mEq/L/hr (1 mmol/L/hr) to a maximum of 10 to 12 mEq/L (10–12 mmol/L/day). Chronic hypernatremia should be corrected gradually because cerebral edema may develop if correction is over rapid. In patients at risk of thrombotic episodes, prophylactic anticoagulation should also be considered.

ACKNOWLEDGMENTS

The authors have nothing to disclose.

REFERENCES

1. **Lindner G, Funk GC.** Hypernatremia in critically ill patients. *J Crit Care.* 2013;28:216.e11– 216.e20.
2. **Kraft MD, Btaiche IF, Sacks GS, Kudsk KA.** Treatment of electrolyte disorders in adult patients in the intensive care unit. *Am J Health Syst Pharm.* 2005;62:1663–1682.
3. **Arampatzis S, Exadaktylos A, Buhl D, Zimmermann H, Lindner G.** Dysnatraemias in the emergency room: undetected, untreated, unknown? *Wien Klin Wochenschr.* 2012;124:181–183.
4. **Arampatzis S, Funk GC, Leichtle AB, et al.** Impact of diuretic therapy-associated electrolyte disorders present on admission to the emergency department: a cross-sectional analysis. *BMC Med.* 2013;11:83.
5. **Miller M.** Fluid and electrolyte homeostasis in the elderly: physiological changes of ageing and clinical consequences. *Baillieres Clin Endocrinol Metab.* 1997;11:367–387.
6. **Crowe MJ, Forsling ML, Rolls BJ, Phillips PA, Ledingham JG, Smith RF.** Altered water excretion in healthy elderly men. *Age Ageing.* 1987;16:285–293.
7. **Adrogue HJ, Madias NE.** Hypernatremia. *N Engl J Med.* 2000;342:1493–1499.
8. **Baylis PH, Thompson CJ.** Osmoregulation of vasopressin secretion and thirst in health and disease. *Clin Endocrinol (Oxf).* 1988;29:549–576.
9. **McKenna K, Thompson C.** Osmoregulation in clinical disorders of thirst appreciation. *Clin Endocrinol (Oxf).* 1998;49:139–152.
10. **Gill G, Baylis P, Burn J.** A case of "essential" hypernatraemia due to resetting of the osmostat. *Clin Endocrinol (Oxf).* 1985;22:545–551.
11. **Thompson CJ, Freeman J, Record CO, Baylis PH.** Hypernatraemia due to a reset osmostat for vasopressin release and thirst, complicated by nephrogenic diabetes insipidus. *Postgrad Med J.* 1987;63:979–982.
12. **Schaff-Blass E, Robertson GL, Rosenfield RL.** Chronic hypernatremia from a congenital defect in osmoregulation of thirst and vasopressin. *J Pediatr.* 1983;102:703–708.
13. **Crowley RK, Sherlock M, Agha A, Smith D, Thompson CJ.** Clinical insights into adipsic diabetes insipidus: a large case series. *Clin Endocrinol (Oxf).* 2007;66:475–482.
14. **Sherlock M, Agha A, Crowley R, Smith D, Thompson CJ.** Adipsic diabetes insipidus following pituitary surgery for a macroprolactinoma. *Pituitary.* 2006;9:59–64.

15. **Smith D, McKenna K, Moore K, et al.** Baroregulation of vasopressin release in adipsic diabetes insipidus. *J Clin Endocrinol Metab.* 2002;87:4564–4568.
16. **Hammond DN, Moll GW, Robertson GL, Chelmicka-Schorr E.** Hypodipsic hypernatremia with normal osmoregulation of vasopressin. *N Engl J Med.* 1986;315:433–436.
17. **Thompson CJ, Baylis PH.** Thirst in diabetes insipidus: clinical relevance of quantitative assessment. *Q J Med.* 1987;65:853–862.
18. **Moeller HB, Rittig S, Fenton RA.** Nephrogenic diabetes insipidus: essential insights into the molecular background and potential therapies for treatment. *Endocr Rev.* 2013;34:278–301.
19. **Schrier RW, Gross P, Gheorghiade M, et al.** Tolvaptan, a selective oral vasopressin V2-receptor antagonist, for hyponatremia. *N Engl J Med.* 2006;355:2099–2112.
20. **Berl T, Quittnat-Pelletier F, Verbalis JG, et al.** Oral tolvaptan is safe and effective in chronic hyponatremia. *J Am Soc Nephrol.* 2010;21:705–712.
21. **Sherlock M, Thompson CJ.** The syndrome of inappropriate antidiuretic hormone: current and future management options. *Eur J Endocrinol.* 2010; 162(suppl 1):S13–S18.
22. **Thompson C, Hoorn EJ.** Hyponatraemia: an overview of frequency, clinical presentation and complications. *Best Pract Res Clin Endocrinol Metab.* 2012;26 (suppl 1):S1–S6.
23. **Young WF.** Primary aldosteronism: renaissance of a syndrome. *Clin Endocrinol (Oxf).* 2007;66:607–618.
24. **Mulatero P, Stowasser M, Loh KC, et al.** Increased diagnosis of primary aldosteronism, including surgically correctable forms, in centers from five continents. *J Clin Endocrinol Metab.* 2004;89:1045–1050.
25. **Gregoire JR.** Adjustment of the osmostat in primary aldosteronism. *Mayo Clin Proc.* 1994;69:1108–1110.
26. **Torpy DJ, Mullen N, Ilias I, Nieman LK.** Association of hypertension and hypokalemia with Cushing's syndrome caused by ectopic ACTH secretion: a series of 58 cases. *Ann N Y Acad Sci.* 2002;970:134–144.
27. **Edwards CR.** Renal 11-beta-hydroxysteroid dehydrogenase: a mechanism ensuring mineralocorticoid specificity. *Horm Res.* 1990;34:114–117.
28. **Walker BR, Edwards CR.** Licorice-induced hypertension and syndromes of apparent mineralocorticoid excess. *Endocrinol Metab Clin North Am.* 1994;23: 359–377.
29. **Arora SK.** Hypernatremic disorders in the intensive care unit. *J Intensive Care Med.* 2013;28:37–45.
30. **AlOrainy IA, O'Gorman AM, Decell MK.** Cerebral bleeding, infarcts, and presumed extrapontine myelinolysis in hypernatraemic dehydration. *Neuroradiology.* 1999;41:144–146.
31. **Clark WR.** Diffuse demyelinating lesions of the brain after the rapid development of hypernatremia. *West J Med.* 1992;157:571–573.
32. **Knochel JP.** Neuromuscular manifestations of electrolyte disorders. *Am J Med.* 1982;72:521–535.
33. **Komjati M, Kastner G, Waldhausl W, Bratusch-Marrain P.** Detrimental effect of hyperosmolality on insulin-stimulated glucose metabolism in adipose and muscle tissue in vitro. *Biochem Med Metab Biol.* 1988;39:312–318.
34. **Bratusch-Marrain PR, DeFronzo RA.** Impairment of insulin-mediated glucose metabolism by hyperosmolality in man. *Diabetes.* 1983;32:1028–1034.
35. **Kamijo Y, Soma K, Hamanaka S, Nagai T, Kurihara K.** Dural sinus thrombosis with severe hypernatremia developing in a patient on long-term lithium therapy. *J Toxicol Clin Toxicol.* 2003;41:359–362.
36. **Berneis K, Ninnis R, Haussinger D, Keller U.** Effects of hyper- and hypoosmolality on whole body protein and glucose kinetics in humans. *Am J Physiol.* 1999;276(1 Pt 1):E188–E195.
37. **Druml W, Kleinberger G, Lenz K, Laggner A, Schneeweiss B.** Fructose-induced hyperlactemia in hyperosmolar syndromes. *Klin Wochenschr.* 1986;64: 615–618.
38. **Abramovici MI, Singhal PC, Trachtman H.** Hypernatremia and rhabdomyolysis. *J Med.* 1992;23:17–28.
39. **Darmon M, Timsit JF, Francais A, et al.** Association between hypernatraemia acquired in the ICU and mortality: a cohort study. *Nephrol Dial Transplant.* 2010;25:2510–2515.
40. **Hannon MJ, Crowley RK, Behan LA, et al.** Acute glucocorticoid deficiency and diabetes insipidus are common after acute traumatic brain injury and predict mortality. *J Clin Endocrinol Metab.* 2013;98:3229–3237.
41. **Hannon MJ, Behan LA, O'Brien MM, et al.** Hyponatremia following mild/moderate subarachnoid hemorrhage is due to SIAD and glucocorticoid deficiency and not cerebral salt wasting. *J Clin Endocrinol Metab.* 2014;99:291–298.
42. **Ekpebegh C, Longo-Mbenza B.** Mortality in hyperglycemic crisis: a high association with infections and cerebrovascular disease. *Minerva Endocrinol.* 2013;38:187–193.
43. **Lindner G, Funk GC, Lassnigg A, et al.** Intensive care-acquired hypernatremia after major cardiothoracic surgery is associated with increased mortality. *Intensive Care Med.* 2010;36:1718–1723.
44. **Arampatzis S, Frauchiger B, Fiedler GM, et al.** Characteristics, symptoms, and outcome of severe dysnatremias present on hospital admission. *Am J Med.* 2012;125:1125.e1–1125.e7.
45. **Hoorn EJ, Tuut MK, Hoorntje SJ, van Saase JL, Zietse R, Geers AB.** Dutch guideline for the management of electrolyte disorders—2012 revision. *Neth J Med.* 2013;71:153–165.
46. **Mohmand HK, Issa D, Ahmad Z, Cappuccio JD, Kouides RW, Sterns RH.** Hypertonic saline for hyponatremia: risk of inadvertent overcorrection. *Clin J Am Soc Nephrol.* 2007;2:1110–1107.
47. **Hoorn EJ, Carlotti AP, Costa LA, et al.** Preventing a drop in effective plasma osmolality to minimize the likelihood of cerebral edema during treatment of children with diabetic ketoacidosis. *J Pediatr.* 2007;150:467–473.
48. **Haringhuizen A, Tjan DH, Grool A, van Vugt R, van Zante AR.** Fatal cerebral oedema in adult diabetic ketoacidosis. *Neth J Med.* 2010;68:35–37.
49. **Hannon MJ, Sherlock M, Thompson CJ.** Pituitary dysfunction following traumatic brain injury or subarachnoid haemorrhage—in "Endocrine Management

in the Intensive Care Unit." *Best Pract Res Clin Endocrinol Metab.* 2011;25:783–798.

50. **Thompson CJ.** Polyuric states in man. *Baillieres Clin Endocrinol Metab.* 1989;3:473–497.

51. **Verbalis JG, Goldsmith SR, Greenberg A, et al.** Diagnosis, evaluation, and treatment of hyponatremia: expert panel recommendations. *Am J Med.* 2013;126(10 suppl 1):S1–S42.

CHAPTER 37

Emergency Management of Acute and Chronic Hyponatremia

Joseph G Verbalis

ABSTRACT

Severely symptomatic hyponatremia does not occur often, but its importance lies in the high morbidity and mortality rates characteristic of this metabolic disorder. Most cases of severely symptomatic hyponatremia occur when the hyponatremia has developed acutely, but even more chronic forms of hyponatremia can have significant neurological symptomatology and occasionally life-threatening manifestations. This chapter will focus on the evaluation and treatment of symptomatic hyponatremia in hospitalized patients in order to provide symptom relief and prevent or minimize the many adverse outcomes associated with this disorder.

INTRODUCTION

Severely symptomatic hyponatremia does not occur often, but its importance lies in the high morbidity and mortality rates characteristic of this metabolic disorder. Most cases of severely symptomatic hyponatremia occur when the hyponatremia has developed acutely, but even more chronic forms of hyponatremia can have significant neurological symptomatology and occasionally life-threatening manifestations (Table 37-1). A recent review proposed comprehensive recommendations by an expert panel for the evaluation and treatment of all types and etiologies of hyponatremia (1); this chapter will not reiterate those recommendations, but rather will focus on the evaluation and treatment that should be initiated promptly for symptomatic hyponatremia in hospitalized patients, in order to provide symptom relief and prevent or minimize the many adverse outcomes that have been independently associated with this disorder (2–4). Determining appropriate treatment choices entails first understanding the classification of different types of hyponatremia and how this relates to the wide spectrum of symptoms of hyponatremia, their pathogenesis, and the morbidity and mortality associated with this metabolic disorder.

CLASSIFICATION OF HYPONATREMIA BY PLASMA TONICITY, EXTRACELLULAR FLUID VOLUME STATUS, AND SEVERITY

Hyponatremia can be classified in a variety of manners. The first is generally by plasma *tonicity*. Patients with hyponatremia can either be hypotonic, isotonic, or hypertonic in terms of their plasma tonicity, which depends on the relationship of the plasma osmolality to the serum sodium concentration. In the most common form, hypotonic hyponatremia, serum sodium concentration ([Na^+]) and plasma osmolality are both low. Examples of this form of hyponatremia include the syndrome of inappropriate antidiuretic hormone secretion (SIADH), heart failure, and cirrhosis. It is important clinically to differentiate hypotonic hyponatremia from isotonic and

Table 37-1. Common Clinical Causes of Symptomatic Hyponatremia in Hospitalized Patients

Acute hyponatremia (≤48-hr duration)
• Water intoxication from psychogenic polydipsia (typically in schizophrenic patients) or excessive forced water ingestion (fraternity hazing)
• Exercise-associated hyponatremia (marathons, ultramarathons, and similar prolonged endurance exercise activities)
• Postoperative hyponatremia
• 3,4-methylenedioxymethamphetamine ("Ecstasy")
Chronic hyponatremia (>48-hr duration)
• Syndrome of inappropriate antidiuretic hormone secretion (SIADH; all etiologies)
• Drug-induced hyponatremia (particularly SSRI antidepressants)
• Hypovolemic hyponatremia (all etiologies, but particularly thiazide-induced hyponatremia)
• Heart failure
• Cirrhosis
• Nephrotic syndrome
• Renal failure

hypertonic hyponatremia. Isotonic hyponatremia occurs when the serum [Na+] is low but the plasma osmolality is normal. This can be seen in hyperglycemia and conditions that are called *pseudohyponatremia* because of hyperlipidemia or hyperproteinemia. Hypertonic hyponatremia also has a low serum [Na+], but in this case, plasma osmolality is high rather than low. This can be seen with severe hyperglycemia with dehydration, as well as with the use of some osmotic agents such as mannitol. These distinctions are important because only hypotonic hyponatremia causes a shift of water from the extracellular fluid (ECF) into cells along osmotic gradients; therefore, it is the only type of hyponatremia that results in alterations of water balance between the extracellular and intracellular fluid.

Once it is confirmed that a patient has hypotonic hyponatremia with a low plasma osmolality, the next level of classification is to determine the ECF volume status of the patient. Patients with hypotonic hyponatremia can be hypovolemic with a decreased ECF volume, euvolemic with a normal clinically determined ECF volume, or hypervolemic with an expanded ECF volume. Hypovolemic patients have the typical signs of volume depletion. The usual causes include gastrointestinal, renal, or cutaneous fluid losses, diuretic therapy, and rarely cerebral salt wasting and primary adrenal insufficiency. In contrast, euvolemic hyponatremia is characterized by an absence of any signs of ECF volume depletion or expansion. Typically, the blood urea nitrogen (BUN): creatinine ratio is normal or low, the serum uric acid is low, and the urine sodium is elevated or reflects dietary sodium intake. This is the pattern encountered with SIADH; rare causes include nonsteroidal anti-inflammatory drug (NSAID) use, secondary adrenal insufficiency, severe hypothyroidism (ie, myxedema), exercise-associated hyponatremia, low solute intake, and polydipsia. Finally, hypervolemic hyponatremia patients are those who have edema, ascites, pulmonary congestion, or edema-forming disorders that typically include heart failure, cirrhosis, kidney failure, and the nephrotic syndrome. Classification by ECF volume status is important because virtually all algorithms for the treatment of hypotonic hyponatremia involve an initial determination of the ECF volume status to determine whether the patient has a decreased, normal, or increased ECF volume. This determination dictates the next steps in terms of both diagnostic and treatment decisions, and for that reason it is important to carefully assess the ECF volume status before making treatment decisions for a hyponatremic patient.

Finally, hyponatremia is also classified by severity, which is indicated mainly by neurological symptomatology (Figure 37-1). Severe hyponatremia generally is defined by a lower serum [Na+] (typically <125 mmol/L) and by symptoms indicating significant neurological dysfunction such as coma, obtundation, seizures, respiratory distress, and unexplained vomiting. The typical duration of these cases is short, and it generally represents a more acute form of hyponatremia (Table 37-1). Moderate hyponatremia is also characterized by a low serum [Na+]; however, the serum [Na+] is generally not quite as low as in severe hyponatremia (but it can be), and generally is in the range of <130 mmol/L. The neurological symptoms of moderate hyponatremia, while still present, are not as marked as with severe hyponatremia and include altered mental status, disorientation, confusion, unexplained nausea,

	Serum Sodium	Neurological Symptoms	Typical Duration of Hyponatremia
Severe	<125 mmol/L	Vomiting; seizures; obtundation; respiratory distress; coma	Acute (<24–48 hr)
Moderate	<130 mmol/L	Nausea; confusion; disorientation; altered mental status; unstable gait/falls	Intermediate or chronic (>24–48 hr)
Mild	<135 mmol/L	Headache; irritability; difficulty concentrating; altered mood; depression	Chronic (several days to many weeks/months)

Figure 37-1. Classification of hyponatremia according to severity of presenting symptoms.

unstable gait, and increased falls. Typically these patients have a duration of hyponatremia that is intermediate or chronic, usually greater than 24 to 48 hours but generally not weeks or months in duration. Finally, mild hyponatremia can have any serum [Na^+], including up to 134 mmol/L, and is characterized by very mild and often nonspecific neurological symptoms, including difficulty concentrating, irritability, altered mood, depression, and unexplained headache. Typically patients with this level of severity of hyponatremia have been hyponatremic for several days to many weeks to months; so mild hyponatremia typically is a manifestation of chronic hyponatremia. As explained in the next section, the severity of neurological symptoms is more dependent on the degree of brain adaptation to the hyponatremia than on the level of serum [Na^+]. That is why in the serum [Na^+] column in Figure 37-1, there is a wide range of [Na^+] values that can encompass the various severity levels of hyponatremia. It is crucial to assess the severity of the hyponatremia because most treatment algorithms use the severity of hyponatremia, as determined by the degree of neurological symptoms, to determine the initial therapy.

HYPONATREMIA SYMPTOMS, MORBIDITY, AND MORTALITY

Symptoms of hyponatremia correlate both with the magnitude and rate of the decrease in the serum [Na^+] and with the chronicity of the hyponatremia. Most clinical manifestations of hyponatremia usually begin at serum [Na^+] <130 mmol/L. Although gastrointestinal symptoms often occur early, the majority of the manifestations are neurological, including lethargy, confusion, disorientation, obtundation, and seizures, designated as *hyponatremic encephalopathy* (5). Many of the symptoms of hyponatremic encephalopathy are caused by cerebral edema. In its most severe form, the cerebral edema can lead to tentorial herniation; in such cases, death can occur as a result of brain stem compression with respiratory arrest. The cerebral edema can also cause a neurogenic pulmonary edema and hypoxemia (6), which can, in turn, increase the severity of brain swelling (7). The most severe life-threatening clinical features of hyponatremic encephalopathy are generally seen in cases of acute hyponatremia, defined as <48 hours in duration, but in most cases <24 hours in duration (Table 37-1). The development of neurological symptoms also depends on the age and gender of the patient, and the magnitude and acuteness of the process. Elderly persons and young children with hyponatremia are most likely to develop symptoms. Neurological complications also appear to occur more frequently in menstruating women (7).

The observed central nervous system symptoms of severe hyponatremia are most likely related to the cellular swelling and cerebral edema that result from acute lowering of ECF osmolality, which leads to movement of water into cells. Such cerebral edema occasionally causes brain herniation, as has been noted in postmortem examination of both humans and experimental animals. The increase in brain water is, however, much less marked than would be predicted from the decrease in tonicity were the brain to operate as a passive osmometer. The volume regulatory responses that protect against cerebral edema, and which occur to varying degrees throughout the body, have been extensively studied and reviewed (8); studies of rats demonstrate a prompt loss of both electrolyte and organic osmolytes from the brain after the onset of hyponatremia (9) (Figure 37-2). The rate at which the brain restores the lost electrolytes and osmolytes when hyponatremia is corrected is also of pathophysiological importance. Na^+ and Cl^- recover quickly and even overshoot normal brain contents; however, the reaccumulation of osmolytes is considerably delayed (10). This process is likely to account for the more remarked cerebral dehydration that accompanies the correction in previously adapted animals (11).

The mortality of acute symptomatic hyponatremia has been noted to be as high as 55% and as low as 5% (12,13). The former reflects

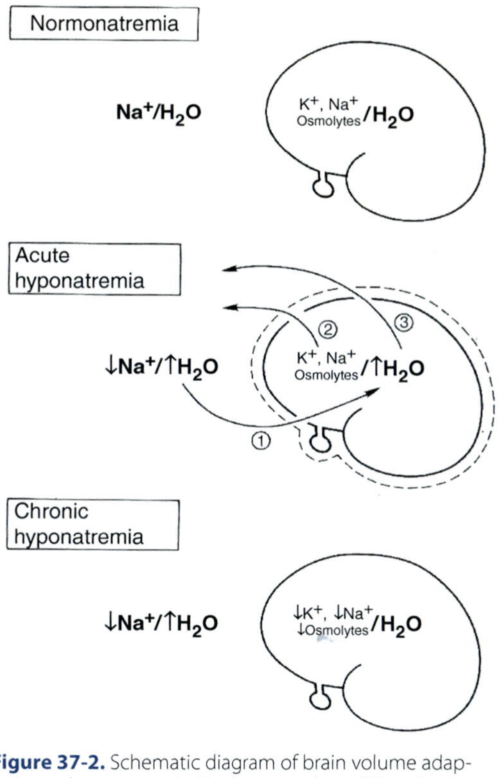

Figure 37-2. Schematic diagram of brain volume adaptation to hyponatremia. Under normal conditions brain osmolality and extracellular fluid (ECF) osmolality are in equilibrium (top panel; for simplicity the predominant intracellular solutes are depicted as K^+ and organic osmolytes and the extracellular solute as Na^+). Following the induction of ECF hypo-osmolality, water moves into the brain in response to osmotic gradients producing brain edema (dotted line, middle panel, #1). However, in response to the induced swelling the brain rapidly loses both extracellular and intracellular solutes (middle panel, #2). As water losses accompany the losses of brain solute, the expanded brain volume then decreases back toward normal (middle panel, #3). If hypo-osmolality is sustained, brain volume eventually normalizes completely and the brain becomes fully adapted to the ECF hyponatremia (bottom panel).

the observation of few symptomatic hyponatremic patients in a consultative setting, the latter the estimate from a broad-based literature survey. The mortality associated with chronic hyponatremia is generally lower and has been reported to be between 14% and 27% (14,15). The contribution of the hyponatremia to the observed mortality in hyponatremic patients remains uncertain. In a survey of hospitalized hyponatremic patients (serum [Na^+] <128 mmol/L), 46% had central nervous system symptoms, and 54% were asymptomatic (16). However, the authors judged that the hyponatremia was the cause of the symptoms in only 31% of the symptomatic patients. In this subgroup of symptomatic patients, the mortality was no different from that of asymptomatic patients (9%–10%). In contrast, the mortality of patients whose central nervous system symptoms were not caused by hyponatremia was high (64%), suggesting that the mortality of these patients is more often due to the associated disease than to the electrolyte disorder itself. This is in agreement with the early report of Anderson (17), who noted a 60-fold increase in mortality in hyponatremic patients over that of normonatremic control subjects, but in the hyponatremic patients, death frequently occurred after the serum [Na^+] was returned toward normal and was generally felt to be due to progression of severe underlying disease. These and other studies suggest that hyponatremia may be more an indicator of severe disease and poor prognosis, rather than a causal factor contributing to mortality. In opposition to this presumption, an increasing number of recent studies indicate that even mild hyponatremia is an independent predictor of higher mortality across a wide variety of disorders, including patients with acute ST-segment elevation myocardial infarctions, heart failure, and liver disease (4,18), as well as all hospitalized medical (2) and surgical (19) patients. Therefore, the degree to which hyponatremia actually causes adverse outcomes rather than simply being associated with underlying comorbidities remains undetermined at the present time (20).

In contrast to acute hyponatremia, chronic hyponatremia is much less symptomatic, and the reason for the profound differences between the symptoms of acute and chronic hyponatremia is now well-understood to be due to the process of *brain volume regulation* described previously (21) (Figure 37-2). Despite this powerful adaptation process, chronic hyponatremia is frequently associated with neurological symptomatology, albeit milder and more subtle in nature. Even in patients adjudged to be "asymptomatic" by virtue of a normal neurological exam, accumulating evidence suggests that there may be previously unrecognized adverse effects as a result of chronic hyponatremia. In one study, 16 patients with hyponatremia secondary to SIADH in the range of 124–130 mmol/L demonstrated a significant gait instability that normalized after correction of the hyponatremia to normal ranges (22). The functional significance of the gait instability was illustrated in a study of 122 patients with a variety of levels of hyponatremia, all judged to be "asymptomatic" at the time of visit to an emergency department (ED). These patients were compared with 244 age-, sex-, and disease-matched controls also presenting to the ED during the same time period. Researchers found that 21% of the hyponatremic patients presented to the ED because of a recent fall, compared with only 5% of the controls; this difference was highly significant and remained so after multivariable adjustment (22). Consequently, this study clearly documented an increased incidence of falls in so-called "asymptomatic" hyponatremic patients. The clinical significance of the gait instability and fall data have been indicated by multiple independent studies that have demonstrated increased rates of bone fractures in patients with hyponatremia (3,23–25). More recently, published studies have shown that hyponatremia is associated with increased bone loss in experimental animals and a significant increased odds ratio for osteoporosis of the femoral neck (OR, 2.87; $p < 0.003$) in humans over the age of 50 years in the NHANES III database (26). Thus, the major clinical significance of chronic hyponatremia may lie in the increased morbidity and mortality associated with falls and fractures in our elderly population.

TREATMENT OF SYMPTOMATIC HYPONATREMIA: GENERAL PRINCIPLES

Correction of hyponatremia is associated with markedly improved neurological outcomes in patients with severely symptomatic hyponatremia. In a retrospective review of patients who presented with severe neurological symptoms and serum [Na^+] <125 mmol/L, prompt therapy with isotonic or hypertonic saline resulted in a correction in the range of 20 mEq/L over several days and neurological recovery in almost all cases; in contrast, in patients who were treated with fluid restriction alone, there was very little correction over the study period (<5 mEq/L over 72 hr), and the neurological outcomes were much worse, with most of these patients either dying or entering a persistently vegetative state (27). Consequently, based on this and many similar retrospective analyses, prompt therapy to rapidly increase the serum [Na^+] represents the standard-of-care for treatment of patients presenting with severe life-threatening symptoms of hyponatremia.

Brain herniation, the most dreaded complication of hyponatremia, is seen almost exclusively in patients with acute hyponatremia (usually <24 hr) or in patients with intracranial pathology (28–30). In postoperative patients, patients with self-induced water intoxication associated with marathon running, patients with psychosis, or those with a history of "Ecstasy" (3,4-methylenedioxymethamphetamine or MDMA) use, nonspecific symptoms like headache, nausea, and vomiting or confusion can rapidly progress to seizures, respiratory arrest, and ultimately to death or to a permanent vegetative state as a complication of severe cerebral edema (31). Hypoxia from noncardiogenic pulmonary edema and/or hypoventilation can exacerbate brain swelling caused by the low serum [Na^+] (6,7). Seizures can complicate both severe chronic hyponatremia and acute hyponatremia. Although usually self-limited, hyponatremic seizures may be refractory to anticonvulsants.

As discussed earlier, chronic hyponatremia is much less symptomatic as a result of the process of brain volume regulation. Because of this adaptation process, chronic hyponatremia is arguably a condition that clinicians feel they may not need to be as concerned about, which has been reinforced by the common usage of the descriptor "asymptomatic hyponatremia" for many such patients. However, as discussed previously, it is clear that such patients very often do have neurological symptoms, even if milder and more subtle in nature, including headaches, nausea, mood disturbances, depression, difficulty concentrating, slowed reaction times, unstable gait, increased falls, confusion, and disorientation (22). Consequently, all patients with hyponatremia who manifest any neurological symptoms that could possibly be related to the hyponatremia should be considered candidates for treatment of the hyponatremia, regardless of the chronicity of the hyponatremia or the level of serum [Na^+]. An additional reason to treat even asymptomatic hyponatremia effectively is to prevent a lowering of the serum [Na^+] to more symptomatic and dangerous levels during treatment of underlying conditions (eg, increased fluid administration via parenteral nutrition, treatment of heart failure with loop diuretics).

CURRENTLY AVAILABLE THERAPIES FOR TREATMENT OF SYMPTOMATIC HYPONATREMIA

Conventional management strategies for hyponatremia range from saline infusion and fluid restriction to pharmacological measures to adjust fluid balance. Although the number of available treatments for hyponatremia is large, some are not appropriate for correction of symptomatic hyponatremia because they work too slowly or inconsistently to be effective in hospitalized patients (eg, demeclocycline, mineralocorticoids). Consideration of treatment options should always include an evaluation of the benefits as well as the potential toxicities of any therapy, and must be individualized for each patient (32). It should always be remembered that sometimes simply stopping treatment with an agent that is associated with hyponatremia is sufficient to correct a low serum [Na^+].

Hypertonic Saline

Acute hyponatremia presenting with severe neurological symptoms is life-threatening, and should be treated promptly with hypertonic solutions, typically 3% NaCl ([Na^+] = 513 mmol/L), as this represents the most reliable method to quickly raise the serum [Na^+]. A continuous infusion of hypertonic NaCl is usually utilized in inpatient settings. Various formulas have been suggested for calculating the initial rate of infusion of hypertonic solutions (28), but until now there has been no consensus regarding optimal infusion rates of 3% NaCl. One of the simplest methods to estimate an initial 3% NaCl infusion rate utilizes the following relationship (32): patient's weight (kg) × desired correction rate (mEq/L/hr) = infusion rate of 3% NaCl (mL/hr).

Depending on individual hospital policies, the administration of hypertonic solutions may require special considerations (eg, placement in the intensive care unit [ICU], sign-off by a consultant), which each clinician needs to be aware of in order to optimize patient care.

An alternative option for more emergent situations is administration of a 100-mL bolus of 3% NaCl, repeated every 30 minutes up to 2 times if there is no clinical improvement, which has been recommended by a consensus conference organized to develop guidelines for prevention and treatment of exercise-induced hyponatremia, an acute and potentially lethal condition (33), and adopted as a general recommendation by an expert panel (1). Injecting this amount of hypertonic saline intravenously raises the serum [Na^+] by an average of 2–4 mmol/L, which is well below the recommended maximal daily rate of change of 10–12 mmol/24 hr or 18 mmol/48 hr (34). Because the brain can only accommodate an average increase of approximately 8% in brain volume before herniation occurs, quickly increasing the serum [Na^+] by as little as 2–4 mmol/L in acute hyponatremia can effectively reduce brain swelling and intracranial pressure (35).

Isotonic Saline

The treatment of choice for depletional hyponatremia (ie, hypovolemic hyponatremia) is isotonic saline ([Na^+] = 154 mmol/L) to restore ECF volume and ensure adequate organ perfusion. This initial therapy is appropriate for patients who either have clinical signs of hypovolemia, or in whom a spot urine Na^+ concentration is <20–30 mEq/L (1). However, this therapy is ineffective for dilutional hyponatremias such as SIADH (36), and continued inappropriate administration of isotonic saline to a euvolemic patient may worsen his or her hyponatremia (37) and/or cause fluid overload. Although isotonic saline may improve the serum [Na^+] in some patients with hypervolemic hyponatremia, their volume status will generally worsen with this therapy, so unless the hyponatremia is profound, isotonic saline should be avoided.

Fluid Restriction

For patients with chronic hyponatremia, fluid restriction has been the most popular and most widely accepted treatment. When SIADH is present, fluids should generally be limited to 500–1,000 mL/24 hr. Because fluid restriction increases the serum [Na^+] largely by under-replacing the excretion of fluid by the kidneys, some have advocated an initial restriction to 500 mL less than the 24-hour urine output (38). When instituting a fluid restriction, it is important for the nursing staff and the patient to understand that this includes all fluids that are consumed, not just water (Table 37-2). Generally the water content of ingested food is not included in the restriction because this is balanced by insensible water losses (perspiration, exhaled air, feces, etc.), but caution should be exercised with foods that have high fluid concentrations (such as fruits and soups). Restricting fluid intake can be effective when properly applied and managed in selected patients, but serum [Na^+] is generally increased only slowly (1–2 mmol/L/day) even with severe fluid restriction (36). In addition, this therapy is often poorly tolerated because of an associated increase in thirst leading to poor compliance with long-term therapy. However, it is economically favorable, and some patients do respond well to this option.

Table 37-2. General Recommendations for Employment of Fluid Restriction and Predictors of the Increased Likelihood of Failure of Fluid Restriction (1)

General recommendations
• Restrict *all* intake that is consumed by drinking, not just water
• Aim for a fluid restriction that is 500 mL/day *below* the 24-hour urine volume
• Do *not* restrict sodium or protein intake unless indicated
Predictors of the likely failure of fluid restriction
• High urine osmolality (>500 mOsm/kg H_2O)
• Sum of the urine Na^+ and K^+ concentrations exceeds the serum [Na^+] concentration
• 24-hour urine volume <1,500 mL/day
• Increase in serum sodium concentration ([Na^+]) <2 mmol/L/day in 24 to 48 hours on a fluid restriction of ≥1 L/day

Fluid restriction should not be used with hypovolemic patients and is particularly difficult to maintain in hospitalized patients with very elevated urine osmolalities secondary to high plasma arginine vasopressin (AVP) levels; if the sum of urine Na^+ and K^+ exceeds the serum [Na^+], most patients will not respond to a fluid restriction because an electrolyte-free water clearance will be difficult to achieve (39–41). This and other known predictors of failure of fluid restriction are summarized in Table 37-2; the presence of any of these factors in hospitalized patients with symptomatic hyponatremia makes this less than ideal as an initial therapy. In addition, fluid restriction is not practical for some patients, particularly patients in intensive care settings who often require administration of significant volumes of fluids as part of their therapies. Consequently, such patients are candidates for more effective pharmacological or saline treatment strategies.

Arginine Vasopressin Receptor Antagonists

Conventional therapies for hyponatremia, although effective in specific circumstances, are suboptimal for many different reasons, including variable efficacy, slow responses, intolerable side effects, and serious toxicities. But perhaps the most striking deficiency of most conventional therapies is that most of these therapies do not directly target the underlying cause of most dilutional hyponatremias, namely inappropriately elevated AVP levels. A new class of pharmacological agents, *vasopressin receptor antagonists*, also known as "vaptans," that directly block AVP-mediated receptor activation have recently been approved for treatment of euvolemic (United States and European Union) and hypervolemic (United States) hyponatremia (42).

Conivaptan is approved by the Food and Drug Administration (FDA) in the United States for euvolemic and hypervolemic hyponatremia in hospitalized patients. It is available only as an intravenous preparation and is given as a 20-mg loading dose over 30 minutes, followed by a continuous infusion of 20 or 40 mg/day (43). Generally, the 20-mg continuous infusion is used for the first 24 hours to gauge the initial response. If the correction

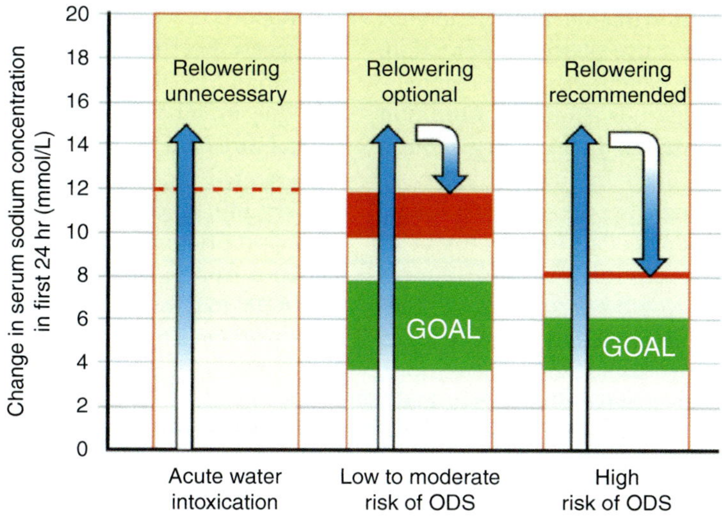

Figure 37-3. Recommended goals (green) and limits (red) for correction of hyponatremia based on risk of producing osmotic demyelination syndrome and recommendations for relowering of serum sodium concentration ($[Na^+]$) to goals for patients presenting with serum $[Na^+]$ <120 mmol/L who exceed the recommended limits of correction in the first 24 hours.

of serum $[Na^+]$ is felt to be inadequate (eg, <5 mmol/L), then the infusion rate can be increased to 40 mg/day. Therapy is limited to a maximum duration of 4 days because of drug-interaction effects with other agents metabolized by the CYP3A4 hepatic isoenzyme. Importantly, for conivaptan and all other vaptans, it is critical that the serum $[Na^+]$ concentration is measured frequently during the active phase of correction of the hyponatremia—a minimum of every 6 to 8 hours for conivaptan but more frequently in patients with risk factors for the osmotic demyelination syndrome (ODS) (32). If the correction exceeds 10 to 12 mmol/L in the first 24 hours, the infusion should be stopped and the patient monitored closely. Consideration should be given to administering sufficient water, either orally or as intravenous 5% dextrose in water, to avoid a correction of >12 mmol/L/day. The maximum correction limit should be reduced to 8 mmol/L over the first 24 hours in patients with risk factors for ODS (1) (Figure 37-3). The most common side effects of conivaptan include headache, thirst, and hypokalemia (44).

Tolvaptan, an oral vasopressin receptor antagonist, is also FDA-approved for the treatment of euvolemic and hypervolemic hyponatremia. In contrast to conivaptan, the availability of tolvaptan in tablet form allows both short- and long-term use (45). Similar to conivaptan, tolvaptan treatment must be initiated in the hospital so that the rate of correction can be monitored carefully. In the United States, patients with a serum $[Na^+]$ <125 mmol/L are eligible for therapy with tolvaptan as primary therapy; if the serum $[Na^+]$ is ≥125 mmol/L, tolvaptan therapy is only indicated if the patient has symptoms that could be attributable to the hyponatremia, and the patient is resistant to attempts at fluid restriction (46). In the European Union, tolvaptan is approved only for the treatment of euvolemic hyponatremia, but any symptomatic euvolemic patient is eligible for tolvaptan therapy regardless of the level of hyponatremia or response to previous fluid restriction. The starting dose of tolvaptan is 15 mg on the first day, and the dose can be titrated to 30 mg and 60 mg at 24-hour intervals if the serum $[Na^+]$ remains <135 mmol/L, or the increase in serum $[Na^+]$ has been <5 mmol/L in the previous 24 hours. As with conivaptan, it is essential that the serum $[Na^+]$ concentration is measured frequently during the active phase of correction of the hyponatremia, at a minimum of every 6 to 8 hours, particularly in patients with risk factors for ODS. Goals and limits for safe correction of hyponatremia and methods to compensate for overly rapid corrections are the same as described previously for conivaptan (Figure 37-3). One additional factor that helps to avoid overly rapid correction with tolvaptan is the recommendation that fluid restriction not be used during the active phase of correction, thereby allowing the patient's thirst to compensate for an overly vigorous aquaresis. Common side effects of tolvaptan include dry mouth, thirst, increased urinary frequency, dizziness, nausea, and orthostatic hypotension (45,46).

Vaptans are not needed for treatment of hypovolemic hyponatremia, because simple volume expansion would be expected to abolish the nonosmotic stimulus to AVP secretion and lead to a prompt aquaresis. Furthermore, inducing increased renal fluid excretion via either a diuresis or an aquaresis can cause or worsen hypotension in such patients. This possibility has resulted in the labeling of these drugs as contraindicated for hypovolemic hyponatremia (32). Importantly, clinically significant hypotension was not observed in either the conivaptan or tolvaptan clinical trials in euvolemic and hypervolemic hyponatremic patients. Although vaptans are not contraindicated with decreased renal function, these agents generally will not be effective if the serum creatinine is 3.0 mg/dL.

Urea

Urea has been described as an alternative oral treatment for SIADH and other hyponatremic disorders. The mode of action is to correct hypo-osmolality not only by increasing solute-free water excretion but also by decreasing urinary sodium excretion. Doses of 15 to 60 g/day are generally effective; the dose can be titrated in increments of 15 g/day at weekly intervals as necessary to achieve normalization of the serum [Na^+]. It is advisable to dissolve the urea in orange juice or some other strongly flavored liquid to camouflage the bitter taste. Even if completely normal water balance is not achieved, it is often possible to allow the patient to maintain a less strict regimen of fluid restriction while receiving urea. The disadvantages associated with the use of urea include poor palatability (though some clinicians feel that this has been exaggerated), the development of azotemia at higher doses, and the unavailability of a convenient or FDA-approved form of the agent. Data suggest that blood urea concentrations may double during treatment (47), but it is important to remember that this does not represent renal impairment.

Reports of retrospective, uncontrolled studies suggest that the use of urea has been effective in treating SIADH in patients with hyponatremia due to subarachnoid hemorrhage and in critical care patients (48), and case reports have documented success in infants with chronic SIADH (49) and the nephrogenic syndrome of inappropriate antidiuresis (50). More recent evidence from a short study in a small cohort of SIADH patients suggests that urea may have a comparable efficacy to vaptans in reversing hyponatremia due to chronic SIADH (51).

Furosemide and NaCl

The use of furosemide (20 to 40 mg/day) coupled with a high salt intake (200 mEq/day), which represents an extension of the treatment of acute symptomatic hyponatremia (52) to the management of chronic euvolemic hyponatremia, has also been reported to be successful in selected cases (53). However, the efficacy of this approach to correct symptomatic hyponatremia both promptly and within accepted goals limits (Figure 37-3) is unknown.

HYPONATREMIA TREATMENT GUIDELINES BASED ON SYMPTOM SEVERITY

Although various authors have published recommendations on the treatment of hyponatremia (1,28,30,32,54,55), no standardized treatment algorithms have yet been universally accepted. For all treatment recommendations, the initial evaluation includes an assessment of the ECF volume status of the patient, because treatment recommendations differ in hypovolemic, euvolemic, and hypervolemic hyponatremic patients. Recommendations for hypovolemic and hypervolemic patients have been updated recently (1). Euvolemic patients, mainly including patients with SIADH, represent a unique challenge because of the multiplicity of causes and presentations of patients with SIADH. A synthesis of existing recommendations for treatment of hyponatremia is illustrated in Figure 37-4. This algorithm is based primarily on the neurological symptomatology of hyponatremic patients rather than the serum [Na^+] or on the chronicity of the hyponatremia, the latter of which is often difficult to ascertain. A careful neurological history and assessment

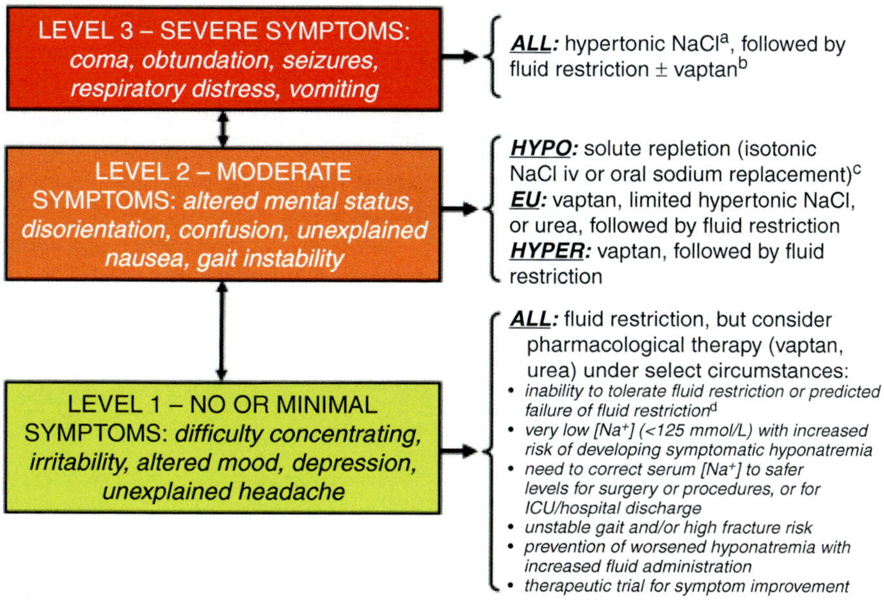

Figure 37-4. Algorithm for treating patients with euvolemic hyponatremia based on their presenting symptoms. The arrows between the symptom boxes indicate movement of patients between different symptom levels. HYPO = hypovolemic hyponatremia; EU = euvolemic hyponatremia; HYPER = hypervolemic hyponatremia; ALL = all types of hypotonic hyponatremia (67).

[a] Some authors recommend simultaneous treatment with desmopressin to limit speed of correction.

[b] No active therapy should be started within 24 hours of hypertonic saline to decrease the risk of overly rapid correction of $[Na^+]$ and risk of ODS.

[c] With isotonic NaCl infusion, serum $[Na^+]$ must be followed closely to prevent overly rapid correction and risk of ODS due to secondary water diuresis.

[d] See Table 37-2 for predictors of failure of fluid restriction.

should always be done to identify potential causes for the patient's symptoms other than hyponatremia, although it will not always be possible to exclude an additive contribution from the hyponatremia to an underlying neurological condition. In this algorithm, patients are divided into 3 groups based on their presenting symptoms (Table 37-1).

Level 1 Symptoms

Level 1 symptoms include coma, obtundation, seizures, respiratory distress or arrest, and unexplained vomiting, and usually imply a more acute onset or worsening of hyponatremia requiring immediate active treatment. Therapies that will quickly raise serum $[Na^+]$ are required to reduce cerebral edema and decrease the risk of potentially fatal brain herniation.

Level 2 Symptoms

Level 2 symptoms are more moderate and include altered mental status, disorientation, confusion, unexplained nausea, gait instability, and falls. These symptoms can be either chronic or acute, but allow more time to elaborate a deliberate approach to choice of treatment.

Level 3 Symptoms

Level 3 symptoms range from minimal symptoms such as difficulty concentrating, irritability, altered mood, depression, and unexplained headache, to a virtual absence of discernable symptoms, and indicate that the patient may have chronic or slowly evolving hyponatremia. These symptoms necessitate a cautious approach, especially when patients have underlying comorbidities.

Patients with severe symptoms (level 1) should be treated with hypertonic (3%) NaCl as first-line therapy, followed by fluid restriction with or without vaptan therapy. Because overly rapid correction of serum $[Na^+]$ occurs in >10% of patients treated with hypertonic NaCl (56), such patients are at risk for ODS unless carefully monitored. For this reason, some authors have proposed simultaneous treatment with desmopressin to reduce the rate of correction to only that produced by the hypertonic NaCl infusion itself (57,58). Whether sufficient clinical data eventually prove that this approach is both effective and safe in larger numbers of patients remains to be determined. Although no cases of ODS have yet been reported in patients receiving vaptans alone as monotherapy, 2 abstracts have been reported where ODS occurred when vaptans were used directly following hypertonic saline administration within the same 24-hour period (1). Consequently, no active hyponatremia therapy should be administered until at least 24 hours following successful increases in serum [Na^+] using hypertonic NaCl.

The choice of treatment for patients with moderate symptoms (level 2) will depend on their ECF volume status (Figure 37-4). Hypovolemic patients should be treated with solute repletion, either via isotonic NaCl infusion or oral sodium replacement (1). Euvolemic patients, typically with SIADH, will benefit from vaptan therapy, limited hypertonic saline administration, or in some cases urea, where available. This can then be followed by fluid restriction or long-term vaptan therapy when the etiology of the SIADH is expected to be chronic (1). In hypervolemic patients with heart failure, vaptans are usually the best choice because fluid restriction is rarely successful in this group, saline administration can cause fluid retention with increased edema, and urea can lead to ammonia build-up in the gastrointestinal tract if hepatic function is impaired. Although moderate neurological symptoms can indicate that a patient is in an early stage of acute hyponatremia, they more often indicate a chronically hyponatremic state with sufficient brain volume adaptation to prevent marked symptomatology from cerebral edema. Because most patents with moderate hyponatremic symptoms have a more chronic form of hyponatremia, guidelines for goals and limits of correction should be followed closely (Figure 37-3), and close monitoring of these patients in a hospital setting is warranted until the symptoms improve or stabilize.

Patients with no or minimal symptoms should be managed initially with fluid restriction, although treatment with pharmacological therapy, such as vaptans or urea, may be appropriate for a wide range of specific clinical conditions (Figure 37-4), foremost of which is a failure to improve the serum [Na^+] despite reasonable attempts at fluid restriction, or the presence of clinical characteristics associated with poor responses to fluid restriction (Table 37-2).

A special case is when spontaneous correction of hyponatremia occurs at an undesirably rapid rate as a result of the onset of a water diuresis. This can occur following cessation of desmopressin therapy in a patient who has become hyponatremic, replacement of glucocorticoids in a patient with adrenal insufficiency, replacement of solutes in a patient with diuretic-induced hyponatremia, or spontaneous resolution of transient SIADH. Brain damage from ODS can clearly ensue in this setting if the preceding period of hyponatremia has been of sufficient duration (usually ≥48 hr) to allow brain volume regulation to occur. If the previously discussed correction parameters have been exceeded, and the correction is proceeding more rapidly than planned (usually because of continued excretion of hypotonic urine), the pathological events leading to demyelination can be reversed by administration of hypotonic fluids, with or without desmopressin. Efficacy of this approach is suggested both from animal studies (59) as well as case reports in humans (30,60) even when patients are overtly symptomatic (61). However, relowering the serum [Na^+] after an initial overly rapid correction is only strongly recommended in patients who are at high risk of ODS (Table 37-3), is considered optional in patients with low to moderate risk of ODS, and is unnecessary in patients with acute water intoxication (Figure 37-3).

Although this classification is based on presenting symptoms at the time of initial evaluation, it should be remembered that in some cases patients initially exhibit more moderate symptoms because they are in the early stages of hyponatremia. In addition, some patients with minimal symptoms are prone to develop more symptomatic hyponatremia during periods of increased fluid ingestion. In support of this, approximately 70% of 31 patients presenting to a university hospital with symptomatic hyponatremia and a mean serum [Na^+] of 119 mmol/L had preexisting "asymptomatic" hyponatremia as the most common risk

Table 37-3. Factors Conferring Increased Risk of Osmotic Demyelination Syndrome That Necessitate Slower Correction of Hyponatremia (1)

• Serum sodium concentration ≤105 mmol/L
• Hypokalemia[a]
• Alcoholism[a]
• Malnutrition[a]
• Advanced liver disease[a]

[a] Unlike the increase in serum sodium concentration, neither the precise level of the serum potassium concentration nor the degree of alcoholism, malnutrition, or liver disease that alters the brain's tolerance to an acute osmotic stress has been rigorously defined.

factor identified (62). Consequently, therapy of hyponatremia should also be considered to prevent progression from lower to higher levels of symptomatic hyponatremia, particularly in patients with a past history of repeated presentations for symptomatic hyponatremia.

MONITORING THE SERUM [NA⁺] IN HYPONATREMIC PATIENTS

The frequency of serum [Na^+] monitoring depends on both the severity of the hyponatremia and the therapy chosen. In all hyponatremic patients neurological symptomatology should be carefully assessed very early in the diagnostic evaluation to assess the symptomatic severity of the hyponatremia and to determine whether the patient requires more urgent therapy. All patients undergoing active treatment with hypertonic saline for level 1 or 2 symptomatic hyponatremia should have frequent monitoring of serum [Na^+] and ECF volume status (every 2–4 hr) to ensure that the serum [Na^+] does not exceed the limits of safe correction during the active phase of correction (32), because overly rapid correction of serum sodium will increase the risk of ODS (63). Patients treated with vaptans for level 2 or 3 symptoms should have serum [Na^+] monitored every 6–8 hours during the active phase of correction, which will generally be the first 24–48 hours of therapy. Active treatment with hypertonic saline or vaptans should be stopped when the patient's symptoms are no longer present; a safe serum [Na^+] (usually >120 mmol/L) has been achieved; or the rate of correction has reached maximum limits of 12 mmol/L within 24 hours, 18 mmol/L within 48 hours (32,34), or 8 mmol/L over any 24-hour period in patients at high risk of ODS (Table 37-3). In patients with a stable level of serum [Na^+] treated with fluid restriction or therapies other than hypertonic saline, measurement of serum [Na^+] daily is generally sufficient, because levels will not change that quickly in the absence of active therapy or large changes in fluid intake or administration.

COMMON CLINICAL QUESTIONS ABOUT INITIAL THERAPY OF SYMPTOMATIC HYPONATREMIA

1. *What is the best method to assess the ECF volume status in patients who appear euvolemic by clinical examination?* In most cases the urine sodium concentration is the best discriminator of effective ECF volume (64,65). Although different authors have proposed different cut-off values for this measure, most agree that a urine sodium <20–30 mmol/L is low and indicates hypovolemia. An exception is patients with heart failure or cirrhosis, who have a low urine sodium because of renal hypoperfusion despite ECF volume expansion.
2. *Can the urine sodium be used in patients on diuretic therapy?* The urine sodium should always be measured prior to initiating therapy in symptomatic patients. If the urine sodium is low, it indicates hypovolemia unless the patient has heart failure or cirrhosis. If the urine sodium is >30 mmol/L, it cannot be determined whether this is due to a contracted ECF volume or to the diuretic until the effect of the diuretic therapy has dissipated (generally 24 hr). Alternatives are measurement of the fractional urine uric acid excretion (65), although it usually takes more than 24 hours to obtain results of this measurement, or a trial infusion of isotonic NaCl to see whether the serum [Na^+] improves (1).
3. *What is the best initial therapy of hyponatremia in patients in whom the ECF volume is indeterminate?* If the patient has severe hyponatremia

by symptoms, infusion of hypertonic NaCl is indicated and will correct both the serum [Na^+] as well as expand the ECF volume. If the patient has moderately symptomatic hyponatremia, the best initial therapy is a trial infusion of isotonic saline to see whether the serum [Na^+] improves (1). Generally 1 L will suffice to make this determination. If no improvement in serum [Na^+] occurs, the infusion should be discontinued, because continued infusion of isotonic NaCl in patents with SIADH can lower the serum [Na^+] via a process called "desalination" (37).

4. *Is measurement of urine sodium concentration valid in patients who have already received saline administration prior to consultation?* The urine sodium reflects the current ECF volume status of the patient. Therefore, it remains useful to differentiate hyponatremia from euvolemia even if patients have already received a saline infusion, which typically occurs in the ED regardless of the etiology of the hyponatremia. However, once the serum [Na^+] begins to correct, the urine sodium is not as useful because many patients with SIADH enter a phase of sodium retention to correct total body sodium deficiency that develops during adaptation to hyponatremia (66).
5. *Should a trial of fluid restriction be tried if the patient manifests predictors of failure of fluid restriction?* The predictors of failure of fluid restriction (Table 37-2) only indicate the relative likelihood of failure of fluid restriction rather than an absolute certainty. However, if fluid restriction is attempted in the presence of 1 or more of these factors, the stringency should be increased to have the best chance of success (ie, maximum fluid of 500–800 mL/day).
6. *Given recent FDA warnings, should liver function tests be monitored in patients receiving a vaptan?* Liver function abnormalities in patients receiving vaptans occurred in clinical trials using 3–5 times the dose of tolvaptan recommended for treatment of hyponatremia for >3 months (1). While it is, therefore, appropriate to avoid tolvaptan use in patients with known liver disease, it is not necessary to closely monitor liver function tests in patients treated with tolvaptan at FDA-approved doses (15–60 mg/day) for shorter periods (<30 day).

ACKNOWLEDGMENTS

JGV has served as a consultant and advisory board and speaker bureau member and has received both research grants and travel support from Otsuka Pharmaceuticals for the development and educational programs related to the use of tolvaptan for the treatment of hyponatremia. He has also served as a consultant and provided expert testimony on behalf of Cornerstone Pharmaceuticals related to their application to the FDA for approval of lixivaptan for the treatment of hyponatremia.

REFERENCES

1. **Verbalis JG, Goldsmith SR, Greenberg A, et al.** Diagnosis, evaluation, and treatment of hyponatremia: expert panel recommendations. *Am J Med.* 2013;126(10 suppl 1):S1–S42.
2. **Wald R, Jaber BL, Price LL, Upadhyay A, Madias NE.** Impact of hospital-associated hyponatremia on selected outcomes. *Arch Intern Med.* 2010;170:294–302.
3. **Hoorn EJ, Rivadeneira F, van Meurs JB, et al.** Mild hyponatremia as a risk factor for fractures: the Rotterdam Study. *J Bone Miner Res.* 2011;26:1822–1828.
4. **Corona G, Giuliani C, Parenti G, et al.** Moderate hyponatremia is associated with increased risk of mortality: evidence from a meta-analysis. *PLoS ONE.* 2013;8:e80451.
5. **Fraser CL, Arieff AI.** Epidemiology, pathophysiology, and management of hyponatremic encephalopathy. *Am J Med.* 1997;102:67–77.
6. **Ayus JC, Varon J, Arieff AI.** Hyponatremia, cerebral edema, and noncardiogenic pulmonary edema in marathon runners. *Ann Intern Med.* 2000;132:711–714.
7. **Ayus JC, Arieff AI.** Pulmonary complications of hyponatremic encephalopathy: noncardiogenic pulmonary edema and hypercapnic respiratory failure [see comments]. *Chest.* 1995;107:517–521.
8. **Pasantes-Morales H, Franco R, Ordaz B, Ochoa LD.** Mechanisms counteracting swelling in brain cells during hyponatremia. *Arch Med Res.* 2002;33:237–244.
9. **Lien YH, Shapiro JI, Chan L.** Study of brain electrolytes and organic osmolytes during correction of

chronic hyponatremia. Implications for the pathogenesis of central pontine myelinolysis. *J Clin Invest.* 1991;88:303–309.

10. **Verbalis JG, Gullans SR.** Rapid correction of hyponatremia produces differential effects on brain osmolyte and electrolyte reaccumulation in rats. *Brain Res.* 1993;606:19–27.
11. **Berl T.** Treating hyponatremia: damned if we do and damned if we don't. *Kidney Int.* 1990;37:1006–1018.
12. **Sterns RH.** Severe symptomatic hyponatremia: treatment and outcome. A study of 64 cases. *Ann Int Med.* 1987;107:656–664.
13. **Berl T.** Treating hyponatremia: what is all the controversy about? [see comments]. [Review]. *Ann Int Med.* 1990;113:417–419.
14. **Sterns RH.** The treatment of hyponatremia: first, do no harm. *Am J Med.* 1990;88:557–560.
15. **Tierney WM, Martin DK, Greenlee MC, Zerbe RL, McDonald CJ.** The prognosis of hyponatremia at hospital admission. *J Gen Intern Med.* 1986;1:380–385.
16. **Baran D, Hutchinson TA.** The outcome of hyponatremia in a general hospital population. *Clin Nephrol.* 1984;22:72–76.
17. **Anderson RJ, Chung HM, Kluge R, Schrier RW.** Hyponatremia: a prospective analysis of its epidemiology and the pathogenetic role of vasopressin. *Ann Int Med.* 1985;102:164–168.
18. **Upadhyay A, Jaber BL, Madias NE.** Incidence and prevalence of hyponatremia. *Am J Med.* 2006;119(7 suppl 1):S30–S35.
19. **Leung AA, McAlister FA, Rogers SO Jr, Pazo V, Wright A, Bates DW.** Preoperative hyponatremia and perioperative complications. *Arch Intern Med.* 2012;172:1474–1481.
20. **Hoorn EJ, Zietse R.** Hyponatremia and mortality: how innocent is the bystander? *Clin J Am Soc Nephrol.* 2011;6:951–953.
21. **Verbalis JG.** Brain volume regulation in response to changes in osmolality. *Neuroscience.* 2010;168:862–870.
22. **Renneboog B, Musch W, Vandemergel X, Manto MU, Decaux G.** Mild chronic hyponatremia is associated with falls, unsteadiness, and attention deficits. *Am J Med.* 2006;119:71.
23. **Gankam KF, Andres C, Sattar L, Melot C, Decaux G.** Mild hyponatremia and risk of fracture in the ambulatory elderly. *QJM.* 2008;101:583–588.
24. **Sandhu HS, Gilles E, DeVita MV, Panagopoulos G, Michelis MF.** Hyponatremia associated with large-bone fracture in elderly patients. *Int Urol Nephrol.* 2009;41:733–737.
25. **Kinsella S, Moran S, Sullivan MO, Molloy MG, Eustace JA.** Hyponatremia independent of osteoporosis is associated with fracture occurrence. *Clin J Am Soc Nephrol.* 2010;5:275–280.
26. **Verbalis JG, Barsony J, Sugimura Y, et al.** Hyponatremia-induced osteoporosis. *J Bone Miner Res.* 2010;25:554–563.
27. **Ayus JC.** Diuretic-induced hyponatremia [editorial]. *Arch Intern Med.* 1986;146:1295–1296.
28. **Adrogue HJ, Madias NE.** Hyponatremia. *N Engl J Med.* 2000;342:1581–1589.
29. **Sterns RH, Hix JK, Silver S.** Treatment of hyponatremia. *Curr Opin Nephrol Hypertens.* 2010;19:493–498.
30. **Sterns RH, Nigwekar SU, Hix JK.** The treatment of hyponatremia. *Semin Nephrol.* 2009;29:282–299.
31. **Arieff AI.** Hyponatremia, convulsions, respiratory arrest, and permanent brain damage after elective surgery in healthy women. *N Eng J Med.* 1986;314:1529–1535.
32. **Verbalis JG, Goldsmith SR, Greenberg A, Schrier RW, Sterns RH.** Hyponatremia treatment guidelines 2007: expert panel recommendations. *Am J Med.* 2007;120(11 suppl 1):S1–S21.
33. **Hew-Butler T, Ayus JC, Kipps C, et al.** Statement of the Second International Exercise-Associated Hyponatremia Consensus Development Conference, New Zealand, 2007. *Clin J Sport Med.* 2008;18:111–121.
34. **Sterns RH, Cappuccio JD, Silver SM, Cohen EP.** Neurologic sequelae after treatment of severe hyponatremia: a multicenter perspective. *J Am Soc Nephrol.* 1994;4:1522–1530.
35. **Battison C, Andrews PJ, Graham C, Petty T.** Randomized, controlled trial on the effect of a 20% mannitol solution and a 7.5% saline/6% dextran solution on increased intracranial pressure after brain injury. *Crit Care Med.* 2005;33:196–202.
36. **Schwartz WB, Bennett S, Curelop S, Bartter FC.** A syndrome of renal sodium loss and hyponatremia probably resulting from inappropriate secretion of antidiuretic hormone. *Am J Med.* 1957;23:529–542.
37. **Steele A, Gowrishankar M, Abrahamson S, Mazer CD, Feldman RD, Halperin ML.** Postoperative hyponatremia despite near-isotonic saline infusion: a phenomenon of desalination [see comments]. *Ann Intern Med.* 1997;126:20–25.
38. **Robertson GL.** Regulation of arginine vasopressin in the syndrome of inappropriate antidiuresis. *Am J Med.* 2006;119(7 suppl 1):S36–S42.
39. **Furst H, Hallows KR, Post J, et al.** The urine/plasma electrolyte ratio: a predictive guide to water restriction. *Am J Med Sci.* 2000;319:240–244.
40. **Decaux G.** The syndrome of inappropriate secretion of antidiuretic hormone (SIADH). *Semin Nephrol.* 2009;29:239–256.
41. **Berl T.** Impact of solute intake on urine flow and water excretion. *J Am Soc Nephrol.* 2008;19:1076–1078.
42. **Greenberg A, Verbalis JG.** Vasopressin receptor antagonists. *Kidney Int.* 2006;69:2124–2130.
43. Vaprisol (conivaptan hydrochloride injection) prescribing information. Deerfield, IL: Astellas Pharma US, Inc.; 2006.
44. **Zeltser D, Rosansky S, van Rensburg H, Verbalis JG, Smith N.** Assessment of the efficacy and safety of intravenous conivaptan in euvolemic and hypervolemic hyponatremia. *Am J Nephrol.* 2007;27:447–457.
45. **Schrier RW, Gross P, Gheorghiade M, et al.** Tolvaptan, a selective oral vasopressin V2-receptor antagonist, for hyponatremia. *N Engl J Med.* 2006;355:2099–2112.
46. Samsca (tolvaptan) prescribing information. Tokyo, Japan: Otsuka Pharmaceutical Co; 2009.
47. **Coussement J, Danguy C, Zouaoui-Boudjeltia K, et al.** Treatment of the syndrome of inappropriate secretion of antidiuretic hormone with urea in critically ill patients. *Am J Nephrol.* 2012;35:265–270.
48. **Decaux G, Andres C, Gankam KF, Soupart A.** Treatment of euvolemic hyponatremia in the intensive care unit by urea. *Crit Care.* 2010;14:R184.

49. **Chehade H, Rosato L, Girardin E, Cachat F.** Inappropriate antidiuretic hormone secretion: long-term successful urea treatment. *Acta Paediatr.* 2012;101:e39–e42.
50. **Levtchenko EN, Monnens LA.** Nephrogenic syndrome of inappropriate antidiuresis. *Nephrol Dial Transplant.* 2010;25:2839–2843.
51. **Soupart A, Coffernils M, Couturier B, Gankam-Kengne F, Decaux G.** Efficacy and tolerance of urea compared with vaptans for long-term treatment of patients with SIADH. *Clin J Am Soc Nephrol.* 2012;7:742–747.
52. **Hantman D, Rossier B, Zohlman R, Schrier R.** Rapid correction of hyponatremia in the syndrome of inappropriate secretion of antidiuretic hormone. An alternative treatment to hypertonic saline. *Ann Int Med.* 1973;78:870–875.
53. **Decaux G, Waterlot Y, Genette F, Mockel J.** Treatment of the syndrome of inappropriate secretion of antidiuretic hormone with furosemide. *N Eng J Med.* 1981;304:329–330.
54. **Ellison DH, Berl T.** Clinical practice. The syndrome of inappropriate antidiuresis. *N Engl J Med.* 2007;356:2064–2072.
55. **Verbalis JG.** Hyponatremia and hypo-osmolar disorders. In: Greenberg A, Cheung AK, Coffman TM, Falk RJ, Jennette JC, eds. *Primer on Kidney Diseases.* Philadelphia. PA: Saunders Elsevier; 2009: 52–59.
56. **Mohmand HK, Issa D, Ahmad Z, Cappuccio JD, Kouides RW, Sterns RH.** Hypertonic saline for hyponatremia: risk of inadvertent overcorrection. *Clin J Am Soc Nephrol.* 2007;2:1110–1117.
57. **Perianayagam A, Sterns RH, Silver SM, et al.** DDAVP is effective in preventing and reversing inadvertent overcorrection of hyponatremia. *Clin J Am Soc Nephrol.* 2008;3:331–336.
58. **Sterns RH, Hix JK, Silver S.** Treating profound hyponatremia: a strategy for controlled correction. *Am J Kidney Dis.* 2010;56:774–779.
59. **Soupart A, Penninckx R, Crenier L, Stenuit A, Perier O, Decaux G.** Prevention of brain demyelination in rats after excessive correction of chronic hyponatremia by serum sodium lowering. *Kidney Int.* 1994;45:193–200.
60. **Goldszmidt MA, Iliescu EA.** DDAVP to prevent rapid correction in hyponatremia. *Clin Nephrol.* 2000;53:226–229.
61. **Oya S, Tsutsumi K, Ueki K, Kirino T.** Reinduction of hyponatremia to treat central pontine myelinolysis. *Neurology.* 2001;57:1931–1932.
62. **Bissram M, Scott FD, Liu L, Rosner MH.** Risk factors for symptomatic hyponatraemia: the role of pre-existing asymptomatic hyponatraemia. *Intern Med J.* 2007;37:149–155.
63. **Sterns RH, Riggs JE, Schochet SS Jr.** Osmotic demyelination syndrome following correction of hyponatremia. *N Eng J Med.* 1986;314:1535–1542.
64. **Chung HM, Kluge R, Schrier RW, Anderson RJ.** Clinical assessment of extracellular fluid volume in hyponatremia. *Am J Med.* 1987;83:905–908.
65. **Fenske W, Stork S, Koschker AC, et al.** Value of fractional uric acid excretion in differential diagnosis of hyponatremic patients on diuretics. *J Clin Endocrinol Metab.* 2008;93:2991–2997.
66. **Verbalis JG.** Whole-body volume regulation and escape from antidiuresis. *Am J Med.* 2006;119(7 suppl 1):S21–S29.
67. **Verbalis JG.** Managing hyponatremia in patients with syndrome of inappropriate antidiuretic hormone secretion. *Endocrinol Nutr.* 2010;57(suppl 2): 30–40.

SECTION XI

Obesity and Clinical Lipidology

SECTION INTRODUCTION

Emergent Management Related to Obesity and Clinical Lipidology

Robert H Eckel

Obesity is an excess of adipose tissue defined by a body mass index (BMI) of ≥30 kg/m^2. Severe obesity defined as a BMI ≥40 kg/m^2 is now present in 5% of Americans. Over the past 20-plus years an obesity "epidemic" has impacted the developed world as well as the developing world. Moreover in India, Southeast Asia, and other populations around the world the prevalence of obesity has increased less but the distribution of excess adipose tissue is more abdominal (often visceral), a location that contributes to insulin resistance and a higher risk of type 2 diabetes and cardiovascular disease (CVD). Obesity is associated with a plethora of other sequelae including cancer (eg, breast, uterus, cervix, colon, esophagus, pancreas, kidney, prostate, and thyroid), hypertension, obstructive sleep apnea, pulmonary thromboembolism, pulmonary hypertension, nonalcoholic fatty liver disease, cholelithiasis, degenerative joint disease, oligomenorrhea/infertility, erectile dysfunction, and cognitive impairment.

The best treatment of obesity is prevention, and an increased effort in pediatrics and primary care is needed. The 2013 American Heart Association/American College of Cardiology Task Force on Practice Guidelines and The Obesity Society (AHA/ACC/TOS) Guideline for the Management of Overweight and Obesity in Adults (1) indicates that overweight (BMI ≥25 but <30 kg/m^2) and obese patients need to be counseled about CVD risk factors (high blood pressure, hyperlipidemia, hyperglycemia); that lifestyle changes that produce even modest, sustained weight loss of 3%–5% produce clinically meaningful health benefits; and that greater weight loss produces greater benefits. With dietary intervention techniques aimed at reducing daily energy intake by at least 500 kcal daily, a range of 4–12 kg at 6 months is typical with a slow weight regain to follow. In general, there is no ideal diet for weight loss and no superiority for any particular diet. Thus, choosing a diet composition based on the patient's preferences and health status is best done with the assistance of a dietician when possible. For weight loss maintenance, face-to-face or telephone-delivered weight loss maintenance programs that provide regular contact (monthly or more frequent) with a trained interventionist are evidence-based, and a high level of physical activity (ie, 3–5 hours/week) is recommended. In this setting, an obsessive/compulsive behavior with frequent weighing predicts a more successful outcome.

For severe obesity or a BMI ≥35 kg/m^2 with comorbidities a surgical procedure may be best. Presently, metabolic surgery is the only obesity therapy proven to prolong life, a benefit attributable to reductions in cancer as well as CVD-related mortality. Increasing evidence also indicates the value of metabolic surgery in treating patients with type 2 diabetes, with many patients free of diabetes medications and some postoperative patients with normal levels of glycosylated hemoglobin A1c rendered nondiabetic. In experienced hands, surgical mortality is now <0.3%.

CLINICAL LIPIDOLOGY

Dyslipidemia is defined as an increase in low-density lipoprotein cholesterol (LDL-C) and triglycerides and/or reductions in high-density lipoprotein cholesterol (HDL-C). An increase in the proatherogenic particle lipoprotein (a) could be included, but presently this risk factor has been omitted from CVD risk screening because specific therapies are not available to document the value of lipoprotein (a) lowering. Nevertheless, when atherosclerotic CVD occurs in the absence of other risk factors and the family history is positive, elevations in lipoprotein (a) should be considered.

Evidence for reducing triglycerides or increasing HDL-C is equivocal at best, and more recent randomized clinical trials wherein drugs have been used in adjunct to statins in high-risk patients have not shown added benefit. Yet most of these trials have suffered from design problems and inadequate power. Nevertheless, support for a fibrate such as fenofibrate in addition to a statin has been suggested when fasting triglycerides are >200 but <500 mg/dL (>2.3 but <5.6 mmol/L), but not when given to patients with triglycerides <200 mg/dL (<2.3 mmol/L). The Veterans Administration Fenofibrate Intervention Trial appears postured to address this important question. For patients with atherosclerotic CVD (ASCVD) or high risk with lower levels of HDL-C, extended release niacin and the cholesteryl ester transfer protein (CETP) inhibitor dalcetrapib added to existing statin therapy have failed to reduce CVD events. Additional CETP inhibitors trials are ongoing.

The 2013 ACC/AHA Guideline on the Treatment of Blood Cholesterol provides updated evidence for the benefit of LDL-C reductions and CVD outcomes (2). In addition to counseling patients about a heart-healthy lifestyle that includes a diet reduced in saturated and *trans* fats and increased in physical activity, 4 indications for statin therapy have evolved. For adults at any age this includes patients with known ASCVD or a LDL-C >190 mg/dL (4.9 mmol/L), and high intensity statins; for example, 40–80 mg atorvastatin daily or 20–40 mg rosuvastatin daily should be used. Patients with diabetes between the ages of 40 and 75 years should be treated with at least a moderate intensity statin, as should patients with a calculated 10-year ASCVD event risk of ≥7.5%. This risk utilizes a risk calculator that now includes risk assessments for African-Americans in addition to Caucasians. For patients with a 5.0%–7.5% 10-year risk, other factors such as a positive family history of premature ASCVD, a LDL-C ≥160 mg/dL (4.1 mmol/L), hs-CRP ≥2.0 mg/L, and/or subclinical atherosclerosis defined as a coronary artery calcification score ≥300 or >75th percentile for age, gender, ethnicity, or an ankle brachial index (ABI) of <0.9 can be helpful in deciding to put patients on a statin. For this group, individualization of statin therapy needs important consideration, and adverse effects need to be carefully discussed.

Other important topics covered in this section include the emergent management of statin-induced myositis and rhabdomyolysis (3), and the role of severe hypertriglyceridemia in pancreatitis (4).

ACKNOWLEDGMENTS

The author has nothing to disclose.

REFERENCES

1. **Jensen MD, Ryan DH, Apovian CM, et al.** 2013 AHA/ACC/TOS Guideline for the Management of Overweight and Obesity in Adults: A Report of the American College of Cardiology/American Heart Association Task Force on Practice Guidelines and The Obesity Society [published online ahead of print November 7, 2013]. *J Am Coll Cardiol.*

2. **Stone NJ, Robinson J, Lichtenstein AH, et al.** 2013 ACC/AHA Guideline on the Treatment of Blood Cholesterol to Reduce Atherosclerotic Cardiovascular Risk in Adults: A Report of the American College of Cardiology/American Heart Association Task Force on Practice Guidelines [published online ahead of print November 12, 2013]. *Circulation.*
3. **Eckel RH.** Approach to the patient who is intolerant of statin therapy. *J Clin Endocrinol Metab.* 2010;95:2015–2022.
4. **Brown WV, Brunzell JD, Eckel RH, Stone NJ.** Severe hypertriglyceridemia. *J Clin Lipidol.* 2012;6: 397–408.

CHAPTER 38

Acute Emergencies Related to Bariatric Surgery

Michael A Via and Jeffrey I Mechanick

INTRODUCTION

Worldwide rates of obesity and associated conditions including hypertension and type 2 diabetes continue to rise (1). Bariatric surgical procedures represent an important therapeutic option to induce weight loss and to treat comorbid conditions in select obese patients. For individual patients who are considering bariatric surgery, careful deliberation of risks imposed by these procedures should be weighed against potential benefits. Postoperatively, patients will need lifelong follow-up. Clinicians who monitor these patients should be aware of possible adverse events that may develop following bariatric surgery. This chapter provides a review of common acute emergencies that patients who undergo bariatric surgery may experience.

SURGICAL EMERGENCIES

The establishment and identification of Bariatric Surgery Centers of Excellence recognized by the Centers for Medicare & Medicaid Services (CMS) in the United States and the use of laparoscopic techniques generally have led to a dramatic improvement in surgical outcomes following bariatric procedures (2). Perioperative mortality as low as 0.25%–0.5% has been consistently reported in case series (3). The need for reoperation or surgical revision following bariatric surgery is 5% for Roux-en-Y gastric bypass (RYGB), 1% for laparoscopic adjustable gastric banding (LAGB), and 3% for laparoscopic sleeve gastrectomy (LSG). Rates of hospital readmission following bariatric surgery are 6% for RYGB, 2% for LAGB, and 5% for LSG (4). The most common reasons for hospital readmission after surgery are summarized in Table 38-1 and include intestinal obstruction, infection, bleeding, and anastomotic leak (4). Although these conditions are uncommon, clinical evaluation for them should be undertaken in appropriate patients.

The CMS recently released an updated policy that as of September 24, 2013, patients are no longer required to undergo bariatric surgery at a designated Center of Excellence (5). This change in policy may affect the rates of adverse surgical outcomes in the immediate postoperative period within the United States (2).

DIARRHEA AND DUMPING SYNDROME

The observed prevalence of diarrhea and fecal incontinence in preoperative obese individuals has been reported to be approximately 20%–35% (6), which may be related to pelvic floor dysfunction and increased intra-abdominal pressure (7). Following bariatric surgery, the prevalence of fecal incontinence is observed to reduce to approximately 10%–15% (6).

Aside from obesity-related pelvic floor dysfunction, surgical alteration of the gastrointestinal (GI) tract can lead to an increase in frequency of bowel movements. In extreme cases, dumping syndrome may develop following RYGB, biliopancreatic diversion with a duodenal switch (BPDDS), or LSG as a result of impaired stomach relaxation (8).

Patients with dumping syndrome experience sudden and large volume diarrhea secondary to rapid passage of chyme from

Table 38-1. Acute Surgical Morbidity Rates, Given as Percentages, Following Bariatric Surgery Performed at CMS Centers of Excellence from July 2007 Through September 2010 (4)

	LAGB	LSG	RYGB[a]
Stricture formation and obstruction	0.13	0.42	1.4
Intestinal obstruction without stricture	0.03	0	0.95
Infection	0.14	0.64	0.36
Bleeding	0.05	0.64	1.1
Anastomotic leak	0	0.74	0.78

[a] *Includes data from patients with RYGB performed laparoscopically.*

the stomach to the small intestine (9). Other symptoms associated with dumping syndrome include abdominal pain and cramping, nausea, flushing, diaphoresis, tachycardia, and lightheadedness. These and other symptoms of hypoglycemia, including sudden hunger, irritability, and reduced cognition, may develop approximately 3 hours postprandially due to an exaggerated incretin hormone response and disproportionate release of insulin (10). Meals containing high amounts of carbohydrates can exacerbate dumping by exerting increased osmotic pressure in the intestinal lumen and by further inducing excessive insulin release (11).

Patients may present acutely, or, if left untreated, dehydration, autonomic dysfunction, and failure to thrive may develop (11). Supportive therapy with intravenous (IV) fluids and restriction of oral dietary intake may be required.

Longer term treatment of dumping syndrome includes reduction in dietary carbohydrates, especially sugar-containing beverages (11). Separation of liquid and solid foods during a meal may also be beneficial (11). These dietary interventions may be all that is necessary to control dumping syndrome. If symptoms persist, the administration of an alpha-glucosidase inhibitor such as acarbose or miglitol with meals may provide symptomatic relief (12). In severe cases, the therapeutic use of somatostatin analogs (eg, octreotide, lanreotide) delays stomach emptying and improves the condition (13).

HYPOGLYCEMIA

Separate from dumping syndrome, patients who undergo bariatric surgery may develop postprandial hypoglycemia without any of the other related symptoms of abdominal pain or nausea. This phenomenon may also be associated with sudden significant increases in incretin activity (14). Indeed, the anatomic alterations in RYGB, LSG, and BPDDS procedures yield significant increased insulin sensitivity and pancreatic beta-cell function. Many diabetic patients demonstrate dramatic improvements in their glycemic control immediately following bariatric surgical procedures, including RYGB, LSG, and BPDDS (15,16). Aside from increased incretin function, other proposed mechanisms for this may include increased circulating levels of bile acids, reduced systemic inflammation, vagal nerve dysfunction, and dietary changes that occur postoperatively (17,18).

In some cases, the pancreatic beta-cell response is exaggerated after bariatric surgery, leading to an increased number of beta-cells and/or overactive beta-cell function in a condition known as nesidioblastosis (14). In these cases, patients experience hypoglycemia approximately 1–3 hours following meals, especially after the ingestion of a high carbohydrate load. Hypoglycemia events may be severe: blood glucose levels of 15–40 mg/dL (0.8–2.2 mmol/L) have been reported and can cause seizures, altered mental status, or loss of consciousness. Insulin and C-peptide levels are inappropriately elevated during these hypoglycemic periods.

The use of octreotide scanning or computerized tomography (CT) can help to rule out other causes of hyperinsulinemia, such as insulin secreting tumors, as a cause of hypoglycemia (14). A careful history should be taken to rule out iatrogenic or factitious causes of hypoglycemia (19). Calcium-stimulated selective mesenteric venous sampling can also confirm diffuse hyperactivity of pancreatic beta-cells in this condition (14).

Nesidioblastosis has been reported following RYGB and BPDDS procedures (14). In most cases, strict adherence to a low carbohydrate diet mitigates the exaggerated insulin response in nesidioblastosis. For refractory cases, the use of alpha-glucosidase inhibitors, such as acarbose or miglitol, or calcium channel blockers can reduce the rate of hypoglycemia (20). The administration of either diazoxide or octreotide has been suggested as a treatment alternative, though only a few reports of their use in nesidioblastosis have been published (21,22). For patients with persistent hypoglycemia despite dietary and medical optimization, distal pancreatectomy may be considered.

MALABSORPTION

In RYGB and BPDDS procedures, effective weight loss is achieved, in part, by intentionally creating a state of malabsorption. In some cases, the surgically created reduction in active small intestinal absorptive surface area yields clinically significant deficiencies in micronutrient or macronutrient absorption. Severe protein-calorie malnutrition necessitating nutritional support has been observed in approximately 1% of RYGB patients annually, with a 5% lifetime risk (23). For patients who undergo BPDDS, the risk of severe protein-calorie malnutrition is reported to be approximately 20%–30%, highlighting the significant malabsorption that is induced by this procedure (24).

For typical patients undergoing bariatric surgical procedures, the greatest amount of weight loss is achieved in the first 18 months of the postoperative period (25). Protein-calorie malnutrition should be suspected in patients who continue to lose weight for 2 or more years after surgery. Other clinical signs that should raise suspicion include fatigue, weakness, muscle wasting, frequent loose and oily bowel movements, and persistent micronutrient deficiencies. The diagnosis of protein-calorie malnutrition should be made on a clinical basis and may be supported through measurement of serum markers of protein synthesis such as albumin, prealbumin, or retinol binding protein.

Treatment options for protein-calorie malnutrition may include the use of high-calorie oral supplements, the placement of enteral feeding tubes, the use of parenteral nutrition, or surgical revision (19).

MICRONUTRIENT MALABSORPTION

The reduction of intestinal absorptive surface area following RYGB and BPDDS procedures increases the risk of micronutrient malabsorption and deficiency. The reduction in gastric acid production in LSG may affect liberation and dissolution of vitamins and essential trace metals. Reduction in gastric secretion of intrinsic factor in RYGB, BPDDS, and LSG procedures can lead to B_{12} deficiency.

Postoperatively, patients are advised to take vitamin supplements and are periodically monitored for deficiency (19). Despite these measures, micronutrient deficiency is common following these procedures and can lead to clinically significant morbidity (26).

Common micronutrient deficiencies (Table 38-2) include iron, thiamin (B_1), folate, copper, and cobalamin (B_{12}). High rates of vitamin D insufficiency are also observed (27). Lipid soluble vitamin deficiencies are common after BPDDS procedures (28). Micronutrient deficiencies rarely present as medical emergencies. Deficiency of B_1, copper, and B_{12}, however, may cause acute syndromes that are reviewed later in this chapter. Patients may also present with anemia due to iron deficiency.

Thiamin

Thiamin (B_1) is a water soluble vitamin that serves as an important cofactor for several steps in glucose metabolism, amino acid synthesis, and the pentose phosphate shunt pathway. The majority of thiamin is obtained through dietary sources, while a small amount may be synthesized by enterocolonic bacteria (29). Deficiency states of thiamin include wet and dry beriberi, as well as Wernicke encephalopathy, which may develop if less than adequate amounts of thiamin are consumed or absorbed. Mild cases of thiamin deficiency may lead to symptoms of intractable nausea, vomiting, or neuropathy.

Dietary thiamin generally exists in a phosphorylated form that must be hydrolyzed prior to absorption. The majority of intestinal phosphatases that act on thiamin phosphate and thiamin pyrophosphate are located in the proximal intestine, which is bypassed in RYGB and BPDDS procedures (29). As a result of decreased hydrolysis and diminished intestinal absorptive surface, thiamin deficiency may develop after these procedures and has been reported in 10%–15% of patients following RYGB (30). Patients should be screened regularly and provided with a vitamin supplementation regimen that includes thiamin. Thiamin deficiency should be suspected in patients with symptoms of Wernicke encephalopathy, beriberi, heart failure, unexplained vomiting, or neuropathy (31). Patients with an acute thiamin deficiency state should be treated with 500 mg/d intravenous thiamin for 3 to 5 days, followed by 250 mg/d for 3 to 5 days or until symptoms resolve (19). Continued supplementation with at least 100 mg/d oral thiamin should be maintained indefinitely.

Copper

Copper is an essential trace metal that functions at the active site of enzymes that catalyze redox reaction and serve in diverse biochemical pathways that include neurotransmitter synthesis, superoxide synthesis, respiratory oxidation, and iron metabolism (32). GI absorption of copper takes place mainly in the duodenum, which is bypassed in the malabsorptive bariatric procedures. Deficiency of copper has been reported in up to 70% of BPDDS patients.

Patients with copper deficiency may experience painful neuropathy, anemia, fatigue, and iron deficiency. Although regular surveillance is not currently recommended for patients who have undergone malabsorptive bariatric surgery, patients who develop symptoms of copper deficiency or those with other signs of severe malabsorption may benefit from measurement of serum copper and ceruloplasmin levels (19). Acute severe neuropathy that includes cerebellar, spinal, and peripheral neuropathy due to copper deficiency has been reported following RYGB (33). Supplementary copper should be administered, either orally or parenterally, in deficient patients.

Cobalamin

Deficiency of cobalamin (B_{12}) is common following bariatric surgical procedures (26). This is partly due to the complex absorptive process of B_{12} that depends on functional physiology of the GI tract. Dietary cobalamin is bound to intrinsic factor, a peptide released from parietal cells located in the gastric antrum and fundus, for protection from the harsh acid environment. As gastric chyme progresses through the intestinal tract, dietary B_{12} is liberated from intrinsic factor for absorption in the distal ileum. Alteration of stomach anatomy in RYGB, LSG, and BPDDS procedures reduces gastric parietal cell mass, potentially leading to B_{12} malabsorption and deficiency. B_{12} deficiency also has been reported at increased rates following LAGB surgery. Symptoms of B_{12} deficiency may range from subtle to severe in nature and include neuropathy, muscle weakness, fatigue, anemia, and mood disorders. Acute presentations of B_{12} deficiency may include neuropathic pain, reduced cognition, and anemia. Rates of B_{12} deficiency are reported to be approximately 20% following LSG, 30%–60% following RYGB, 20%–40% following BPDDS, and 5%–15% following LAGB.

Empiric supplementation with multiple vitamins that contain B_{12} is currently recommended. Regular screening for B_{12} deficiency and supplementing with high-dose B_{12} oral preparations or parenteral B_{12} injections are also recommended following malabsorptive bariatric procedures (19).

Iron

Dietary iron is present as chelated structures and may be classified as either heme or nonheme forms. The acid environment of the stomach maintains ingested iron moieties in the ferric (3+) state in both of these forms, for improved solubility. After transit to the duodenum, ferroreductase activity reduces iron to the ferrous state, which is required for absorption (34,35).

Many of the bariatric surgical procedures, including RYGB, BPDDS, and LSG, diminish stomach acid production, reducing the efficiency of iron absorption (26). The bypassed duodenum in RYGB and BPDDS procedures limits the exposure of ingested iron to ferroreductase, which contributes to reduced iron absorption. Consequently, relatively high rates of iron deficiency are reported following these procedures (Table 38-2).

Patients with clinically significant iron deficiency experience fatigue, microcytic anemia, hair loss, brittle nails, and/or angular cheilosis (35). Iron deficiency can lead to significant morbidity following malabsorptive bariatric procedures, especially in patients with underlying cardiovascular or pulmonary disease. Regular testing for serum iron levels at 6-month intervals and appropriate supplementation are recommended (19).

OSTEOPOROSIS AND BONE FRACTURES

Several factors contribute to the high rate of bone turnover that is observed following

Table 38-2. Prevalence of Micronutrient Deficiencies Following Bariatric Surgery

	LAGB	LSG	RYGB	BPDDS
Thiamin (B_1)	0	0	12%	10%–15%
Folate	10%	22%	15%	15%
Cobalamin (B_{12})	10%	22%	30%–50%	22%
Vitamin A	10%	-	10%–50	60%–70%
Vitamin D (<30 ng/dL)	30%	30%	30%–50%	40%–100%
Iron	0%–32%	14%	25%–50%	25%
Copper	–	–	10%	70%

All data given as percentages. Dashes indicate no data available.

bariatric surgery. Reduced calcium absorption is observed following malabsorptive bariatric procedures and commonly causes secondary hyperparathyroidism (36,37). Moreover, vitamin D insufficiency is reported in 50%–60% of postoperative individuals, despite supplementation (38). This contributes to bone loss and may worsen secondary hyperparathyroidism. The weight loss itself reduces mechanical load on musculature and bones leading to decreased bone density and bone strength. A rise in circulating serotonin following RYGB may also contribute to bone loss (39). Malabsorption of other micronutrients, such as B_{12}, as well as protein malabsorption, may also contribute to bone loss following bariatric surgery.

The result of the above factors is a significant loss in bone density and bone strength. A 2- to 3-fold increase in fracture risk has been reported after RYGB (40). Acute presentations of bone fractures following RYGB are commonly reported at the hip, spine, and wrist (40).

Treatment for bone loss associated with bariatric surgery is preventive in nature. Postoperative supplementation with calcium is currently recommended for all patients (19). Calcium citrate is the preferred form of calcium for supplementation, owing to its superior absorption in conditions of reduced stomach acid production, including surgical alteration of the stomach following LSG, RYGB, LAGB, and BPDDS.

Vitamin D supplementation is also recommended, targeting a circulating 25-hydroxyvitamin D level of 30 ng/dL or greater (19). Current guidelines recommend oral vitamin D supplementation of at least 3,000 International units daily (19). Patients who have undergone malabsorptive procedures, including RYGB and BPDDS, may require increasing doses of vitamin D supplementation to achieve target levels.

The use of bone antiresorptive agents, such as bisphosphonates, is not currently recommended for all patients, but may be considered on an individual basis, especially in patients who sustain fractures (19).

OXALATE NEPHROLITHIASIS

Patients who undergo malabsorptive bariatric procedures are at increased risk for the development of calcium oxalate nephrolithiasis (41–43). In 1 matched comparison study, a 7.6% incidence of nephrolithiasis was noted in 4,636 subjects after undergoing RYGB with 5 years of follow-up, in contrast to an incidence of only 4.5% in obese controls (42). Both plasma and urine oxalate levels are increased in patients who have undergone RYGB and BPDDS, consistent with these findings (44). Increased rates of nephrolithiasis have not been described following LABG or LSG (45–47). An increase in intestinal oxalate absorption may result indirectly from fat malabsorption. The excess of unconjugated fatty acids in the intestinal lumen leads to increased luminal calcium-fatty acid salt formation. This diminishes the sequestration of luminal oxalate by ingested calcium, leading to greater oxalate absorption (44).

Generally, there is no modification for the clinical presentation and treatment of nephrolithiasis in patients who have undergone malabsorptive bariatric procedures. Hydration, stone collection, and urological intervention are employed as necessary.

Prevention of stone formation with oral calcium supplementation reduces oxalate absorption in patients who have undergone RYGB or BPDDS and is currently recommended in these patients (19,48). For patients who have developed oxalate nephrolithiasis, a low oxalate diet that limits tea, nuts, and chocolate intake may reduce the risk of future oxalate stone formation. The use of probiotics may increase intraluminal metabolism of oxalate and also reduce stone formation (49).

INTESTINAL ADAPTATION AND PHARMACOLOGY

In response to malabsorption by any etiology, including following malabsorptive bariatric surgery, the intestinal epithelium adapts to increase the absorptive surface area and to upregulate the expression and function of channel proteins responsible for the absorption of nutrients. This phenomenon of intestinal adaptation may be partly responsible for weight regain following malabsorptive bariatric surgery (50). Another consequence of intestinal adaptation is an alteration of the intestinal absorption of pharmacological agents and alcohol, which can change significantly in the postoperative period of malabsorptive procedures.

Several mechanisms are responsible for these changes that occur after malabsorptive surgery. In many cases the decrease in intestinal absorptive surface area reduces bioavailability of orally ingested drugs. For example, absorption of levothyroxine and of sertraline following RYGB or BPDDS is greatly reduced. Patients may require higher doses to achieve normal circulating levels (51,52).

Following RYGB and BPDDS, there is a decreased transit time to the distal ileum, which reduces the time to peak serum levels of medications that are absorbed in this region, including opiates (53).

Intestinal cytochrome P450 activity serves as an important step in the first pass metabolism of some pharmacological agents, such as atorvastatin. As a result of decreased intestinal cytochrome P450 activity following these procedures, circulating atorvastatin levels may increase (54).

Over time, circulating levels of metformin and acetaminophen (paracetamol) have been observed to increase following malabsorptive surgery, likely due to intestinal adaptation (53).

These few examples demonstrate the diverse set of changes in pharmacokinetics that occur after malabsorptive bariatric surgery. Prescribers must carefully monitor medication use in patients who have undergone these procedures to avoid both toxicity and insufficient medication dosing.

CONCLUSIONS

The significant changes in GI physiology following bariatric surgery greatly impact patients who have undergone these procedures. Increased use of laparoscopic techniques and recognized Centers of Excellence such as those in the United States have diminished rates of surgery-related morbidity in the immediate postoperative period in recent years. Many of the acute emergencies that commonly occur as a result of bariatric surgery are metabolic in nature and are related to either hormonal changes or malabsorption induced by the procedure. Clinical follow-up of patients who have undergone bariatric surgery includes measures for prevention, as well as recognition and treatment of dumping syndrome, nesidioblastosis, protein-calorie malnutrition, micronutrient deficiency, osteoporosis, nephrolithiasis, and altered pharmacokinetic profiles of various medications. The risk of these conditions remains high, necessitating lifelong follow-up.

ACKNOWLEDGMENTS

The authors have nothing to disclose.

REFERENCES

1. **Ezzati M, Riboli E.** Behavioral and dietary risk factors for noncommunicable diseases. *N Engl J Med.* 2013;369:954–964.
2. **Dimick JB, Nicholas LH, Ryan AM, Thumma JR, Birkmeyer JD.** Bariatric surgery complications before vs after implementation of a national policy restricting coverage to centers of excellence. *JAMA.* 2013;309:792–799.
3. **Buchwald H, Estok R, Fahrbach K, Banel D, Sledge I.** Trends in mortality in bariatric surgery: a systematic review and meta-analysis. *Surgery.* 2007;142: 621–632; discussion 632–635.
4. **Hutter MM, Schirmer BD, Jones DB, et al.** First report from the American College of Surgeons Bariatric Surgery Center Network: laparoscopic sleeve gastrectomy has morbidity and effectiveness positioned between the band and the bypass. *Ann Surg.* 2011;254:410–420; discussion 420–422.
5. http://www.cms.gov/Medicare/Medicare-General-Information/MedicareApprovedFacilitie/Bariatric-Surgery.html.
6. **Foster A, Laws HL, Gonzalez QH, Clements RH.** Gastrointestinal symptomatic outcome after

laparoscopic Roux-en-Y gastric bypass. *J Gastrointest Surg.* 2003;7:750–753.

7. **Greer WJ, Richter HE, Bartolucci AA, Burgio KL.** Obesity and pelvic floor disorders: a systematic review. *Obstet Gynecol.* 2008;112(2 Pt 1):341–349.
8. **Tack J, Piessevaux H, Coulie B, Caenepeel P, Janssens J.** Role of impaired gastric accommodation to a meal in functional dyspepsia. *Gastroenterology.* 1998;115:1346–1352.
9. **Tack J, Arts J, Caenepeel P, De Wulf D, Bisschops R.** Pathophysiology, diagnosis and management of postoperative dumping syndrome. *Nat Rev Gastroenterol Hepatol.* 2009;6:583–590.
10. **Toft-Nielsen M, Madsbad S, Holst JJ.** Exaggerated secretion of glucagon-like peptide-1 (GLP-1) could cause reactive hypoglycaemia. *Diabetologia.* 1998;41:1180–1186.
11. **Rohof WO, Bisschops R, Tack J, Boeckxstaens GE.** Postoperative problems 2011: fundoplication and obesity surgery. *Gastroenterol Clin North Am.* 2011;40:809–821.
12. **van der Kleij FG, Vecht J, Lamers CB, Masclee AA.** Diagnostic value of dumping provocation in patients after gastric surgery. *Scand J Gastroenterol.* 1996;31:1162–1166.
13. **Arts J, Caenepeel P, Bisschops R, et al.** Efficacy of the long-acting repeatable formulation of the somatostatin analogue octreotide in postoperative dumping. *Clin Gastroenterol Hepatol.* 2009;7:432–437.
14. **Ceppa EP, Ceppa DP, Omotosho PA, Dickerson JA 2nd, Park CW, Portenier DD.** Algorithm to diagnose etiology of hypoglycemia after Roux-en-Y gastric bypass for morbid obesity: case series and review of the literature. *Surg Obes Relat Dis.* 2012;8:641–647.
15. **Mingrone G, Panunzi S, De Gaetano A, et al.** Bariatric surgery versus conventional medical therapy for type 2 diabetes. *N Engl J Med.* 2012;366:1577–1585.
16. **Schauer PR, Kashyap SR, Wolski K, et al.** Bariatric surgery versus intensive medical therapy in obese patients with diabetes. *N Engl J Med.* 2012;366:1567–1576.
17. **Via MA, Mechanick JI.** The role of bariatric surgery in the treatment of type 2 diabetes: current evidence and clinical guidelines. *Curr Atheroscler Rep.* 2013;15:366.
18. **Haluzik M.** Bariatric surgery and the mechanisms of diabetes remission: are we getting there? *J Clin Endocrinol Met.* 2013;98:4336–4338.
19. **Mechanick JI, Youdim A, Jones DB, et al.** Clinical practice guidelines for the perioperative nutritional, metabolic, and nonsurgical support of the bariatric surgery patient—2013 update: cosponsored by American Association of Clinical Endocrinologists, The Obesity Society, and American Society for Metabolic & Bariatric Surgery. *Endocr Pract.* 2013;19:337–372.
20. **Moreira RO, Moreira RB, Machado NA, Goncalves TB, Coutinho WF.** Post-prandial hypoglycemia after bariatric surgery: pharmacological treatment with verapamil and acarbose. *Obes Surg.* 2008;18:1618–1621.
21. **Myint KS, Greenfield JR, Farooqi IS, Henning E, Holst JJ, Finer N.** Prolonged successful therapy for hyperinsulinaemic hypoglycaemia after gastric bypass: the pathophysiological role of GLP1 and its response to a somatostatin analogue. *Eur J Endocrinol.* 2012;166:951–955.
22. **Arao T, Okada Y, Hirose A, Tanaka Y.** A rare case of adult-onset nesidioblastosis treated successfully with diazoxide. *Endocr J.* 2006;53:95–100.
23. **Faintuch J, Matsuda M, Cruz ME, et al.** Severe protein-calorie malnutrition after bariatric procedures. *Obes Surg.* 2004;14:175–181.
24. **Fox SR.** The use of the biliopancreatic diversion as a treatment for failed gastric partitioning in the morbidly obese. *Obes Surg.* 1991;1:89–93.
25. **Sjostrom L, Lindroos AK, Peltonen M, et al.** Lifestyle, diabetes, and cardiovascular risk factors 10 years after bariatric surgery. *N Engl J Med.* 2004;351:2683–2693.
26. **Coupaye M, Puchaux K, Bogard C, et al.** Nutritional consequences of adjustable gastric banding and gastric bypass: a 1-year prospective study. *Obes Surg.* 2009;19:56–65.
27. **Gudzune KA, Huizinga MM, Chang HY, Asamoah V, Gadgil M, Clark JM.** Screening and diagnosis of micronutrient deficiencies before and after bariatric surgery. *Obes Surg.* 2013;23:1581–1589.
28. **Marinari GM, Murelli F, Camerini G, et al.** A 15-year evaluation of biliopancreatic diversion according to the Bariatric Analysis Reporting Outcome System (BAROS). *Obes Surg.* 2004;14:325–328.
29. **Said HM.** Intestinal absorption of water-soluble vitamins in health and disease. *Biochem J.* 2011;437:357–372.
30. **Matrana MR, Vasireddy S, Davis WE.** The skinny on a growing problem: dry beriberi after bariatric surgery. *Ann Intern Med.* 2008;149:842–844.
31. **Bhardwaj A, Watanabe M, Shah JR.** A 46-yr-old woman with ataxia and blurred vision 3 months after bariatric surgery. *Am J Gastroenterol.* 2008;103:1575–1577.
32. **van den Berghe PV, Klomp LW.** New developments in the regulation of intestinal copper absorption. *Nutr Rev.* 2009;67:658–672.
33. **Rounis E, Laing CM, Davenport A.** Acute neurological presentation due to copper deficiency in a hemodialysis patient following gastric bypass surgery. *Clin Nephrol.* 2010;74:389–392.
34. **Conrad ME, Cortell S, Williams HL, Foy AL.** Polymerization and intraluminal factors in the absorption of hemoglobin-iron. *J Lab Clin Med.* 1966;68:659–668.
35. **Han O.** Molecular mechanism of intestinal iron absorption. *Metallomics.* 2011;3:103–109.
36. **Jin J, Robinson AV, Hallowell PT, Jasper JJ, Stellato TA, Wilhem SM.** Increases in parathyroid hormone (PTH) after gastric bypass surgery appear to be of a secondary nature. *Surgery.* 2007;142:914–920; discussion 914–920.
37. **Youssef Y, Richards WO, Sekhar N, et al.** Risk of secondary hyperparathyroidism after laparoscopic gastric bypass surgery in obese women. *Surg Endosc.* 2007;21:1393–1396.
38. **Aarts E, van Groningen L, Horst R, et al.** Vitamin D absorption: consequences of gastric bypass surgery. *Eur J Endocrinol.* 2011;164:827–832.
39. **Karsenty G, Yadav VK.** Regulation of bone mass by serotonin: molecular biology and therapeutic implications. *Annu Rev Med.* 2011;62:323–331.

40. **Nakamura KM, Haglind EG, Clowes JA, et al.** Fracture risk following bariatric surgery: a population-based study [published online ahead of print August 3, 2013]. *Osteoporos Int.*
41. **Lieske JC, Kumar R, Collazo-Clavell ML.** Nephrolithiasis after bariatric surgery for obesity. *Semin Nephrol.* 2008;28:163–173.
42. **Matlaga BR, Shore AD, Magnuson T, Clark JM, Johns R, Makary MA.** Effect of gastric bypass surgery on kidney stone disease. *J Urol.* 2009;181: 2573–2577.
43. **Nelson WK, Houghton SG, Milliner DS, Lieske JC, Sarr MG.** Enteric hyperoxaluria, nephrolithiasis, and oxalate nephropathy: potentially serious and unappreciated complications of Roux-en-Y gastric bypass. *Surg Obes Relat Dis.* 2005;1:481–485.
44. **Kumar R, Lieske JC, Collazo-Clavell ML, et al.** Fat malabsorption and increased intestinal oxalate absorption are common after Roux-en-Y gastric bypass surgery. *Surgery.* 2011;149:654–661.
45. **Semins MJ, Matlaga BR, Shore AD, et al.** The effect of gastric banding on kidney stone disease. *Urology.* 2009;74:746–749.
46. **Penniston KL, Kaplon DM, Gould JC, Nakada SY.** Gastric band placement for obesity is not associated with increased urinary risk of urolithiasis compared to bypass. *J Urol.* 2009;182:2340–2346.
47. **Semins MJ, Asplin JR, Steele K, et al.** The effect of restrictive bariatric surgery on urinary stone risk factors. *Urology.* 2010;76:826–829.
48. **Mechanick JI, Kushner RF, Sugerman HJ, et al.** American Association of Clinical Endocrinologists, The Obesity Society, and American Society for Metabolic & Bariatric Surgery Medical guidelines for clinical practice for the perioperative nutritional, metabolic, and nonsurgical support of the bariatric surgery patient. *Endocr Pract.* 2008;14(suppl 1):1–83.
49. **Okombo J, Liebman M.** Probiotic-induced reduction of gastrointestinal oxalate absorption in healthy subjects. *Urol Res.* 2010;38:169–178.
50. **Norholk LM, Holst JJ, Jeppesen PB.** Treatment of adult short bowel syndrome patients with teduglutide. *Expert Opin Pharmacother.* 2012;13:235–243.
51. **Rubio IG, Galrao AL, Santo MA, Zanini AC, Medeiros-Neto G.** Levothyroxine absorption in morbidly obese patients before and after Roux-en-Y gastric bypass (RYGB) surgery. *Obes Surg.* 2012;22: 253–258.
52. **Roerig JL, Steffen K, Zimmerman C, Mitchell JE, Crosby RD, Cao L.** Preliminary comparison of sertraline levels in postbariatric surgery patients versus matched nonsurgical cohort. *Surg Obes Relat Dis.* 2010;8:62–66.
53. **Edwards A, Ensom MH.** Pharmacokinetic effects of bariatric surgery. *Ann Pharmacother.* 2012;46: 130–136.
54. **Skottheim IB, Stormark K, Christensen H, et al.** Significantly altered systemic exposure to atorvastatin acid following gastric bypass surgery in morbidly obese patients. *Clin Pharmacol Ther.* 2009;86:311–318.

CHAPTER 39

Acute Medical Aspects Related to Obesity

Andrea Pucci and Nick Finer

ABSTRACT

The rise in obesity is transforming the prevalence of obesity-related disease as well as its presentation and management even in the acute setting. Two examples exemplify this: headache and breathlessness. In the obese person, headache may relate to intracranial hypertension, obstructive sleep apnea, and increased risk of migraine. The differential diagnosis of a patient presenting with breathlessness differs if they are obese rather than lean, and the obesity may pose specific diagnostic and technical barriers to investigation. Clinicians should recognize that diagnostic algorithms and probabilities may be altered by obesity.

INTRODUCTION

The seemingly inexorable rise in the prevalence of obesity is transforming not only the prevalence of obesity-related diseases, but also the way in which they present or should be managed (1). Like the nonobese, persons with obesity may present to clinicians or emergency departments with acute medical illness; however, their presenting symptoms or signs (Table 39-1), their *a priori* altered probability of having a particular disease, and their added difficulty in accessing certain diagnostic procedures (eg, some forms of imaging), may all be influenced by their excessive body weight. Consequently, all of these factors can make diagnosis problematic.

Although the cardiovascular and metabolic consequences of obesity and their impact on longevity are all well-known, in this chapter we consider 2 areas in which the effects of obesity on symptoms and disease are less well-recognized.

HEADACHE

Headache is a common presenting symptom of emergency patients. The differential diagnosis is wide and requires urgent exclusion or confirmation of conditions such as meningitis and cerebral or subarachnoid hemorrhage. An association of obesity with chronic pain, most notably fibromyalgia and osteoarthritis, is increasingly recognized (Table 39-1). The link is partly due to higher mechanical load on joints, but there are now emerging findings about an association between chronic pain and obesity in non-weight-bearing areas such as the abdomen, head, and neck. Migraine is considered by the World Health Organization as one of the world's 20-most-disabling disorders. Traditionally considered as a chronic episodic disorder with a benign course (episodic migraine [EM]), a subgroup of subjects progress to a chronic state, affecting them daily (chronic migraine [CM]), impairing drastically their quality of life (2). Irrespective of the above subtypes, obesity and migraine are linked. Two large population-based studies found that obesity increased the frequency and severity of migraine attacks (3,4). A body mass index (BMI) greater >30 kg/m^2 carries a 5 times higher risk of developing chronic headaches compared to the lean group (5).

Table 39-1. Symptoms Directly Related to—or at Increased Frequency in—Obesity

Symptom or Sign	Additional Obesity-Related Diagnoses to Be Considered	Increased Frequency in Obesity
Leg swelling	Lymphedema, lipedema	Venous thromboembolic disease, congestive heart failure
Amenorrhea	Therapeutic weight loss, unrecognized pregnancy, bulimia, hypothalamic disorder, genetic syndromes (eg, Prader-Willi)	Polycystic ovary syndrome, central (hypothalamic or pituitary) or peripheral (corpus luteum) defects within the hypothalamic-pituitary-ovarian axis
Jaundice	Nonalcoholic fatty liver disease	Gall stones, pancreatic cancer
Chest pain	Fibromyalgia	Reflux esophagitis, ischemic heart disease
Bone pain		Osteoarthritis, vitamin D deficiency, nerve entrapment syndromes
Hypertension	Obstructive sleep apnea	"Essential"
Weight loss	Intentional	Nonintentional due to development of type 2 diabetes, cancer
Hypoglycemia	Postbypass incretin-mediated late "dumping" syndrome	Failure to down-titrate insulin and noninsulin antihypoglycemic agents with diet and weight loss

Other more recent studies have found a clear relationship between obesity and CM but not with chronic tension-type headache (6,7). The available literature supports the concept that obesity is an exacerbating factor for migraine but not for simple headaches overall, particularly in those with abdominal obesity. It also has been suggested that obesity-related psychological comorbidities, such as depression and anxiety, could have an additive effect on the risk of migraine progression (2). The pathogenetic mechanisms of migraine are complex but are believed to be due to an impaired interaction between central and peripheral events resulting in an improper sensory conduction and higher inflammatory response. In this regard, obesity could influence the severity of migraine peripherally as a proinflammatory state or centrally with the impaired secretion of neuropeptides involved in the nociceptive processing as well in energy homeostasis.

So obesity can increase migraine severity, resulting in increased morbidity and impairing the quality of life. In addition, the "International Classification of Headache Disorders" (ICHD-3) from the International Headache Society (2013) classifies at least 2 other categories of headache that are also associated with obesity and can present emergently (8): 1) sleep apnea-related headache; and 2) headache attributed to idiopathic intracranial hypertension (IIH).

Obstructive sleep apnea syndrome (OSAS) is very common in the obese person. OSAS is linked to resistant hypertension and an increased risk of stroke (9). Daytime sleepiness and/or fatigue is reported and could expose workers in certain jobs (eg, building and construction, driving) to particular risk (10). Morning headache is increased 3- to 10-fold in the obese with OSAS compared to the general population. In comparison, up to 42% of patients with morning headache have been found to have OSAS using polysomnography, especially in women (11). The exact mechanisms of headache pathogenesis in OSAS remain controversial, but several hypotheses have been proposed, including nighttime fluctuations of oxygen saturation with hypercapnia; vasodilatation; increased intracranial pressure; disturbances of cerebral blood flow autoregulation; excessive neck movements; bruxism; and increased muscle activation and impaired sleep quality and shorter percentage of time in rapid eye movement (REM) sleep (11). All these mechanisms could have an effect in brain regions involved in sleep regulation and nociception, resulting in a dysfunction of central pain-inhibitory activity.

IIH is a disorder characterized by increased intracranial pressure (ICP) of unknown cause, mostly seen in young and obese women. A diagnosis of IIH requires the exclusion of all other causative factors, such as intracranial space occupying lesions, vascular disorders, and metabolic, toxic, or hormonal causes of intracranial hypertension, all together with the demonstration of an increased ICP by lumbar puncture. Together with visual disturbances, headache is a key symptom of IIH, usually it is the most common symptom at presentation, and it is more reported by women. The headache of IIH is usually progressive, with diffuse and/or constant (nonpulsating) pain, with daily occurrence. Holocranial, it can be worse after waking, and it may be exacerbated by coughing or straining. If headache is predominantly due to raised ICP, it can improve dramatically following a lumbar puncture or a cerebrospinal fluid (CSF) diversion procedure. Only a modest degree of weight loss is usually required for improvement in such symptoms and signs as headaches and papilledema (12).

BREATHLESSNESS

Breathlessness is another common symptom that can present as an emergency. Obesity is a very common cause of breathlessness on exertion: 80% of obese patients reported dyspnea after climbing 2 flights of stairs (13). Obese patients report their breathlessness differently than normal-weight individuals, describing incomplete respiration and a need for deep inspiration, wheezing, and air hunger more commonly at rest and in response to exercise (14). Asthma is more prevalent, more severe, and associated with less favorable response to therapy with regard to symptoms, level of forced expiratory volume in 1 second (FEV1), fraction of exhaled nitric oxide, and airway responsiveness in the obese (15). However, misdiagnosis of asthma in the obese is common. Pulmonary venous thromboembolic (VTE) disease is an important cause of breathlessness and occurs more commonly in obesity (Table 39-1), yet diagnostic clues may mislead or be problematic (16), especially if one adds the common lack of large bore scanners and poor image quality when the obese patient undergoes ventilation/perfusion (V/Q) scanning (Table 39-2) (17).

These 2 examples (and the others listed in Table 39-1) highlight the need for clinicians to understand the impact of obesity on disease occurrence and presentation, and how in the acute setting the diagnostic algorithms and probabilities may be altered.

Table 39-2. Common Physiological Alterations Complicating a Diagnosis of Pulmonary Embolism (16)

Suggestive Diagnostic Criteria for PE	Common Physiological Alterations in Obese and Morbidly Obese Patients
Dyspnea	Respiratory rates up to 40% higher than normal
Tachycardia	Heart rate increases as BMI increases
Signs of DVT	Leg edema and chronic skin changes
Hypoxemia	PaO_2 inversely related to waist circumference
Elevated blood natriuretic peptide	Complex BNP alterations with both decreases and elevations seen
Elevated D-dimer	D-dimer is commonly elevated
Pulmonary hypertension	RVSP up to 40 mm Hg may be normal in obesity

Abbreviations: BNP = elevated blood natriuretic peptide; DVP = deep vein thrombosis; PE = pulmonary embolism; RVSP = right ventricular systolic pressure.

ACKNOWLEDGMENTS

The authors have nothing to disclose.

REFERENCES

1. **Jensen M, Ryan DH, Apovian CM, et al.** 2013 AHA/ACC/TOS Guideline for the Management of Overweight and Obesity in Adults: a report of the American College of Cardiology/American Heart Association Task Force on Practice Guidelines and The Obesity Society. *J Am Coll Cardiol.* pii: S0735-1097(13)06030-0. doi: 10.1016/j.jacc.2013.11.004. [Epub ahead of print].
2. **Bigal ME, Rapoport AM.** Obesity and chronic daily headache. *Curr Pain Headache Rep.* 2012;16:101–109.
3. **Bigal ME, Liberman JN, Lipton RB.** Obesity and migraine: a population study. *Neurology.* 2006;67:246–251.
4. **Winter AC, Berger K, Buring JE, Kurth T.** Body mass index, migraine, migraine frequency and migraine features in women. *Cephalalgia.* 2013;33:130–135.
5. **Scher AI, Stewart WF, Ricci JA, Lipton RB.** Factors associated with the onset and remission of chronic daily headache in a population-based study. *Pain.* 2003;106:81–89.
6. **Bigal ME, Lipton RB, Holland PR, Goadsby PJ.** Obesity, migraine, and CM: possible mechanisms of interaction. *Neurology.* 2007;68:1851–1861.
7. **Bigal ME, Tsang A, Loder E, Serrano D, Reed ML, Lipton RB.** Body mass index and episodic headaches: a population-based study. *Arch Intern Med.* 2007;167:1964–1970.
8. **Headache Classification Committee of the International Headache Society (IHS).** The International

Classification of Headache Disorders. 3rd ed. (beta version). *Cephalalgia.* 2013;33:629–808.

9. **Barone DA, Krieger AC.** Stroke and obstructive sleep apnea: a review. *Curr Atheroscler Rep.* 2013;15:334.
10. **Provini F, Vetrugno R, Lugaresi E, Montagna P.** Sleep-related breathing disorders and headache. *Neurol Sci.* 2006;27:S149–S152.
11. **Ohayon MM.** Prevalence and risk factors of morning headaches in the general population. *Arch Intern Med.* 2004;164:97–102.
12. **Thurtell MJ, Bruce BB, Newman NJ, Biousse V.** An update on idiopathic intracranial hypertension. *Rev Neurol Dis.* 2010;7:e56–e68.
13. **Gibson GJ.** Obesity, respiratory function and breathlessness. *Thorax.* 2000;55(suppl 1):S41–S44.
14. **Essalhi M, Gillaizeau F, Chevallier JM, et al.** Cross-sectional assessment of the roles of comorbidities in resting and activity-related dyspnea in severely obese women. *J Asthma.* 2013;50:565–572.
15. **Scott S, Currie J, Albert P, Calverley P, Wilding JP.** Risk of misdiagnosis, health-related quality of life, and BMI in patients who are overweight with doctor-diagnosed asthma. *Chest.* 2012;141:616–624.
16. **Hawley PC, Hawley MP.** Difficulties in diagnosing pulmonary embolism in the obese patient: a literature review. *Vasc Med.* 2011;16:444–451.
17. **Uppot RN, Sahani DV, Hahn PF, Gervais D, Mueller PR.** Impact of obesity on medical imaging and image-guided intervention. *Am J Roentgenol.* 2007;188:433–440.

CHAPTER 40

Chylomicronemia Syndrome

Very Severe Hypertriglyceridemia and Acute Pancreatitis

John D Brunzell and Alan Chait

ABSTRACT

Pancreatitis is a life-threatening complication of very severe hypertriglyceridemia. Moreover, the pancreatitis often is recurrent if hypertriglyceridemia is not appreciated to be the cause of the pancreatitis and if triglyceride levels are not adequately treated. All patients are at increased risk of developing acute, recurrent pancreatitis with triglyceride level above 1,000 mg/dL (11.2 mmol/L). Although pancreatitis usually ensues only with values >2,000 mg/dL (22.4 mmol/L), levels can rapidly exceed this level in patients with values >1,000 mg/dL (11.2 mmol/L). Causes of the chylomicronemia syndrome have been divided into familial chylomicronemia syndrome (FCS) and "multifactorial chylomicronemia syndrome" (MFCS). MFCS patients have an underlying familial form of hypertriglyceridemia and secondary cause(s) of hypertriglyceridemia. In MFCS, the secondary cause(s) of hypertriglyceridemia need to be identified and treated. Certain drugs are known to cause very severe hypertriglyceridemia and pancreatitis and should ideally be avoided or discontinued. Fibrate therapy is indicated for long-term therapy in patients with MFCS who have persistent hypertriglyceridemia above 1,000 mg/dL (11.2 mmol/L).

INTRODUCTION

Milky plasma (lipemia) was first reported in 1799 and eruptive xanthomata in 1851 (1,2). These xanthomata were termed xanthomata diabeticorum in the early 1900s because of their appearance in untreated persons with diabetes and milky plasma. Familial chylomicronemia was described in 1932 by Burger and Grutz (1) and found to be due to lipoprotein lipase (LPL) deficiency in 1960 (3). The association of severe hypertriglyceridemia with acute pancreatitis was first reported by Speck in 1865 (2). Interest in hypertriglyceridemia-associated pancreatitis was renewed in the 1970s by Cameron and associates (4).

The modern era of lipid metabolism began with the classic series of papers by Fredrickson, Levy, and Lees (5), in which they classified hypertriglyceridemia into types dependent on the pattern of lipoproteins on paper electrophoresis and the presence or absence of very low density lipoprotein (VLDL) and/or chylomicrons in fasting plasma. Types IV and V hyperlipoproteinemia had increased VLDL levels while Types 1 and V had chylomicronemia. They recognized that acute pancreatitis and eruptive xanthomata occurred in the presence of chylomicronemia as in Types I and V hyperlipoproteinemia. Chylomicrons are usually present in fasting plasma with triglyceride levels above 1,000 mg/dL (11.2 mmol/L) and absent below that value (6). In a prospective study of patients admitted with acute pancreatitis and plasma triglycerides measured at the peak of the pain, the distribution of plasma triglycerides was bimodal (Figure 40-1) (6). Triglyceride levels less than 885 mg/dL (10 mmol/L) were associated with gallbladder disease and chronic alcoholism, while those above 2,000 mg/dL (22.4 mmol/L) were associated with the simultaneous presence of a familial form of hypertriglyceridemia with secondary forms of hypertriglyceridemia (7). Hypertriglyceridemia-associated pancreatitis has been reported with triglyceride levels lower than 2,000 mg/dL (22.4 mmol/L) (8,9), but in our experience this only occurs when hypertriglyceridemic patients stopped eating some time before the blood was drawn. However, subjects with triglyceride levels greater than 1,000 mg/dL (11.2 mmol/L) are at significantly increased risk of pancreatitis.

The term chylomicronemia syndrome was first used in 1981 to describe a constellation of clinical findings that occurred in association with very high triglyceride levels (10). Causes of the chylomicronemia syndrome have been divided into familial chylomicronemia syndrome (FCS) related to autosomal recessive disease of the LPL complex, and nonfamilial chylomicronemia syndrome (11). The term nonfamilial chylomicronemia syndrome may be misleading because there is always a genetic component to the very severe hypertriglyceridemia. Type V hyperlipoproteinemia is also not appropriate because many, if not most, Type V patients have triglyceride levels between 1,000 and 2,000 mg/dL (11.2–22.4 mmol/L), that is, levels below which pancreatitis occurs. For this chapter we will use the term "multifactorial chylomicronemia syndrome" (MFCS) to describe patients who are not classified as having FCS. Terms for the levels of hypertriglyceridemia were first defined by the National Cholesterol Education Program Adult Treatment Panel (NCEP ATP) in 2000 and more recently by the Endocrine Society (12) (Table 40-1). Here we will use the term moderate hypertriglyceridemia for triglyceride levels between 200 and 999 mg/dL (2.3–11.2 mmol/L), the term severe hypertriglyceridemia for 1,000 to 1,999 mg/dL (11.2–22.4 mmol/L), and very severe hypertriglyceridemia for values >2,000 mg/dL (22.4 mmol/L).

Plasma triglyceride level with abdominal pain

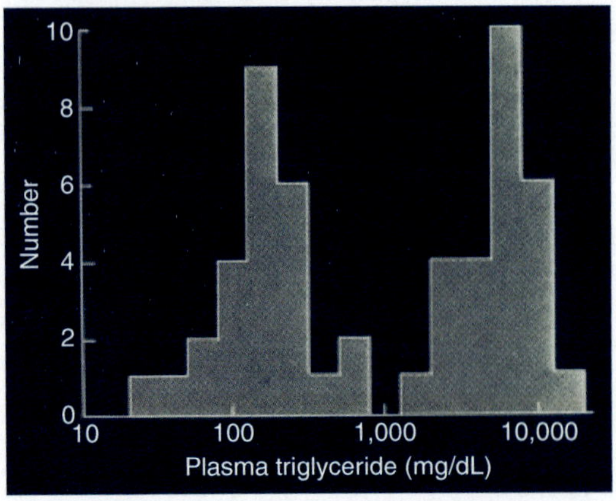

TG <800 mg/dL or >2,000 mg/dL

Figure 40-1. Frequency distribution of plasma triglyceride levels in patients with probable pancreatitis. Note bimodal distribution of triglyceride levels: highest triglyceride level in lower mode was 759 mg/dL (8.6 mmol/L), lowest in higher mode was 1,925 mg/dL (21.7 mmol/L) (6).

The prevalence of very severe hypertriglyceridemia with triglyceride levels above 2,000 mg/dL (22.4 mmol/L) was 7 out of 39,090 individuals (1.8/10,000) in the Lipid Research Clinics population-based prevalence study in 1980 (1). In National Health and Nutrition Examination Survey (NHANES), 2001 to 2006, the prevalence was similar at 3 out of 5,680 individuals (5.3/10,000) (13). FCS makes up a small portion of very severe hypertriglyceridemia with a population prevalence of about 1 per million in the United States and Europe. Mutations in LPL genes leading to LPL deficiency are much more common than defects in the other genes (eg, apolipoprotein CII, GPIHDLBP1, apolipoprotein A5, and lipase modulating factor-1 [LMF1]) that facilitate LPL functionality (14). MFCS would then be estimated to be several hundred times more prevalent than FCS (1). Overall, the prevalence of severe hypertriglyceridemia in the general population is thus very low.

Conversely, very severe hypertriglyceridemia has been reported in 12%–20% of patients with acute pancreatitis (4,15). This number may reflect some referral bias, but in the absence of gallbladder disease and chronic alcoholism, very severe hypertriglyceridemia is a common cause of acute pancreatitis. Moreover, the pancreatitis often is recurrent if

Table 40-1. Criteria Proposed for Clinical Diagnosis of Elevated Triglyceride Levels Under Fasting Conditions (12)

NCEP-ATP III			Endocrine Society Guidelines		
Normal	<150 mg/dL	<1.7 mmol/L	Normal	<150 mg/dL	<1.7 mmol/L
Borderline-high triglycerides	150–199 mg/dL	1.7–2.3 mmol/L	Mild hypertriglyceridemia	150–199 mg/dL	1.7–2.3 mmol/L
High triglycerides	200–499 mg/dL	2.3–5.6 mmol/L	Moderate hypertriglyceridemia	200–999 mg/dL	2.3–11.2 mmol/L
Very high triglycerides	≥500 mg/dL	≥5.6 mmol/L	Severe hypertriglyceridemia	1,000–1,999 mg/dL	11.2–22.4 mmol/L
			Very severe hypertriglyceridemia	≥2,000 mg/dL	≥22.4 mmol/L

The criteria developed for the Endocrine Society Guidelines (12) focused on the ability to assess risk for premature cardiovascular disease (CVD) versus risk for pancreatitis. The designation of mild and moderate hypertriglyceridemia corresponded to the range of levels predominant in risk assessment for premature CVD, and this range contains the vast majority of patients with hypertriglyceridemia. Severe hypertriglyceridemia carries susceptibility for intermittent increases in levels above 2,000 mg/dL (22.4 mmol/L) and subsequent risk of pancreatitis; very severe hypertriglyceridemia is indicative of high risk for pancreatitis. In addition, these levels suggest different etiologies. The presence of mild or moderate hypertriglyceridemia is commonly due to a dominant underlying cause in each patient, whereas severe or very severe hypertriglyceridemia is more likely due to several contributing factors.

hypertriglyceridemia is not appreciated to be the cause of the pancreatitis and if triglyceride levels are not adequately treated.

PATHOPHYSIOLOGY

In FCS, the severe defect in plasma chylomicron and VLDL triglyceride hydrolysis leads to the accumulation of dietary fat as chylomicrons even after an overnight fast. VLDL levels do not seem to be greatly elevated since hepatic triglyceride production is suppressed. However, if a situation occurs that leads to increased triglyceride production in these patients, the secreted VLDL appears to compete with the remaining plasma triglyceride removal mechanisms and aggravates the underling chylomicronemia. In MFCS, it is more complicated. Here, mild-to-moderate hypertriglyceridemia can be due to hepatic over-secretion of triglyceride into plasma, or to defects in LPL-related triglyceride hydrolysis, or both. Because the removal system is saturable (16), drugs or conditions that affect either triglyceride appearance or clearance can make the removal of the prior day's absorbed fat more difficult, thereby leading to the development of chylomicronemia. In both FCS and MFCS, the pancreatitis may be related to microvascular ischemia as a result of chylomicron clusters plugging pancreatic capillaries followed by cell necrosis, with release of pancreatic lipase.

ETIOLOGY

Familial Chylomicronemia Syndrome

Most FCS patients are homozygous or compound heterozygous for 2 defective LPL alleles. Over 100 gene variants have been described leading to LPL deficiency (14,17). Many of these patients have missense variants, sometimes in catalytically important sites and sometime in regions that predispose to instability in the homodimeric structure of LPL required for enzyme activity (18). Even less often defects are due to insertions/deletions and premature stop codons. Many common LPL gene variants have been described that have no clinical effects (19). Much rarer forms of the FCS can be due to major gene defects in other proteins, such as apolipoprotein CII, GPIHDLBP1, apolipoprotein A5, and LMF1. Each of these proteins plays an important role in assisting LPL function (14). Homozygous mutations in each of these related proteins can lead to very severe hypertriglyceridemia and pancreatitis. The lipoprotein phenotype in these rarer disorders is similar to that in LPL deficiency.

Multifactorial Chylomicronemia Syndrome

MFCS is much more common than FCS (1). Most, if not all, patients with MFCS have a genetic form of moderate hypertriglyceridemia in their families; in addition, almost all have a second defect causing hypertriglyceridemia (7) (see section Clinical Features, MFCS below). Following treatment of the secondary form of hypertriglyceridemia in MFCS, triglyceride levels usually decrease to levels seen in their moderately hypertriglyceridemic relatives (Figure 40-2) (7). Recently Johansen and Hegele have reported many common variants with small effects in patients with severe hypertriglyceridemia that account for about 20% of the triglyceride elevation (20). How this relates to the coexistence of a familial and a secondary form hypertriglyceridemia, which in our experience is the usual cause of very severe hypertriglyceridemia, is unknown. Perhaps an additional single nucleotide variant is required in addition to the familial and secondary forms of hypertriglyceridemia noted above in order to develop triglyceride levels above 2,000 mg/dL (22.4 mmol/L) and acute pancreatitis (21).

CLINICAL FEATURES

Pancreatitis is a life-threatening complication of very severe hypertriglyceridemia. Patients with this complication often present with similar symptoms and signs as patients with other etiologies. However, there may be additional features in the history and physical examination that suggest the diagnosis of hypertriglyceridemia-associated pancreatitis.

Familial Chylomicronemia Syndrome

FCS often presents in early childhood. The diagnosis is often made in infancy because of the presence of severe colic or failure to thrive, accompanied by a laboratory report of lipemic plasma. Later in childhood, the detection of lipemic plasma in an asymptomatic child can be the initial presentation. Acute, recurrent pancreatitis is a severe manifestation of FCS at all ages. Although LPL deficiency often presents with abdominal pain and pancreatitis in childhood, apolipoprotein CII deficiency may present at an older age. Rarely, FCS can initially present when the patient enters adolescence, related to use of estrogen-based oral contraceptives or alcohol that increase hepatic VLDL triglyceride production (16). A history of consanguinity may be present, particularly in inbred populations. In this situation, other homozygous abnormalities not related to triglyceride metabolism also can occur. Each LPL variant often is restricted to one family, due to unique, identical rare gene variants shared by the parents. Major gene defects such as insertions, deletions, and premature stop codons occur commonly in the FCS patients who have defects other than LPL deficiency. Genetic confirmation of the functional genetic defect can be performed. However, in children with lipemic plasma a clinical diagnosis can be reliable. If the child has no diabetes, is on no lipid-raising medications, and

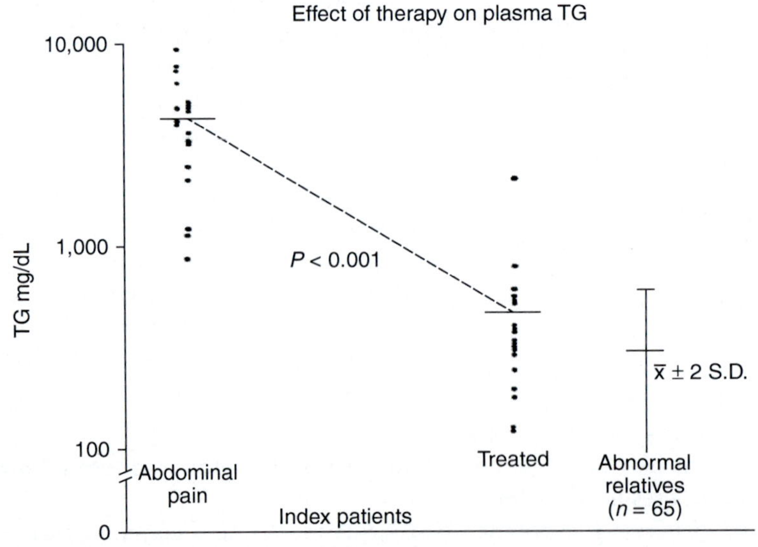

Figure 40-2. Plasma triglycerides in patients with MFCS before and after removal of secondary causes of hypertriglyceridemia, compared with triglyceride levels of their hypertriglyceridemia relatives (7).

does not have glycogen storage disease (Type I), the likelihood that the diagnosis of the FCS is reliable is high without genetic confirmation. The medications of consequence are estrogen-based oral contraceptives, the leukemia medication asparaginase, and protease inhibitors used for human immunodeficiency virus/acquired immunodeficiency syndrome (HIV/AIDS) (2). With chronic chylomicronemia, FCS patients may develop eruptive xanthomata and acute abdominal pain, often due to acute pancreatitis. The obligate heterozygote parents often present with mild-to-moderate hypertriglyceridemia (22).

Multifactorial Chylomicronemia Syndrome

MFCS often initially presents with acute abdominal pain. The other most common presentation is a laboratory report of lipemic plasma. Rarer presentations occur with the recognition of lipemia retinalis by ophthalmologists, eruptive xanthomata (Figure 40-3) by dermatologists, or acute recent memory loss noted by the patient (10). These patients almost always have relatives with common forms of hypertriglyceridemia, such as familial combined hyperlipidemia (FCHL), monogenic familial hypertriglyceridemia, familial low HDL syndrome with hypertriglyceridemia, and remnant removal disease (Type III) (23). Often the patient is unaware of his or her underlying moderate dyslipidemia and presents with very severe hypertriglyceridemia after the development of a secondary cause of hypertriglyceridemia (Table 40-2). In the past, this most commonly coincided with the onset of marked hyperglycemia of untreated diabetes. Since the clinical utilization of glycosylated hemoglobin (HgbA1c), this degree of hyperglycemia and very severe hypertriglyceridemia appears to be less common. With treatment of the diabetes and the reduction in plasma triglyceride levels, the addition of beta-adrenergic blocking agents (selective and nonselective) and/or diuretics (thiazides and loop-diuretics such as furosemide) for hypertension and/or heart failure can be associated with the return of very severe hypertriglyceridemia. Further, unsuccessful maintenance of weight loss has been associated with increasing triglyceride levels during weight regain. More recently, MFCS commonly results from the addition of specific drugs in patients with an underlying familial form of dyslipidemia. In addition to beta blockers and diuretics, such drugs include retinoid therapy, oral estrogen therapy, selective estrogen receptor modulators (SERMs, particularly raloxifene) protease inhibitors, atypical antipsychotic drugs, and possibly sertraline (1). The need for protease inhibitors and atypical antipsychotic agents can be complicated by the development of the MFCS in the absence of suitable alternative agents. Very severe hypertriglyceridemia also can be seen in Kobberling syndrome (type 1 partial lipodystrophy) where control of both hypertriglyceridemia and type 2 diabetes can be difficult (24,25). In patients with underlying hypertriglyceridemia, pancreatitis due to very

Table 40-2. Causes of Hypertriglyceridemia (12)

Primary hypertriglyceridemia
Familial combined hyperlipidemia (FCHL)
Familial hypertriglyceridemia (FHTG)
Familial Type III (remnant removal disease)
Familial hypoalphalipoproteinemia (FHA)
Familial chylomicronemia and related disorders
Primary genetic susceptibility
Metabolic syndrome
Treated type 2 diabetes
Secondary hypertriglyceridemia
Excess alcohol intake
Drug-induced (eg, thiazides, beta blockers, estrogens, isotretinoin, glucocorticoids, bile acid-binding resins, antiretroviral protease inhibitors, immunosuppressants, antipsychotics)
Untreated or poorly controlled diabetes mellitus
Endocrine diseases
Renal disease
Liver disease
Pregnancy
Autoimmune disorders

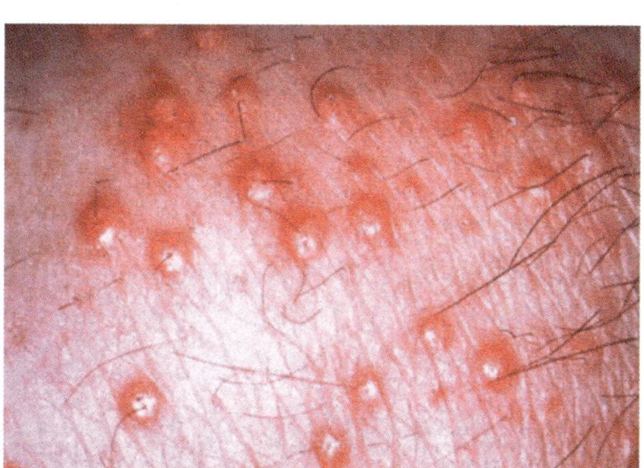

Figure 40-3. Photograph of cutaneous eruptive xanthomata on the buttock, which is the most common pressure point for their development.

severe hypertriglyceridemia may occur during infusions with lipid emulsions for parenteral feeding (26). This also may occur during infusions of anesthetic propofol, which is infused in a 10% fat emulsion (27). Finally, very severe hypertriglyceridemia can develop during pregnancy, particularly during the third trimester, in a subset of women who have moderate or severe hypertriglyceridemia before conception. Acute pancreatitis can develop in this situation (28).

As with FCS, patients with MFCS can present with eruptive xanthomata, acute memory loss, abdominal pain, and acute pancreatitis. The pancreatitis often is recurrent, but does not become relapsing. With long-term multiple episodes of acute, recurrent pancreatitis, exocrine pancreatic insufficiency or insulin deficient secondary diabetes may occur. Of note, this form of acute pancreatitis is often associated with normal amylase and lipase levels (4), even in patients with hemorrhagic pancreatitis at laparoscopy or by computer tomography (CT) scan or magnetic resonance imaging (MRI). Abdominal pain also may be the result of rapid expansion of the liver by fat, since fatty liver occurs commonly in all forms of severe hypertriglyceridemia (1).

INVESTIGATIONS

In the emergent setting of acute pancreatitis work-up, nonfasting triglyceride levels are appropriate. However, in other settings the diagnosis and degree of hypertriglyceridemia is suggested to be based on fasting levels where the length of fast is recommended to be 12 hours (12). During this time period, intake of liquids without caloric content is acceptable. Once hypertriglyceridemia is diagnosed, secondary causes should be excluded (Table 40-2). Diagnostic tests for DNA variants can also be performed. If available, postheparin plasma LPL activity may be measured. Usually this is not necessary because of the differences in clinical presentation between FCS and MFCS related to other causes of hypertriglyceridemia. As noted above, hypertriglyceridemia-associated pancreatitis is often associated with normal amylase and lipase levels (4). Abdominal imaging is the definitive test for pancreatitis in these circumstances.

TREATMENT

General supportive acute care for the patient admitted for hypertriglyceridemia-associated pancreatitis is initially identical to that for other causes of acute pancreatitis (eg, analgesia, intravenous [IV] fluids, nothing-by-mouth [NPO]). However, as the patient begins oral intake (usually after pain is controlled), chylomicronemia syndrome patients need to avoid oral fat intake. In addition, IV hyperalimentation with fat emulsions is also contraindicated. Secondary causes should be addressed and precipitating drugs should be stopped.

Lipid-Specific Therapies

FCS. In infants presenting with abdominal pain or failure to thrive, discontinuation of breast feeding with replacement by very low fat formula feeding will cause a marked decrease in triglyceride levels and decrease in symptoms. Later in childhood, dietary fat calories (saturated, monounsaturated, and unsaturated long-chain fatty acids) should be restricted to the extent that is required for control of the very severe hypertriglyceridemia and abdominal pain. As a result dietary fat may only provide ~5% to 15% of total daily calories. Children quickly learn which foods to avoid and how to avoid acute pancreatitis by immediately decreasing fat and calorie intake for a day or two after the onset of abdominal pain. Dietary indiscretion is more common during adolescence. Long chain fatty acids may be replaced by medium-chain triglycerides (MCT). MCTs are a source of calories that do not enter the thoracic duct as chylomicrons, but rather are taken up directly by the liver after absorption by the enterocytes. Omega 3 fatty acids lower plasma triglyceride levels in MFCS, but may actually aggravate the severe hypertriglyceridemia of FCS. Therefore, omega 3 fatty acids are contraindicated in LPL deficiency (29,30). Similarly, fibrates do not seem to be beneficial in LPL deficiency (1), perhaps because hepatic triglyceride secretion is low and LPL activity is absent.

During adolescence, use of oral estrogen contraceptives and alcohol intake can precipitate very severe hypertriglyceridemia and acute pancreatitis. Until 20 years ago, a successful pregnancy was very uncommon. With near-total fat restriction, perhaps accompanied by fibrate treatment such as gemfibrozil, successful pregnancies have become more common (31,32). Although near total fat restriction can theoretically result in essential fatty deficiency, the problem does not seem to arise in this situation (31). Polyunsaturated fatty acids have been administered cutaneously as a potential source of essential fatty acids (33).

MFCS. The primary goal of treatment of MFCS is to prevent the development of acute pancreatitis. The initial presentation of MFCS often is severe, requiring hospitalization in an intensive care unit. The diagnosis of hypertriglyceridemia-induced pancreatitis is strongly suggested by plasma triglyceride levels above 2,000 mg/dL (22.4 mmol/L) on admission. Values sometimes can be as high as 30,000 mg/dL (340 mmol/L). Acute therapy is the same as for pancreatitis due to other diseases, although lipid emulsions should not be used for parenteral feeding, because their use will exacerbate the hypertriglyceridemia. CT scan or MRI should be performed early to confirm pancreatitis. With clinical improvement oral feeding may begin with total removal of all fat from the diet.

It is important to appreciate that patients with MFCS usually have multiple causes of hypertriglyceridemia, including a common familial form of moderate hypertriglyceridemia and a secondary cause. The patient often is unaware of the background lipid disorder. The challenge is to determine both the primary and secondary cause(s) of the very severe hypertriglyceridemia that preceded the acute pancreatitis. In the past the secondary cause often was the initial presentation of very out-of-control type 2 diabetes. With therapy for the hyperglycemia and moderate dietary fat restriction, plasma triglyceride levels can decrease significantly in these patients. However, the diabetes-related defect in adipose tissue LPL that occurs in these very hyperglycemic patients may take as long as 3 months to correct (34), leading to continuing severe hypertriglyceridemia during this time period. In such patients we usually start fibrate drugs (fenofibrate or gemfibrozil) and continue a low fat diet with a total fat content of 20% to 30% of calories. The dietary fat restriction can be eased after 3 months and the need for fibrates reassessed. With the treatment of the diabetes and avoidance of triglyceride-raising drugs, most patients with diabetes and MFCS will have triglyceride levels below 1,000 mg/dL (11.2 mmol/L) under these circumstances. An exception are women who have Kobberling partial lipodystrophy, in whom glucose and triglyceride control can be difficult (24,25). Apheresis is seldom required and heparin infusions (which can enhance LPL activity) are ineffective.

Against a background of a familial form of hypertriglyceridemia, many drugs have been associated with very severe hypertriglyceridemia and MFCS (2,6). Oral estrogens have been associated with MFCS in women with underlying familial forms of hypertriglyceridemia who developed acute pancreatitis. This is less common today because of less frequent use of postmenopausal estrogens, the use of skin patches for estrogen replacement therapy, and the use of lower dose estrogen in birth control pills or alternative methods of contraception. SERMs can have similar effects to oral estrogens. Alcohol has been recognized as a cause of acute and chronic relapsing pancreatitis due to the direct toxic effects of alcohol on the pancreas. However, alcohol also can lead to very severe hypertriglyceridemia and triglyceride-induced pancreatitis in patients with an underlying lipid disorder. Retinoid therapy for severe acne raises triglyceride levels and is contraindicated in patients with baseline triglyceride levels above 500 mg/dL (5.6 mmol/L) because of the concern for risk of acute pancreatitis. Oral estrogen therapy, glucocorticoid therapy, continuing alcohol intake, and retinoid therapy are sometimes possible by adding fibrate therapy.

With the development of new drug therapies, additional causes of adult MFCS have been reported (2). Protease inhibitors for HIV/AIDS and atypical antipsychotic drug therapy can be associated with very severe hypertriglyceridemia. It has not been determined whether an underlying familial form of dyslipidemia is required. In some individuals with background moderate hypertriglyceridemia, sertraline therapy has led to MFCS (1). Rarer causes of very severe hypertriglyceridemia include autoimmune disease (sometimes with LPL-specific antibodies), asparaginase therapy

Table 40-3. Major Points in the Treatment of Very Severe Hypertriglyceridemia

1. Familial chylomicronemia, for example, LPL deficiency, is very rare but is associated with very severe hypertriglyceridemia onset in early childhood. It should be treated with strict dietary fat restriction to decrease triglyceride levels to those at which abdominal pain does not occur.
2. All patients are at increased risk of developing acute, recurrent pancreatitis with triglyceride level above 1,000 mg/dL (11.2 mmol/L). Although pancreatitis usually ensues only with values >2,000 mg/dL (22.4 mmol/L), levels can rapidly exceed this in patients with values >1,000 mg/dL (11.2 mmol/L).
3. MFCS patients have underlying familial form of hypertriglyceridemia and secondary cause(s) of hypertriglyceridemia (Table 40-2).
4. In MFCS the secondary cause(s) of hypertriglyceridemia need to be identified and treated (Table 40-2).
5. Certain drugs are known to be the cause of very severe hypertriglyceridemia and pancreatitis and should ideally be avoided or discontinued.
6. Fibrate therapy is indicated for long-term therapy in patients with MFCS who have persistent hypertriglyceridemia above 1,000 mg/dL (11.2 mmol/L).

for acute lymphoblastic leukemia, and bexarotene, a RXR agonist used in the treatment of cutaneous T cell lymphoma (2). As noted above, IV fat emulsions, including propofol in 10% fat emulsion, can be problematic. Obesity is often associated with the familial forms of hypertriglyceridemia, but alone is not sufficient to lead to very severe hypertriglyceridemia.

If fasting plasma triglyceride levels remain above 1,000 mg/dL (11.2 mmol/L) after treating or removing the precipitating cause of the very severe hypertriglyceridemia, fibrate or omega 3 fatty acid therapy (3 to 4 grams per day) is indicated. It is not certain which patients with a familial form of moderate hypertriglyceridemia will develop very severe hypertriglyceridemia and MFCS. Therefore, life-long fibrate therapy might be considered. A secondary goal of therapy is the prevention of cardiovascular disease (CVD) in some MFCS patients. This in particular pertains to those individuals in whom FCHL is the genetic disorder underlying the MFCS. A presumptive diagnosis of FCHL often can be made by the presence of premature CVD in multiple family members, determined after taking a careful and detailed family history. In such cases, statin therapy and lifestyle changes aimed at reducing the risk of CVD should be undertaken in addition to strategies to maintain reduced triglyceride levels (12,35).

Emerging Therapies

Newer therapies are on the horizon for FCS. Drugs that block pancreatic lipase and cause fat malabsorption lower plasma triglycerides, but the gastrointestinal side effects associated with fat malabsorption often are not tolerable. Gene therapy for LPL deficiency has been approved for adults in Europe with significant restrictions. The patient has to be 18 years of age or older, have a defect in LPL with some LPL protein present, and have unmanageable recurrent acute pancreatitis (36). Experimental drugs that block chylomicron synthesis in the gut are also being explored. Plasma apheresis is not indicated in FCS because it has no advantage over the marked and rapid decrease in plasma triglycerides that occurs with total dietary fat restriction.

CONCLUSIONS

Pancreatitis is a life-threatening complication of very severe hypertriglyceridemia. The approach to treatment of very severe hypertriglyceridemia is summarized in Table 40-3.

ACKNOWLEDGMENTS

JDB is an advisory board member for uniQure and ISIS Pharmaceuticals. AC has consulted for Uniqure in the past 2 years.

REFERENCES

1. **Brunzell JD, Deeb S.** Familial lipoprotein lipase deficiency, apo cii deficiency and hepatic lipase deficiency. In: Scriver CS, Beudet AL, Sly WS, et al, eds. *The Metabolic and Molecular Basis of Inherited Disease.* 8th ed. New York: McGraw-Hill Book Co.; 2001:2789–2816.
2. **Yadav D, Pitchumoni CS.** Issues in hyperlipidemic pancreatitis. *J Clin Gastroenterol.* 2003;36:54–62.
3. **Havel RJ, Gordon RS Jr.** Idiopathic hyperlipemia: metabolic studies in an affected family. *J Clin Invest.* 1960;39:1777–1790.

4. **Cameron JL, Capuzzi DM, Zuidema GD, Margolis S.** Acute pancreatitis with hyperlipemia: the incidence of lipid abnormalities in acute pancreatitis. *Ann Surg.* 1973;177:483–489.
5. **Fredrickson D, Levy R, Lees R.** Fat transport and lipoproteins—an integrated approach to mechanisms and disorders. *N Engl J Med.* 1967;276:32,94,148,215,273.
6. **Brunzell JD, Bierman EL.** Chylomicronemia syndrome. Interaction of genetic and acquired hypertriglyceridemia. *Med Clin North Am.* 1982;66: 455–468.
7. **Brunzell JD, Schrott HG.** The interaction of familial and secondary causes of hypertriglyceridemia: role in pancreatitis. *J Clin Lipidol.* 2012;6:409–412.
8. **Tremblay K, Methot J, Brisson D, Gaudet D.** Etiology and risk of lactescent plasma and severe hypertriglyceridemia. *J Clin Lipidol.* 2011;5:37–44.
9. **Lloret Linares C, Pelletier AL, Czernichow S, et al.** Acute pancreatitis in a cohort of 129 patients referred for severe hypertriglyceridemia. *Pancreas.* 2008;37:13–22.
10. **Chait A, Robertson HT, Brunzell JD.** Chylomicronemia syndrome in diabetes mellitus. *Diabetes Care.* 1981;4:343–348.
11. **Gaudet D, Signorovitch J, Swallow E, et al.** Medical resource use and costs associated with chylomicronemia. *J Med Econ.* 2013;16:657–666.
12. **Berglund L, Brunzell JD, Goldberg AC, et al.** Evaluation and treatment of hypertriglyceridemia: an Endocrine Society Clinical Practice Guideline. *J Clin Endocrinol Metab.* 2012;97:2969–2989.
13. **Christian JB, Bourgeois N, Snipes R, Lowe KA.** Prevalence of severe (500 to 2,000 mg/dL) hypertriglyceridemia in United States adults. *Am J Cardiol.* 2011;107:891–897.
14. **Surendran RP, Visser ME, Heemelaar S, et al.** Mutations in LPL, APOC2, APOA5, GPIHBP1 and LMF1 in patients with severe hypertriglyceridaemia. *J Intern Med.* 2012;272:185–196.
15. **Farmer RG, Winkelman EI, Brown HB, Lewis LA.** Hyperlipoproteinemia and pancreatitis. *Am J Med.* 1973;54:161–165.
16. **Brunzell JD, Hazzard WR, Porte D Jr, Bierman EL.** Evidence for a common saturable triglyceride removal mechanism for chylomicrons and very low density lipoproteins in man. *J Clin Invest.* 1973;52:1578–1585.
17. **Rahalkar AR, Giffen F, Har B, et al.** Novel LPL mutations associated with lipoprotein lipase deficiency: two case reports and a literature review. *Can J Physiol Pharmacol.* 2009;87:151–160.
18. **Peterson J, Ayyobi AF, Ma Y, et al.** Structural and functional consequences of missense mutations in exon 5 of the lipoprotein lipase gene. *J Lipid Res.* 2002;43:398–406.
19. **Nickerson DA, Taylor SL, Weiss KM, et al.** DNA sequence diversity in a 9.7-kb region of the human lipoprotein lipase gene. *Nat Genet.* 1998;19:233–240.
20. **Johansen CT, Hegele RA.** Allelic and phenotypic spectrum of plasma triglycerides. *Biochim Biophys Acta.* 2012;1821:833–842.
21. **Rosenthal E RJ, Cosslin DR, Burt A, et al.** Joint linkage and association analysis with exome sequence data implicates SLC25A40 in hypertriglyceridemia. *Am J Hum Genet.* 2013;93(6):1035–1045.
22. **Hokanson JE, Brunzell JD, Jarvik GP, Wijsman EM, Austin MA.** Linkage of low-density lipoprotein size to the lipoprotein lipase gene in heterozygous lipoprotein lipase deficiency. *Am J Hum Genet.* 1999;64: 608–618.
23. **Chait A, Brunzell JD.** Severe hypertriglyceridemia: role of familial and acquired disorders. *Metabolism.* 1983;32:209–214.
24. **Herbst KL, Tannock LR, Deeb SS, Purnell JQ, Brunzell JD, Chait A.** Kobberling type of familial partial lipodystrophy: an underrecognized syndrome. *Diabetes Care.* 2003;26:1819–1824.
25. **Strickland LR, Guo F, Lok K, Garvey WT.** Type 2 diabetes with partial lipodystrophy of the limbs: a new lipodystrophy phenotype. *Diabetes Care.* 2013;36:2247–2253.
26. **Mirtallo JM, Dasta JF, Kleinschmidt KC, Varon J.** State of the art review: intravenous fat emulsions: current applications, safety profile, and clinical implications. *Ann Pharmacother.* 2012;688–700.
27. **Devaud JC, Berger MM, Pannatier A, et al.** Hypertriglyceridemia: a potential side effect of propofol sedation in critical illness. *Intensive Care Med.* 2012;38:1990–1998.
28. **Goldberg AS, Hegele RA.** Severe hypertriglyceridemia in pregnancy. *J Clin Endocrinol Metab.* 2012;97:2589–2596.
29. **Rouis M, Dugi KA, Previato L, et al.** Therapeutic response to medium-chain triglycerides and omega-3 fatty acids in a patient with the familial chylomicronemia syndrome. *Arterioscler Thromb Vasc Biol.* 1997;17:1400–1406.
30. **Brunzell JD.** Familial lipoprotein lipase deficiency. *GeneReviews at GeneTests: Medical Genetics Information Resource.* 2011:1997–2010.
31. **Tsai EC, Brown JA, Veldee MY, Anderson GJ, Chait A, Brunzell JD.** Potential of essential fatty acid deficiency with extremely low fat diet in lipoprotein lipase deficiency during pregnancy: a case report. *BMC Pregnancy Childbirth.* 2004;4:27.
32. **Al-Shali K, Wang J, Fellows F, Huff MW, Wolfe BM, Hegele RA.** Successful pregnancy outcome in a patient with severe chylomicronemia due to compound heterozygosity for mutant lipoprotein lipase. *Clin Biochem.* 2002;35:125–130.
33. **Press M, Hartop PJ, Prottey C.** Correction of essential fatty-acid deficiency in man by the cutaneous application of sunflower-seed oil. *Lancet.* 1974;1:597–598.
34. **Brunzell JD, Porte D Jr, Bierman EL.** Abnormal lipoprotein lipase mediated plasma triglyceride removal in untreated diabetes mellitus associated with hypertriglyceridemia. *Metabolism.* 1979;28:897–903.
35. **Hegele RA, Ginsberg HN, Chapman MJ, et al. on behalf of the European Atherosclerosis Society Consensus Panel.** The polygenic nature of hypertriglyceridaemia: implications for definition, diagnosis, and management [published online December 23, 2013]. *Lancet Diabetes Endocrinol.* doi: 10.1016/S2213-8587(13)70191-8.
36. **Carpentier AC, Frisch F, Labbe SM, et al.** Effect of alipogene tiparvovec (AAV1-LPL(S447X)) on postprandial chylomicron metabolism in lipoprotein lipase-deficient patients. *J Clin Endocrinol Metab.* 2012;97:1635–1644.

CHAPTER 41

Statin-Related Myositis and Rhabdomyolysis

Carmelo V Venero and Paul D Thompson

ABSTRACT

Statins are the most effective and commonly prescribed medication used to lower low-density lipoprotein cholesterol (LDL-C) levels. Statins are well-tolerated by most patients, but 3% to 10% of patients develop myalgia with these drugs, and fatal rhabdomyolysis has been estimated to occur in approximately 1.5 per 10 million statin prescriptions. Preventive and emergent management of severe statin-related muscle complications is outlined.

INTRODUCTION

3-Hydroxy-3-methyl-glutaryl coenzyme A (HMG-CoA) reductase inhibitors (statins) are the most effective and commonly prescribed medication used to lower low-density lipoprotein cholesterol (LDL-C) levels. Multiple studies have documented that statins reduce cardiovascular events (1–4). Statins are well-tolerated by most patients, but 3% (5) to 10% (6) of patients develop myalgia with these drugs, and fatal rhabdomyolysis has been estimated to occur in approximately 1.5 per 10 million statin prescriptions (7). Statins can produce a variety of myopathic complaints, including myalgia, muscle cramps, weakness, elevated creatine kinase (CK) levels with or without symptoms, and rarely rhabdomyolysis with renal compromise.

DEFINITION OF TERMS

How the various forms of statin myopathy are described varies among different medical groups and trials. The American College of Cardiology/American Heart Association/National Heart, Lung and Blood Institute (ACC/AHA/NHLBI) Clinical Advisory on statins used the following definition of terms:

1. Myopathy—general term for any disease of muscle
2. Myalgia—muscle ache or weakness without CK elevation
3. Myositis—muscle symptoms with increased CK levels
4. Rhabdomyolysis—muscle symptoms with marked CK levels (typically >10× ULN) and with creatinine elevation

The National Lipid Association (NLA) Muscle Safety Expert Panel suggested the following terminology:

1. Myopathy—general term for every potential muscle problem
   - Asymptomatic myopathy: serum CK elevation without myalgia or weakness
   - Symptomatic myopathy: presence of myalgia, weakness, or cramps

2. Rhabdomyolysis—evidence of muscle cell injury evidenced by an increase in serum CK levels
   - Mild CK increase: CK levels > normal but <10× ULN
   - Moderate CK increase: CK levels ≥10× ULN, but <50× ULN
   - Marked CK increase: CK levels ≥50× ULN

There is, however, no consensus on how these muscle abnormalities should be defined.

THE INCIDENCE OF STATIN-RELATED MYOPATHY

Fatal rhabdomyolysis has been estimated at 1.5 deaths per 10 million prescriptions using the Federal Drug Administration (FDA) Adverse Event Reports System (AERS) and a national prescription auditing system (7). Deaths associated with cerivastatin were 21-fold more frequent than for the class in total, which prompted cerivastatin's withdrawal from the market. Rhabdomyolysis is rare in statin clinical trials and in clinical practice. The incidence of rhabdomyolysis in clinical trials, defined as CK ≥10× ULN or ≥2,000 U/L, was calculated to be 4.4 versus 2.8 per 100,000 person-years in the statin and placebo groups, respectively, a nonsignificant difference (8). A combined analysis of 2 clinical cohort studies, from the United States (9) and the United Kingdom (10), reported only 3.4 cases of rhabdomyolysis per 100,000 person-years in patients treated with statins other than cerivastatin. This rate was 10-fold higher when statins were combined with gemfibrozil.

Myositis is rare in clinical trials. Myositis, defined either by the study investigators or as a CK >10× ULN, occurred in 49 participants treated with statins and 44 persons with placebo among 42,323 and 41,435 clinical trial subjects, respectively (5).

Minor muscle complaints are more frequent, but also relatively rare in clinical trials. Among 74,102 subjects enrolled in 35 trials with statin therapy (excluding cerivastatin), the absolute risk of myalgia, CK elevation, or rhabdomyolysis was not significantly increased. Specifically, the risk difference per every 1,000 treated patients was 2.7 higher than placebo for myalgia, 0.2 higher than placebo for CK elevations (defined by varying laboratory parameters), and 0.4 higher than placebo for rhabdomyolysis (defined as CK elevations ≥10× ULN) (11). In contrast to these controlled clinical trials, the PRIMO (Prediction of Muscular Risk in Observational conditions) study reported muscular complaints in 10.5% of 7,924 unselected patients treated with fluvastatin 80 mg, atorvastatin 40–80 mg, pravastatin 40 mg, or simvastatin 40–80 mg for at least 3 months (6). The Effect of Statins on Skeletal Muscle Function and Performance (STOMP) study provides additional insights into PRIMO's findings. In STOMP, 9.3% of 203 healthy volunteers randomly assigned to 80 mg of atorvastatin for 6 months developed myalgia versus 4.6% of 217 subjects assigned to placebo ($P = 0.05$). There were no differences in STOMP in muscle strength or exercise performance between the 2 subject groups (12). The STOMP results suggest that the true incidence of myalgia in clinical practice related to statins is approximately 5%, at least during short-term treatment. It is not clear, but likely, that the incidence of myalgia increases with time.

RISK FACTORS FOR STATIN MYOPATHY

Factors that increase the risk of statin myopathy include conditions or drugs that increase statin serum and muscle concentration and factors that increase muscle susceptibility to injury (Table 41-1).

Statin concentration increases with drug dose, advanced age, debilitation, reduced body size, female gender, decreased renal and hepatic function, hypothyroidism, and concomitant medications (12). Statin serum concentration can be affected by other compounds that alter statin hepatic or intestinal catabolism. Lovastatin, simvastatin, and atorvastatin are catabolized primarily by cytochrome P450 (CYP)3A4, whereas fluvastatin, and to a lesser degree rosuvastatin and pitavastatin, are metabolized by CYP2C9 (Table 41-2) (13,14). Interactions with drugs (Table 41-3) and certain tropical juices such as grapefruit, star fruit, and pomegranate that interfere with statins' CYP metabolism can increase statin levels and the risk of muscle injury (14).

The CYP system does not explain all drug interactions with statins. Gemfibrozil inhibits glucuronidation, which is part of the statins' phase II metabolism. Gemfibrozil increases all

Table 41-1. Risk Factors Associated with Statin-Induced Myopathy (14)

1. Factors related to an increase in statin serum level
a. Statin dose
b. Small body frame
c. Decreased statin metabolism and excretion
i. Drug-drug interactions
ii. Grapefruit juice (possibly also pomegranate and star fruit)
iii. Hypothyroidism and diabetes mellitus
iv. Advanced age
v. Liver disease
vi. Renal disease
vii. Genetic predisposition SLCO1B1 variants
2. Factors related to muscle predisposition
a. Alcohol consumption
b. Drug abuse (cocaine, amphetamines, heroin)
c. Heavy exercise
d. Baseline muscular disease:
i. Multisystemic diseases: diabetes mellitus, hypothyroidism, vitamin D deficiency
ii. Inflammatory or inherited metabolic muscle defects
iii. Genetic predisposition: CoQ2 and GATM locus variants

Abbreviations: SLCO1B1 = solute carrier organic anion transporter family member 1B1; GATM = glycine amidinotransferase.

statin concentrations except fluvastatin. In contrast, fenofibrate does not appear to affect the glucuronidation of statins, and appears to be safer from this perspective when used with statins (14).

Skeletal muscle genetic and metabolic variants probably also increase the risk of myopathy. These patients may present with increased CK levels prior to statin therapy or persistent CK elevations 2–3 months after stopping the drug. Up to 10% of patients with presumed statin myopathy, who were willing to undergo a muscle biopsy, were found to be heterozygous or homozygous for mutations causing myophosphorylase deficiency or McArdle's disease, carnitine palmitoyltransferase II deficiency, or myoadenylate deaminase deficiency (14). Other genetic variants linked to increased risk for statin myotoxicity include a polymorphism in the solute carrier organic anion transporter family member 1B1 (SLCO1B1) gene, which encodes the organic anion-transporting polypeptide (OATP1B1) that regulates the hepatic uptake of statins (15); CoQ2 gene variants, which reduce the production of coenzyme Q10 (CoQ10), a mitochondrial transport protein (16); and variants in GATM (glycine amidinotransferase), which is essential for creatine synthesis and muscle energy storage (17).

Table 41-2. Pharmacokinetic Characteristics of Statins (13,14)

Statin	Absorption (%)	Bioavailability (%)	Lipophilicity	Primary Metabolic Pathways	Elimination Half-Life (hr)	Urinary Excretion (%)
Atorvastatin	30	12	Yes	CYP3A4	15–30	2
Fluvastatin XL	95	6	Yes	CYP2C9	4.7	6
Lovastatin[a]	30	5[b]	Yes	CYP3A4	2.9	10
Pitavastatin	80	60	Yes	Minimal metabolism[c]	10–13	N/A
Pravastatin	34	18	No	Sulfation	1.3–2.8	20
Rosuvastatin	50	20	No	Minimal hepatic metabolism[d]	20.8	10
Simvastatin	60–80	5	Yes	CYP3A4	2–3	13

Abbreviations: CYP = cytochrome P450 superfamily; N/A = not available.

[a] *Administered as inactive prodrug requiring activation by liver metabolism.*

[b] *Immediate-release lovastatin should be administered with food to increase bioavailability.*

[c] *Minimal metabolism by CYP2C9.*

[d] *<10% metabolism by CYP2C9 and CYP2C19.*

Table 41-3. Drugs Affecting Statin Metabolism (14)

Drug(s)	Statin(s) Affected	Comments
Glucuronidation inhibitor		
Gemfibrozil	All except fluvastatin	Fenofibrate preferred fibrate to combine with statin, especially when statin used beyond its starting dose
CYP3A4 inhibitors		
Itraconazole, ketoconazole	Atorvastatin, lovastatin, simvastatin	Avoid concomitant use if possible
Macrolide antibiotics	Atorvastatin, lovastatin, simvastatin, pravastatin	Avoid concomitant use if possible
Protease inhibitors	Lovastatin, simvastatin affected more than atorvastatin Rosuvastatin	- Pravastatin and fluvastatin can be used at usual doses - Atorvastatin may be used at lowest possible dose - Rosuvastatin should be limited to 10 mg daily in patients using lopinavir/ritonavir
Amlodipine, verapamil, diltiazem	Simvastatin, lovastatin, atorvastatin	Recommended maximal dose of simvastatin 20 mg/d and lovastatin 40 mg/d when used in patients receiving concomitant verapamil or amlodipine
Amiodarone	Simvastatin, lovastatin, atorvastatin	Recommended maximal dose of simvastatin 20 mg/d and lovastatin 40 mg/d
CYP2C9 inhibitors		
Fluconazole, ketoconazole	Fluvastatin>>rosuvastatin	Avoid concomitant use if possible
Various mechanisms		
Cyclosporine	All except fluvastatin	- Fluvastatin has no drug interaction with cyclosporine - Rosuvastatin does not increase cyclosporine level but highest dose should be 5 mg/d - Pitavastatin is contraindicated - Other statins require lowest possible dose with monitoring of cyclosporine levels
Colchicine	Lovastatin, simvastatin affected more than atorvastatin, pravastatin, fluvastatin	Fluvastatin, pravastatin, rosuvastatin, and atorvastatin are less likely to interact with colchicine

All patients treated with statin and the above-mentioned drugs are at increased risk for myotoxicity and should be monitored for myopathy.

Physical activity has been associated with increased CK levels and symptoms during statin treatment (14). Exercise itself can increase CK levels, and in the PRIMO study, patients who participated in some "intense form of sport" reported muscle symptoms during statin therapy 38% more frequently than those performing less vigorous activities (6).

PATHOPHYSIOLOGICAL MECHANISMS OF STATIN-INDUCED MYOPATHY

The cause of statin-induced myopathy is unknown and it is not certain that the same metabolic changes produce the entire spectrum of statin complaints. Statins block cholesterol synthesis early in its metabolic pathway at a step that not only reduces cholesterol synthesis but also the production of other important metabolites, including ubiquinone or coenzyme Q10, dolichols, and other prenylated isoprenoids required for normal functioning of the skeletal myocyte (14). Decreased cholesterol production has been associated with malfunctioning of the myocyte cellular membrane or intracellular entrapment of very low density lipoprotein (VLDL) and LDL leading to fat myopathy (14). A reduction of the isopentenylation of selenocysteine tRNA, the isoprenoids, dolichols, and ubiquinone (CoQ10), and the guanosine triphosphate (GTP)-binding proteins Rho, Ras, and Rac affect processes essential for myogenesis and myoregeneration (14).

Several studies have suggested that changes in the ubiquitin proteasome pathway (UPP), which catabolizes muscle during such conditions as cancer cachexia, diabetes, uremia, and sepsis, may contribute to statin myopathy (14). Some patients present with persistent CK elevations and progressive weakness despite stopping statins. Many of these patients have skeletal muscle genetic variations as described previously, but a few have a statin-associated necrotizing autoimmune myopathy. The classic presentation is persistence of muscle weakness and CK elevations after stopping statin therapy. The pathophysiological process in this condition includes the development of antibodies against HMG-CoA reductase, which provokes myofiber degeneration and necrosis in the absence of a significant lymphocytic infiltrate (18). This entity must be diagnosed early because it often requires immunosuppressive therapy and untreated can cause persistent muscle weakness (19).

THE MANAGEMENT OF STATIN MYOPATHY

The management of statin myopathy includes preventing symptoms in the first place, monitoring patients with symptoms or CK elevations, using novel strategies to lower lipids in statin-intolerant patients, and constantly evaluating the risk and benefits of these agents in individual patients (Table 41-4).

Muscle complaints and frank rhabdomyolysis generally increase with increasing statin doses so that patients should be treated with the lowest dose necessary to achieve their therapeutic goal. This approach has not changed for most clinicians despite the 2013 ACC/AHA cholesterol treatment guidelines, which de-emphasize goal-oriented care (20). Concomitant therapy with gemfibrozil should be avoided, and fenofibrate should be the fibrate of choice when needed to combine with statins. We tend to select rosuvastatin, atorvastatin, pravastatin, fluvastatin, or pitavastatin for therapy in patients at high risk for myopathy because of age or concomitant medications because these agents appear well-tolerated (7), and all except atorvastatin, undergo little metabolism by the CYP3A4 system and should, therefore, be well-tolerated with most concomitant medications (Table 41-2).

Patients should be gently warned about the symptoms of myotoxicity, and clinicians should not ignore unexplained systemic complaints in patients on high-dose statin therapy. The diagnosis of rhabdomyolysis may be delayed because patients report a flu-like illness. We recommend discontinuing statins for 5 days prior to extreme exertion such as marathon running given the magnified muscle injury produced by exercise during statin therapy (21).

CK Measurement

Baseline CK measurements before statin therapy are useful and recommended by the National Cholesterol Education Program—Adult Treatment Panel III (NCEP—ATP III). Many patients have baseline CK elevations, and a baseline level helps differentiate statin from endogenous CK increases. Routine surveillance of CK levels is not required except for patients at high risk for myopathy, such as those with hepatic or renal disease or on medications that could interfere with statin metabolism.

Increases in CK levels are common during statin therapy and may be due to other factors, most notably unusual physical activity. Consequently, asymptomatic increases in CK should prompt a query about recent exercise, hypothyroidism, and a search for other muscle toxins such as alcohol or cocaine use. Once other causes of increased CK are excluded, we recommend that patients with asymptomatic CK increases $<5\times$ ULN be reassured and asked to report symptoms, that patients with asymptomatic CK increase ≥ 5, but $<10\times$ ULN be monitored for symptoms and have periodic CK determinations monthly or bimonthly, and that asymptomatic patients with CK $\geq 10\times$ ULN have the statin stopped or carefully evaluated for the risks and benefits of further treatment.

Rhabdomyolysis is typically described by the clinical triad of muscle pain, weakness, and dark urine, but more than 50% of patients may not present muscular symptoms (22) and many

Table 41-4. Statin-Related Myopathy Management Recommendations (14)

1. Asymptomatic patients
   a. Routine surveillance of CK levels is not required except in high-risk patients
   b. If CK measured
      i. CK <5× ULN: reassurance
      ii. CK ≥5 but <10× ULN: monitor for symptoms and periodical CK determination
      iii. CK ≥10× ULN: stop statin and reconsider risks and benefits of statin treatment
         1. Patients with CK >5,000 U/L: fluid resuscitation and management according to the rhabdomyolysis recommendations described in the text
2. Symptomatic patients
   a. Reconsider risks and benefits of statin treatment
   b. Tolerable symptoms
      i. Follow recommendations per above-mentioned CK guidelines
      ii. May try tonic water or coenzyme Q10 supplementation
   c. Intolerable symptoms or serum CK values ≥10× ULN, stop statin
      i. Patients with associated acute renal failure or CK >5,000 U/L
         1. Fluid administration and management according to the rhabdomyolysis recommendations described in the text
         2. Once recovered, benefit-risk of statin therapy needs to be reconsidered; careful use of alternative lipid lowering agent recommended
      ii. Other patients, once symptoms and CK returned to baseline can:
         1. Rechallenge same statin and dose to evaluate reproducibility of symptoms
         2. Switch to statin-containing regimen tried in patients intolerant to daily statin
            a. 80 mg fluvastatin XL and 10 mg EZT daily
            b. 10 mg atorvastatin BIW and 10 mg EZT daily
            c. 2.5–10 mg rosuvastatin 2 or 3 times a week
            d. 10–40 mg atorvastatin 3 times a week
         3. Try coenzyme Q10 supplementation
         4. Unable to tolerate or unwilling to retry statins requires use of alternative lipid lowering agents (including red yeast rice) or LDL apheresis for qualified patients

When CK increases, search for causes of CK elevation, such as increased physical activity, trauma/falls, infections, hypothyroidism, alcohol or cocaine use.

Abbreviations: CK = creatine kinase; ULN = upper limit of normal; EZT = ezetimibe; BIW = twice a week.

present nonspecific symptoms like malaise, fever, tachycardia, nausea, and vomiting (23). Increased serum CK levels and urine myoglobin levels are the major laboratory findings that lead to the diagnosis of rhabdomyolysis. Serum myoglobin levels are not mandatory for the diagnosis of rhabdomyolysis because it is cleared more rapidly than CK and, therefore, is less sensitive for detecting rhabdomyolysis (24). Laboratory testing should also search for acute kidney injury (AKI), hyperkalemia, hyperphosphatemia, hypocalcemia, and hyperuricemia.

The management of rhabdomyolysis involves limiting additional skeletal damage, prevention of AKI, and early identification of life-threatening complications. Rhabdomyolysis in patients taking statins involves stopping the statin and searching for alternative etiologies or precipitating factors such as trauma, extreme exertion (especially in the untrained individual), electrolyte abnormalities, concomitant use of prescription or illicit drugs that increase the risk for statin myopathy, and systemic or muscular metabolic disarrangement.

The next step in the management of rhabdomyolysis is the prevention of AKI, which happens in 10%–60% of patients (24). Possible renal toxins such as nonsteroidal medications should be discontinued. Patients with a stable CK below 5,000 U/L do not require intravenous (IV) fluid because the risk for AKI is low (25), whereas in patients with CK above 5,000 U/L, a large amount of IV fluid within the first 24 hours is associated with improved outcomes (24). Most recommendations for fluid resuscitation are based on small retrospective observational studies, as well as case reports or series without randomized controlled trials. The goal of therapy is to maintain a urine output of 200–300 mL/h, which usually is achieved with 6–12 L daily of IV fluids. The type of IV fluid used is controversial but in general, 0.9% normal saline IV fluids should suffice. Alkalinization of the urine to decrease precipitation of myoglobin in the renal tubules is commonly done but without robust clinical evidence. An international consensus in intensive care medicine suggested that sodium bicarbonate infusion was not superior to normal saline to increase the urine pH (26). Additionally, alkalinization of the plasma is associated with hypocalcemia, which requires calcium levels to be monitored closely. Despite these limitations, bicarbonate infusion is frequently used, especially in patients with CK above 5,000 U/L associated with severe muscle injury or a rising serum CK. The bicarbonate infusion is prepared by mixing 3 amps of 8.4% sodium bicarbonate with 1 L of 5% dextrose or water. The initial rate is usually 200 mL/h, with adjustment of the rate to achieve a urine pH above 6.5. Calcium and arterial pH should be monitored every 2 hours and the bicarbonate infusion discontinued if symptomatic hypocalcemia develops, arterial pH exceeds 7.5, or if serum bicarbonate increases beyond 30 mEq/L (30 mmol/L). The routine use of mannitol is not recommended, and the use of loop diuretics to convert anuria or oliguria to nonoliguria is based on limited clinical evidence. Calcium and potassium levels need close monitoring if loop diuretics are used because loop diuretics can aggravate hypocalcemia and hypokalemia. Loop diuretics could be used in the management of patients with hyperkalemia. Finally, renal replacement therapy may be necessary if renal failure does not respond to fluid resuscitation maneuvers and the patient develops severe hyperkalemia, metabolic acidosis, volume overload, anuria, or azotemia (24).

Symptomatic Patients

We continue symptomatic patients on the statin if therapy is justified by a risk/benefit analysis, and if the patient deems the symptoms tolerable, while using the CK guidelines previously outlined. If the symptoms are intolerable, we stop the statin until the patient feels normal. This can take up to 2 months (27), but often the patients report symptomatic improvement within 2 weeks of drug discontinuation. We then restart the statin at a lower dose or try a different statin. If the patient can only tolerate a lower dose, we will add ezetimibe, niacin, or bile sequestrants to achieve a lower LDL level. Patients with severe familial hypercholesterolemia or at very high risk for cardiovascular events can be treated with the new agents mipomersen or lomitapide, but we have little experience with these drugs and are concerned about steatohepatitis with both compounds, so use these as agents of last resort. If no statin is tolerated, we will use another lipid-lowering class of medication or LDL apheresis for qualified patients (14). We await additional studies with the proprotein convertase subtilisin/kexin type 9 (PCSK9) inhibitors. One such inhibitor, AMG145, a monoclonal antibody to PCSK9, was used in the GAUSS randomized trial (28) to treat 160 statin-intolerant patients. Subjects were randomized to 10 mg ezetimibe alone, 280 mg AMG145, 350 mg AMG145, 420 mg AMG145, or 420 mg AMG145/10 mg ezetimibe. AMG145 was administered by injection every 4 weeks for a total of 12 weeks. LDL cholesterol decreased 40.8%–50.7% (CI 32.9–58.6%). Myalgia was reported by 7.4% of patients in the AMG145 alone groups and by 3.1% of patients taking ezetimibe (28).

We also have had apparent clinical success with atypical treatment regimens, although only some of these are published in peer-reviewed journals. Some patients deemed intolerant of statins can successfully use over-the-counter red yeast rice, which has lovastatin among its active ingredients (14). Two 600-mg tablets with the evening meal can reduce LDL-C 21%–27% (29,30). We have also used atorvastatin or rosuvastatin every other day (31,32) or rosuvastatin twice weekly (33) in statin-intolerant patients with good tolerance and LDL reductions. Fluvastatin XL with or without ezetimibe (14), and twice-a-week atorvastatin combined with daily ezetimibe (14), are also effective. Some statin-intolerant patients can tolerate statins for brief periods of time, for example, 8 weeks. If these patients definitely require statin therapy, we will treat them using what we call "pulse therapy," meaning that we treat them but stop 1 to 2 weeks prior to the usual start of their pain. We then give them a week or two off therapy before restarting treatment. This approach is based on the belief that some time with lower cholesterol levels is more beneficial than consistently higher levels.

We have had apparent clinical success advising patients with statin-related leg cramps to consume 12 ounces of tonic water, which contains quinine, at bedtime. We also occasionally use coenzyme Q10 supplements, and some patients appear to benefit, possibly from a placebo effect. Finally, those patients with progressive weakness and CK elevation despite statin withdrawal should be evaluated for genetic skeletal muscle metabolic disorders as well as for testing for statin-associated necrotizing autoimmune myopathy. If the latter autoimmune myopathy is identified, treatment with immunosuppressive therapy is necessary, which typically involves prednisone in combination with an additional immunosuppressive agent such as methotrexate.

ACKNOWLEDGMENTS

PDT has received research support from Genomas, Roche, Sanolfi, Regeneron, Esperion, Amarin, and Pfizer; has served as a consultant for Amgen, Astra Zenica, Regeneron, Merck, Genomas, Runners World, Sanolfi, Esperion, Amarin, and Novartis; has received speaker honoraria from Merck, Astra Zenica, Kowa, and Amarin; owns stock in Abbvie, Abbott Labs, General Electric, and Johnson & Johnson; and has provided expert legal testimony on exercise-related cardiac events and statin myopathy. CV has nothing to disclose.

REFERENCES

1. **Scandinavian Simvastatin Survival Study Group.** Randomised trial of cholesterol lowering in 4444 patients with coronary heart disease: the Scandinavian Simvastatin Survival Study (4S). *Lancet.* 1994;344:1383–1389.
2. **Downs JR, Clearfield M, Weis S, et al.** Primary prevention of acute coronary events with lovastatin in men and women with average cholesterol levels: results of AFCAPS/TexCAPS. Air Force/Texas Coronary Atherosclerosis Prevention Study. *JAMA.* 1998;279:1615–1622.
3. **Sacks FM, Pfeffer MA, Moye LA, et al.** The effect of pravastatin on coronary events after myocardial infarction in patients with average cholesterol levels. Cholesterol and Recurrent Events Trial investigators. *N Engl J Med.* 1996;335:1001–1009.
4. **Shepherd J, Cobbe SM, Ford I, et al.** Prevention of coronary heart disease with pravastatin in men with hypercholesterolemia. West of Scotland Coronary Prevention Study Group. *N Engl J Med.* 1995;333:1301–1307.
5. **Thompson PD, Clarkson P, Karas RH.** Statin-associated myopathy. *JAMA.* 2003;289:1681–1690.
6. **Bruckert E, Hayem G, Dejager S, Yau C, Begaud B.** Mild to moderate muscular symptoms with high-dosage statin therapy in hyperlipidemic patients—the PRIMO study. Sponsored by the International Society of Cardiovascular Pharmacotherapy. *Cardiovasc Drugs Ther.* 2005;19:403–414.
7. **Staffa JA, Chang J, Green L.** Cerivastatin and reports of fatal rhabdomyolysis.*N Engl J Med.* 2002;346:539–540.
8. **Law M, Rudnicka AR.** Statin safety: a systematic review. *Am J Cardiol.* 2006;97:52C–60C.
9. **Graham DJ, Staffa JA, Shatin D, et al.** Incidence of hospitalized rhabdomyolysis in patients treated with lipid-lowering drugs. *JAMA.* 2004;292:2585–2590.
10. **Black C, Jick H.** Etiology and frequency of rhabdomyolysis. *Pharmacotherapy.* 2002;22:1524–1526.
11. **Kashani A, Phillips CO, Foody JM, et al.** Risks associated with statin therapy: a systematic overview of randomized clinical trials. *Circulation.* 2006;114:2788–2797.
12. **Parker BA, Capizzi JA, Grimaldi AS, et al.** Effect of statins on skeletal muscle function. *Circulation.* 2013;127:96–103.
13. **Neuvonen PJ, Niemi M, Backman JT.** Drug interactions with lipid-lowering drugs: mechanisms and clinical relevance. *Clin Pharmacol Ther.* 2006;80:565–581.
14. **Venero CV, Thompson PD.** Managing statin myopathy. *Endocrinol Metab Clin North Am.* 2009;38:121–136.
15. **Group SC, Link E, Parish S, et al.** SLCO1B1 variants and statin-induced myopathy—genomwide study. *N Engl J Med.* 2008;359:789–799.
16. **Oh J, Ban MR, Miskie BA, Pollex RL, Hegele RA.** Genetic determinants of statin intolerance. *Lipids Health Dis.* 2007;6:7.
17. **Mangravite LM, Engelhardt BE, Medina MW, et al.** A statin-dependent QTL for GATM expression is associated with statin-induced myopathy. *Nature.* 2013;502:377–380.
18. **Mohassel P, Mammen AL.** Statin-associated autoimmune myopathy and anti-HMGCR autoantibodies. *Muscle Nerve.* 2013;48:477–483.

19. **Padala S, Thompson PD.** Statins as a possible cause of inflammatory and necrotizing myopathies. *Atherosclerosis.* 2012;222:15–21.
20. **Stone NJ, Robinson J, Lichtenstein AH, et al.** 2013 ACC/AHA Guideline on the Treatment of Blood Cholesterol to Reduce Atherosclerotic Cardiovascular Risk in Adults: A Report of the American College of Cardiology/American Heart Association Task Force on Practice Guidelines [published online ahead of print November 12, 2013]. *Circulation.*
21. **Parker BA, Augeri AL, Capizzi JA, et al.** Effect of statins on creatine kinase levels before and after a marathon run. *Am J Cardiol.* 2012;109:282–287.
22. **Gabow PA, Kaehny WD, Kelleher SP.** The spectrum of rhabdomyolysis. *Medicine.* 1982;61:141–152.
23. **Giannoglou GD, Chatzizisis YS, Misirli G.** The syndrome of rhabdomyolysis: pathophysiology and diagnosis. *Eur J Intern Med.* 2007;18:90–100.
24. **Zimmerman JL, Shen MC.** Rhabdomyolysis. *Chest.* 2013;144:1058–1065.
25. **de Meijer AR, Fikkers BG, de Keijzer MH, van Engelen BG, Drenth JP.** Serum creatine kinase as predictor of clinical course in rhabdomyolysis: a 5-year intensive care survey. *Intensive Care Med.* 2003;29:1121–1125.
26. **Brochard L, Abroug F, Brenner M, et al.** An Official ATS/ERS/ESICM/SCCM/SRLF Statement: Prevention and Management of Acute Renal Failure in the ICU Patient: an international consensus conference in intensive care medicine. *Am J Respir Crit Care Med.* 2010;181:1128–1155.
27. **Thompson PD, Clarkson PM, Rosenson RS, National Lipid Association Statin Safety Task Force Muscle Safety Expert P.** An assessment of statin safety by muscle experts. *Am J Cardiol.* 2006;97:69C–76C.
28. **Sullivan D, Olsson AG, Scott R, et al.** Effect of a monoclonal antibody to PCSK9 on low-density lipoprotein cholesterol levels in statin-intolerant patients: the GAUSS randomized trial. *JAMA.* 2012;308:2497–2506.
29. **Becker DJ, Gordon RY, Halbert SC, French B, Morris PB, Rader DJ.** Red yeast rice for dyslipidemia in statin-intolerant patients: a randomized trial. *Ann Intern Med.* 2009;150:830–839, W147–149.
30. **Venero CV, Venero JV, Wortham DC, Thompson PD.** Lipid-lowering efficacy of red yeast rice in a population intolerant to statins. *Am J Cardiol.* 2010;105: 664–666.
31. **Backes JM, Venero CV, Gibson CA, et al.** Effectiveness and tolerability of every-other-day rosuvastatin dosing in patients with prior statin intolerance. *Ann Pharmacother.* 2008;42:341–346.
32. **Juszczyk MA, Seip RL, Thompson PD.** Decreasing LDL cholesterol and medication cost with every-other-day statin therapy. *Prev Cardiol.* 2005;8:197–199.
33. **Gadarla M, Kearns AK, Thompson PD.** Efficacy of rosuvastatin (5 mg and 10 mg) twice a week in patients intolerant to daily statins. *Am J Cardiol.* 2008;101:1747–1748.

SECTION XII

Inherited Metabolic Disorders

SECTION INTRODUCTION

Emergent Management of Inherited Metabolic Disorders in Adults

Timothy M Cox

Latterly it has become trivial to refer to the importance of studying rare diseases, such as the inborn errors of metabolism: the political and human importance of rare diseases has been the subject of a spectacular renaissance. Since attention was first drawn to the importance of studying unusual and rare manifestations of disease by the early clinical investigator in Western medicine, William Harvey, stepwise recognition that he was right has increased over four centuries. Moreover, there exists a huge incentive to understand and introduce treatments for rare disorders through the orphan medicinal legislation—now, in the United States, 30 years old (1). With this has come benefits for patients, as well as biopharmaceutical companies and their investors.

Therapeutic investment in orphan diseases has brought with it improved scientific focus on the nature of the inborn in diverse genetic diseases and of the pressing need to describe and quantify gene–environment effects. But more than anything, investigators now realize, building on the work of Harvey, Francis Galton, William Bateson, and Archibald Garrod, that understanding very rare conditions will, sooner or later, contribute to scientific understanding in the round and provide penetrating insights into common disorders. In a recent essay, "The Battlefield of Rare Diseases Where Uncommon Insights Are Common," William Gahl gives vivid examples of how understanding the critical pathways and mechanisms that emerge from investigating rare genetic disorders provides universal truth (2). Perhaps the most facile example is familial hypercholesterolemia due to mutations in the low-density lipoprotein (LDL) receptor: this condition occurs with a frequency of just 1 in 1,000,000 live births, but provided the inspiration for Akira Endo's discovery of the statins—now global blockbusters that decrease the risk of major killer diseases such as coronary heart disease and stroke.

Inherited metabolic disorders are not only fascinating and instructive, they are rewarding to treat (3). For the non-aficionado, inborn errors of metabolism often serve as a haunting reminder of undergraduate biochemistry never understood, and some might appear to intimidate by their complexity. For those who have little experience with or attraction for the treatment of patients suffering from chronic diseases, many metabolic conditions may latterly have appealed to a restricted band of professionals only—and rather like Wagner operas, there might be long (and sometimes boring) half hours, but these are punctuated by a very exciting 5 minutes!

A list of disorders with challenging acute disturbances on a background of inherited disorders of metabolism in adults would be very long (4,5). Nonetheless, the following conditions should certainly be part of that lexicon: acute porphyrias; organic acidemias; amino acidemias; hyperammonemia in urea-cycle defects, including type

2 citrullinemia and cobalamin defects; glycogen-storage diseases; and acute metabolic decompensation in many mitochondrial diseases. In the succeeding section, we have a conspectus of acute medicine within the context of inherited metabolic diseases that present in the emergent situation. Here, frequent abnormalities in the urea cycle are discussed, of which ornithine transcarbamoylase deficiency is of considerable importance, particularly in adult women. Severe hyperammonemia in the acute situation is often triggered by intercurrent disease or stress almost at any time in life; at the same time, life-changing deterioration develops insidiously to yield a dramatic clinical presentation, which if overlooked or not promptly treated to remove and prevent the accumulation of ammonia, leads to irreversible neurological injury and cognitive loss. Nitrogen scavenging drugs and other supplements, together with long-term management by dietary means and restriction of protein using specialized formula diets, are key to management and are life-saving. An unusual X-linked inheritance pattern poses challenges for diagnosis, and identification of affected at-risk relatives and their management by appropriate therapy are an essential component of overall management.

Hyperammonemia occurs as a consequence of several disorders, including the acute acidoses that complicate the organic acidemias and inborn errors of amino acid metabolism, especially methylmalonic acidemia—often caused by defects in vitamin B_{12} metabolism and supply. Although these demonstrate the complexity and interrelation of metabolic pathways, at the same time, they demonstrate the readiness with which they might be corrected. Propionic aciduria, methylmalonic aciduria, and defects of branch chain amino acid metabolism including maple syrup urine disease are but a few metabolic conditions that present in acute crises in adults and which can be cured or at least rescued by timely intervention with rigorous nutritional adjustment—and vitamin supplementation where appropriate.

Clinicians who practice metabolic medicine are not alone in wishing to have prowess in the field of diagnosis and treatment for all-comers in acute or general medicine. It is noteworthy that numerous disorders in this category may develop acute decompensation requiring urgent intervention (eg, stroke, arterial and venous thrombosis including myocardial infarction, and blindness in pyridoxine-responsive homocystinemia—a disease that can be ameliorated in the long-term by appropriate vitamin supplementation). Many diverse inborn errors affecting organelles, such as the peroxisome and lysosome, for example, can be complicated by acute deterioration—cardiovascular (Fabry, MPS I and II, and Danon diseases), skeletal (osteonecrosis in Gaucher disease), renal (hyperoxalurias, cystinosis and Fabry disease), respiratory obstruction (eg, in mucopolysaccharidoses). The interdependence of metabolic processes of catabolism and anabolism, continuously active in the daily life of the living human, mandates a level of curiosity and understanding of all doctors—or at least a willingness to learn. Presented with an acutely deteriorating patient, it is surprising how facile the treatment of many inborn errors of metabolism can be, even though it can be life-saving.

The short section that follows vividly illustrates the interaction between cofactors, including vitamins and minerals, dietary components, and illness; these conspire in the individual either to rescue a maladapted inborn error of metabolism or favor unmitigated clinical catastrophe. The management of acute crises in inborn errors of metabolism is not restricted to the pundits: clear thinking and prompt action—with the application of basic principles of human biochemistry and clinical practice—very often save the day.

ACKNOWLEDGMENTS

The author has nothing to disclose.

REFERENCES

1. **Braun MM, Farag-El-Massah S, Xu K, Coté R.** Emergence of orphan drugs in the United States: a quantitative assessment on the first 25 years. *Nat Rev Drug Discov.* 2010;9:519–522.
2. **Gahl, WA.** The battlefield of rare diseases: where uncommon insights are common. *Sci Transl Med.* 2012; 4:154ed7.
3. **Cox TM.** Alkaptonuria: leading to the treasure in exceptions. *JIMD Rep.* 2012;5:49–57.
4. **Hoffmann GF, Zschocke J, Nyhan WL.** *Inherited Metabolic Diseases. A Clinical Approach.* Berlin Heidelberg: Springer-Verlag; 2010.
5. **Saudubray J-M, van den Berghe G, Walter JH.** *Inborn Metabolic Diseases.* Berlin Heidelberg: Springer-Verlag; 2012.

CHAPTER 42

Acute Presentations of Inherited Metabolic Disease in Adulthood

Elaine Murphy and Robin H Lachmann

ABSTRACT

The majority of adults with an inherited metabolic disease (IMD) who present to emergency services will already have a known diagnosis, usually made in childhood. They may bring with them specific information and/or guidelines for emergency management of their condition. Affected individuals can also present for the first time in adulthood. It is important for clinicians working in the adult sector to be aware of these disorders, not only to manage survivors of childhood but also to recognize patients presenting in adulthood. This chapter describes some acute clinical scenarios in which IMDs need to be considered. Because they are genetic diseases, missing the diagnosis may have implications both for the affected individuals and for their families. Not all diagnostic tests are readily available in the emergency setting, or even outside specialist laboratories, so appropriate samples (ideally including deoxyribonucleic acid [DNA]) should be collected and stored in the acute setting.

INTRODUCTION

The majority of adults with an inherited metabolic disease (IMD) who present to emergency services will already have a known diagnosis, usually made in childhood. They may bring with them specific information and/or guidelines for emergency management of their condition. In some countries nationally agreed guidelines may be accessible via the Internet (eg, the British Inherited Metabolic Disease Group Guidelines, www.BIMDG.org.uk).

Other patients may present for the first time in adulthood, and while, quite correctly, the emphasis is on diagnosing acquired conditions such as infection or poisoning, the possibility of a late presentation of an IMD should always be considered for patients presenting with encephalopathy (which can be a psychiatric presentation in adults), disturbances of acid-base balance, atypical stroke, psychiatric features, or rhabdomyolysis—particularly if these episodes are recurrent and there is no other obvious underlying cause. Hypoglycemia is a fairly unusual initial presentation of IMD in adulthood. Due to compensatory mechanisms adults can maintain their blood glucose levels despite significant metabolic disturbance, and thus presentation with hypoglycemia often represents a late event in a severe metabolic decompensation (eg, in fatty acid oxidation disorders or organic acidemias). Typically acute decompensations can be triggered by metabolic "stress" (fasting, intercurrent infection, major surgery, gastrointestinal illness, excessive alcohol or exercise), but a precise underlying precipitant is not always identified.

This chapter deals with some of the more frequent acute presentations of adults with IMDs and their emergency management. Table 42-1 summarizes these conditions. It is important for adult clinicians to be aware of these disorders as effective treatments are

Table 42-1. Summary of Potential Inherited Metabolic Diseases Presenting as an Emergency in Adulthood

Disorder	Emergency Presentation	Useful Laboratory Tests	Treatment Options
Glycogen storage disorders	Rhabdomyolysis Cardiomyopathy	Creatine kinase	Modified diet Exercise advice
Fatty acid oxidation disorders	Rhabdomyolysis Cardiomyopathy	Creatine kinase Acylcarnitine profile Urine organic acids Fibroblast FAO studies Plasma ketones	IV dextrose Modified diet Exercise advice Bezafibrate L-carnitine
Urea cycle defects	Encephalopathy Stroke-like episode Psychiatric features	Ammonia Plasma amino acids Urine orotic acid	IV dextrose Hemofiltration Arginine Sodium benzoate Sodium phenylbutyrate
Organic acidemias	Encephalopathy Cardiac disease Renal impairment Metabolic acidosis	Blood gases Ammonia Acylcarnitine profile Urine organic acids	IV dextrose Hemofiltration L-carnitine
Homocystinuria	Thrombosis Lens dislocation Psychiatric features	Plasma amino acids	Pyridoxine Folate B_{12} Betaine
Lysosomal storage disorders	Cardiomyopathy Psychiatric features Stroke	White cell enzyme activities Filipin staining of fibroblasts	Enzyme replacement therapy Substrate reduction therapy
Adrenoleukodystrophy	Adrenal insufficiency Spastic paraparesis	Very long chain fatty acid levels Short ACTH stimulation test	Adrenal replacement therapy Consider bone marrow transplant
Mitochondrial disease	Cardiomyopathy Stroke-like episode Lactic acidosis	See text	See text
Acute porphyrias	Abdominal pain Psychiatric features Neuropathy	Urine porphobilinogen	Heme arginate infusion
Hereditary fructose intolerance	Hypoglycemia Liver/renal impairment	Liver function tests and coagulation Blood gases	Eliminate all sources of fructose Organ support (HDU/ITU)

available for many, and, because the disorders are genetic, making the diagnosis has implications both for the affected patients and their relatives. Not all diagnostic tests are readily available in the emergency setting, or even outside specialist laboratories, so appropriate samples (ideally including deoxyribonucleic acid [DNA]) should be collected and stored in the acute setting.

RHABDOMYOLYSIS

Muscle has high energy requirements, particularly during exercise. Stored glycogen is metabolized to pyruvate, which enters mitochondria. Long-chain fatty acids are transported across the mitochondrial membrane by a process mediated by acylcarnitine translocase and carnitine palmitoyltransferases 1 and 2. In the mitochondria, these substrates are then used to generate acetyl CoA, which feeds into the Krebs cycle, ultimately delivering electrons to the mitochondrial respiratory chain to produce energy in the form of adenosine triphosphate (ATP). Inherited defects of glycogen metabolism or fatty acid oxidation are, therefore, frequently associated with muscle pathology.

The most common metabolic causes of exercise-induced rhabdomyolysis in adulthood include disorders of glycogen metabolism (eg, glycogen storage disease [GSD] types V or VII) and the fatty acid oxidation disorders (eg, carnitine palmitoyltransferase 2 [CPT2] and very long chain acyl-CoA dehydrogenase [VLCAD] deficiencies). At presentation, patients may give a history of previous episodes of less severe muscle pain precipitated by exercise or illness, or a family history of others with muscle pain.

GSD V (McArdle Disease)

GSD V (McArdle disease) is characterized by muscle pain that typically comes on within a few minutes of starting exercise (1). Exercise tolerance (reduction in heart rate) may improve after 7–10 minutes if aerobic exercise (eg, jogging, cycling) is continued but at a slower, gentler pace—this is called the second-wind phenomenon. Static or isometric exercise (eg, bench press, shoulder raises, carrying heavy shopping) is poorly tolerated, as is sprinting. Some older patients may have evidence of a fixed proximal myopathy with wasting.

Diagnosis. Laboratory tests will show elevated creatine kinase, urate, and myoglobinuria and, in severe cases, renal impairment. In up to 85% of patients from Northern Europe, a common mutation R50X can be detected, and so, in patients with a typical clinical history, genetic mutation analysis may be used as a first-line diagnostic test. GSD V can also be confirmed by muscle biopsy, which shows an excess of glycogen and absence of muscle phosphorylase. The ischemic forearm exercise test, with measurement of lactate and ammonia, the traditional screening test for muscle disorders of carbohydrate metabolism, is less often performed now—because it is painful for the patient, not specifically diagnostic for GSD V, and has been largely superseded by genetic testing.

Management. Acute severe rhabdomyolysis should be treated with prompt fluid replacement (normal saline) and renal support as required. Intravenous (IV) dextrose during acute crises and oral sucrose prior to exercise may also be helpful. Patients should be given advice on safe forms of exercise and how to achieve the second-wind phenomenon.

Fatty Acid Oxidation Disorders

Fatty acid oxidation disorders such as CPT2 or VLCAD deficiencies can present for the first time in adolescence/adulthood (2). The presentation is typically with symptoms of myalgia/muscle stiffness/rhabdomyolysis after more prolonged exercise, such as playing sports or marathon running. Prolonged fasting, cold exposure, intercurrent infection, or even emotional stress are other well-recognized precipitants. Symptoms may last for a number of weeks following an acute attack, but patients may be completely asymptomatic, with normal muscle strength on examination, between attacks.

Diagnosis. If there is a strong suspicion of a fatty acid oxidation disorder, then a muscle biopsy may be avoided. Instead, an acylcarnitine profile (plasma or blood spot) may suggest the condition, which can then be confirmed by measurements of fatty acid oxidation and/or CPT2 enzyme activity in skin fibroblasts (grown from a punch skin biopsy). Genetic testing allows screening of other potentially affected family members.

Management. Acute severe rhabdomyolysis should be treated with prompt fluid (saline) replacement, IV dextrose, and renal support as required. Other measures that may be helpful in preventing recurrent symptoms include restriction of dietary long-chain fat, with substitution by medium-chain triglyceride (MCT) and carbohydrate. The lipid-lowering agent, bezafibrate (200 mg three times daily), has been shown to increase CPT II enzyme activity in muscle and reduce the number of attacks of rhabdomyolysis, although a recent randomized study has not confirmed these findings (3,4). Note that patients with fatty acid oxidation disorders cannot achieve the second-wind phenomenon.

ENCEPHALOPATHY

Acute encephalopathy is a rapid decrease in consciousness level (over hours or days), not secondary to ictal or syncopal episodes. In adult patients with IMDs, encephalopathy may be intermittent, fluctuating, or rapid and fulminant progressing to coma. Patients may present with reduced cognition/concentration, a change in personality (often agitated/aggressive), lethargy, vomiting, or decreased consciousness/coma. Neurological findings may include secondary seizures, abnormal posturing, abnormal gait, and poor coordination. Symptoms are often reversible with early treatment, and consideration of a metabolic cause should be given to any adult who presents with encephalopathy. Late-onset "attenuated" forms of IMD in adults can often be precipitated by intercurrent infection, as well as alcohol or drug (mis)use, and so clinicians should be wary of attributing all encephalopathic symptoms to these, particularly if patients are not responding as expected to standard treatments. Information about previous unusual behaviors, such as protein aversion or unexplained episodes of confusion or agitation, should be sought from family and friends.

All adults who present with acute or acute-on-chronic encephalopathy in whom there is no obvious cause (eg, recent trauma or hypoxia) should have a plasma ammonia level measured promptly.

By far the most common cause of hyperammonemia in adults is hepatic disease, often associated with portosystemic shunting. Once this has been excluded as a cause then consideration should be given to other primary causes, and defects of the urea cycle are important among these (5). Hyperammonemia can also occur in fatty acid oxidation disorders or organic acidemias (2,6)—but in these conditions presentation usually occurs in infancy/childhood rather than in adulthood. An important secondary cause of elevated ammonia is valproate therapy, which has been well-described to precipitate hyperammonemia, including in individuals with a previously unknown urea cycle defect.

While the precise underlying cause of the hyperammonemia may take some time to elucidate, it is essential to start treatment immediately in order to avoid death or long-term neurological damage. The aims of treatment are to reduce catabolism and ammonia production and to lower plasma ammonia before cerebral edema develops.

Diagnosis

Definitive diagnosis should not delay immediate treatment but appropriate samples should be taken, preferably during the acute presentation, in order that chronic management can be tailored and genetic counselling can be given to both the index patient and other potentially affected family members.

The following tests should be taken as a minimum, but others may be required depending on the specific presentation:

Routine chemistry

- Liver function tests
- Complete (full) blood count
- Lactate, glucose, creatine kinase
- Blood gas analysis
- Blood and urine cultures
- Toxicology

Specialist chemistry

- Plasma amino acids
- Urine amino acids
- Urine organic acids (specifically for orotic acid)
- Acylcarnitine profile
- Store DNA for future mutation analysis

These tests should be discussed with your local specialist laboratory to ensure the correct sample conditions and transport. It is very important to avoid hemolysis and delayed separation of samples.

Management

In severe hyperammonemia with marked encephalopathy, seizures, or coma, hemodialysis is the most efficient way to reduce plasma ammonia (peritoneal dialysis is not as efficient and should be avoided). Vascular access should be secured and hemodialysis started as soon as possible in the high dependency unit (HDU) or intensive care unit (ICU) setting.

Protein intake should be stopped for 24–48 hours, and a hypercaloric solution (IV 10% dextrose; Intralipid) started, with insulin if needed to enhance anabolism. Intravenous arginine and ammonia scavengers (sodium benzoate and sodium phenylbutyrate) will promote the excretion of nonurea nitrogen-containing metabolites in the urine.

Long-term management will require input from a specialist center to ensure appropriate dietary advice (including supplementation of vitamins and minerals in those on a restricted diet) and titration of oral medications to ensure optimal metabolic control.

ACUTE ADRENAL CRISIS

This may be the first presentation in a male patient with an *ABCD1* gene mutation (adrenomyeloneuropathy/adrenoleukodystrophy) (7). All male patients presenting in adrenal crisis should, therefore, have adrenal autoantibodies measured and be asked about a family history of leukodystrophy and/or spastic paraparesis (this condition has X-linked inheritance).

Diagnosis

If there is no evidence of autoimmunity or another secondary cause, then diagnosis is made by measuring a very long chain fatty acid profile, and confirmed by mutation analysis of the *ABCD1* gene.

Management

Immediate management of the adrenal crisis is carried out as per standard guidelines.

METABOLIC "STROKE"

Stroke or stroke-like events can occur in a number of metabolic disorders including Fabry disease, homocystinuria, mitochondrial disorders, organic acidemias, and urea cycle defects.

Fabry Disease

Fabry disease is an X-linked disorder caused by deficiency of the enzyme alpha-galactosidase A (α-Gal A). Pain (acroparesthesia), renal disease, and cardiovascular disease are the major sources of morbidity and mortality. Male patients typically have more severe symptoms at an earlier age than heterozygote females. A characteristic angiokeratomatous rash is sometimes present.

Strokes or transient ischemic attacks (TIA) have been reported to occur in approximately 13% of affected individuals (15% males, 11.5% females) (8). Cerebrovascular manifestations result primarily from multifocal small vessel involvement and may include thrombosis, TIA, basilar artery ischemia and aneurysm, seizures, hemiplegia, hemianesthesia, aphasia, labyrinthine disorders, or frank cerebral hemorrhage (9).

Diagnosis. Diagnosis in males is made by measuring α-Gal A enzyme activity in plasma, isolated leukocytes, and/or cultured cells. In heterozygote females enzyme activity is unreliable, and the diagnosis must be confirmed by finding a pathogenic mutation in the *GLA* gene.

Management. Two enzyme replacement therapies (Fabrazyme [agalsidase beta] and Replagal [agalsidase alfa]) are now available. Patients should be strongly encouraged to stop smoking. Symptomatic paresthesia and renal and cardiac disease are treated as per standard guidelines.

Homocystinuria

Homocystinuria is an autosomal recessive condition caused by deficiency of the enzyme cystathione β-synthase (CBS). Classical clinical manifestations involve the eye, skeleton, and central nervous and vascular systems, but the age of onset, severity, and type of clinical involvement can vary widely among affected individuals.

In a large study of the natural history of 629 individuals with homocystinuria, just over a third had suffered a thromboembolic event—with cerebrovascular accidents accounting for a third of these (10). The chance of having any thromboembolic event was about 50% by age 29 years, and was a significant causative or contributory factor to death in nearly 80% of the 64 patients who had died. Pregnancy is a particular risk factor for cerebral thrombosis in women with homocystinuria. Cerebral thrombosis may be the first and only manifestation of homocystinuria in an adult (particularly in patients who are pyridoxine responsive—pyridoxine is a cofactor for the CBS enzyme).

Diagnosis. Diagnosis is made biochemically on a plasma amino acid profile (increased total homocysteine and free homocystine, increased methionine, decreased cysteine). Confirmation is by demonstration of reduced cystathione β-synthase activity in skin fibroblasts and/or mutation analysis of the *CBS* gene.

Management. Anticoagulation as per local guidelines. Ensure adequate vitamin B_{12} and folate status. Test for pyridoxine responsiveness. If patient is not pyridoxine responsive, then consider betaine supplementation and a low-protein, methionine-restricted diet.

Mitochondrial Disorders

Mitochondrial disorders should be considered as a possible cause of stroke in a patient who presents with a stroke or encephalopathy and involvement of 2 additional systems (eg, eye, ear, cardiac, renal, endocrine, or gastrointestinal). These disorders are caused by a disruption in the generation of energy by oxidative phosphorylation. There is considerable overlap in the clinical presentation of different mitochondrial disorders.

Diagnosis. There is no single diagnostic test for mitochondrial disease—so the clinical features and biochemical assays are used to direct genetic testing. Input from a specialist center is advised to direct testing. Tests may include measurement of

- Complete (full) blood count
- Tests of endocrine function
- Lactic acid (plasma and cerebrospinal fluid [CSF])
- Lactate:pyruvate ratio
- Plasma amino acid profile
- Acylcarnitine profile
- Biotinidase activity
- Mononuclear coenzyme Q10 level
- Plasma/urine thymidine and deoxyuridine
- Urine organic acids
- CSF amino acids, protein, and neurotransmitters
- Muscle biopsy for histology, respiratory chain enzyme analysis, and molecular genetic testing

Management. Management is largely supportive, apart from a small number of potentially treatable conditions caused by specific deficiencies (eg, of coenzyme Q10 or riboflavin). Citrulline and arginine have been suggested as possible useful therapies in the management of mitochondrial encephalomyopathy, lactic acidosis, and stroke-like episodes (MELAS) syndrome (11).

CARDIAC DISEASE

Acute presentations of cardiac disease (cardiomyopathy, arrhythmias, sudden death) secondary to an underlying metabolic disorder can occur in a number of conditions and may be the first presenting feature in adulthood (Table 42-2) (8,12–14).

Diagnosis

Diagnosis depends on the clinical features (note that the cardiac disease may be isolated) and family history, which will direct the biochemical and/or genetic testing. If a cardiac biopsy is taken, then histological analysis should include assessment of glycogen storage—*PRKAG2* gene mutations can cause isolated cardiomyopathy with glycogen storage.

Management

Management is largely as for standard cardiac disease. Patients may require a cardiac pacemaker or an implantable cardioverter defibrillator (ICD). Dietary manipulation and treatment of acute metabolic decompensation may be helpful in the management of the cardiomyopathy of glycogen storage disease type III, fatty acid oxidation disorders, and the organic acidemias. Carnitine supplementation is recommended in carnitine transporter deficiency.

PSYCHIATRIC PRESENTATIONS

Table 42-3 lists IMDs that can potentially present with psychiatric features or behavioral/

Table 42-2. Metabolic Disorders Associated with Cardiac Disease

Arrhythmias, conduction defects
Fatty acid oxidation defects
Congenital disorder of glycosylation
Fabry disease
Cardiomyopathy
Fabry disease
Fatty acid oxidation defects
Glycogen storage disorders (AGL, PRKAG2, LAMP2, RBCK1 mutations)
Organic acidemias (methylmalonic and propionic)
Mucopolysaccharidoses
Mitochondrial disorders (eg, Barth syndrome)
Refsum disease
Valvular disease
Mucopolysaccharidoses
Mucolipidoses

Table 42-3. Metabolic Disorders Associated with Psychiatric Features

Urea cycle defects
Disorders of B_{12}/folate/homocysteine metabolism
Methylene tetrahydrofolate reductase deficiency
Intracellular cobalamin (B_{12}) processing defects
Homocystinuria
Lysosomal storage disorders
Metachromatic leukodystrophy
Krabbe disease
Niemann-Pick C disease
Acute porphyria
Wilson disease
Cerebral adrenoleukodystrophy (ABCD1 gene mutation)

personality changes. Psychiatric features may be isolated for some time before other organ involvement is noted—particularly if the possibility of organic disease is not considered during the initial presentation (15,16).

Nonetheless, when the family history is suggestive of recessive or X-linked inheritance; or when the clinical signs are triggered by situations such as intercurrent infection, surgery, or prolonged fasting; or when neurological signs, such as cognitive or motor dysfunction, or other organ involvement, are present, then an IMD should be considered.

Treatment can be very effective—particularly for the urea cycle defects, disorders of B_{12}/folate and homocysteine metabolism, Wilson disease, and the acute porphyrias. Hence, any patient in whom an underlying metabolic cause is suspected should have the following measured as a minimum:

- Plasma amino acid profile
- Serum copper and ceruloplasmin
- Urine organic acids, copper, and porphobilinogen

More specialist investigations, depending on the family history and clinical picture (and brain magnetic resonance imaging [MRI] findings), should include the following:

- Very long chain fatty acid levels
- White cell enzyme activities (for metachromatic leukodystrophy and Krabbe disease)
- Filipin staining of fibroblasts (for Niemann-Pick disease type C)

PREGNANCY

Pregnancy is not in itself an acute emergency. However, women with certain metabolic conditions may be at increased risk of metabolic decompensation during pregnancy and the puerperium (17–19). Early pregnancy, if complicated by morning sickness, can be a difficult time for women with inherited disorders of energy metabolism, such as fatty acid oxidation disorders, glycogen storage diseases, urea cycle defects, and disorders of ketone body metabolism. Nausea and vomiting lead to problems in taking supplements and medications, which may result in episodes of metabolic decompensation.

Pregnancy is also a prothrombotic period, and presentation of hypercoagulable conditions (eg, homocystinuria) during pregnancy, often with cerebral venous sinus thrombus, is well-described. In all conditions with a known thrombotic risk, anticoagulation (usually with subcutaneous heparin) during pregnancy and the postpartum period needs to be considered.

Labor and delivery are times of increased energy requirement, and women may require additional energy supplementation (usually IV dextrose) during this time. Following delivery, there is a well-recognized risk period for acute decompensation of some disorders, particularly those of protein metabolism (eg, the urea cycle defects). Classically this decompensation occurs between day 3 and 14 postpartum. The reasons for this are not entirely clear but are thought to relate to the relative metabolic stress of the changes of the puerperium and an increased protein load for catabolism following involution of the uterus. Care must be taken not to confuse the behavioral changes of hyperammonemia for symptoms of postpartum psychosis or depression.

Risks to the Fetus

Aside from the risks secondary to acute maternal decompensation, a number of inherited metabolic conditions are thought to be directly teratogenic to the developing fetus. The most well-described of these is the maternal phenylketonuria (PKU) syndrome (20). Children exposed to high levels of maternal phenylalanine *in utero* are at risk of developmental delay, microcephaly, cardiac defects, and dysmorphic features. With good maternal control of phenylalanine levels this syndrome can be prevented (21). Hence, women with PKU who present pregnant or are planning pregnancy need to be referred for specialist counselling and management as a matter of urgency.

CONCLUSIONS

Inherited metabolic disorders can present acutely to a number of different specialities. Although individually these conditions are rare, if they are not considered in the differential diagnosis, then a potentially treatable condition can be missed, with devastating consequences for the individual and their family.

Any patient identified as being at risk of acute decompensation should be advised to wear a medical alert bracelet and to carry information with contact details of their treating medical team and an emergency treatment guideline. This should include information on who to contact for advice in the event of emergency/elective surgery or pregnancy.

ACKNOWLEDGMENTS

The authors have nothing to disclose.

REFERENCES

1. **Quinlivan R, Buckley J, James M, et al.** McArdle disease: a clinical review. *J Neurol Neurosurg Psychiatry.* 2010;81:1182–1188.
2. **Spiekerkoetter U, Lindner M, Santer R, et al.** Treatment recommendations in long-chain fatty acid oxidation defects: consensus from a workshop. *J Inherit Metab Dis.* 2009;32:498–505.
3. **Ørngreen MC, Madsen KL, Preisler N, et al.** Bezafibrate in skeletal muscle fatty acid oxidation disorders: a randomized clinical trial. *Neurology.* 2014; 82(7):607–613.
4. **Bonnefont JP, Bastin J, Laforêt P, et al.** Long-term follow-up of bezafibrate treatment in patients with the myopathic form of carnitine palmitoyltransferase 2 deficiency. *Clin Pharmacol Ther.* 2010;88(1): 101–108.
5. **Walker V.** Severe hyperammonaemia in adults not explained by liver disease. *Ann Clin Biochem.* 2012;49(Pt 3):214–228.
6. **Grünert SC, Müllerleile S, De Silva L, et al.** Propionic acidemia: clinical course and outcome in 55 pediatric and adolescent patients. *Orphanet J Rare Dis.* 2013;8:6.
7. **Steinberg SJ, Moser AB, Raymond GV.** X-Linked adrenoleukodystrophy. In: Pagon RA, Adam MP, Bird TD, Dolan CR, Fong CT, Stephens K, eds. *GeneReviews.* Seattle: University of Washington; 1993–2013.
8. **Ginsberg L, Manara R, Valentine AR, et al.** Magnetic resonance imaging changes in Fabry disease. *Acta Paediatr.* 2006;95(suppl):57–62.
9. **Mehta A, Hughes DA.** Fabry disease. In: Pagon RA, Adam MP, Bird TD, Dolan CR, Fong CT, Stephens K, eds. *GeneReviews.* Seattle: University of Washington; 1993–2013.
10. **Mudd SH, Skovby F, Levy HL, et al.** The natural history of homocystinuria due to cystathionine beta-synthase deficiency. *Am J Hum Genet.* 1985;37: 1–31.
11. **El-Hattab AW, Emrick LT, Chanprasert S, Craigen WJ, Scaglia F.** Mitochondria: role of citrulline and arginine supplementation in MELAS syndrome [published online ahead of print January 8, 2014]. *Int J Biochem Cell Biol.* pii: S1357-2725(13)00378-6.
12. **Austin SL, Proia AD, Spencer-Manzon MJ, et al.** Cardiac pathology in glycogen storage disease type III. *JIMD Rep.* 2012;6:65–72.
13. **Prada CE, Al Jasmi F, Kirk EP, et al.** Cardiac disease in methylmalonicacidemia. *J Pediatr.* 2011;159: 862–864.
14. **Lee TM, Addonizio LJ, Barshop BA, Chung WK.** Unusual presentation of propionic acidaemia as isolated cardiomyopathy. *J Inherit Metab Dis.* 2009;32(suppl 1):S97–S101.
15. **Sedel F, Baumann N, Turpin JC, et al.** Psychiatric manifestations revealing inborn errors of metabolism in adolescents and adults. *J Inherit Metab Dis.* 2007;30:631–641.
16. **Ahmed RM, Murphy E, Davagnanam I, et al.** A practical approach to diagnosing adult onset leukodystrophies [published online ahead of print January 15, 2014]. *J Neurol Neurosurg Psychiatry.* doi: 10.1136/jnnp-2013-305888.
17. **Langendonk JG, Roos JC, Angus L, et al.** A series of pregnancies in women with inherited metabolic disease. *J Inherit Metab Dis.* 2012;35:419–424.
18. **Peterson DE.** Acute postpartum mental status change and coma caused by previously undiagnosed ornithine transcarbamylase deficiency. *Obstet Gynecol.* 2003;102(5 Pt 2):1212–1215.
19. **Arn PH, Hauser ER, Thomas GH, et al.** Hyperammonemia in women with a mutation at the ornithine carbamoyltransferase locus. A cause of postpartum coma. *N Engl J Med.* 1990;322:1652–1655.
20. **Mabry CC, Denniston JC, Nelson TL, Son CD.** Maternal phenylketonuria. A cause of mental retardation in children without the metabolic defect. *N Engl J Med.* 1963;269:1404–1408.
21. **Lenke RR, Levy HL.** Maternal phenylketonuria and hyperphenylalaninemia. An international survey of the outcome of untreated and treated pregnancies. *N Engl J Med.* 1980;303:1202–1208.

Index

Note: Page numbers followed by *f* and *t* indicate figures and tables, respectively.

D

G

I

R